U0232963

THE PHARMACEUTICAL INDEX

Biologics: Monoclonal Antibody

Volume I

A collection of drug information and research data

on worldwide approved monoclonal antibodies

Edited by 药渡 Pharmacodia

CHINA MEDICAL SCIENCE PRESS

图书在版编目（CIP）数据

世界新药概览单克隆抗体卷 I. 药渡经纬信息科技（北京）有限公司主编.
—北京：中国医药科技出版社，2018.5
ISBN 978-7-5214-0317-6

Ⅰ. ①世⋯ Ⅱ. ①药⋯ Ⅲ. ①生物制品–单克隆抗体–研究–英文
Ⅳ. ①R977

中国版本图书馆 CIP 数据核字（2018）第 111399 号

The Pharmaceutical Index Biologicals-Monoclonal Antibody Volume 1

Compiled by Pharmacodia (Beijing) Co., LTD

Room 105, Haohai Building, No.7, 5th Street, Shangdi, Haidian District, Beijing, P.R. China, 100085

ISBN 978-7-5214-0317-6

Executive Editor: Jin Ma

Cover Designer: Junqi Chen

Format Designer: Lu Zhang

Published by China Medical Science Press, 2018.1

A-22 Northern Wenhuiyuan Road, Haidian District, Beijing, China, 100082

Printed in the People's Republic of China

编写委员会

吴辰冰　　　　　上海岸迈生物科技有限公司

陆　丹　　　　　Kadmon公司

陈宜顶　　　　　北京百普赛斯生物科技有限公司

孟　坤　　　　　盛诺基医药集团

俞德超　　　　　信达生物制药（苏州）有限公司

夏　瑜　　　　　中山康方生物医药有限公司

钱雪明　　　　　迈博斯生物医药（苏州）有限公司

徐　霆　　　　　苏州康宁杰瑞生物科技有限公司

唐艳旻　　　　　启明创投

黄　浩　　　　　江苏恒瑞医药股份有限公司

曹一孚　　　　　兴盟生物医药有限公司

曹国庆　　　　　明慧医药有限公司

龚兆龙　　　　　思路迪医药科技有限公司

药渡编委成员

刘　恕　　徐　军　　武幸幸　　顾雪菲

Editorial Board

Qianye Karen Liu	3E Bioventures Capital, Beijing
Jing Li	WuXi Biologics, Shanghai
Baiyong Li	Akeso Biopharma, Inc., Guangdong
Chenbing Wu	Shanghai EpimAb Biotherapeutics Co., Ltd., Shanghai
Dan Lu	Kadmon Corporation
Mike Chen	ACROBiosystems, Beijing
Kun Meng	Shenogen Pharma Group, Beijing
Dechao Yu	Innovent Biologics (Suzhou) Co., Ltd., Jiangsu
Yu Xia	Akeso Biopharma, Inc., Guangdong
Xueming Qian	MabSpace Biosciences (Suzhou) Co., Ltd., Jiangsu
Ting Xu	Alphamab Co., Ltd., Jiangsu
Yanmin Tang	Qiming Venture Partners, Beijing
Hao Huang	Jiangsu Hengrui Medicine Co., Ltd., Jiangsu
Yifu Cao	Synermore Biologics Co., Ltd., Jiangsu
Guoqing Cao	Minghui Pharmaceutical, Shanghai
Zhaolong Gong	3D Medicines, Shanghai

Contributors in Pharmacodia

Shu Liu   Jun Xu   Xingxing Wu   Xuefei Gu

专家简介

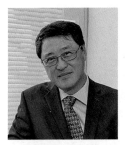

现任美国耶鲁大学 UTC 癌症研究讲席教授，免疫学、肿瘤内科学和皮肤病学教授，耶鲁癌症中心免疫学部主任。主要从事基础免疫学、肿瘤免疫和免疫疾病治疗的研究。首次揭示 PD-L1/PD-1 通路在肿瘤微环境免疫逃逸中的作用并首创以抗体阻断 PD-1/PD-L1 通路治疗癌症的方法。以此发现为基础而发展起来的肿瘤免疫治疗方法已经对癌症治疗产生革命性的转变。先后荣获国际免疫学 William Coley 奖、美国免疫学家协会 AAI-Steinman 奖、中国生物物理学会贝时璋奖，Warren Alpert 基金会奖。

陈列平 博士
著名免疫学家、
首创以抗体阻断
PD-1/PD-L1 通路
治疗癌症的方法

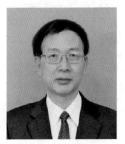

现任四川大学华西医院临床肿瘤中心主任与生物治疗国家重点实验室主任，中国医药生物技术协会理事长，国家生物治疗协同创新中心负责人，国家综合性新药研究开发技术大平台负责人，*Signal Transduction and Targeted Therapy* 共同主编，*Human Gene Therapy* 副主编，*Current Molecular Medicine* 副主编，负责 *Current Cancer Drug Targets* 亚洲地区编委，教育部"长江学者奖励计划"第二批特聘教授，十五"863"生物与农业技术领域生物工程技术主题专家组组长，十二五"863"生物与医学领域生物技术药物主题专家组成员。曾任四川大学副校长，原中华医学会副会长，原教育部科学技术委员会生物医学学部常务副主任。主要从事肿瘤生物治疗的基础研究、关键技术开发、产品研发及临床治疗等，相关研究结果已在多种国际杂志上发表，SCI 论文 300 多篇，申请专利 60 余项，研发了多个创新药，转让给企业后联合开发。

魏于全 博士
中国科学院院士

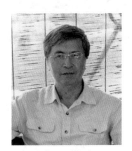

现任吉林大学基础医学院免疫学教授，博士生导师，同写意新药英才俱乐部理事长；兼任国家新药咨询委员会成员，国家自然科学基金委生命科学部专家评审组成员，药渡战略总师等；《药学进展》副主编，尚城资本特聘医药专家等。原白求恩医科大学副校长。主要从事免疫学、分子生物学研究及医药领域投资。先后主持或参与承担国家自然科学基金、卫生部等资助的课题 20 多项，国内外发表论文 200 多篇，主编及参与编写专著和教材 20 余部；指导培养研究生及博士后人员 80 余名。1993 年享受国务院政府特殊津贴；先后荣获"全国中青年医学科技之星"称号、"世川医学奖学金优秀归国进修人员奖"、"全国优秀留学回国人员"，并于 2000 年入选教育部"高等学院骨干教师资助计划"及"跨世纪优秀人才培养计划"。

朱迅 博士
著名免疫学家

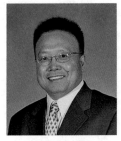

现任嘉和生物药业有限公司总裁，同时担任中国药学会药物生物技术理事会特邀副理事长，中国蛋白质药物质量联盟发起人和第一届主席，ISPE（国际制药工程协会）生物药产品与工艺中国区发起人和第一届主席，Amgen 中国校友会发起人和第一届会长。曾任全球最大生物制药公司 Amgen 工艺开发科学总监，北京大学国际药物工程管理硕士项目客座教授。

周新华 博士
"千人计划"专家

专家简介

（以姓氏笔画为序）

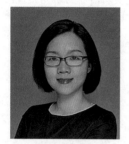

丁红霞 博士

现任 Pharmacodia（药渡）CEO，拥有 12 年以上创新药物研发项目工作经验。2013 年，联合创办药渡，打造了中国第一个独创的"全球药物研发大数据平台-药渡数据"。曾任职 Shenogen（盛诺基医药）化学部高级研发总监，BioDuro（保诺科技）资深组长。在过去的 8 年中，特邀撰写全球每年上市新药综述文章 *Synthetic Approaches to Year's New Drugs*，并发表于 *Journal of Medicinal Chemistry* 和 *Bioorganic & Medicinal Chemistry* 等杂志，该综述连续 5 年成为该杂志中下载量最高的期刊文章。

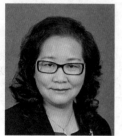

马璟 博士
研究员

现任国家上海新药安全评价研究中心主任，博士生导师，中国药理学会毒理专业委员会主任，中国毒理学会常务理事兼副秘书长，中国药学会药物安全评价专业委员会副主任，上海市药理学会副理事长、毒理专业委员会主任，原国家食品药品监督管理总局（CFDA）药品审评专家及 GLP 检查专家，担任《中国医药工业杂志》《中国药理与毒理学杂志》《中国药理学通报》《中国不良反应杂志》等杂志编委。主要从事药物的药理、毒理学研究，先后主持承担国家"863"、"十一五"、"十二五"重大新药创制重大专项、国家自然科学基金等 20 多项课题，发表论文 100 余篇。曾获国务院政府特殊津贴、全国"五一"劳动奖章、全国优秀科技工作者称号、上海市科学进步二等奖、上海市浦东新区科学技术奖一等奖、上海市领军人才称号、上海市巾帼创新奖等。

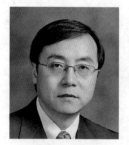

王劲松 博士

现任和铂医药创始人、董事长兼首席执行官，中国抗癌协会肿瘤精准治疗专业委员会常务委员，药物信息协会（DIA）中国区顾问委员会主席，宾夕法尼亚大学医学院内科风湿免疫科客座助理教授。曾任赛诺菲中国研发中心总裁和亚太区转化医学负责人，百时美施贵宝药物发现和临床药理总监等，惠氏制药转化医学部炎症免疫、肌肉骨骼性疾病以及妇女健康等部门的负责人。曾担任中国国家自然科学基金重点及国际重大合作项目的评审专家，英国医学研究委员会、英国国家卫生研究院及国民医疗服务机构的评审专家。在国际权威学术期刊发表论文数十篇，并参与撰写多本教科书中有关转化医学、炎症与自身免疫疾病的章节。

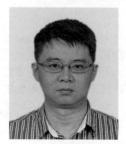

王笑非 博士

现任佛山安普泽生物医药股份有限公司首席科学家，生物药物药学研究和中试平台（与广东省科学院下辖广东省生物资源应用研究所合作共建）负责人。曾在 Avigen、Amgen 公司担任项目科学家，负责工程细胞株构建、中试工艺放大以及生产线扩建等工作。2015 年入选广东省第五批"珠江人才计划"领军人才。

专家简介

（以姓氏笔画为序）

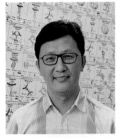

卢宏韬 博士
"千人计划" 专家

现任科望医药（礼来亚洲基金独家投资）共同创始人和首席科学官，生物医药产业著名免疫学家。在美期间在 Berlex/Bayer Schering Pharma 负责对自身免疫病和肿瘤新靶点的鉴定和验证；曾任葛兰素史克高级总监和首任全球神经免疫部门负责人，主导 GSK 中国研发中心神经免疫研发的战略和执行；曾任再鼎医药 CEO，为再鼎建立了研发团队和完整的产品线，并且完成多个重磅品种的引进。

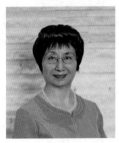

丛杰

现任北京佰荣泰华生物医药科技有限公司 CEO。曾是美国昆泰中国代表处第一批经理人。在新药注册和临床试验领域拥有丰富的实操经验和项目管理经验，主持过 50 余项新药注册及临床试验项目，是创新药临床申报和早期临床研究策略专家。

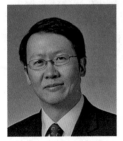

朱祯平 博士
"千人计划" 专家

现任三生制药集团研发总裁兼首席科学官。曾任 Kadmon 公司执行副总裁，ImClone Systems 公司研发副总裁，Novartis 生物制药研发副总裁兼蛋白质科学和药物设计全球总管；曾兼任中国医学科学院/北京协和医学院血液学研究所客座教授。参与及领导研发出多种 FDA 批准上市的治疗性抗肿瘤抗体，包括 cetuximab（Erbitux®，爱必妥）、ramucirumab（Cyramza®，雷莫芦）、necitumumab（Portrazza®）和 olaratumab（Lartruvo®），是 ramucirumab 和 necitumumab 的专利发明人。有超过 30 年在治疗性抗体领域研发的经历，包括 25 年在美国和欧洲大型国际生物制药企业研发和管理的经验。至今在国际刊物发表学术论文 190 余篇，包括第一或通讯作者 100 余篇。已申请或获得美国和其他国家专利 100 余项。

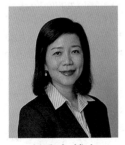

刘千叶 博士

现任本草资本（一家专注于中美医疗健康行业的投资基金）创始合伙人。曾任开物投资合伙人、崇德投资董事总经理。拥有哈佛大学免疫学博士、哈佛医学院医学科学硕士、康奈尔大学生物化学理学学士以及长江商学院 EMBA 学位。从 2005 年开始从事医疗投资，是中国医疗行业最早的投资人之一。一直负责领导生物医药项目投资并已参与投资二十几个医疗项目，领域涉及新药开发，医疗器械，临床诊断，宠物健康等等多个细分行业。

专家简介

（以姓氏笔画为序）

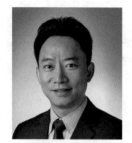

李竞 博士

现任药明生物技术有限公司高级副总裁。曾任美国惠氏制药公司（现辉瑞制药公司）高级研究员和项目负责人，美国诺华制药公司肿瘤研究部试验室负责人兼项目负责人，及诺华生物制药中心生物新药研发战略合作高级主管。曾获耶鲁大学管理学院工商管理硕士学位。拥有 20 年以上抗体工程的专业经验和 18 年以上生物新药研发的工业界经验，2015 年入选江苏双创人才计划。

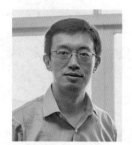

李百勇 博士

现任中山康方生物医药有限公司副总裁及首席科学官。主持研发的肿瘤免疫治疗抗体 AK107 成功授权给美国默沙东，公司在研新药项目 29 个，其中 8 个项目已进入临床试验阶段。曾任美国辉瑞公司肿瘤研究部研发总监，成功领导了多项用于癌症免疫调节治疗的单克隆抗体研发并获得了美国的 IND 临床批文。拥有 20 余年学术界和生物制药工业界的从业经历，是免疫学和抗体新药研发专家。

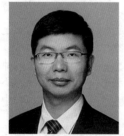

李超凡

现任超凡知识产权服务股份有限公司副总裁、数据与咨询事业部总经理。主要从事专利挖掘、布局、组合设计以及专利分析方法研究。精通专利信息检索以及竞争情报挖掘。曾任国家知识产权局原副处长/审查员，国家知识产权局第一批高层次人才，国家知识产权局专利分析带头人，学术委员会文献专业委员会委员，知识产权示范城市专利分析与布局指导专家，重大经济科技知识产权评议指导专家。

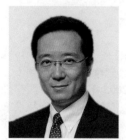

吴辰冰 博士
"千人计划"专家

现任上海岸迈生物科技有限公司总裁。曾任职于雅培制药公司生物研究中心、上海睿智化学研究有限公司、上海中信国健药业股份有限公司（首席科学官兼研究院院长）。主要从事分子免疫及抗体药物研究工作，有多篇首席作者论文发表在 *Nature Immunology* 和 *Nature Biotechnology* 等国际一流学术期刊上，并有多项国际专利授权和 50 多项国际专利申请。曾带领多个项目从早期研究开始成功进入到临床申报。目前带领团队开发出新一代的双特异性抗体平台技术 "FIT-Ig"，并有多种由该技术开发出来的新型抗体进入临床申报阶段。

专家简介

（以姓氏笔画为序）

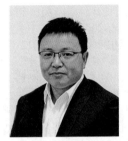

陈宜顶

现任 ACROBiosystems（百普赛斯）董事长兼 CEO。曾担任 Thermo Fisher 工业项目应用科学家。拥有超过 15 年在制药相关及生物技术公司产品开发、运营管理及国际市场拓展经验。

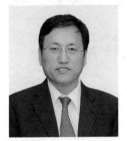

孟坤 博士
"千人计划"专家

现任盛诺基医药集团创始人兼 CEO；为国务院特殊津贴专家，北京市"海聚人才"、"百名领军人才"及山东"泰山学者"等。拥有 20 年以上分子生物学、小分子药物和药理学方面的研究经验，发表了 30 多篇学术论文，拥有几十项新药发明专利。十年以上药物研发和管理经验，始终致力于创新药物的研发，所开发的抗肿瘤 I 类新药阿可拉定已进入临床III期，后续产品抗体、抗体偶联及小分子药物也即将陆续进入临床。凭借多年的科研和管理经验，深刻了解药物开发从科研到临床、从市场营销到资本市场的全过程。

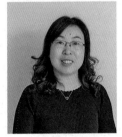

赵小平 博士

现任上海益诺思生物技术有限公司（国家上海新药安全评价研究中心）药代及生物分析总监，副研究员。曾任职于上海恒瑞医药有限公司、保诺科技（北京）有限公司。超过 10 年的药物代谢研究经验，主要从事小分子药物和生物技术药物的生物分析、PK/TK，PK-PD，临床药理及转化医学等研究。负责及参与多项国家十二五、十三五重大新药创制课题，北京、上海市多项课题。在药物分析、药物代谢动力学方向发表论文 20 余篇，SCI 文章超过 15 篇。

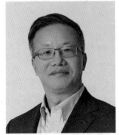

俞德超 博士
"千人计划"专家

现任信达生物制药（苏州）有限公司董事长兼总裁。国内外刊物上发表了 60 多篇 SCI 论文和专著，70 多项专利（包括 38 项美国专利）发明人。发明了世界上第一个上市的肿瘤溶瘤免疫治疗类抗肿瘤药物"安柯瑞"，开创了人类利用病毒治疗肿瘤的先河；共同发明和领导开发了中国第一个拥有全球知识产权的单克隆抗体新药"康柏西普"。先后荣获 2013 年"国家生命科学领域最具影响力的海归人才"、2014 年"创新中国十大年度人物"、2015 年"安永企业家"奖、2016 年"江苏省优秀企业家"、"国家 2016 年度科技创新人物"、"2017 中国医药经济年度人物"、"2017 生命科学领域最具影响力的十大年度人物"等。

专家简介

（以姓氏笔画为序）

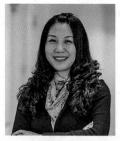

夏瑜 博士
"千人计划"专家

现任中山康方生物医药有限公司董事长、总裁兼首席执行官。曾任职德国拜耳、美国 PDL 生物制药（现雅培制药）、美国 Celera Genomics 等欧美制药公司；2008 年担任中美冠科生物技术有限公司生物制药部资深副总裁，辉瑞-亚洲癌症研究中心负责人；2012 年联合创建中山康方生物医药有限公司。国家"千人计划"、科技部"创新创业人才"、广东省"特支计划"创业人才、广东省"双创人才"。拥有 20 余年学术界和生物制药工业界的从业经历，是抗体药物发现、生产工艺开发及规模化生产专家。曾成功领导了全球第一例跨国制药公司抗体新药研发在中国的整体合作项目；国内首例由创新型生物科技公司将完全自主研发的单克隆抗体新药授权给全球制药巨头美国默沙东，实现国产创新抗体药物在海外市场的新突破。

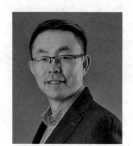

钱雪明 博士
"千人计划"专家

现任迈博斯生物创始人及首席执行官。苏州工业园区领军人才，苏州市姑苏人才和第十二批国家"千人计划"创业人才，百华协会会员和新药创始人俱乐部会员。曾在美国安进公司任职 12 年，参与及领导开发了多个抗体新药项目。

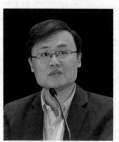

徐霆 博士
"千人计划"专家

现任苏州康宁杰瑞生物科技有限公司总裁。曾担任 Archemix、Serono 和 Biogenldec 公司资深首席研究员等职位，先后成立苏州康宁杰瑞生物科技有限公司、康宁杰瑞（吉林）生物科技有限公司和苏州丁孚靶点生物技术有限公司。拥有对蛋白质药物筛选、表达、纯化、分析、质控及动物药理毒理方面丰富的经验和独特的见解，发表了多篇关于蛋白质化学的具有重要创新性的研究论文，参与开发的多个蛋白质工程药物已经在欧美上市或处在临床阶段。目前已建立多个自有知识产权的研发平台，转让生物类似药项目近 30 个，大多进入临床开发，自主申报创新药临床批件 9 项，6 个项目进入临床开发。申请专利 20 多项，获得专利授权 7 项。

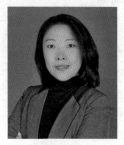

唐艳旻

现任启明创投投资合伙人、暨南大学生物工程硕士研究生实践指导教师。生物化学与分子生物学专业硕士，长江商学院工商管理学硕士。曾就职于葛兰素史克制药公司，从事新药注册公司长达 7 年；自 2002 年担任晨兴创投北京办公室总经理，开始了新药投资生涯，至今已有 16 年。在此期间，独立投资数十家生物医药公司，任多家公司董事，深度参与投后管理及项目退出。

专家简介

（以姓氏笔画为序）

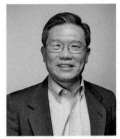

曹一孚 博士

现任美国密歇根大学生物化学工程特聘教授，兴盟生物医药有限公司总裁。曾任 MedImmune 公司副总裁。精通于细胞系和培养基优化、生物反应器流程设计、蛋白质纯化、工艺放大及 cGMP 生产。在美国的 25 年，直接参与负责 8 个生物大分子药物生产基地、涉及 18 个临床试验药物和 4 个上市药物的生产。近年曾任多家生物医药公司顾问，并负责比尔盖茨基金会旗下的 Aeras 的工艺开发、生产、质控和设施设计等细菌和病毒疫苗技术运营。于 2008 年加入晨兴投资集团，专注于指导帮助晨兴相关投资公司生物大分子药物的产业化。于 2013 年创立兴盟制药建设生物药研发生产基地，全权主管平台的设计、规划、建设和技术团队整合。

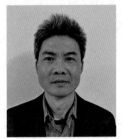

曹国庆 博士
"千人计划"专家

现任明慧医药有限公司董事长及首席执行官。曾在美国礼来从事新药研发，后加入江苏恒瑞医药集团任副总经理。

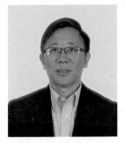

龚兆龙 博士
美国 FDA 新药审评员
（1998–2008）

现任思路迪医药 CEO，中国医药创新促进会药物临床研究专业委员会委员，《中国新药杂志》编委，《药学进展》编委，AAALAC 理事会成员，同写意俱乐部理事。曾任美国 FDA 新药审评员（1998-2008）。2008 年回国后先后担任昭衍新药首席技术官，莱博药业 CEO 和百济神州新药开发和药政副总裁。近 20 年中，从 FDA、CRO 和新药研发企业等不同角度参与新药研发，在新药全球开发战略规划、非临床和临床试验方案设计、GLP 及 GCP 法规、新药项目选择及成药性评估、协调推进非临床试验和临床试验以及项目推进中的风险评估等方面积累了丰富的经验。

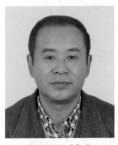

程远国 博士
研究员

现任上海益诺思生物技术有限公司（国家上海新药安全评价研究中心）副总裁，首席科学官，博士生导师，上海市生物技术药物 PK-PD 工程技术中心主任，原国家食品药品监督管理总局新药审评专家，全国药物代谢专业委员会委员。曾任军事医学科学院微生物流行病研究所生物技术药物 PK-PD 研究室主任。主要从事生物技术药物代谢及分子药理研究，在生物技术药物代谢动力学及其相关领域的研究中积累了丰富的经验。近几年，先后申请并承担国家与"新药药物 PK-PD 及相关技术研究"相关的"十五"科技攻关课题 1 项，重大新药创制课题 2 项，国家"863"计划重大课题 2 项，国家自然基金课题 4 项，北京市自然基金课题 3 项，与科研院、所及企业合作课题 150 余项。目前共发表论文 30 余篇，其中 SCI 论文 20 篇。

Foreword I

Monoclonal Antibody: The Crown Jewel of Biologic Drugs

The last two decades have witnessed dramatic progress in the medical applications of monoclonal antibody (mAb) which is undoubtedly taking center stage in pharmaceutical industry. In the 1990s, it was even hard to believe that mAb could become drug. In fact, upon initial excitement in the 1980s to successfully produce recombinant mAb, major pharmaceutical companies dramatically decreased their efforts on mAb-based drug development, largely due to its high cost, limited understanding of its biological behavior in the human body, and a competition from the boom in small molecule drugs. During this "dark" time, however, scientists who believed in mAb, continued their work to significantly improve technology. Impactful advancements in mAb technology in the last 15-20 years have led to high-yield production of genetic engineering of recombinant mAb as well as the success of several therapeutic mAbs in medical applications, which is serving to revive and raise awareness in the field once again.

Why and how can a mAb become good drug? The foremost aspects depend on its specificity. The interaction of a mAb and its target protein is highly specific, which relies on a complicated and less understood process, but involves matching two sophisticated protein structures on their interface. Conformational recognition structures and multiple anchor points all contribute to this specificity. The mAb-target protein interaction is non-covalent in an on- and off-mode which assures and re-assures binding specificity. The second critical feature of a mAb is high affinity for target protein. The affinities of mAbs may vary but the majority of them is at least one or two logs higher than the intrinsic interactions of proteins. This allows efficient interference and manipulation of physiological interactions of intrinsic protein interactions. Commonly used IgG mAbs are also dimeric, which facilitates binding with avidity. The third feature is favorable pharmacokinetics and pharmacodynamics of mAbs in the human body. An IgG molecule is large with a molecular weight of 150-170 kDa and the Fc portion of an antibody also binds Fc receptors which are widely available in the body. These features ensure that an antibody could be retained in the body and give most mAbs long serum half-life in comparison with other small molecules and chemicals.

Nothing is perfect and the mAb has its own challenges as a drug. Although one can generate mAbs against virtually any protein using current technologies, antibodies do not normally penetrate cell membrane to interact with intracellular proteins due to their large size and a lack of cell internalization mechanisms in general. Therefore, the targets of antibodies are limited to a fraction of all proteins. In the human genome, ~ 35,000 coding genes are estimated to produce proteins with ~8,000 encoding cell surface proteins and ~1,500 soluble proteins. Therefore, only ~1/3-1/4 human proteins can be recognized by mAbs and serve as mAb targets. Another issue is an antibody's immunogenicity. While antibodies represent host-defense tools that recognize the non-self and eventually remove them from the body, an antibody itself could also be recognized as the foreign by the immune system, such as by other antibodies and T lymphocytes, and because of this recognition, be removed from the body. While a naturally produced antibody could be considered completely self, its idiotype could still be recognized by other B-cells and therefore other antibodies. Repeated antibody administration could elicit neutralizing antibodies, due to incomplete tolerance during the development of the immune system. Finally, engineered proteins, which may alter the sequence and order of amino acids, could be recognized by the immune system and therefore, the induction of neutralizing antibodies. With the advancement of antibody engineering technologies, it is likely that all these issues could be overcome in the near future.

As an immunologist using mAb daily as a research tool and for drug discovery, the mAb is a large part of my life. I am glad to see the Pharmaceutical Index publish this landmark book, Biologics: Monoclonal Antibodies, and I applaud its success.

Lieping Chen, M.D., Ph.D.
United Technologies Corporation Professor in Cancer Research
Professor of Immunobiology, Dermatology and Medicine
Director of Cancer Immunology Program
Yale University School of Medicine
New Haven, Connecticut, USA
January 2018

Foreword II

即使明知药物研发工作需要按部就班地进行，不能一蹴而就，但每个科学家在情感上都希望能马上研发出可以对指定疾病有效的药物，因为在当下正有成千上万的患者承受病痛折磨并翘首以待最好的药物治疗方法和产品，这种动力和紧迫感，会驱动科学家们不断尝试用一切可能的方法去开展探索，以期缩短发现最好治疗方法和治疗药物的时间。数据时代的来临，为科学家的梦想提供了新的可能。

从 2003 年开始，存储技术和运算能力的发展速度超出了人类自身的想象，巨大的网络沉淀下来的无穷尽的珍贵数据，让我们史无前例的认识到，那是人类的思想和行为宝藏。科学本就是探索从偶然性到必然性之规律，大数据时代让我们更加理性和科学地预测和规划我们的未来。而将药物研发工作放在大数据时代的背景下，必定会给我们的研发工作带来新的思考和新的契机，虽然目前并没有明确的案例证明，以大数据驱动的药物筛选和设计方法能缩短发现新疗法和新产品的时间，但大数据在其他领域取得的瞩目成就以及在药物研发领域的实验性探索，让我们有理由对药物研发的大数据时代充满期待。

作为一名科研工作者，如何与时俱进的建立大数据思维方式，或许是成为你们脱颖而出的因素之一。科学没有定义和规定我们要必须遵从某种共同的研究模式开展科学研究工作，科学研究方法必须足够多样，人类的智慧之花才能绚烂多彩。科学家要具有怀疑精神，但所有的怀疑都建立在规律之上，而不是凭空想象。透过更多的数据来源并加以分析，必定会让科学家们在掌握更多信息的情况下，以科学精神将信息转化为知识并发现可能的创新，这一点毋庸置疑。

无论怎样，今天从事药物研发的科学家，比以往任何时候都需要更多精准的多学科数据为药物研发工作提供智力支持。药物研发工作需要和化学、生物、医学、数学、计算机等学科高速融合和发展，药物研发的全球化知识共享时代已经到来。

从 1975 年 Kohler 和 Milstein 创立了体外杂交瘤技术，得到了鼠源单克隆抗体，为抗体大规模应用于疾病治疗奠定了基础，开创了单克隆抗体技术的新时代，Kohler 和 Milstein 也因此获得 1984 年诺贝尔医学奖。随着分子生物学技术、抗体库技术、转基因技术的发展，单克隆抗体经历了嵌合单抗、人源化单抗、全人源单抗几个阶段。单克隆抗体以其特异性、均一性、可大量生产等优点，已经广泛用于疾病的治疗。相关数据显示，国内单抗药物复合增长率远高于其他医药细分子行业。目前全球已有 85 个抗体类药物获批，年销售额接近千亿美元；全球销售排名前十位的产品中有 6 个是抗体类药物。国内单抗药品总体市场规模小、增速快，对中国药物研发从业者来说，随着中国药物研发政策的不断利好，单抗药物研发的创新活力将以前所未有的形式迸发，并驱动中国单抗药物研发以满足更广阔的刚性需求。而创新的知识源和动力源必须依靠信息和数据。

"药渡"（Pharmacodia）主编的《世界新药概览单克隆抗体卷 I》图书，涵盖了 1997-2016 年最具有代表性、体现领域多样性以及对未来研发有重要影响的单抗药物。我非常高兴地看到由"药渡"完成的首部抗体药物数据工具图书《世界新药概览单克隆抗体卷 I》即将出版发行，这部图书分别从靶点生物学，抗体药物基本信息（包括氨基酸序列、作用机制图、批准的适应症及用量、上市后的每年销量等），临床前药理、药代、毒理试验数据，临床疗效与安全性试验数据，及关键专利信息几个方面进行了详实、精准的数据汇整；同时也给出了相关专利、文献和资料以及数据的来源。这些数据和相关信息线索，可大为节省科研工作者文件检索和有效信息的筛选时间，特别是为从事 biosimilar、biobetter 及创新性抗体药物的研发人员提供有价值的参考。

我有幸受邀做这个序，也为药渡这家致力于为中国药物研发提供大数据支撑的创业团队感到骄傲和敬佩。这是机遇，也是挑战。这是中国药物研发的大时代，其中卓越的药物研发数据支撑能力，是中国的药物研发水平在新的历史契机中弯道超车并屹立于世界之林的硬指标之一。

祝《世界新药概览单克隆抗体卷 I》发行成功。

魏于全
中国科学院院士
中国医药生物技术协会 理事长
四川大学生物治疗国家重点实验室主任

yu-quan Wei

Preface I

Current Global mAb Market Landscape and Current Blockbuster Agents

The global monoclonal antibody (mAb) therapeutic market reached about $62.3bn in 2015, up from revenues of $44.6 bn (USD) in 2010 due to great global sales of many blockbuster mAb therapeutics (Table 1). A recent report thus by Visiongain, a London-based business information company, forecasts that the monoclonal antibody drug market will expand steadily through 2021. There will be sales growth in established and emerging markets, especially in the U.S., Japan, China and India. The future of mAb technologies is promising, with high demand for novel treatments for cancer, autoimmune diseases and eye disorders in particular.

Monoclonal antibody therapeutic shows great treatment for autoimmune diseases where chimeric and humanized mAb are produced and used in clinical application due to the extremely efficacious clinical effects observed (Figure 1). In comparison, mAb agents designed for oncology including Rituxin®, Herceptin® and Avastin® showed limited clinical effects. The data showed that statistically, treatments with these drugs only prolonged the patient's life by 6 to 8 months. However, recent breakthroughs in check-point mAb development revealed great insight to treat the most threating tumor diseases-Melanoma. After treatment with PD-1 mAb, a patient who may have prolonged her or his life by 2-3 months now has a prognosis of 4-6 years. Mr. Jimmy Carter, the previous U.S. President, is a successful case for using new immunotherapy drugs to prolong the life of a patient. The therapeutic power of mAb released T-cells of human immunologic system and cured his disease for now. These facts have pushed the research and development of novel antibody therapeutics to the forefront. Treatment effects through check-point mAb or CAR-NK cells/macrophages to fight with tumor tissues will reveal bright new avenues of therapy in comparison with the treatment by using small molecule drugs, E. coli derived recombinant proteins and even targeted naked mAbs (Figure 1).

Development History of mAb as Therapeutics to Cure Human Diseases

At least four scientists have received Nobel Prizes due to their excellent work on discovery of antibodies and immunology systems.

Paul Ehrlich initially described the concept of antibodies as therapeutic agents in his seminal 1891 manuscript "Experimental Studies on Autoimmunity," in which he introduced the term "antik¨orper," German for antibody. He also introduced the concept of Zaberkugel (magic bullet) therapeutics. He and Élie Metchnikoff received the 1908 Nobel Prize for Physiology or Medicine for this work, which led to an effective syphilis treatment by 1910. In 1972, Gerald M. Edelman from the United States and Rodney R. Porter from United Kingdom received the Nobel Prize for their discoveries concerning the chemical structure of antibodies. In 1975, Georges Köhler and César Milstein succeeded in making fusions of myeloma cell lines with B cells to create hybridomas that could produce antibodies, specific to known antigens and were immortalized. They shared the Nobel Prize in Physiology or Medicine in 1984 for the discovery. In 1987, Susumu Tonegawa from Japan received Nobel Prize for his discovery of the genetic principle for generation of antibody diversity.

Although these great findings provided solid foundation for antibodies and human immunology, the application of so-called "magic bullet" in human diseases has undergone nearly two to three decades. In 1980s, initial clinical trial using mouse antibody caused great immunogenic problems. To fix the severe damage on human patients, four major historic milestones have been achieved in the past 20 some years that mAb generation platform nowadays led to fully human mAb from mouse mAb, chimeric mAb and then human-ized mAb. The fully human mAb is designed and produced attempt to solve the dangerous issue of im-munogenicity which is sometimes deadly for the patient.

As a feasible clinical agent, the amount of mAb produced to meet patients is very critical. The titer in early 1990s was only about 10-50 mg/L produced in expensive cell culture media, so producing it was more costly than mining for gold. In following decade, "crazy" scientists found the way out to make titer from 1g/L to today's 5-10 g/L (Figure 2). Advanced technology also led to significant improvements in up-stream processes and downstream processes. In the upstream process, stable cell culture today can be employed for 6-8 months instead of the cells surviving for just 200 hrs. The media cost has been signifi-cantly reduced to current price of $2-5/L depending on the amount used. These achievements make new application of Alternative Tangential Filtration (ATF) concentrated fed batch or ATF perfusion that can present high titer up to 10 g/L routinely. In downstream process, column unit operation has been reduced from a previous 5-step process to a 3-step or even 2-step operation with extensive usage of filters that reduce manufacturing time from 15 to 5 days, and total average recovery yield of 70%.

A high titer production of mAb therapeutics makes the high dosage of mAb in clinical application possible. For example, for a recent PD-L1 mAb in one injection, 1.2 g is needed for oncology patients. The high titer of mAb makes ADC (Antibody Drug Conjugate) feasible as well, and several ADC therapeutic mole-cules have been launched in the market for oncology indications (Figure 2).

Due to a high production titer, large 15,000-25,000 L stainless steel bioreactors with automated systems are not the industry preferred technology anymore. Instead, Single Use Systems (SUS) have become pop-ular (Figure 2). These plastic bioreactor bags can easily handle the mass up to 2,000 L and 10 g/L with ATF technology is expected. In this new manufacturing arena, the modern facility has the characteristic of flexibility and can handle multi-product processes for cost effective production (Figure 2).

Drug Perspectives: Biologics in the Future

In this edition of the mAb index, what we have listed as references in the book is current mAb therapeutics. Some of them are blockbuster drugs with global sales of over 6 billion US dollars. The rest of the new-comers have global sales at least over a few million US dollars, which will likely increase to a few billion US dollar market. Meanwhile newly developed therapeutic mAbs for different indications will be updated in later editions.

Therapeutic mAb has advanced the treatment of autoimmune diseases and recent effective therapies for oncology patients with check-point mAbs after three decades of innovation and development in this arena. There are still many challenges for the mAb market.
1. High potency of mAb significantly to reduce dosage that seems crucial. In the current application of mAb therapeutics a high dosage is always needed for cancer patients. A just approved PD-L1 mAb re-quires a dosage of 1.2 g of injection per patient. This can cause potential challenges on manufacturing capacity, product impurity, worries for immunogenicity issues and drug stability.
2. New formulation development is great requirement arena. In the future, s.c. administration is becoming popular, less volume handling (<1 mL per injection) is needed thus a high concentration of mAb in a stable form in syringe is required.
3. The high cost of mAb therapeutics needs to be addressed. It seems that mAb biosimilars and newly

developed novel mAbs request highly efficient bioprocess and continuous bioprocess is expected to solve the cost issue; but there are still many years to come for solving continuous process dilemma.

4. Extensive selection of sensitive and robust biomarker is perhaps another area for future precision medicine application particularly for mAb therapeutics. Great biomarker can speed up clinical trials and increase successful rate remarkably.

In order for entire industry to overcome these issues, advanced technology in drug design, bioprocess including USP and DSP, modern facility design should be our focus. In addition, new target validation for even much powerful mAb discovery is expected. In our next edition, a new generation of mAb therapeutics will exhibit the much progress in the industry.

Table 1 Global: Continuous Growing Trend of Biologics Top 16-Best Selling in 2013: mAbs

Drug Name	Company	2013 (Billion $)	2012 (Billion $)	Change, %	Class
Humira	Abbvie/Abbot	10.66	9.27	14.99	mAb
Remicade	JNJ, Merck	8.94	8.22	8.76	mAb
Rituxan/MabThera	Roche, Biogen Idec	8.92	8.65	3.12	mAb
Advair/Seretide	GSK	8.78	8.40	4.52	Small mol.
Enbrel	Amgen, Pfizer	8.33	7.96	4.65	mAb
Lantus (Insulin Glargine)	Sanofi	7.85	6.65	18.05	rProtein
Avastin (Bevacizumab)	Roche	7.04	6.49	8.47	mAb
Herceptin (Trastuzumab)	Roche	6.84	6.62	3.32	mAb
Crestor (Rosuvastatin Cal.)	AstraZeneca	5.99	6.62	-9.52	Small mol.
Abilify (Aripiprazole)	Otsuka, BMS	5.27	4.09	28.85	Small mol.
Cymbalta (Duloxetine)	Eli Lilly, Shionogi	5.19	5.08	2.17	Small mol.
Gleevec (Imatinib mesylate)	Novartis	4.69	4.68	0.21	Small mol.
Lyrica/pregabalin	Pfizer	4.60	4.16	10.58	Small mol.
Neulasta (Pegfilgrastim)	Amgen	4.39	4.09	7.33	rProtein
Copaxone	Teva	4.33	4.00	8.25	Polypeptide
Revlimid (Lenalidomide)	Celgene	4.28	3.77	13.53	Small mol.

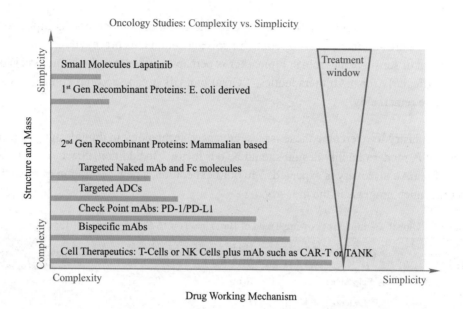

Figure 1   Comparison of Molecule's Size vs. Drug's Working Mechanism Demonstrates Efficacy in Oncology Studies
(Y-axis presents the structure and mass of therapeutics, x-axis presents working mechanism of therapeutics,
and colour depth from left to right presents treatment efficacy.)

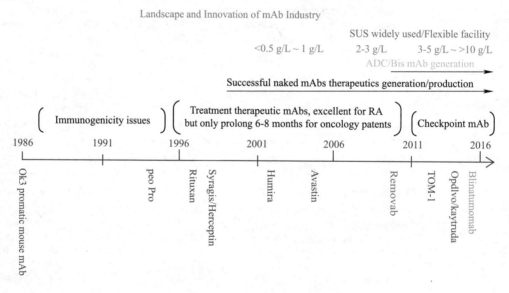

Figure 2   Landscape and Innovation of mAb Industry

Joe Zhou, PhD
Genor Biopharma Co. Ltd., CEO
La Jolla, California, USA
December, 2015

Contents

This first volume of the book series, "The Pharmaceutical Index Biologics: Monoclonal Antibodies", includes detailed information for ten blockbuster antibody drugs that were approved between 1997-2016 with annual sales reaching over one billion USD.

Stay tuned for more of the "The Pharmaceutical Index Biologics: Monoclonal Antibodies" book series. The second volume of the book series will soon be published. It also includes ten approved monoclonal antibody drugs: adalimumab, denosumab, evolocumab, infliximab, nivolumab, palivizumab, pembrolizumab, ramucirumab, secukinumab, and ustekinumab.

CHAPTER

1

Ado-trastuzumab Emtansine

Ado-trastuzumab Emtansine

(Kadcyla®)

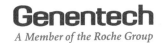
Genentech
A Member of the Roche Group

Research code: PRO-132365, R-3502, RG-3502, RO-5304020, T-DM1

1 Target Biology

The HER2 Receptor

❖ The human epidermal growth factor receptor 2 (HER2, also known as Neu, ErbB-2, CD340 or p185) is a member of the epidermal growth factor receptor (EGFR/ErbB) family encoded by the ERBB2 gene.   The family also includes the endothelial growth factor receptor (EGFR/ErbB-1), HER3, and HER4 receptors.   These receptors function by forming homo- and hetero-dimers with members of the family, with HER2 as the preferred binding partner.[1]

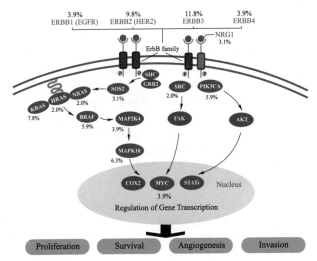

❖ HER2 binds to other members of EGF receptor family to form a heterodimer, which acts as co-receptor or a shared signaling unit, leading to stabilized ligand binding, prolonged and enhanced downstream signaling (i.e. MAPK and PI3K pathways), which regulates cell differentiation, growth and proliferation.

❖ Sequence homology of HER2 proteins can be found in Chapter *Trastuzumab*.[2]

❖ Overexpression and amplification of HER2 is present in approximately 20.0%-25.0% of human breast cancers.[3] Due to its kinase activity, HER2/neu overexpression results in enhanced tyrosine phosphorylation activities, and an increase in the proliferative stimuli associated with HER2, leading to increased tumor growth.

❖ Five HER2-targeting drugs have been approved and marketed (Gilotrif®, Kadcyla®, Perjeta®, Tykerb®, and Herceptin®).

Tubulin and Microtubules

❖ Tubulin is the protein that polymerizes into long chains that form microtubules, a major component of the eukaryotic cytoskeleton, found throughout the cytoplasm.[4]

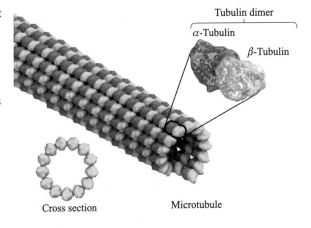

Tubulin dimer
α-Tubulin
β-Tubulin

Cross section   Microtubule

❖ With the ability to shift through various formations, microtubules function in several essential cellular processes, including mitosis.   Microtubules are the major constituents of mitotic spindles and are involved in chromosome separation, facilitating cell division.[5]

❖ Tubulins are targets for anticancer drugs like Taxol®, tesetaxel and the "vinca alkaloid" drugs such as vinblastine and vincristine.   Taxol® prevents a cell from dividing by binding to tubulin and causing the proteins to lose its flexibility.[6]   In clinical, it is an effective treatment for a number of cancers including breast, lung and ovarian.

2   General Information

Kadcyla®

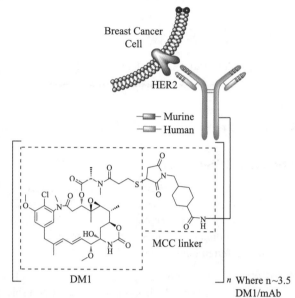

❖ Kadcyla® (Ado-trastuzumab emtansine) is an antibody-drug conjugate (ADC).   It is composed of the cytotoxic agent $N^{2'}$-deacetyl-$N^{2'}$-(3-mercapto-1-oxopropyl)-maytansine (DM1) conjugated to trastuzumab via a linker molecule succin-imidyl-*trans*-4-[*N*-maleimidomethyl]cyclohexane-1-carboxylate (SMCC).   The ADC is abbreviated as T-DM1. The average drug to antibody ratio is approximately 3.5:1 with a maximum ratio of 8:1.[7]

- **Trastuzumab**: A recombinant DNA-derived humanized monoclonal antibody that targets the extracellular domain of the ErbB-2/Her2/neu receptor, sold under the brand name Herceptin®.   Detailed information on trastuzumab can be found in Chapter *Trastuzumab*.[2]
- **DM1**: A thiol-containing derivative of cytotoxic agent, also called Mertansine®.   DM1 blocks the polymerization of tubulin, arrests the cell cycle at G2/M phase, and inhibits mitosis.   DM1 has a similar mechanism of action to the vinca alkaloids, however, it is 20-100 times more potent than vincristine, 24-270 times more potent than paclitaxel, and 2-3 times more potent than doxorubicin.
- **SMCC**: A non-cleavable linker, containing two functional groups: a succinimide ester and a maleimide.   The succin-imide ester group of SMCC reacts with lysine residue in the trastuzumab molecule to form trastuzumab-MCC via an amide bond.   The maleimide moiety then links to the free sulfhydryl group of DM1, forming trastuzumab-MCC-DM1 (T-DM1) via a thioether bond.
- **Emtansine**: The moiety of MCC-DM1.

❖ Kadcyla® binds to HER2 with an affinity similar to that of trastuzumab, which is required for its anti-tumor activity.   It is hypothesized that after binding to HER2, ado-trastuzumab emtansine undergoes receptor-mediated internalization, fol-lowed by intracellular release of DM1 and subsequent cyto-toxic killing of tumor cells.[7]

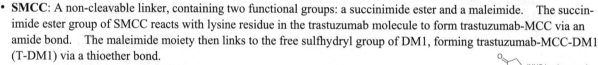

❖ Kadcyla® is provided as a single-use lyophilized formulation in a colorless 20 mL Type I glass vial.   Upon reconstitution, the resulting product contains 20 mg/mL ado-trastuzumab emtansine, 10 mM sodium succinate, pH 5.0, 6.0% (*W/V*) (i.e., 60 mg/mL) sucrose, and 0.020% (*W/V*) polysorbate 20.   Each 20 mL vial allows delivery of 160 mg ado-trastuzumab emtansine.   The reconstituted product contains no preservative and is intended for single use only.[7]

❖ The total sales of 839 million US$ for 2016; No sales data as of 2017.

Mechanism of Action[3, 7]

❖ The mechanism of action of Kadcyla® consists of a multi-step process:

- Binding of T-DM1 to HER2-overexpressing tumor cell disrupts the interaction between HER2 and other ligand-bound members of the EGFR family, thus interfering with the transduction of HER2-mediated growth signals.
- Recognition of the trastuzumab Fc region by Fc receptors present on immune cells, such as macrophages or natural killer cells, triggers antibody-dependent cell-mediated cytotoxicity (ADCC) targeting the HER2-expressing tumor cell.
- Binding of T-DM1 favors internalization of the HER2-ADC complex.   The following lysosomal proteolysis degrada-tion of the antibody moiety slowly releases Lys-MCC-DM1 molecules, an active derivative of DM1, in the cytoplasm of the tumor cell.   These activated compounds bind tubulin molecules and inhibit microtubule polymerization and mitotic division.

Sponsor

❖ Kadcyla® (Ado-trastuzumab emtansine) was developed and marketed by Genentech, Inc., a subsidiary of Roche.

World Sales[8]

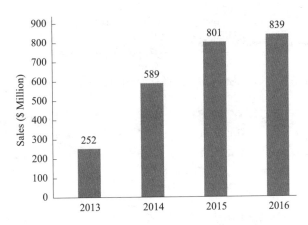

Figure 1   World Sales of Ado-trastuzumab Emtansine since 2013

Approval and Indication[8, 9]

Table 1   Summary of the Approval of Kadcyla®[8, 9]

	US (FDA)	Japan (PMDA)	EU (EMA)
First approval date	02/22/2013	09/20/2013	11/15/2013
Application or approval No.	BLA125427	22500AMX01816 22500AMX01817	EMEA/H/C/002389
Brand name	Kadcyla®	Kadcyla®	Kadcyla®
Indication	MBC	MBC	MBC
Authorization holder	Genentech (Roche)	Chugai (Roche)	Roche

Till Jan 2018, it had not been approved by CFDA (China).   MBC: Metastatic breast cancer.

Table 2   Indication and Administration[9]

No.	Administration	Indication
1	3.6 mg/kg given as an intravenous infusion every 3 weeks (21-day cycle) until disease progression or unacceptable toxicity.	Metastatic HER2-overexpressing breast cancer.

Sourced from US FDA drug label information.

HER2 Antagonist

Table 3　Other Marketed HER2-targeting Drugs[8]

Drug	Trade	Sponsor	Type	Approval	Indication
Trastuzumab	Herceptin®	Genentech (Roche)	HER2-targeting mAb	09/1998-FDA 08/2000-EMA 04/2001-PMDA 12/2015-FDA	BC, ABC, MBC, MGC, EBC
Pertuzumab	Perjeta®	Genentech (Roche)	HER2-targeting mAb	06/2012-FDA 03/2013-EMA 06/2013-PMDA	MBC
Afatinib dimaleate	Gilotrif®	Boehringer Ingelheim	EGFR/HER2 pan antagonist	07/2013-FDA 09/2013-EMA 01/2014-PMDA 02/2017-CFDA	NSCLC
Lapatinib ditosylate hydrate	Tykerb®/Tyverb®	GSK	EGFR/HER2 pan antagonist	03/2007-FDA 06/2008-EMA 04/2009-PMDA 11/2013-CFDA	BC

ABC: Adjuvant treatment for breast cancer.　BC: Breast cancer.　EBC: Early breast cancer.　EGFR: Epidermal growth factor receptor.　HER2: Human epidermal growth factor receptor 2.　mAb: Monoclonal antibody.　MBC: Metastatic breast cancer.　MGC: Metastatic gastric cancer.　NSCLC: Non-small cell lung cancer.

ADC Drugs

Table 4　Other Marketed ADC Drugs[8]

Drug	Trade	Sponsor	Type	Approval	Indication
Brentuximab vedotin	Adcetris®	Seattle Genetics Millennium (Takeda)	CD30-targeting mAb with MMAE	08/2011-FDA 10/2012-EMA 01/2014-PMDA	HD, SALCL

ADC: Antibody drug conjugates.　HD: Hodgkin's disease.　mAb: Monoclonal antibody.　MMAE: Monomethyl auristatin E.　SALCL: Systemic anaplastic large cell lymphoma.

3　CMC Profile

Product Profile[7]

Dosage route:　　IV infusion.
Strength:　　100 and 160 mg per vial.
Dosage form:　　Lyophilized powder for IV infusion solution.
Formulation:　　Upon reconstitution, the resulting product contains 20 mg/mL T-DM1, 10 mM sodium succinate, pH 5.0, 6.0% (*W/V*) (i.e., 60 mg/mL) sucrose, and 0.020% (*W/V*) polysorbate 20.
Dissolution:　　Reconstitution with 5 mL (for 100 mg/vial) or 8 mL (for 160 mg/vial) of the appropriate diluent yields a solution containing 20 mg/mL T-DM1 at pH of approximately 5.0.
Stability:　　The proposed shelf life of T-DM1 drug product, 160 mg/vial, is 36 months when stored at 2-8 °C; the proposed shelf life of T-DM1 drug product, 100 mg/vial, is 24 months when stored at 2-8 °C.

Molecular Information

Molecular formula[3, 10]
　　T-DM1:　　$C_{6448}H_{9948}N_{1720}O_{2012}S_{44} \cdot (C_{47}H_{62}ClN_4O_{13}S)_n$ (n: ~3.5; range: 0-8)
　　Trastuzumab:　　Light chain: $C_{1032}H_{1603}N_{277}O_{335}S_6$
　　　　　　Heavy chain: $C_{2192}H_{3387}N_{583}O_{671}S_{16}$
　　Emtansine:　　$C_{47}H_{62}ClN_4O_{13}S$

Ansamitocin P-3

Molecular weight[10]
　　T-DM1:　　~151 kDa
　　Trastuzumab:　　~148 kDa
　　Emtansine:　　~960 Da

Production Process

- ❖ Trastuzumab: CHO cells platform (disulfide and glycosylation profile can be found in Chapter *Trastuzumab*[2]).
- ❖ DM1: Synthesized starting from ansamitocin p-3[11], which was produced and purified from *Actinosynnema pretiosum*.[12]
- ❖ SMCC linker: Commercially available.
- ❖ T-DM1: The succinimide ester group of SMCC reacts with lysine residue in the trastuzumab molecule to form trastuzumab-MCC via an amide bond. The maleimide moiety then links to the free sulfhydryl group of DM1, forming trastuzumab-MCC-DM1 (T-DM1) via a thioether bond.[13]
- ❖ The average drug-to-antibody ratio (DAR) is approximately 3.5:1 with a maximum ratio of 8:1, which was achieved by controlling the ratio of SMCC to trastuzumab and the ratio of DM1 to trastuzumab-MCC during conjugation reactions.[13] DAR was characterized by UV spectroscopic, hydrophobic interaction chromatography and mass analysis.

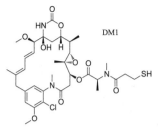

4 Pre-clinical Pharmacodynamics

Summary

Overview of *in vitro* Activities
- ❖ Trastuzumab bound to HER2 receptor in CHO cell: $K_D = 5$ nM.[2]
- ❖ Cells overexpressing HER2 are more sensitive to ado-trastuzumab emtansine than HER2 negative cells.
- ❖ Ado-trastuzumab emtansine decreased the cell proliferation of HER2-overexpressing cells more than trastuzumab, free DM1 toxin, or free MCC-DM1 conjugate.
- ❖ Like trastuzumab alone, binding of ado-trastuzumab emtansine to FcγRIa is notably avid and binding to RII and RIII type is in μg/mL range.
- ❖ No ADCC difference has been observed between the results of ado-trastuzumab emtansine and those for trastuzumab alone.
- ❖ *In vitro* metabolism studies in human liver microsomes suggest that DM1 is metabolised mainly by CYP3A4 and to a lesser extent by CYP3A5.[14]

Overview of *in vivo* Activities
- ❖ Human breast cancer cell MMTV-HER2 Fo5 xenograft mouse models:
  - • Significant tumor growth inhibition and regression at 15-30 mg/kg for 42 days.
- ❖ Human breast cancer cell BT-474 EEI xenograft mouse models:
  - • Significant tumor growth inhibition and regression at ≥10 mg/kg for 42 days.
- ❖ Human breast cancer cell KPL-4 xenograft mouse models:
  - • Significant tumor growth inhibition at 3 mg/kg, i.v. once.

Overview of *in vitro* Activities

Target Binding and Mechanism of Action

Table 5   Decrease in Cellular Viability by T-DM1 at 72 h[3]

Cell Line	Origin Tissue	HER2 Sensitivity	EC$_{50}$ (μg/mL)
SK-BR-3	Human breast cancer	3+	0.0050
BT-474	Human breast cancer	3+	0.15
MCF-7	Human breast cancer	0 (normal)	>5.0
MDA-MB-468	Human breast cancer	Negative	>2.0

Cell-based Activities *in vitro*

Table 6   Anti-proliferative Activity of T-DM1 in Breast Cancer Cell Lines[3]

Cell Line	HER2 Expression	Trastuzumab		T-DM1	
		IC$_{50}$ (nM)	IC$_{50}$ (µg/mL)	IC$_{50}$ (nM)	IC$_{50}$ (µg/mL)
BT-474	3+	1.7	0.25	0.46	0.069
SK-BR-3	3+	0.41	0.059	0.040	0.0060
KPL-4	3+	>70.0	>10.0	0.060	0.0090
HCC1954	3+	>70.0	>10.0	0.29	0.043
BT-474EE1	2+	>70.0	>10.0	0.12	0.018
MCF-7	0	>70.0	>10.0	>70.0	>10.0
MDA-MB-468[a]	0	>70.0	>10.0	13.4	2.0[a]

[a] Estimated value for trastuzumab emtansine from the graph.

Table 7   Comparison of Anti-proliferative Activity[3]

Molecule	Assay 1	Assay 2	Assay 3	Assay 4	Assay 5	Mean	% Activity vs. Trastuzumab-MCC-DM1
Trastuzumab-MCC-DM1 EC$_{50}$ (nM)[a]	0.50	0.50	0.40	0.50	0.50	0.50	100
Trastuzumab EC$_{50}$ (nM)[a]	1.6	1.9	NT	NT	1.9	1.8	28.2
DM1 bound (trastuzumab-MCC-DM1) EC$_{50}$ (nM)[b]	NT	1.6	1.5	1.8	1.6	1.6	100
Free DM1 EC$_{50}$ (nM)	NT	32.3	32.7	35.4	NT	33.5	4.8
Free MCC-DM1 EC$_{50}$ (nM)	NT	NT	NT	114	185	150	1.1

MCC: Maleimidomethyl cyclohexane-1-carboxylate linker as in T-DM1.   NT: Not test.   [a] Molar concentration of antibody.   [b] Molar concentration of bound DM1 in trastuzumab-MCC-DM1.

Fc & FcR Binding and Fc Inducing Function

Table 8   T-DM1 Binding to Fc Receptors (EC$_{50}$ Values)[3]

Fcγ Receptor	Rituxan Control (µg/mL)	Trastuzumab (µg/mL)	Trastuzumab (nM)	T-DM1 (µg/mL)	T-DM1 (nM)
FcγRIa	0.0049	0.0056	0.038	0.0058	0.039
FcγRIIa	1.3	2.8[a]	19.2	0.80[a]	5.4
FcγRIIb	8.9	ND	ND	ND	ND
FcγRIIIa F158	11.6	ND	ND	1.5	10.1
FcγRIIIa V158	1.4	1.2	8.2	0.30	2.0

ND: Not determined.   [a] Estimated value; binding curve did not well define an upper asymptote.

Table 9   Relative Activity of T-DM1 and Trastuzumab Samples from ADCC Assay[3]

Sample	EC$_{50}$ Range (ng/mL)		Relative Activity Range[a]	
	Lower	Upper	Lower	Upper
Trastuzumab	8.7	20.5	0.57	0.90
T-DM1 reference material	6.4	13.2	1.0	1.0
T-DM1 Qual. Lot B107	7.7	17.7	0.70	1.0
T-DM1 Phase 2 Lot	7.0	19.6	0.67	1.1

ADCC: Antibody-dependent cell-mediated cytotoxicity.   Qual.: Qualification.   [a] Relative activity = EC$_{50}$ T-DM1 reference/EC$_{50}$ sample.

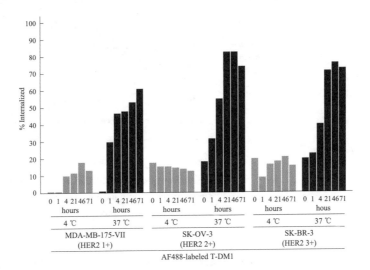

Figure 2   *In vitro* Internalization Assays of T-DM1 on HER2 3+, 2+, and 1+ Tumor Cells[15]

Overview of *in vivo* Activities

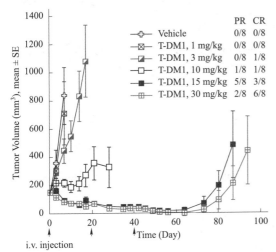

Study: Antitumor activities in MMTV-HER2 Fo5 human breast cancer xenograft mouse model.

Animal: Nude mouse (female).

Model: MMTV-HER2 Fo5 cells were implanted into the s.c. of nude mice.

Administration: i.v., once in 3 weeks for 42 days; T-DM1: 1, 3, 10, 15, or 30 mg/kg; Control: vehicle.

Starting: Tumors reached a size of 0.20 cm³.

Test: Measured tumor volumes.

Result: Tumor growth inhibition in a dose-dependent manner for 1-10 mg/kg, and appeared to plateau at ≥15 mg/kg.   Tumor regression at 3, 10, 15, and 30 mg/kg; and 1/8, 1/8, 3/8, 6/8 were complete regression.

Figure 3   Effects of T-DM1 on Human Breast Cancer MMTV-HER2 Fo5 Cell Xenograft Mouse Model[16]

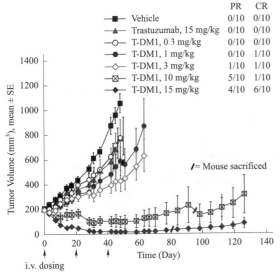

Study: Antitumor activities in BT-474EEI human breast cancer xenograft mouse model.

Animal: Nude mouse (female).

Model: BT-474 EEI cells were implanted into the s.c. of nude mice.

Administration: i.v., once in 3 weeks for 42 days; T-DM1: 0.3, 1, 3, 10, or 15 mg/kg; Control: vehicle; Trastuzumab: 15 mg/kg.

Starting: Tumors reached a size of 0.20 cm³.

Test: Measured tumor volumes.

Result: Tumor growth inhibition in a dose-dependent manner for 0.3-10 mg/kg, and appeared to plateau at ≥10 mg/kg.   Tumor regression at 10 and 15 mg/kg; and 1/10, 6/10 were complete regression.

Figure 4   Effects of T-DM1 on Human Breast Cancer BT-474EEI Cell Xenograft Mouse Model[16]

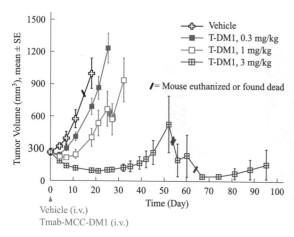

Study: Antitumor activities in KPL-4 human breast cancer xenograft mouse model.

Animal: Nude mouse (female).

Model: KPL-4 cells were implanted into the s.c. of nude mice.

Administration: i.v., once; T-DM1: 0.3, 1, or 3 mg/kg; Control: vehicle.

Starting: Tumors reached a size of 0.20-0.30 cm³.

Test: Measured tumor volumes.

Result: Tumor growth inhibition in a dose-dependent manner for 0.3-3 mg/kg. Tumor regression at 1 and 3 mg/kg; and 1/8, 7/8 were partial regression; No complete regression observed.

Figure 5   Effects of T-DM1 on Human Breast Cancer KPL-4 Cell Xenograft Mouse Model[16]

5   Toxicology

Summary

Non-clinical Single-Dose Toxicology

❖ Acute toxicity in SD rat: No lethality up to 50 mg/kg T-DM1, and 0.2 mg/kg MNLD for DM1 toxin (mortality/morbidity at >0.4 mg/kg).

❖ Acute toxicity in monkeys: Highest non-severely toxic dose up to 30 mg/kg.

Non-clinical Repeated-Dose Toxicology

❖ A series of i.v. repeated-dose toxicology studies were conducted with T-DM1 in Cynomolgus monkeys (up to 6 months).

❖ Minimal toxic response at 30 mg/kg dose, once every 3 weeks for 4 doses.

Safety Pharmacology

❖ No abnormal effect on cardiovascular systems, determined by *in vivo* safety pharmacology studies with Cynomolgus monkeys.

❖ Similar tissue cross-reactivity profiles determined in human and monkey tissues.

Other Toxicology

❖ No evidence of mutagenic activity in the standard Ames bacterial mutagenicity assays at concentrations of up to 5,000 μg/mL.

❖ No evidence of chromosomal damage to rat or monkey bone marrow cells in an *in vivo* micronucleus assays following doses of up to 10 mg/kg T-DM1, or 0.2 mg/kg DM1 toxin.

❖ No hemolysis or compatibility issue observed in human and monkey blood *in vitro*.

❖ T-DM1 impaired megakaryocyte and platelet production, despite no direct effect on platelet function.

Table 10   Single-Dose Toxicity Studies of T-DM1 and Free DM1[17]

Species	Dose (mg/kg)	MNLD (mg/kg)	Finding
Rat (SD)	T-DM1: 10, 25, 50, i.v.	50	T-DM1: 50 mg/kg: transient body weight loss, increased liver enzyme levels (AST, ALT, GGT, total bilirubin), decreased platelet counts.
	DM1: 0.1, 0.2, 0.4, 0.6, 0.8, 1.0, i.v.	0.2	Mortality/morbidity at ≥0.4 mg/kg with clinical signs of uro-genital staining, hind limb paralysis, limping, piloerection, shaking, tremors, and lethargy.
Cynomolgus monkey	T-DM1: 3, 10, 30, i.v.	30	Highest non-severely toxic dose: 30 mg/kg.

AST: Aspartate transaminase.   ALT: Alanine amniotransferase.   DM1: A derivative of maytansine.   GGT: γ-Glutamyl transpeptadase.   T-DM1: Trastuzumab em-tansine.

Non-clinical Multiple-Dose Toxicology

Table 11　Repeated-Dose Toxicity Studies of T-DM1[17]

Species	Duration	Dose [mg/(kg·day)]	NOEL [mg/(kg·day)]	Finding
Rat (SD)	3 weeks	5/F: 10, 26, 52; Days 1, 8, 15	ND	Mortality/morbidity at 52 mg/kg on Day 22 and Day 24 with decreased body weight gain, decreased platelets, and increased liver enzyme levels.
Cynomolgus monkey	6 weeks	Male & female: 29, 34, 51; Days 1, 22	ND	Decreased platelets and reticulocytes; increased liver enzymes (AST and ALT); increased numbers of mitotic cells arrested in metaphase and apoptotic cells in liver parenchyma; diffuse petechiae in lung.
	3 months	Male & female: 3, 10, 30; once every 3 weeks for 4 doses	ND	30 mg/kg: Kupffer cell hypertrophy; increased sinusoidal leukocytes; increased (arrested) mitosis; axonal degeneration; hypertrophy, hyperplasia, Schwann cells.
	6 months	Male & female: 1, 3, 10; once every 3 weeks for 4 doses	ND	30 mg/kg: Increased mitotic figures-mononuclear cells-red pulp; atrophy-hepatocytes focal to multifocal; decreased mucous cells.

ND: Not determined.

Safety Pharmacology

Table 12　Safety Pharmacology Study Summary of T-DM1[3]

Study	System	Dose	Finding
Cardiovascular effect	Monkey (n = 4)	3, 10, 30 mg/kg, i.v.	No effect.
Tissue cross-reactivity	Human and monkey tissues	1, 10 µg/mL	T-DM1 binding to human and Cynomolgus monkey tissue sections consisted primarily of epithelial, spindle, glial, and mononuclear cell staining in several tissues. Binding in monkey tissues was similar to that of human tissues yet less prevalent.

Other Toxicology

Table 13　Genotoxicity Studies of Trastuzumab[14, 17]

Assay	Species/System	Age	Dose	Finding
In vitro reverse mutation assay (Ames)	S. typhimurium: TA98, TA100, TA1535, TA1537 E. coli: WP2 uvrA	-	DM1: 1.6-5,000 µg/mL	Negative.
In vivo micronucleus assay	Rat bone marrow	8-10 weeks	DM1: 0.05, 0.1, 0.2 mg/kg, i.v.	Positive. Free DM1 was cytotoxic to the bone marrow.
	Monkey bone marrow	2-4 years	T-DM1: 1, 3, 10 mg/kg, i.v.	Negative.

DM1: A derivative of maytansine.　T-DM1: Trastuzumab emtansine.

Table 14　Special Toxicology Studies of Trastuzumab[17]

Special Toxicology	Species	Item	Dose (mg/animal/dose)	Finding
Platelet decrease	Human	Platelet-rich plasma	100 µg/mL T-DM1; 0.01-100 µM DM1	Trastuzumab emtansine did not have a direct effect on platelet function, but did impair megakaryocyte and platelet production.
		Hematopoietic stem cells	25 µg/mL T-DM1	
Hemolysis and compatibility	Human or Monkey blood	Hemolytic potential	0, 1.25, 2.5, 5 mg/mL	No T-DM1-related hemolysis in human and monkey blood.
		Blood compatibility	0, 1.25, 2.5, 5 mg/mL	T-DM1 compatible in human and monkey serum and plasma.

DM1: A derivative of maytansine.　T-DM1: Trastuzumab emtansine.

6 Non-clinical Pharmacokinetics/ADME/Toxicokinetics

Summary

❖ In single-dose
- Exhibited non-linear pharmacokinetics in Cynomolgus monkeys, with a pattern of supra-proportional increases in AUC in the dose of 3, 10, 30 mg/kg ado-trastuzumab emtansine.
- Showed a half-life ranging between 11-13 days for trastuzumab, 5-6 days for conjugated T-DM1 in mice, longer than those in Cynomolgus monkeys (5-9 days and 2-5 days, respectively).
- AUC of naked emtansine (DM1) toxin was minimal, comparing to conjugated T-DM1 or trastuzumab.

❖ In multiple-dose studies in Cynomolgus monkeys
- Clearance was 4-9 mL/(h·kg) with terminal half-lives ranging from 4 to 9 days for trastuzumab, and 10-15 mL/(h·kg) with half-lives ranging from 3 to 6 days for conjugated T-DM1.
- Non-linear pharmacokinetics with a pattern of supra-proportional increases in AUC observed in the dose of 3, 10, 30 mg/mg T-DM1.
- AUC of naked emtasine toxin was minimal.

❖ Distribution
- Besides tumor site, uptake of radioactivity was also substantially found in liver, kidney and spleen for ado-trastuzumab (3H-labeled)-emtansine.
- Distribution of naked emtansine toxin was minimal comparing to conjugated T-DM1.

❖ Drug with radioactivity was excreted into urine and feces after 168 hours.

❖ Trastuzumab emtansine conjugate showed stability in human and monkey blood serum within 48 hours at 37 °C.

Non-clinical Pharmacokinetics

Table 15 *In vivo* Pharmacokinetic Parameters of T-DM1 in Mice, Rats and Monkeys after Single-Dose[18]

Species	Route	Dose (mg/kg)	Analyte	T_{max} (Day)	C_{max} (µg/mL)	AUC_{inf} (µg·day/mL)	$t_{1/2}$ (Day)	CL or CL/F [mL/(day·kg)]	V_c (mL/kg)	MRT (Day)
Mouse (female/4)	i.v.	0.3	T	-	5.8	32.6	11.4	8.1	46.0	16.1
			T-DM1	-	5.3	14.3	5.2	18.5	50.1	7.2
	i.v.	3	T	-	53.8	309	11.7	10.0	57.6	16.5
			T-DM1	-	49.3	140	5.3	22.1	62.9	7.4
	i.v.	15	T	-	260	1,890	13.1	8.0	58.2	18.6
			T-DM1	-	267	838	5.6	18.1	56.8	7.9
Sprague-Dawley rat (female/4)	i.v.	0.3[a]	T	-	5.9 ± 0.19	31.7 ± 2.5	10.2 ± 1.2	10.7 ± 0.87	57.4 ± 3.2	14.2 ± 1.6
			T-DM1	-	5.6 ± 0.12	15.3 ± 0.18	5.0 ± 0.19	22.1 ± 0.46	61.0 ± 1.7	6.7 ± 0.21
			DM1	-	-	-	-	-	-	-
	i.v.	3	T	-	54.3 ± 5.4	287 ± 65.8	9.0 ± 1.4	11.5 ± 2.4	58.8 ± 4.2	12.4 ± 1.9
			T-DM1	-	53.1 ± 4.1	151 ± 29.6	4.8 ± 0.41	21.6 ± 3.6	60.0 ± 3.7	6.3 ± 0.38
			DM1	2.5×10^{-3}	0.0042 ± 0.00052	0.00023 ± 0.00021	-	-	-	-
	i.v.	20	T	-	444 ± 22.6	2,000 ± 361	10.5 ± 1.6	10.6 ± 2.5	46.4 ± 2.4	14.0 ± 2.0
			T-DM1	-	449 ± 23.9	1,050 ± 134	5.0 ± 0.47	20.0 ± 3.0	45.9 ± 2.4	6.4 ± 0.55
			DM1	2.2×10^{-3}	0.028 ± 0.0048	0.011 ± 0.0015	-	-	-	-
Cynomolgus monkey (female/6)[b]	i.v.	3	T	-	81.9	325	4.6	9.4	37.1	5.7
			T-DM1	-	75.1	203	2.7	15.0	40.5	3.4
			DM1	-	-	-	-	-	-	-
	i.v.	10	T	-	253 ± 23.1	1,430 ± 231	7.4 ± 0.96	7.0 ± 1.1	39.1 ± 3.5	9.8 ± 1.2
			T-DM1	-	257 ± 36.2	844 ± 121	3.9 ± 0.45	11.8 ± 1.6	38.7 ± 5.1	5.0 ± 0.43
			DM1	3.5×10^{-3}	0.020 ± 0.0020	0.20 ± 0.0074	-	-	-	-
	i.v.	30	T	-	697 ± 59.9	5,580 ± 1,140	9.9 ± 0.24	5.4 ± 1.2	42.3 ± 3.8	13.4 ± 0.62
			T-DM1	-	680 ± 66.8	3,090 ± 693	5.4 ± 0.20	9.9 ± 2.4	43.5 ± 4.4	6.8 ± 0.56
			DM1	3.5×10^{-3}	0.051 ± 0.0090	0.072 ± 0.0076	-	-	-	-

T: Trastuzumab.   [a] $n = 3$ for this analysis.   [b] $n = 3$ for summary statistics because of interim necropsies (scheduled necropsy) in each group.

Table 16　*In vivo* Pharmacokinetic Parameters of T-DM1 after Multiple-Doses in Cynomolgus Monkeys[18]

Species	Schedule	Dose [mg/(kg·dose)]	Analyte	AUC_{inf} (µg·day/mL)	$t_{1/2}$ (Day)	CL [mL/(h·kg)]	V_c (mL/kg)
Cynomolgus monkey (female/6)[a]	i.v., once per 3 weeks for 4 times	3	Trastuzumab	338 ± 41.4	7.1 ± 1.8	8.9 ± 1.0	37.5 ± 1.7
			T-DM1	195 ± 19.8	2.9 ± 0.16	15.3 ± 1.5	38.0 ± 1.4
			DM1	0.0032[b] ± 0.00058	-	-	-
	i.v., once per 3 weeks for 4 times	10	Trastuzumab	1,990 ± 269	12.6 ± 3.1	5.0 ± 0.57	37.4 ± 3.1
			T-DM1	930 ± 125	4.6 ± 0.42	10.7 ± 1.3	37.1 ± 2.7
			DM1	0.023[c] ± 0.0046	-	-	-
	i.v., once per 3 weeks for 4 times	30	Trastuzumab	7,670 ± 697	14.6 ± 1.9	3.9 ± 0.34	37.9 ± 2.9
			T-DM1	3,150 ± 162	5.6 ± 0.24	9.4 ± 0.56	38.2 ± 2.2
			DM1	0.093[c] ± 0.0097	-	-	-

[a] n = 3 for summary statistics because of interim necropsies (scheduled necropsy) in each group.　[b] AUC after dose 4.　[c] AUC_{63-69}.

Table 17　*In vivo* Tissue Distribution of T-DM1 and Free DM1 in Sprague-Dawley Rat[18]

Tissue	Mean Tissue Concentration of Radioactive T-DM1					Tissue Concentration of Radioactive DM1				
	% ID/g					% ID/mL or g				
	1 h	1 d	4 d	7 d	14 d	10 min	1 h	3 h	1 d	5 d
Plasma	12.1 ± 1.7	6.3 ± 0.25	3.6 ± 0.050	2.7 ± 0.22	1.1 ± 0.070	0.12 ± 0.017	0.099 ± 0.021	0.086 ± 0.92	0.023 ± 0.00084	0.0017 ± 0.00097
Liver	2.8 ± 0.14	2.3 ± 0.23	1.8 ± 0.11	1.2 ± 0.15	0.39 ± 0.020	1.9 ± 0.097	1.7 ± 0.39	0.98 ± 0.66	0.53 ± 0.079	0.30 ± 0.076
Kidney	2.0 ± 0.31	2.1 ± 0.18	2.3 ± 0.050	2.0 ± 0.17	0.57 ± 0.080	2.9 ± 0.52	2.8 ± 0.36	1.9 ± 0.19	0.85 ± 0.089	0.26 ± 0.061
Lung	1.6 ± 0.18	1.4 ± 0.41	1.0 ± 0.090	1.0 ± 0.14	0.38 ± 0.030	3.1 ± 1.4	1.3 ± 0.48	0.66 ± 0.025	0.21 ± 0.0075	0.035 ± 0.0084
Heart	0.93 ± 0.23	0.73 ± 0.17	0.56 ± 0.090	0.45 ± 0.030	0.18 ± 0.010	1.1 ± 0.13	0.67 ± 0.057	0.43 ± 0.032	0.087 ± 0.0012	0.019 ± 0.0017
Spleen	1.6 ± 0.27	1.5 ± 0.25	0.84 ± 0.090	0.65 ± 0.070	0.39 ± 0.010	1.8 ± 0.32	1.2 ± 0.13	0.80 ± 0.057	0.29 ± 0.045	0.10 ± 0.020
Thymus	0.18 ± 0.12	0.34 ± 0.12	0.22 ± 0.010	0.22 ± 0.11	0.070 ± 0.010	0.17 ± 0.15	0.21 ± 0.13	0.15 ± 0.015	0.22 ± 0.020	0.11 ± 0.036
Bone marrow	0.84 ± 0.17	0.58 ± 0.040	0.35 ± 0.080	0.29 ± 0.020	0.17 ± 0.020	0.010 ± 0.00026	0.0080 ± 0.0019	0.010 ± 0.0058	0.0028 ± 0.00035	0.0014 ± 0.0033
Stomach	0.25 ± 0.040	0.39 ± 0.040	0.27 ± 0.020	0.17 ± 0.080	0.070 ± 0.020	0.47 ± 0.13	0.46 ± 0.072	0.36 ± 0.16	0.12 ± 0.039	0.038 ± 0.016
Brain	0.10 ± 0.020	0.080 ± 0.080	0.040 ± 0.020	0.030 ± 0.0040	0.010 ± 0.00040	0.020 ± 0.0054	0.015 ± 0.00037	0.018 ± 0.013	0.010 ± 0.0063	0.0053 ± 0.00067

Table 18　Excretion Profiles of T-[³H]DM1 in Rat after Single-Dose Administration of 10 mg/kg[18]

Gender	Dose (mg/kg)	Route	Time	1.0% TFA/ACN Soluble (%)	1.0% TFA/ACN Precipitable (%)
Non-cannulated	10	i.v.	Plasma 15 min-168 h	0.80-2.3	98.0-99.0
			Urine 0-168 h	95.0-99.5	0.50-5.4
			Feces 0-168 h	78.0-86.0	14.0-22.0
Bile duct-cannulated	10	i.v.	Plasma 15 min-168 h	0.80-1.9	98.0-99.0
			Bile 0-168 h	97.0-99.5	0.50-3.1
			Feces 0-168 h	74.0-98.0	1.8-26.0

ACN: Acetonitrile.　TFA: Trifluoroacetic acid.

Table 19　Plasma Stability (37 °C) of T-DM1 in Monkey, Rat and Human[18]

Time (h)	Human			Cynomolgus Monkey			Rat			Buffer		
	T-mab (μg/mL)	T-DM1 (μg/mL)	% Conj.	T-mab (μg/mL)	T-DM1 (μg/mL)	% Conj.	T-mab (μg/mL)	T-DM1 (μg/mL)	% Conj.	T-mab (μg/mL)	T-DM1 (μg/mL)	% Conj.
0	49.6	51.0	103	46.2	48.0	104	45.0	45.9	102	40.5	39.8	98.4
8	47.4	47.5	100	48.6	45.1	92.8	43.2	39.8	92.2	39.9	41.9	105
24	45.9	44.5	96.9	42.8	38.1	89.0	40.2	31.1	77.3	40.9	45.0	110
48	43.8	35.1	80.1	39.4	32.1	81.5	35.3	22.9	64.8	45.8	44.2	96.5
96	37.9	24.1	63.5	37.3	21.3	57.2	32.9	13.8	41.9	40.1	37.7	94.1

Conj.: Conjugated T-DM1.　T-mab: Total antibody (trastuzumab).

7　Clinical Efficacy and Safety

Overview Profile

❖ In 2012, FDA approved ado-trastuzumab emtansine for the treatment of HER2-positive metastatic breast cancer patients who have received prior treatment with trastuzumab and taxane chemotherapy.

❖ In 2013, T-DM1 was also approved for treatment of HER2-overexpressing MBC by EMA.

❖ Chugai filed a regulatory application in Japan in 2013 and received the approval in September 2013 for the treatment of HER2-positive inoperable or recurrent breast cancer.　In 2014, the product was launched in Japan for this indication.

❖ Patients treated with T-DM1 had a median progression-free survival (PFS) of 9.6 months, compared to 6.4 months in patients treated with lapatinib + capecitabine; the median overall survival (OS) was 30.9 months in the T-DM1 group and 25.1 months in the lapatinib + capecitabine group.

❖ T-DM1 was approved with a Boxed Warning that the drug can cause liver toxicity, heart toxicity and death.　Kadcyla® can also cause severe life-threatening birth defects.

Summary of the Key Clinical Studies

Table 20　The Key Clinical Trials of T-DM1[7]

ID	Phase	N	Population	Design	Primary Endpoint
TDM4258g	2	112	Previously treated HER2 + MBC progressed on HER2-directed therapy	Single arm	ORR
TDM4374g	2	110	Previously treated HER2 + MBC, ⩾2 lines of HER2-directed therapy, must have received trastuzumab and lapatinib	Single arm	ORR
TDM4450g	2	104	HER2 + LABC or MBC; no prior MBC treatment	Radomized; T-DM1 vs. trastuzumab + docetaxel	PFS
TDM4370g	3	991	HER2 + MBC must have received trastuzumab and taxane	Randomized T-DM1 vs. capecitabine + lapatinib	PFS, OS

MBC: Metastatic breast cancer.　LABC: Locally advanced breast cancer.　ORR: Objective response rate.　OS: Overall survival.　PFS: Progression-free survival.

Clinical Efficacy

Table 21　Efficacy of Phase 2 Clinical Trials[7]

Trial ID	N	ORR	Median PFS (Month)	Median DOR (Month)
TDM4450g	104	64.0%	14.2	-
TDM4374g	110	32.7% (both by IRF and investigator review)	6.9 by IRF assessment; 5.5 by investigator review	9.7 (by investigator assessment, not reached by IRF assessment)
TDM4258g	112	26.9% by single-reader IRF review; 38.9% by investigator review	4.6 by both single-reader IRF and investigator review	9.4 (by investigator assessment, not reached by IRF assessment)

DOR: Duration of response.　IRF: Independent review committee.　ORR: Objective response rate.　TTP: Time to progression.

Table 22　Efficacy of Phase 3 Clinical Trials for Approval[7]

Trial ID	Study Posology	Control	Endpoint	Efficacy (Median)		
				T-DM1	Control	Hazard Ratio
TDM4370g (EMILIA)	T-DM1 (n = 495)	Lapatinib + Capecitabine (n = 496)	PFS (Month)	9.6	6.4	0.65
			OS (Month)	30.9	25.1	0.68
			DOR (Month)	12.6	6.5	-
			ORR (CR+PR)	43.6%	30.8%	-
			CR	1.0%	0.50%	-
			PR	42.6%	20.3%	-

CR: Complete response.　DOR: Duration of response.　ORR: Objective response rate.　OS: Overall survival.　PFS: Progression-free survival.　PR: Partial response.

Clinical Safety

Table 23　Adverse Events in the Safety Population in Clinical Studies TDM4450g[a, 19]

Adverse Event	Lapatinib + Capecitabine (N = 488)		T-DM (N = 490)	
	Any Grade n (%)	≥ Grade 3 n (%)	Any Grade n (%)	≥ Grade 3 n (%)
Any event	477 (97.7)	278 (57.0)	470 (95.9)	200 (40.8)
Specific events[b]				
Diarrhea	389 (79.7)	101 (20.7)	114 (23.3)	8 (1.6)
Palmar-plantar erythrodysesthesia	283 (58.0)	80 (16.4)	6 (1.2)	0
Vomiting	143 (29.3)	22 (4.5)	93 (19.0)	4 (0.80)
Neutropenia	42 (8.6)	21 (4.3)	29 (5.9)	10 (2.0)
Hypokalemia	42 (8.6)	20 (4.1)	42 (8.6)	11 (2.2)
Fatigue	136 (27.9)	17 (3.5)	172 (35.1)	12 (2.4)
Nausea	218 (44.7)	12 (2.5)	192 (39.2)	4 (0.80)
Mucosal inflammation	93 (19.1)	11 (2.3)	33 (6.7)	1 (0.20)
Anemia	39 (8.0)	8 (1.6)	51 (10.4)	13 (2.7)
Elevated ALT	43 (8.8)	7 (1.4)	83 (16.9)	14 (2.9)
Elevated AST	46 (9.4)	4 (0.80)	110 (22.4)	21 (4.3)
Thrombocytopenia	12 (2.5)	1 (0.20)	137 (28.0)	63 (12.9)

ALT denotes alanine aminotransferase, and AST aspartate aminotransferase.　ALT: Alanine amniotransferase.　AST: Aspartate transaminase.　[a] The safety population included all patients who received at least one dose of the study treatment.　[b] Listed are adverse events of Grade 3 or above with an incidence of 2.0% or higher in either group.

8　Clinical Pharmacokinetics

Summary

❖ The pharmacokinetics of Kadcyla® was evaluated in a phase 1 study and in a population pharmacokinetic analysis for the ado-trastuzumab emtansine conjugate (ADC) using pooled data from 5 trials in patients with breast cancer.

❖ A population PK analysis estimated the TDM1 clearance and terminal elimination half-life as 0.68 L/day and ~4 days, respectively; inter-individual variability of CL is 19.1%.

❖ T-DM1 accumulation was not observed following multiple dosing.

❖ No dose adjustments were required for significant covariates (sum of longest diameter of target lesions by RECIST, albumin, HER2 ECD concentrations, baseline trastuzumab concentrations, AST, and body weight).

❖ Based on the population PK analysis, as well as analysis of Grade 3 or greater adverse drug reactions and dose modifications, dose adjustments are not needed for mild or moderate renal impairment.

❖ The influence of hepatic impairment on the PK of T-DM1 or DM1 has not been determined.
❖ *In vitro* studies indicate that DM1, the cytotoxic component of T-DM1, is metabolized mainly by CYP3A4. Concomitant use of strong CYP3A4 inhibitors with T-DM1 should be avoided due to the potential for an increase in DM1 exposure and toxicity.

Single-Dose Pharmacokinetics

Table 24　The Pharmacokinetics after Single-Dose or Cycle 1 in Multiple-Dose of T-DM1[20]

Dose (mg/kg)	N	Analyte	$t_{1/2}$ (Day)[a]	CL [mL/(day·kg)]	V_d (mL/kg)[a]
0.3	3	T-DM1	1.3 (0.20)	21.1 (4.5)	35.7 (7.5)
		Trastuzumab	4.8 (3.2)	10.1 (8.4)	32.2 (23.2)
0.6	1	T-DM1	1.3 (-)	24.5 (-)	43.8 (-)
		Trastuzumab	8.1 (-)	5.7 (-)	51.1 (-)
1.2	1	T-DM1	1.3 (-)	27.8 (-)	51.8 (-)
		Trastuzumab	1.8 (-)	19.7 (-)	43.7 (-)
2.4	1	T-DM1	2.2 (-)	7.2 (-)	30.7 (-)
		Trastuzumab	5.2 (-)	5.7 (-)	44.0 (-)
3.6	15[b]	T-DM1	3.1 (0.70)	12.7 (3.6)	58.4 (12.4)
		Trastuzumab	9.1 (4.9)	4.9 (3.2)	50.7 (19.7)
4.8	3	T-DM1	4.1 (0.70)	7.1 (0.10)	41.2 (6.2)
		Trastuzumab	8.9 (2.1)	2.7 (1.2)	32.8 (4.5)

[a] Mean ± SD.　[b] Study#: TDM3569g.

Multiple-Dose Pharmacokinetics

Table 25　The Pharmacokinetics[a] of T-DM1 after Multiple-Dose of T-DM1 (3.6 mg/kg, q3w)[20]

Study	Cycle	N	C_{max} (µg/mL)	AUC (µg·day/mL)[b]	$t_{1/2}$ (Day)	CL [mL/(day·kg)]	V_d (mL/kg)
TDM4258g	1	101	80.9 (20.7)	457 (129)	3.5 (0.70)	8.5 (2.7)	28.4 (12.9)
	4	69	68.9 (21.8)	461 (136)	4.4 (1.7)	8.4 (4.3)	45.2 (43.0)
TDM4374g	1	105	79.5 (21.1)	486 (141)	4.0 (1.0)	8.0 (3.0)	31.2 (10.9)
	4	82	78.3 (25.6)	456 (162)	4.3 (0.80)	7.3 (2.5)	39.3 (32.8)
TDM4450g	1	62	84.2 (30.6)	495 (158)	3.5 (0.70)	8.2 (4.0)	30.2 (21.3)
	5	39	79.1 (23.7)	473 (141)	4.2 (0.60)	6.7 (1.6)	33.6 (12.4)
TDM4688g	1	51	75.6 (21.9)	431 (126)	4.0 (0.90)	9.2 (3.0)	41.2 (24.5)
	3	47	80.7 (18.1)	475 (150)	4.5 (0.90)	7.9 (3.3)	43.6 (40.7)
TDM4370g	1	292	83.4 (16.5)	489 (122)	3.7 (0.90)	7.8 (2.2)	29.5 (14.6)
	4	257	85.0 (33.4)	475 (127)	4.2 (0.70)	7.1 (1.9)	33.4 (11.4)

[a] Mean ± SD.　[b] AUC = AUC_{inf} for Cycle 1 and AUC = AUC to last sampling time for Cycles 3, 4 or 5.

Table 26   The Pharmacokinetics[a] of Trastuzumab after Multiple-Dose of T-DM1 (3.6 mg/kg, q3w)[20]

Study	Cycle	N	C_{max} (µg/mL)	AUC (µg·day/mL)[b]	$t_{1/2}$ (Day)	CL [mL/(day·kg)]	V_d (mL/kg)
TDM4258g	1	101	88.0 (30.2)	1,040 (1,030)	9.2 (10.9)	5.6 (6.3)	46.5 (58.4)
	4	69	85.7 (24.7)	888 (294)	11.2 (6.3)	3.5 (2.2)	46.1 (19.9)
TDM4374g	1	105	89.9 (31.3)	1,150 (852)	9.4 (4.9)	4.6 (2.6)	43.2 (16.3)
	4	82	89.2 (29.1)	700 (280)	10.0 (4.8)	3.3 (1.7)	39.6 (13.3)
TDM4450g	1	60	83.3 (20.5)	700 (260)	5.8 (2.0)	6.2 (4.3)	38.6 (11.8)
	5	38	107 (71.0)	788 (323)	8.3 (2.1)	3.1 (0.90)	34.8 (10.5)
TDM4688g	1	51	95.9 (32.3)	1,420 (1,390)	10.3 (6.8)	4.2 (2.4)	41.9 (16.2)
	3	47	98.6 (26.1)	958 (394)	12.0 (6.2)	3.1 (1.7)	43.7 (15.4)
TDM4370g	1	291	86.3 (20.1)	816 (422)	7.8 (4.0)	5.4 (2.3)	45.2 (15.6)
	4	256	87.4 (30.7)	604 (166)	6.9 (2.2)	4.7 (1.9)	41.4 (14.5)

[a] Mean ± SD.   [b] AUC = AUC$_{inf}$ for Cycle 1 and AUC = AUC to last sampling time for Cycles 3, 4, or 5.

Table 27   The Pharmacokinetics[a] of DM1 after Multiple-Dose of T-DM1 (3.6 mg/kg, q3w)[20]

Study	Cycle	N	C_{max} (ng/mL)
TDM4258g	1	105	5.4 (2.0)
	4	83	5.9 (2.2)
TDM4374g	1	104	5.4 (2.6)
	4	81	5.1 (1.9)
TDM4450g	1	63	5.1 (2.3)
	5	50	4.8 (2.3)
TDM4688g	1	51	5.4 (1.6)
	3	47	5.5 (1.9)
TDM4370g	1	287	4.6 (1.6)
	4	267	5.1 (4.1)

[a] Mean ± SD.

Anti-product Antibody (APA) Analysis

❖ With the immunogenicity assays used, the overall incidence of positive anti-therapeutic antibody (ATA) to T-DM1 was determined to be 5.3% in the studies included in the BLA.

❖ The presence of T-DM1 in patient serum at the time of ATA sampling can interfere with the ability of this assay to detect anti-KADCYLA antibodies.

❖ Data may not accurately reflect the true incidence of anti-T-DM1 antibody development.

❖ In addition, neutralizing activity of anti-T-DM1 antibodies has not been assessed.

9   Patent

❖ Ado-transtuzumab emtansine was approved by the U.S. Food and Drug Administration (FDA) in 2013.   It was developed and marketed as Kadcyla® by Genentech Inc., a subsidiary of Roche.

Summary

❖ The patent application (WO0100244A2) related to the anti-ErbB receptor antibody-maytansinoid conjugate (i.e. Ado-trastuzumab Emtansine) was filed by Genentech on Jun 23, 2000.   Accordingly, its PCT counterpart has, among the others, been granted before USPTO (US7097840B2, US7575748B1, US8093358B2 and US8337856B2), EPO (EP2293967B, EP2283867B1 and EP2283866B1), JPO (JP4780633B2 and JP4778101B2) and SIPO (CN100482281B and CN101518653B), respectively.

❖ The patent applications (WO8906692A1 and WO9222653A1) related to the monoclonal antibody specifically binding the extracellular domain of the HER2 receptor (i.e. Trastuzumab) were filed by Genentech in 1989 and 1992. Accordingly, its PCT counterpart has, among the others, been granted by USPTO (US5821337A, US6407213B1 and US6719971B1) and JPO (JP4836147B2 and JP3040121B2), respectively.

Table 28　Originator's Key Patent of Ado-trastuzumab Emtansine in Main Countries and/or Region

Country/Region	Publication/Patent No.	Application Date	Granted Date	Estimated Expiry Date
WO	WO8906692A1	01/05/1989	/	/
JP	JP3040121B2	01/05/1989	03/03/2000	01/05/2009
WO	WO9222653A1	06/15/1992	/	/
US	US5821337A	06/15/1992	10/13/1998	08/21/2012
	US6407213B1	06/15/1992	06/18/2002	06/30/2020
	US6719971B1	06/15/1992	04/13/2004	05/14/2012
JP	JP4836147B2	06/15/1992	12/14/2011	06/18/2028
WO	WO0100244A2	06/23/2000	/	/
US	US7097840B2	03/16/2001	08/29/2006	01/27/2023
	US7575748B1	03/16/2001	08/18/2009	03/16/2021
	US8093358B2	03/16/2001	01/10/2012	07/03/2023
	US8337856B2	03/16/2001	12/25/2012	07/03/2023
EP	EP2293967B1	06/23/2000	05/21/2014	06/23/2020
	EP2283867B1	06/23/2000	05/21/2014	06/23/2020
	EP2283866B1	06/23/2000	02/25/2015	06/23/2020
JP	JP4780633B2	06/23/2000	09/28/2011	06/23/2020
	JP4778101B2	07/16/2010	09/21/2011	07/16/2030
CN	CN100482281C	06/23/2000	04/29/2009	06/23/2020
	CN101518653B	06/23/2000	08/19/2015	06/23/2020

Table 29　Originator's International Patent Protection of Use and/or Method of Ado-trastuzumab Emtansine

Publication No.	Title	Publication Date
Technical Subjects	TREATMENT METHOD	
WO2011069074A2	Methods of treating metastatic breast cancer with trastuzumab-MCC-DM1	06/09/2011
Technical Subjects	DIAGNOSTIC METHOD	
WO2009114711A2	Genetic variations associated with drug resistance	09/17/2009
WO2013033380A1	Diagnostic markers	03/07/2013
Technical Subjects	COMBINATION METHOD	
WO2009117277A2	Combinations of an anti-HER2 antibody-drug conjugate and chemotherapeutic agents, and methods of use	09/24/2009
WO2010120561A1	Anti-FcRH5 antibodies and immunoconjugates and methods of use	10/21/2010
WO2010114940A1	Anti-FcRH5 antibodies and immunoconjugates and methods of use	10/07/2010
WO2012078771A1	Treatment of HER2-positive cancer with paclitaxel and trastuzumab-MCC-DM1	06/14/2012
WO2016097072A1	Tetrahydro-pyrido[3,4-b]indole estrogen receptor modulators and uses thereof	06/23/2016
WO2016196373A2	Methods of treating HER2-positive metastatic breast cancer	12/08/2016
WO2017007846A1	Combination therapy with an anti-HER2 antibody-drug conjugate and a BCL-2 inhibitor	01/12/2017
WO2017059289A1	Pyrrolobenzodiazepine antibody drug conjugates and methods of use	04/06/2017
Technical Subjects	FORMULATION	
WO2011012637A2	Subcutaneous anti-HER2 antibody formulation	02/03/2011

The data was updated until Jan 2018.

10 Reference

[1] Karunagaran D, Tzahar E, Beerli R R, et al. ErbB-2 is a common auxiliary subunit of NDF and EGF receptors: implications for breast cancer [J]. EMBO Journal, 1996, 15(2): 254-264.

[2] Pharmacodia. The Pharmacentical Index Biologics: Monoclonal Antibobqly. Vol 1. Beijing: China Medical Science Press.

[3] U. S. Food and Drug Administration (FDA) Database. http://www.accessdata.fda.gov/drugsatfda_docs/nda/2013/125427 Orig1s000PharmR. pdf.

[4] Gunning P W, Ghoshdastider U, Whitaker S, et al. The evolution of compositionally and functionally distinct actin filaments [J]. Journal of Cell Science, 2015, 128(11): 2009-2019.

[5] Barisic M, Maiato H. The Tubulin Code: a navigation system for chromosomes during mitosis [J]. Trends in Cell Biology, 2016, 26(10): 766-775.

[6] Jordan M A, Wilson L. Microtubules as a target for anticancer drugs [J]. Nature Reviews Cancer, 2004, 4(4): 253-265.

[7] FDA Database. http://www.accessdata.fda.gov/drugsatfda_docs/nda/2013/125427Orig1s000MedR.pdf.

[8] The financial reports of Genentech; http://data.pharmacodia.com/web/homePage/index.

[9] FDA Database. http://www.accessdata.fda.gov/drugsatfda_docs/label/2014/125427s033lbl.pdf.

[10] PMDA Database. http://www.pmda.go.jp/drugs/2013/P201300137/450045000_22500AMX01816_E100_2.pdf.

[11] Chari R, Goldmacher V, Lambert J, et al. Cytotoxic agents comprising maytansinoids and their therapeutic use: US5416064 [P]. 1995-05-16.

[12] Hasegawa T, Izawa M, Nagaokakyo T, et al. Antibiotic C-15003 PHM and production thereof: US4450234 [P]. 1984-05-22.

[13] Steeves R, Lutz R, Chari R, et al. Conjugates of maytansinoid DM1 with antibody trastuzumab, linked through a non-cleavable linker, and its use in the treatment of tumours: EP1689846B1 [P]. 2013-03-27.

[14] European Medicines Agency (EMA) Database. http://www.ema.europa.eu/docs/en_GB/document_library/EPAR_-_ Public_assessment_report/human/002389/WC500158595.pdf.

[15] Van Der L M, Groothuisl P, Ubink R, et al. The preclinical profile of the duocarmycin-based HER2-targeting ADC SYD985 predicts for clinical benefit in low HER2-expressing breast cancers [J]. Molecular Cancer Therapeutics. 2015, 14(3): 692-703.

[16] Pharmaceuticals and Medical Devices Agency (PMDA) Database. http://www.pmda.go.jp/drugs/2013/P201300137/ 450045000_22500AMX01816_H100_2.pdf.

[17] PMDA Database. http://www.pmda.go.jp/drugs/2013/P201300137/450045000_22500AMX01816_J100_2.pdf.

[18] PMDA Database. http://www.pmda.go.jp/drugs/2013/P201300137/450045000_22500AMX01816_I100_2.pdf.

[19] Verma S, Miles D, Gianni L, et al. Trastuzumab emtansine for HER2-positive advanced breast cancer [J]. The New England Journal of Medicine, 2012, 368(25): 1783-1791.

[20] FDA Database. http://www.accessdata.fda.gov/drugsatfda_docs/nda/2013/125427Orig1s000ClinPharmR.pdf.

CHAPTER

2

Atezolizumab

Atezolizumab

(Tecentriq®)

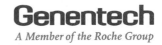

Research code: 52CMI0WC3Y, MPDL3280A, RG7446, RO5541267

1 Target Biology

The PD-L1 Ligand

❖ Programmed death-ligand 1 (PD-L1) is also known as cluster of differentiation 274 (CD274) or B7 homolog 1 (B7-H1). It is expressed by hematopoietic and non-hematopoietic cells, such as activated T cells, B cells, antigen-presenting cells (APCs), and various types of tumor cells.[1]

❖ PD-L1 is a 40 kDa type 1 transmembrane protein that is encoded by the CD274 gene. It is a member of the B7 gene family and consists of an IgV-like and an IgC-like extracellular domain, with a hydrophobic transmembrane domain followed by a short charged cytoplasmic domain (~30 amino acids) that is conserved across species but without any known function.

❖ PD-L1 can bind to PD-1 or B7.1 (CD80) and transmits an inhibitory signal suppressing the immune system by reducing the proliferation, activation of T cells and cytokine production. PD-L1 is also able to control the accumulation of activated T cells through apoptosis.

❖ PD-L1 and its receptors interactions are important for preventing autoimmunity by maintaining homeostasis of the immune response. In tumor microenvironments, this interaction provides an immune escape for tumor cells.[1]

Biology Activity

❖ PD-L1 binds to its receptor PD-1 which is expressed on activated T cells, B cells and myeloid cells to modulate their activation or inhibition.

❖ After PD-L1 and PD-1 engagement: 1) PD-1 clusters and localizes to TCR and inhibit following TCR engagement by inhibiting the phosphorylation of the TCR CD3ζ chains and Zap-70; 2) PD-1 signaling inhibits Ras which is an enhancer of survival and proliferation; 3) PD-1 intracellular ITSM (immunoreceptor tyrosine-based switch motif) will be phosphorylated and recruit SHP-1 and SHP-2 leading to inactivation of PI3K and inhibition of down-stream Akt.[1]

❖ The downstream signaling of PD-1/PD-L1 engagement includes: 1) a decrease in T-cell proliferation; 2) a decrease of inflammatory cytokines including tumor necrosis factor α (TNF-α), interferon γ (IFN-γ), and interleukin 2 (IL-2).[2]

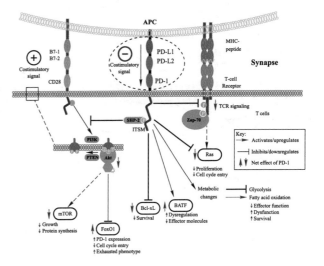

❖ PD-L1/PD-1 engagement can promote and maintain the induced Treg (iTregs) cells development and function via inhibiting the Akt/mTOR signaling cascade, thereby flipping the molecular switch in a naïve CD4+ T-cell to T reg cell development.[3]

❖ PD-1 signaling results in the inhibition of glycolysis and metabolism of amino acids while simultaneously promoting fatty acid oxidation and consistent with an inhibition of effector function.[4]

❖ PD-1/PD-L1 signaling also appears to be self-reinforcing by protecting FoxO1 from degradation leading to increasing PD-1 expression.[5] In the tumor microenvironment PD-1 expression is associated with an exhausted and dysfunctional phenotype. Blockade of PD-1/PD-L1 signaling is able to restore CD8 T-cell function and allows recovery of cytotoxic capabilities form the exhausted phenotype.[4]

2   General Information

Tecentriq®

❖ Tecentriq® (Atezolizumab) is a recombinant humanized monoclonal antibody targeting programmed death-ligand 1 (PD-L1) on antigen-presenting cells or tumor cells.

❖ Tecentriq® was developed and marketed by Genentech, Inc., a subsidiary of Roche.

❖ Biochemical:[6] Tecentriq® targets programmed death-ligand 1 (PD-L1) on antigen-presenting cells or tumor cells.   Upon binding to PD-L1, Tecentriq® prevents interaction with programmed death-1 (PD-1) receptor, which is an inhibitory receptor expressed on T cells.   Interference of PD-L1/PD-1 and PD-L1/B7.1 interactions may enhance the magnitude and quality of the tumor specific T-cell response through increased T-cell priming and expansion.

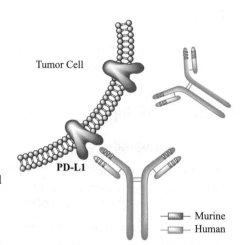

❖ FDA: Accelerated approval for treatment of patients with locally advanced or metastatic urothelial carcinoma.

❖ No sales data as of 2016 and 2017.

❖ Tecentriq® is based on an IgG1 framework that contains heavy chain V_HIII and light chain V_κI subgroup sequences.   A point mutation in the amino acid sequence (N298A) in Fc domain results in the removal of the glycosylation site, thereby limiting binding to human Fcγ receptors and preventing antibody-dependent cell-mediated cytotoxicity (ADCC).[8]

❖ Humanized IgG1κ monoclonal antibody: $C_{6434}H_{9878}O_{1996}N_{1702}S_{42}$, ~144 kDa (calculated molecular mass).   Tecentriq® has been produced from CHO cells and consists of two heavy chains (448 amino acid residues each) and two light chains (214 amino acid residues each).[7]

❖ Tecentriq® is presented as a sterile liquid solution for intravenous injections.   It was developed to deliver a nominal amount of 1,200 mg of atezolizumab per vial, which contains 60 mg/mL atezolizumab in 20 mM histidine acetate, 13 mM glacial acetic acid, 120 mM sucrose, and 0.04 mg/mL (0.040% w/v) polysorbate 20 at pH 5.8.[7, 8]

Table 1   Summary of Tecentriq®[6, 7]

Generic Name	Atezolizumab
CAS registry No.	1380723-44-3
Code name	MPDL3280A, RO5541267, PRO#303280
Chemical name	Humanized anti-PD-L1 IgG1κ monoclonal antibody
Molecular formula	$C_{6434}H_{9878}O_{1996}N_{1702}S_{42}{}^a$
Molecular weight	144 kDa[a]
Pharmacological class	PD-L1 blocking antibody

[a] Peptide chains only, without heavy chain C-terminal lysine residues.

Approval and Indication

❖ FDA: Accelerated approval for treatment of patients with locally advanced or metastatic urothelial carcinoma who have disease progression during or following platinum-containing chemotherapy or have disease progression within 12 months of neoadjuvant or adjuvant treatment with platinum-containing chemotherapy (05/18/2016).

Table 2　The Approval of Tecentriq®[8]

	US (FDA)	EU (EMA)
First approval date	05/18/2016	09/21/2017
Application or approval No.	BLA761034	EMEA/H/C004143
Brand name	Tecentriq®	Tecentriq®
Indication	Second line mUC	NSCLC, carcinoma, transitional cell
Authorization holder	Genentech (Roche)	Roche Registration Limited

Till Jan 2018, it had not been approved by PMDA (Japan) and CFDA (China).　NSCLC: Non-small cell lung cancer.

Table 3　Indication and Administration[8]

No.	Administration	Indication
1	1,200 mg over 60 min i.v. infusion every 3 weeks until disease progression or unacceptable toxicity.　If 1st i.v. is tolerated, all subsequent i.v. may be over 30 min.	Second line therapy for patients with locally advanced or metastatic urothelial carcinoma.

Sourced from US FDA drug label information.

Other PD-1/PD-L1 Antagonist
❖ Two PD-1 targeting mAbs, but no other PD-L1 mAbs have been approved as of 08/2016.

Table 4　Marketing PD-1/PD-L1-targeting Drugs[9-14]

Drug	Trade	Sponsor	Type	Approval	Indication
Nivolumab	Opdivo®	Bristol-Myers Squibb	PD-1 mAb	07/2014-PMDA 12/2014-FDA 06/2015-EMA	Melanoma, NSCLC, RCC, cHL
Pembrolizumab	Keytruda®	Merck & Co.	PD-1 mAb	09/2014-FDA 07/2015-EMA 09/2016-PMDA	Melanoma, NSCLC, HNSCC

cHL: Classical Hodgkin's lymphoma.　EMA: European Medicines Agency.　FDA: Food and Drug Administration.　HNSCC: Head and neck squamous cell carcinoma.　mAb: Monoclonal antibody.　NSCLC: Non-small cell lung cancer.　PMDA: Pharmaceuticals and Medical Devices Agency.　RCC: Renal cell carcinoma.

3　CMC Profile

Product Profile[6, 8]

Dosage form:　　IV infusion.
Strength:　　US: 1,200 mg/20 mL (60 mg/mL).
Formulation:　　60 mg/mL atezolizumab in 20 nM histidine acetate, 120 mM sucrose, and 0.4 mg/mL (0.040% *W/V*) polysorbate 20 at pH 5.8, and was developed to deliver a nominal amount (net quantity) of 1,200 mg of atezolizumab per vial.
Dilution:　　Dilute 20 mL of atezolizumab in a single-dose vial to 250 mL polyvinyl chloride (PVC), polyethylene (PE), or polyolefin (PO) infusion bag containing 0.90% sodium chloride injection, USP.
Storage:　　Administer immediately once prepared.　If diluted atezolizumab infusion solution is not used immediately it can be stored either: At room temperature for no more than 6 h from the time of preparation; Under refrigeration at 2-8 °C for no more than 24 h.　Do not freeze.　Do not shake.

Amino Acid Sequence[6, 15, 16]

❖ Atezolizumab is an Fc-engineered, humanized monoclonal antibody.

❖ Molecular formula: $C_{6434}H_{9878}O_{1996}N_{1702}S_{42}$ (Peptide chains only, without heavy chain C-terminal lysine residues).

```
  1  EVQLVESGGGLVQPGGSLRLSCAASGFTFSDSWIHWVRQAPGKGLEWVAWISPYGGSTYY
 61  ADSVKGRFTISADTSKNTAYLQMNSLRAEDTAVYYCARRHWPGGFDYWGQGTLVTVSSAS
121  TKGPSVFPLAPSSKSTSGGTAALGCLVKDYFPEPVTVSWNSGALTSGVHTFPAVLQSSGL
181  YSLSSVVTVPSSSLGTQTYICNVNHKPSNTKVDKKVEPKSCDKTHTCPPCPAPELLGGPS
241  VFLFPPKPKDTLMISRTPEVTCVVVDVSHEDPEVKFNWYVDGVEVHNAKTKPREEQYAST
301  YRVVSVLTVLHQDWLNGKEYKCKVSNKALPAPIEKTISKAKGQPREPQVYTLPPSREEMT
361  KNQVSLTCLVKGFYPSDIAVEWESNGQPENNYKTTPPVLDSDGSFFLYSKLTVDKSRWQQ
421  GNVFSCSVMHEALHNHYTQKSLSLSPGK
```

Heavy chain sequence: 448 amino acids

```
  1  DIQMTQSPSSLSASVGDRVTITCRASQDVSTAVAWYQQKPGKAPKLLIYSASFLYSGVPS
 61  RFSGSGSGTDFTLTISSLQPEDFATYYCQQYLYHPATFGQGTKVEIKRTVAAPSVFIFPP
121  SDEQLKSGTASVVCLLNNFYPREAKVQWKVDNALQSGNSQESVTEQDSKDSTYSLSSTLT
181  LSKADYEKHKVYACEVTHQGLSSPVTKSFNRGEC
```
⬜ : Variable Region. ⬜ : CDR.

Light chain sequence: 214 amino acids

Production Process

❖ Production platform: CHO cells platform.

❖ Protein yield: NA.

❖ Protein purity: NA.

4 Pre-clinical Pharmacology

Overview of *in vitro* Activities[15]

❖ Binding and inhibitory activity of atezolizumab and chimeric antibodies were evaluated in the following assays:
  - *In vitro*, MPDL3280A bound to human, Cynomolgus monkey, and murine PD-L1 with subnanomolar affinity, indicating that all three species are pharmacologically relevant.
  - Chimeric antibodies bound to PD-L1 with subnanomolar affinity, which was comparable to MPDL3280A.
  - MPDL3280A blocked PD-L1 binding to its receptors, PD-1 and B7-1, with picomolar inhibitory activity and enhance the tumor-specific T-cell response.
  - MPDL3280A showed minimal binding to Fcγ receptors. EC_{50} values were >100 μg/mL.

❖ Atezolizumab has reduced ADCC activity by mutation at N298A in the Fc domain which results in removal of the glycosylation site.

❖ Atezolizumab did not stimulate cytokine release from unstimulated human peripheral blood mononuclear cells (PBMCs) *in vitro*.

Table 5　Binding of Atezolizumab and Chimeric Antibodies to Human, Cynomolgus Monkey and Murine PD-L1[15]

	Equilibrium Binding Assay (K_d, nM) ($N = 2$)		ELISA Binding Assay (EC_{50}, nM)		
	Human PD-L1	Murine PD-L1	Activated Human T Cells	Activated Monkey T Cells	HEK293 Cells Expressing Murine PD-L1
MPDL3280A	0.43, 0.40	0.13, 0.12	0.40	0.70	0.52
PRO304397	0.37, 0.34	0.15, 0.19	-	-	0.41
PRO314483	-	-	-	-	0.43

PRO304397 and PRO314483 are murine chimeric antibody of MPDL3280A.　-: Not available.

Table 6   Inhibitory Activity of Atezolizumab A and Murine Chimeric Antibodies[15]

| | Blockade of Receptor/Ligand Binding (IC$_{50}$, pM) | | | |
| | Human | | Mouse | |
	B7-1/PD-L1	PD-1/PD-L1	B7-1/PD-L1	PD-1/PD-L1
MPDL3280A	48.4	82.8	75.6	104
PRO304397	47.5	77.5	79.4	113
PRO314483	41.0	78.9	96.6	125

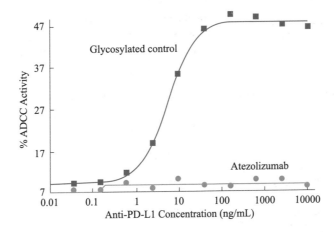

Figure 1   ADCC Activity of Atezolizumab[15]

Overview of *in vivo* Activities[15]

❖ Atezolizumab demonstrated excellent anti-tumor activities in syngeneic mouse models of melanoma and colorectal cancer.
  • Tumor growth inhibition: From 76.0% to complete inhibition.
  • For *in vivo* efficacy studies, murine/human chimeric antibodies of atezolizumab was generated to minimize immunogenicity in mice.

Table 7   Anti-tumor Efficacy of Atezolizumab in Syngeneic Mouse Model[15]

| SC Syngeneic Model | | | Drug | Dose (i.p., mg/kg) | Schedule | Finding |
Cell Line	Model	Animal				
MC38.OVA	Mouse colorectal cancer	Female C57BL/6 mice	PRO314483	10	qiw for 1, 2, 3 weeks	All mice receiving 10 mg/kg anti-PD-L1 had complete responses.
CT26	Mouse colorectal cancer	Balb/c mice	PRO314483	10	qiw × 3	Reduced tumor growth by >90.0% and prolonged the time to progression by approximately two weeks compared to controls.
S91	Mouse melanoma	DBA/2 mice	PRO314483	10	qiw × 3	Reduced tumor growth by 78.0% and prolonged time to progression by 6 days compared to controls.
MC38	Mouse colorectal cancer	C57BL/6 mice	PRO314483	10 10 10	qiw × 1 qiw × 2 qiw × 3	TGI = 76.0%; 1 PR. TGI = 98.0%; 3 CR + 3 PR. TGI = 103%; 3 CR + 3 PR.

PRO314483 are a murine chimeric antibody of MPDL3280A.   Anti-gp120 antibody was used as a control in all studies.   CR: Complete response.   qiw: Three times per week.   PR: Partial response.   TGI: Percent tumor growth inhibition at Day 25.

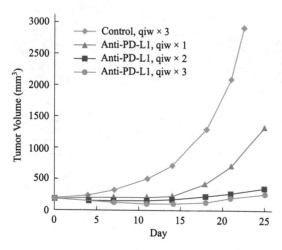

Study: Evaluation of the anti-tumor efficacy of anti-PD-L1 monoclonal antibody in the syngeneic MC38 colorectal model in C57BL/6 mice.

Animal: C57BL/6 mice.

Model: MC38 cells were mixed 50:50 with Matrigel and injected s.c. into the right flank of female C57BL/6 mice.

Administration: i.p. three times per week for 1, 2, 3 weeks; PRO314483: 10 mg/(kg·day); Control: anti-gp120 antibody, 10 mg/kg.

Starting: Tumors reached a size of 200 mm³.

Test: Measured tumor volumes.

Result: Anti-PD-L1 reduced tumor growth by 76.0%, 98.0%, and 103% following treatment of one, two, and three cycles, respectively. Time to progression was also prolonged with each increase in treatment length. There were no treatment-related effects on body weight.

Figure 2　Anti-tumor Activity of Anti-PD-L1 Antibody in a Syngeneic Mouse Model of MC38 Colorectal Cancer[15]

5　Toxicology

Summary

Single-Dose Toxicology

❖ No data or information available.

Repeated-Dose Toxicology[15]

❖ Mice received doses up to 50 mg/(kg·week) i.v. atezolizumab for three doses:
- Minimal sciatic neuropathy (vacuolation and lymphocytic infiltration) at doses ≥10 mg/kg i.v. observed in mice at the end of dosing and recovery period.
- All mice were positive for ATAs, which significantly reduced drug exposure by Day 17.

❖ Cynomolgus monkeys received atezolizumab at doses up to 50 mg/(kg·week) given s.c. for 8 weeks or administered i.v. for up to 26 weeks:
- The major toxicological finding was minimal to mild multifocal arteritis/periarteritis in multiple organs in Cynomolgus monkeys. Arteritis/periarteritis were noted in animals administered ≥15 mg/kg s.c. and 50 mg/kg i.v. atezolizumab. The findings were reversible following a 3-month recovery period.
- During the study, the majority of animals were positive for ATAs.

Safety Pharmacology[17]

❖ There were no test article-related effects on blood pressure, ECG, respiratory rate, or neurological parameters at doses up to 50 mg/(kg·week) administered for up to 26 weeks.

❖ All animals survived to scheduled necropsy.

❖ Body weight gain in males was slightly reduced at all dose levels compared to controls. There were no test article-related effects in female monkeys.

❖ Females administered 50 mg/kg MPDL3280A showed elevated leukocyte counts, correlating with microscopic findings of arteritis/periarteritis in multiple organs.

❖ Organ weight changes were observed in the ovary, thymus, and thyroid/parathyroid without microscopic correlates.

❖ Females administered 50 mg/kg MPDL3280A experienced irregular menstruation during the dosing period, including an increase in mean menstrual cycle length compared to controls.

Reproductive Toxicology[17]

❖ No reproductive and developmental toxicology studies with atezolizumab were conducted.

❖ The pharmacology/toxicology team agreed that a non-product specific literature-based assessment was appropriate to characterize the potential risk of embryo-fetal toxicity:
- Nonclinical studies demonstrate that PD-L1 blockade leads to a loss of fetal tolerance and an increased risk of immune-mediated abortion.
- The allogenic pregnancy models did not evaluate offspring for teratogenicity or adverse developmental effects.

Other Toxicology[17]

❖ A concentration of 125 mg/mL MPDL3280A did not cause hemolysis of human or Cynomolgus monkey blood.

❖ Tissue cross-reactivity of MPDL3280A:
- Membrane staining was reported only in syncytiotrophoblasts of human placenta. Cytoplasmic staining was observed in human lymph node, thymus, and tonsils.
- Staining of Cynomolgus monkey tissues was reported only in the lymph node (1-3+ cytoplasmic staining of sinusoidal cells; rare to frequent).

❖ No carcinogenicity studies were performed.

❖ No genetic toxicology studies were performed.

Anti-therapeutic Antibody Profile[17]

❖ The number of ATA-positive monkeys decreased with increasing atezolizumab dose.

❖ It is recognized that the sensitivity of the detection system of anti-atezolizumab antibodies could be compromised by the presence of high concentration of atezolizumab in the serum samples of the monkeys.

Repeated-Dose Toxicology

Table 8　Repeated-Dose Toxicity Studies of Atezolizumab[17]

Species	Duration	Dose [mg/(kg·day)]	Finding
C57BL/6 mouse	15 days; 4 weeks recovery	Male & female: 0, 10, 50; Days 1, 8, 15	All mice survived to scheduled necropsy. Minimal sciatic neuropathy (vacuolation and lymphocyte infiltration). All positive for ATA on Day 18 or 43. Mean C_{max} on Day 17 was reduced by 90.0% vs. Day 1.
CD-1 mouse	15 days; 4 weeks recovery	Male & female: 0, 50; Days 1, 8, 15	All mice survived to scheduled necropsy. No adverse findings. All positive for ATA on Day 18 or 43. Mean C_{max} on Day 17 was reduced by 75.0% vs. Day 1.
Cynomolgus monkey	8 weeks; 12 weeks recovery	Male & female: 0, 5, 15, 50; i.v. or s.c. weekly	All animals survived to scheduled necropsy. Minimal to mild multifocal arteritis/periarteritis in multiple organs. ATA were present in the majority of the animals.
	26 weeks; 13 weeks recovery	Male & female: 0, 5, 15, 50; i.v. weekly	All animals survived to scheduled necropsy. Minimal to mild multifocal arteritis/periarteritis in multiple organs. Organ weight changes were observed in the ovary, thymus, and thyroid/parathyroid without microscopic correlates. ATA were present in the majority of the animals.

ATA: Anti-therapeutic antibody.

Table 9　Summary of Organ Weights in Cynomolgus Monkeys at End of Dosing Necropsy (% Change Relative to Control)[17]

Organ	Weight	5 mg/kg		15 mg/kg		50 mg/kg	
		Male	Female	Male	Female	Male	Female
Ovary	A		-		↓35.9		↓35.9
	R/BW		-		-		↓41.7
Ovary (cysts excluded)	A		-		↓27.3		↓35.9
	R/BW		-		-		↓41.7
Thymus	A	-	-	-	26.5	-	44.7
	R/BW	-	-	-	41.9	-	31.0
Thyroid/ Parathyroid	A	-	↓43.8	-	↓35.8	-	↓28.5
	R/BW	-	↓35.2	-	↓26.1	-	↓32.7

There were no statistically significant findings. A: Absolute weight. R/BW: Relative per body weight. -: No test article-related change. ↓: Decrease.

Table 10 Summary of Hematology Parameters (% Change Relative to Controls)[17]

Parameter	Day	5 mg/kg		15 mg/kg		50 mg/kg	
		Male	Female	Male	Female	Male	Female
Leukocytes	60	-	-	-	-	-	36.4
	116	-	-	-	-	-	54.5a
Neutrophils	3	-	-	-	↓31.6	-	↓37.6
	116	↓32.8	-	↓41.3	↓22.4	↓25.8	40.5
	183	-	-	-	↓37.5	-	↓35.8
Lymphocytes	3	-	-	-	-	-	25.8
	60	-	-	-	-	-	67.6
	116	-	-	-	-	-	57.8
	183	-	-	-	-	-	39.9
	185	-	-	-	-	-	57.6
Eosinophils	60	-	-	-	-	-	123
	116	-	-	-	-	-	327

Significant finding. -: No test article-related change. ↓: Decrease. a P <0.050.

Anti-therapeutic Antibody Profile

Table 11 Immunogenicity Results from Cynomolgus Monkeys Receiving MPDL3280A Weekly[17]

	5 mg/(kg·dose)	15 mg/(kg·dose)	50 mg/(kg·dose)
Total No. of ATA-positive monkeys	10/10	8/10	3/10
Day 8	-	-	1/10
Day 15	10/10	8/10	-
Day 57	10/10	5/10	2/10
Day 113	10/10	4/10	2/10
Day 183	10/10	4/10	1/10
Day 225	4/4	2/4	-
Day 267	4/4	3/4	2/4
Findings	All anaphylaxis	Almost all anaphylaxis; APA emerged and decreased post multiple-dose	Low anaphylaxis at high dose

APA: Aminopenicillanic acid. -: No test article-related change.

Special Toxicology

Table 12 Special Toxicology Studies of Atezolizumab[17]

Special Toxicology	Species	Dose (mg/mL)	Finding
Hemolysis	Human or Cynomolgus monkey blood	125	No hemolysis.
Cross-reactivity	Human or Cynomolgus monkey tissue *ex vivo*	0.25, 1.25 (Biotin-labeled)	Atezolizumab bound to the cell membrane of syncytiotrophoblasts in human placenta and within the cytoplasm of human and monkey lymph nodes and human thymus and tonsils.

6 Non-clinical Pharmacokinetic/ADME/Toxicokinetics

Summary

Non-clinical Pharmacokinetics[6, 17]

❖ General toxicology studies evaluated atezolizumab in mice for two weeks and in Cynomolgus monkeys for up to 26 weeks. Atezolizumab was immunogenic in mice, resulting in significantly reduced exposures by Week 3.
❖ In single-dose
  • C_{max} and AUC increased with increasing dose and were slightly greater than dose proportional across the dose range tested.
  • In the two-compartment model, clearance of MPDL3280A ranged from 4.6 to 8.9 mL/(day·kg).   Mean volume at steady-state was 70.9 mL/kg.   Mean terminal half-life was 8.6 days.
  • In the non-compartment analysis, mean clearance and volume at steady-state were 3.8 mL/(day·kg) and 53.2 mL/kg, respectively.   Mean terminal half-life was 7.4 days.
❖ In repeated-dose studies in Cynomolgus monkeys
  • Systemic exposure in the 5 mg/kg dose group was greatly reduced due to formation of ATAs.
  • C_{max} and AUC increased in monkeys receiving 15 and 50 mg/kg MPDL3280A and were dose proportional at these dose levels.
  • Systemic exposure was greater on Day 182 compared to Day 1 in animals receiving 15 and 50 mg/kg antibody, indicating accumulation following repeat dosing.
  • Terminal half-life ranged from 11.8-23.5 days for recovery animals.
❖ Distribution
  • No data or information available.
❖ Drug-Drug interaction
  • No data or information available.

Non-clinical Pharmacokinetics

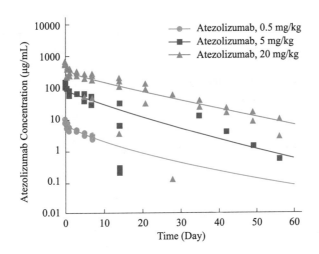

Figure 3   Single-Dose Pharmacokinetic Study of Atezolizumab Administered by Intravenous Injection to Cynomolgus Monkeys[17]
(Observed and Predicted Serum Concentration-Time Profiles)

Table 13   *In vivo* Pharmacokinetic Parameters of MPDL3280A in Cynomolgus Monkeys after Single Intravenous[17]

Dose Level (mg/kg) (N = 4/group)	$t_{1/2, beta}$ (Day)	C_{max} (µg/mL)	AUC_{inf} (µg·day/mL)
Non-compartmental analyses			
0.5	8.3	8.6	62.0
5	7.3	123	830
20	10.1	610	4,680
Two compartmental analyses			
5/20	11.5	NC	4,080

NC: Not calculated.

Table 14　Mean Toxicokinetic Parameters in Monkeys Administered Intravenous MPDL3280A[17]

	Sex	Dose mg/(kg·week)	C_{max} (µg/mL)	C_{max}/D (µg/mL)/D	AUC_{0-t} (µg·day/mL)	AUC_{0-t}/D (µg·day/mL)/D
Day 1	Male	5	139	27.8	263	52.6
		15	351	23.4	758	50.5
		50	1,290	25.8	2,880	57.6
	Female	5	107	21.4	224	44.8
		15	251	16.7	629	41.9
		50	1,110	22.2	2,690	53.8
Day 182	Male	5	7.3	1.5	NA	NA
		15	1,220	81.3	4,250	283
		50	4,060	81.2	10,100	202
	Female	5	116	23.2	378	75.6
		15	1,350	90.0	2,810	187
		50	3,300	66.0	6,740	135

Limited data were available for the 5 mg/kg dose level due to anti-therapeutic antibody formation in all animals.　Female means in the 5 mg/kg group were calculated from 2 of 3 animals.　Following a single-dose, AUC was estimated from Day 0 to 3.　For TK analysis on Day 182, AUC was estimated from Day 182 to 185.　NA: Not applicable.

7　Clinical Efficacy and Safety

Overview Profile

❖ Atezolizumab started clinical trials in the US in 2011.　There are more than 80 clinical trials in activity with atezolizumab antibody as monotherapy or combinatorial therapy on indications, such as bladder cancer, lung cancer, breast cancer (Clinicaltrials.gov).

❖ Breakthrough Therapy Designation (BTD) was previously granted by FDA for metastatic urothelial carcinoma (mUC) and NSCLC on 05/22/2014 and 01/28/2015, respectively.

❖ FDA granted Tecentriq® accelerated approval for patients with second line therapy for patients with locally advanced or metastatic urothelial carcinoma on May 18, 2016, based on the results from Cohort 2 of the study IMVigor 210.　Atezolizumab has been demonstrated a favorable benefit-risk profile in this study.[18, 19, 20]

❖ According to Medical Review and Clinical Pharmacology Biopharmaceutics Review released by FDA, the clinical studies submitted to support the Biologics License Application (BLA) approval are listed as the following.

Table 15　Clinical Trials of Atezolizumab[18]

ID	Phase	N	Population	Design	Study Posology	Endpoint
PCD4989g (GO27831)	1	481	Solid tumor: 481 mUC: 92	Open, single arm	0.01 to 20 mg/kg and 1,200 mg	Safety, PK, PPK, immunogenicity
JO28944	1	6	Japanese patients with solid tumors	Open, single arm	10 and 20 mg/kg	PK, PPK, immunogenicity
IMvigor 210 (GO29293)[a]	2	429	mUC: 429 Cohort 1 (1L): 118 Cohort 2 (2L+): 311	Open, single arm	1,200 mg/q3w	Safety, PK, PPK, immunogenicity, efficacy (Cohort 2 only)

Cohort 1 was intended to assess the activity and safety of atezolizumab in patients unfit for cisplatin-based chemotherapy and the results were not relevant for the current proposed indication.　1L: First-line treatment.　2L+: Second-line plus treatment.　mUC: Metastatic urothelial carcinoma.　PK: Pharmacokinetics.　PPK: Population pharmacokinetics.　q3w: Every 3 weeks.　[a] Results from Cohort 2 were evaluated in this application.

Clinical Efficacy

❖ GO29293 was a multicenter, open-label, two-cohort study of atezolizumab in patients with locally advanced or metastatic urothelial carcinoma. The key objectives were to evaluate the safety and antitumor activity of the product, as assessed by independent review per RECIST v1.1, and to evaluate the duration of response (DOR) according to the independent review as well as progression-free survival (PFS) and overall survival (OS).

- The overall objective response rate (ORR) was 15.0%, while it was much higher (26.0%) in patients with PD-L1 high expression.
- The durable responses were observed in patients regardless of PD-L1 IC scores, and Ventana PD-L1 (SP142) assay will be included in the atezolizumab package insert as complementary information that can inform prescribers of these results.
- The durability of the responses observed with atezolizumab appeared to be better than available therapy, and the drug was well tolerated in most studied patients.
- Serious risks included hepatitis, pneumonitis, endocrine disorders, colitis, infection, and neurological disorders.

Table 16   Efficacy of Cohort 2 of the Phase 2 IMVigor210 Trials (mUC) for the First Approval[18, 21]

	Efficacy (Median)		
	All Patients (N = 310)	PD-L1 Expression of <5.0% in ICs (IC 0/1) (N = 210)	PD-L1 Expression of ≥5.0% in ICs (IC 2/3) (N = 100)
No. of IRF-assessed confirmed responders per RECIST v1.1	46	20	26
ORR % (95% CI)	14.8% (11.1, 19.3)	9.5% (5.9, 14.3)	26.0% (17.7, 35.7)
Complete response (CR) (%)	5.5%	2.4%	12.0%
Partial response (PR) (%)	9.4%	7.1%	14.0%
DOR, median (Month) (Range)	NR (2.1+, 13.8+)	12.7 (2.1+, 12.7+)	NR (4.2, 13.8+)
No. of patients responding for ≥6 months (%)	37/46 (80.4%)	14/20 (70.0%)	23/26 (88.5%)
No. of patients responding for ≥12 months (%)	6/46 (13.0%)	2/20 (10.0%)	2/26 (15.4%)
PFS[a] of events (%)	266 (85.8%)	228 (88.0%)	93 (77.0%)
PFS, median (Month) (95% CI)	2.1 (2.1, 2.1)	2.1 (2.0, 2.1)	2.2 (2.1, 4.1)
OS[a] of events (%)	204 (65.8%)	154 (73.0%)	50 (50.0%)
OS, median (Month) (95% CI)	7.9 (6.6, 9.3)	6.7 (5.4, 8.0)	11.9 (7.6, NE)
Time to onset of response, median (Min, Max), (Month)	2.1 (1.6, 8.3)	2.1 (1.9, 8.3)	2.0 (1.6, 6.2)
No. of investigator assessed confirmed responders per modified RECIST	60	31	29
ORR, % (95% CI)	19.4% (15.1, 24.2)	14.8% (10.3, 20.2)	29.0% (20.4, 38.9)
CR (%)	5.8%	4.8%	8.0%
PR (%)	13.5%	10.0%	21.0%

NE: Not estimable. NR: Not reached.   [a] PD-L1 expression in tumor-infiltrating cells (ICs).

Clinical Safety

❖ The safety of atezolizumab was primarily evaluated in Trial IMvigor 210, a multi-center, single arm trial of atezolizumab monotherapy in patients with locally advanced or metastatic urothelial bladder cancer. Patients were divided into two cohorts.

❖ This review focused on the 310 patients in cohort 2 treated with atezolizumab with a data cut-off of May 5, 2015.

- The median duration of treatment was 12 weeks (range, 0 to 66).
- All cause, any grade adverse events were reported in 97.0% of patients, with 55.0% of patients experiencing a grade 3-4 event. Sixty-nine percent of patients had a treatment-related adverse event of any grade, and 16.0% of patients had a grade 3-4 related adverse event. Treatment-related serious adverse events were observed in 11.0% of patients.
- There were no treatment-related deaths reported on study.

- The majority of treatment-related adverse events was mild to moderate in nature, with fatigue (30.0%), nausea (14.0%), decreased appetite (12.0%), pruritus (10.0%), pyrexia (9.0%), diarrhea (8.0%), rash (7.0%), and arthralgia (7.0%) among the most common any grade events.
- The incidence of Grade 3-4 treatment-related adverse events was low, with fatigue the most commonly occurring at 2.0% (Table 17). There were no reports of febrile neutropenia.
- Seven percent of patients had an immune-mediated adverse event of any grade, with pneumonitis (2.0%), increased aspartate aminotransferase (1.0%), increased alanine aminotransferase (1.0%), rash (1.0%), and dyspnea (1.0%) being the most common adverse events.

Table 17   AEs in Cohort 2 of IMvigor210[18]

Adverse Reaction	All AEs		Treatment-related AEs	
	Any Grade (%)	Grades 3-4 (%)	Any Grade n (%)	Grade 3-4 n (%)
All Adverse Reactions	95.0	50.0	215 (69.0)	50.0 (16.0)
Gastrointestinal Disorders				
Diarrhea	18.0	1.0	24.0 (8.0)	1.0 (<1.0)
Constipation	21.0	0.0		
Nausea	25.0	0.30	42.0 (4.0)	0.0
Vomiting	17.0	1.0	18.0 (6.0)	1.0 (<1.0)
Abdominal pain	18.0	4.0		
Colitis			3.0 (1.0)	2.0 (1.0)
General Disorders and Administration				
Fatigue	52.0	6.0	93.0 (30.0)	5.0 (2.0)
Pyrexia	21.0	1.0	28.0 (9.0)	1.0 (<1.0)
Peripheral edema	18.0	1.0		
Infections and Infestations				
Urinary tract infection	22.0	9.0		
Metabolism and Nutrition Disorders				
Decreased appetite	26.0	1.0	36.0 (12.0)	2.0 (1.0)
Musculoskeletal and Connective Tissue Disorders				
Back/Neck pain	15.0	2.0		
Arthralgia	14.0	1.0	21.0 (7.0)	2.0 (1.0)
Renal and urinary disorders				
Hematuria	14.0	3.0		
Respiratory, Thoracic and Mediastinal Disorders				
Dyspnea	16.0	4.0	10.0 (3.0)	2.0 (1.0)
Cough	14.0	0.30		
Pneumonitis			7.0 (2.0)	2.0 (1.0)
Skin and Subcutaneous Tissue Disorders				
Rash	15.0	0.30	23 (7.0)	1.0 (<1.0)
Pruritis	13.0	0.30	31 (10.0)	1.0 (<1.0)
Hepatic Adverse Events (All)	15.8	4.2		
AST increased	4.2	0.60	10.0 (3.0)	2.0 (1.0)
ALT increased	3.9	1.0		
AKP increased	3.2	1.3		
Elevated bilirubin/hyperbilirubinemia	2.3	0.30		

Continued

Adverse Reaction	All AEs		Treatment-related AEs	
	Any Grade (%)	Grades 3-4 (%)	Any grade n (%)	Grade 3-4 n (%)
GGT increased	0.30	0.0		
Transaminases increased	1.0	0.0		
Hepatitis	0.30	0.30		
Autoimmune hepatitis	0.30	0.30		
Cholestasis	0.30	0.30		

AEs: Adverse events.

8 Clinical Pharmacokinetics[19]

Summary

❖ Pharmacokinetics: Atezolizumab demonstrated linear pharmacokinetics (PK) at a dose range of 1-20 mg/kg. Based on data from 472 patients who received 1-20 mg/kg of atezolizumab every 3 weeks, the population PK mean estimates were as follows:
  - Clearance, 0.20 L/day.
  - Volume of distribution at steady-state, 6.9 L.
  - Half-life, 27 days.
  - Time to reach steady-state concentrations, 6 to 9 weeks (2 to 3 cycles) after 1,200 mg every 3 weeks and the systemic accumulation of area under the curve (AUC), approximately 1.9-fold.
❖ Population pharmacokinetic analysis: Population PK analyses ($N = 472$) showed that the following factors have no clinically important effect on the PK parameters of atezolizumab administrated at 1,200 mg every 3 weeks: gender, body weight, tumor burden, serum albumin level, anti-therapeutic antibody (ATA) status, mild and moderate renal impairment, and mild hepatic impairment. Therefore, no dose adjustments based on above covariates are needed.
❖ Exposure/Dose-response relationship for efficacy and safety at 1,200 mg q3w: Steady-state exposure (AUC, ss) of atezolizumab was not a significant predictor of either probability of ORR or probability of adverse events in patients.
❖ Immunogenicity: The percentages of evaluable patients tested positive ATA were 41.9% (161/384), 31.7% (139/439) and 16.7% (1/6) in Phase 2 pivotal study IMvigor 210, Phase 1 supportive study PCD4989g, and Phase 1 supportive study JO28944, respectively. The presence of ATAs did not appear to have a clinically significant impact on pharmacokinetics, safety or efficacy.
❖ Drug-Drug interaction (DDI) potential: No DDI studies have been conducted.
❖ QT prolongation: IRT-QTc review team concluded that there is no evidence from nonclinical or clinical data to suggest that atezolizumab has the potential to delay ventricular repolarization.

Single-Dose Pharmacokinetics

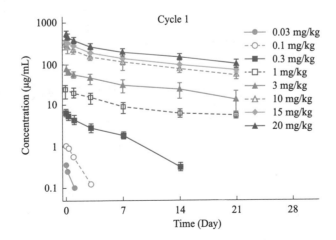

Figure 4   Atezolizumab Mean Serum Concentration vs. Time in Cycle 1 in PCD4989g Trial[22]

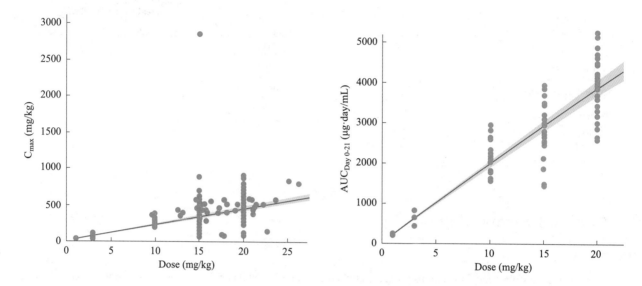

Figure 5　Relationship between Dose and Atezolizumab C_{max} (Left) and $AUC_{Day\ 0\text{-}21}$ (Right) in Cycle 1 (Day 0-21) of Study PCD4989[6]

Table 18　Summary of Atezolizumab Serum PK Parameters in Study PCD4989g Cycle 1[6]

Dose Group	Atezolizumab PK Parameters in Cycle 1 (GM, %CV)				
	C_{max} (μg/mL)	C_{max}/D μg/(mL·mg)	C_{min} (μg/mL)	C_{min}/D μg/(mL·mg)	$t_{1/2}$[a] (Day)
0.01 mg/kg (N = 1)	NA	NA	NA	NA	NA
0.03 mg/kg (N = 1)	0.37	0.16	NA	NA	NA
0.1 mg/kg (N = 1)	0.96	0.14	NA	NA	NA
0.3 mg/kg (N = 3)	6.5 (19) (n = 3)	0.33 (8.3) (n = 3)	NA	NA	NA
1 mg/kg (N = 3)	25.8 (17) (n = 3)	0.35 (26) (n = 3)	3.8 (160) (n = 3)	0.050 (120) (n = 3)	26.6 (n = 1)
3 mg/kg (N = 3)	75.6 (26) (n = 3)	0.27 (24) (n = 3)	12.2 (62) (n = 3)	0.040 (67) (n = 3)	21.8 (n = 1)
10 mg/kg (N = 36)	265 (16) (n = 36)	0.30 (240) (n = 36)	54.1 (25) (n = 34)	0.060 (33) (n = 34)	22.7 (56) (n = 10)
15 mg/kg (N = 235)	332 (53) (n = 232)	0.29 (57) (n = 232)	67.1 (73) (n = 214)	0.060 (76) (n = 214)	18.0 (39) (n = 29)
20 mg/kg (N = 145)	472 (35) (n = 145)	0.31 (37) (n = 145)	91.1 (36) (n = 132)	0.060 (43) (n = 132)	23.7 (36) (n = 28)
1,200 mg (N = 45)	405 (50) (n = 40)	0.34 (50) (n = 40)	95.5 (51) (n = 30)	0.080 (51) (n = 30)	NA

NA: Not available.　[a] The terminal half-life ($t_{1/2}$) was calculated with patient data ranging from Cycle 3 to 36.

Table 19   Summary of Atezolizumab Serum PK Parameters in Study PCD4989g Cycle 1[6]

Dose Group	Atezolizumab PK Parameters in Cycle 1 (GM, %CV)				
	AUC_{0-21} (μg·day/mL)	AUC_{0-21}/D [μg·day/(mL·mg)]	AUC_{0-inf} (μg·day/mL)	CL (L/day)	V_{ss} (L)
0.1 mg/kg (N = 1)	1.6	0.24	1.6	4.2	5.3
0.3 mg/kg (N = 3)	31.5 (8.1) (n = 3)	1.6 (12) (n = 3)	33.0 (7.9) (n = 2)	0.60 (15) (n = 2)	2.8 (13) (n = 2)
1 mg/kg (N = 3)	201 (8.5)	2.7 (27) (n = 3)	225 (2.8) (n = 2)	0.30 (19) (n = 2)	2.7 (53) (n = 2)
3 mg/kg (N = 3)	601 (34) (n = 3)	2.2 (25) (n = 3)	651 (22) (n = 2)	0.42 (10) (n = 2)	5.2 (7.4) (n = 2)
10 mg/kg (N = 36)	2,240 (17) (n = 3)	2.5 (28) (n = 29)	2,780 (22) (n = 9)	0.33 (33) (n = 9)	4.3 (39) (n = 9)
15 mg/kg (N = 235)	2,730 (27) (n = 29)	2.2 (22) (n = 29)	3,280 (35) (n = 17)	0.37 (23) (n = 17)	4.9 (22) (n = 17)
20 mg/kg (N = 145)	3,870 (21) (n = 32)	2.6 (27) (n = 32)	4,860 (23) (n = 10)	0.29 (30) (n = 10)	3.9 (30) (n = 10)

PK parameters were not calculated for the 0.01, 0.03 and 1,200 mg dose groups due to insufficient data. AUC_{0-21}: Area under the curve from Day 1 to Day 21. AUC_{0-21}/D: Dose-normalized AUC from Day 1 to Day 21. AUC_{inf}: AUC form time zero to infinity.   CL: Clearance. V_{ss}: Volume at steady-state.

Table 20   Summary of Atezolizumab Serum PK Parameters in Study JO28944 Cycle 1[6]

Dose group	Atezolizumab PK Parameters in Cycle 1 (GM, %CV)							
	C_{max} (μg/mL)	C_{max}/D μg/(mL·mg)	C_{min} (μg/mL)	$t_{1/2}$ (Day)	AUC_{0-21} (μg·day/mL)	AUC_{0-inf} (μg·day/mL)	CL (L/day)	V_{ss} (L)
10 mg/kg (N = 3)	219 (10.3)	0.41 (22.4)	36.8 (3.6)	11.6 (8.5)	1,670 (3.0)	2,290 (4.5)	0.23 (23.3)	3.6 (29.3)
20 mg/kg (N = 3)	534 (9.1)	0.32 (30.4)	113 (10.1)	13.0 (10.2)	4,480 (8.8)	6,610 (10.4)	0.20 (29.3)	3.8 (18.8)

C_{max}: Maximum serum concentration. C_{max}/D: Dose-normalized C_{max}. C_{min}: Trough or minimum serum concentration. $t_{1/2}$: Half-life.

Multiple-Dose Pharmacokinetics

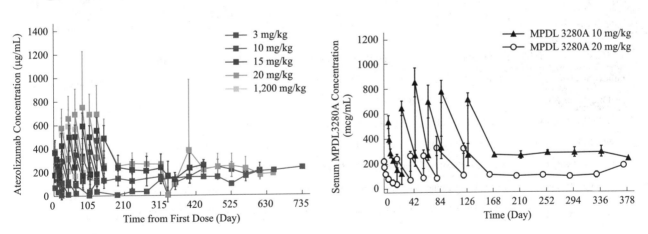

Figure 6   Mean (SD) Serum Atezolizumab (MPDL3280A) Concentration vs. Time Profile for All Cycles by Dose Group for Study PCD4989g (Left) and Study JO28944 (Right)[6]

Table 21   Atezolizumab Accumulation Ratio Based on C_{min} and C_{max} at Each Treatment Cycle
(Patients Receiving 1 mg/kg or Higher) in Study PCD4989g[6]

	Cycle 2	Cycle 3	Cycle 4	Cycle 5	Cycle 6	Cycle 7	Cycle 8
C_{min} (GM, %CV)	1.5 (42) (n = 333)	1.8 (42) (n = 290)	2.1 (42) (n = 165)	2.0 (61) (n = 81)	2.4 (52) (n = 133)	2.4 (68) (n = 100)	NA
C_{max} (GM, %CV)	1.2 (38) (n = 384)	1.3 (34) (n = 307)	1.3 (44) (n = 277)	1.4 (56) (n = 55)	1.4 (43) (n = 70)	1.4 (58) (n = 34)	1.2 (70) (n = 15)

NA: Not available.

9   Patent

❖ Atezolizumab was approved by the U.S. Food and Drug Administration (FDA) on May 18, 2016. It was developed and marketed as Tecentriq® by Genentech Inc., a subsidiary of Roche.

Summary

❖ The patent application (US1263339) related to the anti-PD-L1 antibody (i.e. Atezolizumab), nucleic acid encoding the same and therapeutic compositions thereof was filed by Genentech on Dec 8, 2009. Accordingly, its PCT counterpart has, among the others, been granted before USPTO (US8217149B2), EPO (EP2376535B1), JPO (JP5681638B2) and SIPO (CN102245640B), respectively.

Table 22   Originator's Key Patent of Atezolizumab in Main Countries and/or Region

Country/Region	Publication/Patent No.	Application Date	Granted Date	Estimated Expiry Date
WO	WO2010077634A1	12/08/2009	/	/
US	US8217149B2	12/08/2009	07/10/2012	/
EP	EP2376535B1	12/082009	04/12/2017	/
JP	JP5681638B2	12/08/2009	03/11/2015	/
	JP6178349B2	12/08/2009	08/09/2017	/
CN	CN102245640B	12/08/2009	12/31/2014	12/08/2029
	CN104479018A	12/08/2009	/	/

Table 23   Originator's International Patent Protection of Use and/or Method of Atezolizumab

Publication No.	Title	Publication Date
Technical Subjects	**TREATMENT METHOD**	
WO2010077634A1	Anti-PD-L1 antibodies and their use to enhance T-cell function	12/08/2009
WO2013019906A1	Methods of treating cancer using PD-1 axis binding antagonists and MEK inhibitors	08/01/2012
WO2013181452A1	Methods of treating cancer using PD-L1 axis binding antagonists and VEGF antagonists	05/30/2013
WO2015009856A2	Methods of treating cancer using PD-1 axis binding antagonists and TIGIT inhibitors	07/16/2014
WO20167023875A	Combination therapy of antibodies activating human CD40 and antibodies against human PD-L1	08/11/2015
WO2016079050A1	Combination therapy of T-cell activating bispecific antigen binding molecules CD3 ABD folate receptor 1 (FOLR1) and PD-1 axis binding antagonists	11/16/2015
WO2016179003A1	Masked anti-CD3 antibodies and methods of use	04/29/2016
WO2016183326A1	Therapeutic and diagnostic methods for cancer	05/12/2016
WO2016196381A1	PD-L1 promoter methylation in cancer	05/27/2016
WO2016200835A1	Methods of treating cancer using anti-OX40 antibodies and PD-1 axis binding antagonists	06/07/2016
WO2016205200A1	Anti-CLL-1 antibodies and methods of use	06/14/2016

Continued

Publication No.	Title	Publication Date
WO2016205320A1	Methods of treating locally advanced or metastatic breast cancers using PD-1 axis binding antagonists and taxanes	06/15/2016
WO2017053748A2	Anti-TIGIT antibodies and methods of use	09/23/2016
WO2017087280A1	Methods of treating HER2-positive cancer	11/11/2016
WO2017107979A1	TDO2 inhibitors	12/23/2016
WO2017118675A1	Methods of treating CEA-positive cancers using PD-1 axis binding antagonists and anti-CEA/anti-CD3 bispecific antibodies	01/05/2017
WO2017151502A1	Therapeutic and diagnostic methods for cancer	02/27/2017
WO2017159699A1	Methods of treating cancers using PD-1 axis binding antagonists and anti-GPC3 antibodies	03/14/2017
Technical Subjects	**DIAGNOSTIC METHOD**	
WO2014083178A1	Identification of patients in need of PD-L1 inhibitor cotherapy	11/29/2013
WO2014151006A2	Biomarkers and methods of treating PD-1 and PD-L1 related conditions	03/12/2014
WO2016007235A1	Anti-PD-L1 antibodies and diagnostic uses thereof	05/29/2015
WO2016183326A1	Therapeutic and diagnostic methods for cancer	05/12/2016
WO2017085397A1	Method of identifying immune cells in PD-L1 positive tumor tissue	11/21/2016
Technical Subjects	**FORMULATION**	
WO2015048520A1	Anti-PD-L1 antibody formulations	09/26/2014

The data was updated until Jan 2018.

10　Reference

[1] Chinai J M, Janakiram M, Chen F, et al. New immunotherapies targeting the PD-1 pathway [J]. Trends in Pharmacological Sciences, 2015, 36(9): 587-595.

[2] Freeman G J, Long A J, Iwai Y, et al. Engagement of the PD-1 immunoinhibitory receptor by a novel B7 family member leads to negative regulation of lymphocyte activation [J]. Journal of Experimental Medicine, 2000, 192(7): 1027-1034.

[3] Francisco L M, Salinas V H, Brown K E, et al. PD-L1 regulates the development, maintenance, and function of induced regulatory T cells [J]. Journal of Experimental Medicine, 2009, 206(13): 3015-3029.

[4] Patsoukis N, Bardhan K, Chatterjee P, et al. PD-1 alters T-cell metabolic reprogramming by inhibiting glycolysis and promoting lipolysis and fatty acid oxidation [J]. Nature Communications, 2015, 6: 6692-6704.

[5] Staron M M, Gray S M, Marshall H D, et al. The transcription factor FoxO1 sustains expression of the inhibitory receptor PD-1 and survival of antiviral CD8(+) T cells during chronic infection [J]. Immunity, 2014, 41(5): 802-814.

[6] Food and Drug Administration (FDA) Database.　http://www.accessdata.fda.gov/drugsatfda_docs/nda/2016/761034 Orig1s000ClinPharmR.pdf.

[7] FDA Database.　http://www.accessdata.fda.gov/drugsatfda_docs/nda/2016/761034Orig1s000ChemR.pdf.

[8] FDA Database.　http://www.accessdata.fda.gov/drugsatfda_docs/nda/2016/761034Orig1s000Lbl.pdf.

[9] FDA Database.　https://www.accessdata.fda.gov/drugsatfda_docs/label/2014/125554lbl.pdf.

[10] FDA Database.　https://www.accessdata.fda.gov/drugsatfda_docs/label/2014/125514lbl.pdf.

[11] FDA Database.　https://www.accessdata.fda.gov/scripts/cder/daf/index.cfm?event=overview.process&applno=125514.

[12] European Medicines Agency (EMA) Database.　http://www.ema.europa.eu/ema/index.jsp?curl=pages/medicines/human/medicines/003985/human_med_001876.jsp&mid=WC0b01ac058001d124.

[13] EMA Database.　http://www.ema.europa.eu/ema/index.jsp?curl=pages/medicines/human/medicines/003820/human_med_001886.jsp&mid=WC0b01ac058001d124.

[14] Pharmaceuticals and Medical Devicesran (PMDA) Database.　http://www.pmda.go.jp/english/review-services/reviews/approved-information/drugs/0001.html#select14.

[15] FDA Database.　http://www.accessdata.fda.gov/drugsatfda_docs/nda/2016/761034Orig1s000PharmR.pdf.

[16] Irving B, Chiu H, Maecker H, et al. Anti-PD-L1 antibodies, compositions and articles of manufacture: US8217149B2 [P]. 2012-07-10.

[17] Drug Bank Database.　http://www.drugbank.ca/drugs/DB11595.

[18] FDA Database.　http://www.accessdata.fda.gov/drugsatfda_docs/nda/2016/761034Orig1s000MedR.pdf.

[19] FDA Database.　http://www.accessdata.fda.gov/drugsatfda_docs/nda/2016/761034Orig1s000SumR.pdf.

[20] FDA Database. http://www.accessdata.fda.gov/drugsatfda_docs/nda/2016/761034Orig1s 000RiskR.pdf.

[21] Rosenberg J E, Hoffman-censits J, Powles T, et al. Atezolizumab in patients with locally advanced and metastatic urothelial carcinoma who have progressed following treatment with platinum-based chemotherapy: a single arm, multi-center, Phase 2 trial [J]. The Lancet, 2016, 387(10031): 1909-1920.

[22] Herbst R S, Soria J C, Kowanetz m, et al. Predictive correlates of response to the anti-PD-L1 antibody MPDL 3280A in cancer patients [J]. Nature, 2014, 515(7528): 563-567.

CHAPTER
3
Bevacizumab

Bevacizumab

(Avastin®)

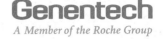

Research code: G180CL, G180CU, G180DL, NSC-704865, R-435, RG-435, rhuMab-VEGF, RO-4876646

1 Target Biology

The VEGF

❖ Vascular endothelial growth factor A (VEGFA, previously known as vascular permeability factor (VPF) identified by Senger and colleagues in 1983), was isolated and sequenced by Ferrara and colleagues in 1989.[1-4]

❖ VEGFA is the prototype member of a family of proteins that includes VEGFB, VEGFC, VEGFD, VEGFE (a virally encoded protein) and placental growth factor (PIGF, also known as PGF).[5]

❖ Multiple isoforms of VEGFA are derived from alternative splicing of exons 6 and 7, including $VEGFA_{121}$, $VEGFA_{165}$, $VEGFA_{189}$ and $VEGF_{206}$. $VEGFA_{165}$ is the most frequently expressed isoform in normal tissues and tumors. $VEGFA_{165}$ has an intermediary behavior between the highly diffusible $VEGFA_{121}$ and the extracellular matrix-bound $VEGFA_{189}$, and is thought to be the most physiologically relevant VEGFA isoform.[6]

❖ VEGFA can bind VEGFR1 and VEGFR2 on endothelial cells *in vivo*. VEGFR2 is the main mediator of the roles of VEGFA in cell proliferation, angiogenesis and vessel permeabilization. VEGFR2 binds to VEGF with a K_d of approximately 75-125 pM and lead to receptor dimerization and autophosphorylation.[7, 8]

Sequence Homology of VEGF Proteins[9-14]

Human: 191aa.   Accession: AAK95847.1.

```
  1  MNFLLSWVHW  SLALLLYLHH  AKWSQAAPMA  EGGGQNHHEV  VKFMDVYQRS  YCHPIETLVD
 61  IFQEYPDEIE  YIFKPSCVPL  MRCGGCCNDE  GLECVPTEES  NITMQIMRIK  PHQGQHIGEM
121  SFLQHNKCEC  RPKKDRARQE  NPCGPCSERR  KHLFVQDPQT  CKCSCKNTDS  RCKARQLELN
181  ERTCRCDKPR  R
```

Pan troglodytes: 191aa.   Accession: XP_016811082.1.

❖ BLAST:
  • Max score: 401; Total score: 401; Query cover: 100%; Identities: 100%.

```
  1  MNFLLSWVHW  SLALLLYLHH  AKWSQAAPMA  EGGGQNHHEV  VKFMDVYQRS  YCHPIETLVD
 61  IFQEYPDEIE  YIFKPSCVPL  MRCGGCCNDE  GLECVPTEES  NITMQIMRIK  PHQGQHIGEM
121  SFLQHNKCEC  RPKKDRARQE  NPCGPCSERR  KHLFVQDPQT  CKCSCKNTDS  RCKARQLELN
181  ERTCRCDKPR  R
```

Macaca mulatta: 191aa.   Accession: AFE64645.1.

❖ BLAST:
  • Max score: 401; Total score: 401; Query cover: 100%; Identities: 100%.

```
  1  MNFLLSWVHW  SLALLLYLHH  AKWSQAAPMA  EGGGQNHHEV  VKFMDVYQRS  YCHPIETLVD
 61  IFQEYPDEIE  YIFKPSCVPL  MRCGGCCNDE  GLECVPTEES  NITMQIMRIK  PHQGQHIGEM
121  SFLQHNKCEC  RPKKDRARQE  NPCGPCSERR  KHLFVQDPQT  CKCSCKNTDS  RCKARQLELN
181  ERTCRCDKPR  R
```

Rattus norvegicus: 190aa.   Accession: AAL07526.1.

❖ BLAST:
  • Max score: 334; Total score: 334; Query cover: 100%; Identities: 90.0%.

```
  1  MNFLLSWVHW  ■LALLLYLHH  AKWSQAAP■■  EG■QK■HEV■  KFMDVYQRSY  C■PIETLVDI
 61  FQEYPDEIEY  IFKPSCVPLM  RC■GCCNDE■  LECVPT■ESN  VTMQIMRIKP  HQ■QHIGEMS
121  FLQHS■CECR  PKKDR■KPEN  ■C■PCSERRK  HLFVQDPQTC  KCSCKNTDSR  CKARQLELNE
181  RTCRCDKPRR
```

Mus musculus: 190aa.　　Accession: EDL23467.1.

❖ BLAST:
  • Max score: 334; Total score: 334; Query cover: 100%; Identities: 90.0%.

```
  1  MNFLLSWVHW  ■LALLLYLHH  AKWSQAAP■■  EG■QKSHEV■  KFMDVYQRSY  C■PIETLVDI
 61  FQEYPDEIEY  IFKPSCVPLM  RC■GCCNDE■  LECVPT■ESN  ITMQIMRIKP  HQ■QHIGEMS
121  FLQHS■CECR  PKKDR■KPEN  ■C■PCSERRK  HLFVQDPQTC  KCSCKNTDSR  CKARQLELNE
181  RTCRCDKPRR
```

Biology Activity

❖ VEGFA is the master regulator of angiogenesis, binding to VEGFR2 to stimulate the proliferation of endothelial cells via the RAS-RAF-MAPK-ERK signaling pathway. VEGFA triggers endothelial cell migration, which is an integral component of angiogenesis.[15]

❖ More recent studies have shown that phosphorylation of VEGFR2 Tyr 1175 (in humans; Tyr1173 in mice) has a crucial role in regulating VEGFA-dependent angiogenesis.[16]

❖ Binding of VEGFA to VEGFR1 is lack of mitogenic effects following VEGFR1 activation, suggest that VEGFR1 may act at least in some circumstances as a decoy receptor, sequestering VEGFA and regulating VEGFR2 activity.[7]

❖ VEGF is a survival factor for endothelial cells both *in vitro* and *in vivo*. *In vivo*, the prosurvival effects of VEGF are developmentally regulated.[17]

❖ VEGF promotes monocyte chemotaxis and induces colony formation by mature subsets of granulocyte-macrophage progenitor cells.[18]

❖ VEGF has the ability to induce vascular leakage, which underlies significant roles of this molecule in inflammation and other pathological circumstances.[19]

❖ VEGF induces vasodilatation *in vitro* in a dose-dependent fashion as a result of endothelial cell-derived nitric oxide, and produces transient tachycardia, hypotension and decrease in cardiac output when injected intravenously in conscious, instrumented rats.[20]

❖ VEGF has been implicated in pathological angiogenesis associated with tumors, intraocular neovascular disorders and other conditions.[6]

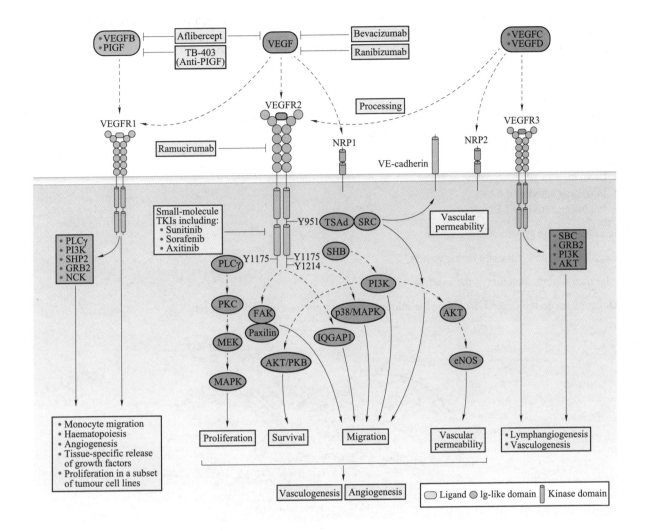

Figure 1　VEGF-VEGFR Signaling[15]

2　General Information

Avastin®[21]

❖ Avastin® (Bevacizumab) is a humanized mouse antibody.　It comprises mutated human IgGl framework regions and antigen-binding complementarity-determining regions from the murine anti-hVEGF monoclonal antibody A4.6.1 that blocks binding of human VEGF to its receptors.　Approximately 93.0% of the amino acid sequence of bevacizumab, including most of the framework regions, is derived from human IgGl, and about 7.0% of the sequence is derived from the murine antibody A4.6.1.

❖ Avastin® is a full-length IgG1κ isotype antibody composed of two identical light chains (214 amino acid residues) and two heavy chains (453 residues) with a total molecular weight of 149 kDa.

❖ Avastin® was originally derived from a murine monoclonal antibody (muMAb A4.6.1), which was produced at Genentech using hybridomas generated from mice immunized with the 165-residue-form of recombinant human vascular endothelial growth factor (rhuVEGF165) conjugated with keyhole limpet hemocyanin.

❖ The humanization of the A4.6.1 antibody involved insertion of the six CDRs of A4.6.1, in place of those of a selected human antibody Fab framework (pEMX1), which has a consensus human kappa subgroup I light chain (domains VL-CL) and a truncated human subgroup III immunoglobulin gamma (IgG1) heavy chain (domains VH-CH1).　A series of framework residue substitutions were made to produce the final humanized version, Fab-12, which contains eight substitutions of the human framework outside of the CDRs.　The V_H and V_L domains of Fab-12 were combined with human IgG1 constant domains CH1-CH2-CH3 and CL, respectively, to produce bevacizumab.

❖ The expression plasmid pSVID5.ID.LLnspeV.xvegf36HC.LC encoding bevacizumab was introduced into Chinese hamster ovary parental cells CHO DP-12 by lipofection and cells were selected in the presence of increasing concentrations of methotrexate (MTX).   Isolates were selected for secretion of active bevacizumab.

❖ The total sales of 6,852 million US$ for 2016; No sales data as of 2017.

Mechanism of Action[22]

❖ Blocking binding of VEGFA to its receptors, inhibiting survival, proliferation, migration and permeability of endothelial cells through the following mechanism:
  • Blocking PI3K/Akt signaling pathway.
  • Blocking MAPK/P38 signaling pathway.
  • Blocking PLC/PKC signaling pathway.
  • Inhibiting activity of FAK.
  • Inhibiting activity of TSAd-Src.

❖ Inhibition of the growth of new vessels.

❖ Regression of newly formed tumor vessels.

❖ Alternation of the function of the vascular bed.

❖ Direct effect on tumor cells, including the inhibition of antiapoptotic autocrine signals.

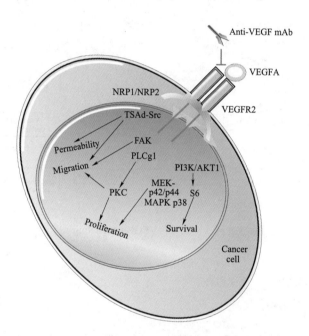

Figure 2   Mechanism of Anti-VEGF mAb[22]

Sponsor

❖ Avastin® (Bevacizumab) was developed and market by Genentech, Inc., a subsidiary of Roche.

World Sales[23]

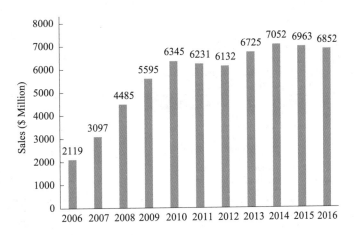

Figure 3   World Sales of Bevacizumab since 2006

Approval and Indication

Table 1   Summary of the Approved Indication[21, 23-27]

Approval (Year)	Agency	Indication
2004	FDA	First-line treatment of metastatic carcinoma of the colon and rectum.
2006	FDA	Second-line treatment of metastatic colorectal cancer; First-line treatment of unresectable, locally advanced, recurrent or metastatic non-squamous, non-small cell lung cancer in combination with carboplatin and paclitaxel.
	EMA	Metastatic carcinoma of the colon or rectum.
2007	EMA	Metastatic breast cancer, unresectable advanced, metastatic or recurrent non-small cell lung cancer.
2008	FDA	Metastatic HER2-negative breast cancer.
	EMA	Advanced and/or metastatic renal cell cancer.
2009	FDA	Glioblastoma with progressive disease following prior therapy; Metastatic renal cell carcinoma in combination with interferon alfa.
2011	EMA	Advanced epithelial ovarian, fallopian tube, or primary peritoneal cancer.
2014	FDA	Metastatic cervical cancer.
2015	FDA	Persisten, recurrent, or metastatic carcinoma of the cervix.

Table 2   Summary of the Approval of Avastin®[21, 23-27]

	US (FDA)	EU (EMA)	Japan (PMDA)	China (CFDA)
First approval date	26/02/2004	12/01/2005	18/04/2007	01/07/2015
Application or approval No.	BLA125085	EMEA/H/C/000582	21900AMX0910 21900AMX00921	S20120068 S20120069
Brand name	Avastin®	Avastin®	Avastin®	Avastin®/安维汀®
Indication	MCC, MBC, NSNSCLC, Glioblastoma, mRCC, prmCC, prrEOFTPPC	Carcinoma, NSCLC, colorectal neoplasms, carcinoma, renal cell, ovarian neoplasms, breast neoplasms	Advanced or recurrent colorectal cancer	Advanced or recurrent MCC
Authorization holder	Genentech (Roche)	Roche	Chugai	Genentech (Roche)

EOFTPPC: Epithelial ovarian, fallopian tube or primary peritoneal cancer.   MBC: Metastatic breast cancer.   MCC: Metastatic colorectal cancer.   mRCC: Metastatic renal cell cancer.   NSNSCLC: Non-squamous non-small cell lung cancer.   prmCC: Persistent, recurrent, or metastatic carcinoma of the cervix.   prrEOFTPPC: Platinum-resistant recurrent epithelial ovarian, fallopian tube or primary peritoneal cancer.

Table 3   Indication and Administration[27, 28]

No.	Administration	Indication
1	5 mg/kg i.v. every 2 weeks with bolus-IFL; 10 mg/kg i.v. every 2 weeks with FOLFOX4; 5 mg/kg i.v. every 2 weeks or 7.5 mg/kg i.v. every 3 weeks with fluoropyrimidine-irinotecan or fluoropyrimidine-oxaliplatin based chemotherapy after progression on a first-line Avastin® containing regimen	Metastatic colorectal cancer
2	15 mg/kg i.v. every 3 weeks with carboplatin/paclitaxel	Non-squamous non-small cell lung cancer
3	10 mg/kg i.v. every 2 weeks	Glioblastoma
4	10 mg/kg i.v. every 2 weeks with interferon alfa	Metastatic renal cell carcinoma
5	15 mg/kg i.v. every 3 weeks with paclitaxel/cisplatin or paclitaxel/topotecan	Persistent, recurrent, or metastatic carcinoma of the cervix
6	10 mg/kg i.v. every 2 weeks with paclitaxel, pegylated liposomal doxorubicin or weekly topotecan; 15 mg/kg i.v. every 3 weeks with topotecan given every 3 weeks	Platinum-resistant recurrent epithelial ovarian, fallopian tube or primary peritoneal cancer
7	10 mg/kg i.v. every 2 weeks with paclitaxel	Metastatic breast cancer

Sourced from US FDA drug label information.   FOLFOX4: Oxaliplatin plus continuous infusional 5-FU/FA.   IFL: Irinotecan plus 5-fluorouracil leucovorin.

Table 4   Marketing VEGF-targeting Drugs[24, 26, 29, 30]

Drug	Trade	Sponsor	Type	Approval	Indication
Ranibizumab	Lucentis®	Genentech, Novartis	Fab fragment	06/2006-FDA 01/2007-EMA 01/2009-PMDA 01/2011-CFDA	AMD, RVO, DME, DR, mCNV
Aflibercept	Zaltrap®	Sanofi-Aventis	Fusion protein	08/2012-FDA 02/2013-EMA 03/2017-PMDA	Metastatic colorectal cancer
Aflibercept	Eylea®	Bayer Pharma	Fusion protein	11/2011-FDA 09/2012-PMDA 09/2012-EMA	wAMD, macular edema due to BRVO or CRVO, DME, myopic CNV
Conbercept	Langmu®/朗沐®	Chengdu KangHong	Fusion protein	11/2013-CFDA	wAMD, CNV

CNV: Choroidal neovascularization.   DME: Diabetic macular edema.   DR: Diabetic retinopathy.   MCC: Metastatic colorectal cancer.   mRCC: Metastatic renal cell cancer.   NSNSCLC: Non-squamous non-small cell lung cancer.   prmCC: Persistent, recurrent, or metastatic carcinoma of the cervix.   prrEOFTPPC: Platinum-resistant recurrent epithelial ovarian, fallopian tube or primary peritoneal cancer.   RVO: Retinal vein occlusion.   wAMD: Wet age-related macular degeneration.

3   CMC Profile

Product Profile[21, 27]

Dosage route: IV infusion.

Strength: 100 mg, 400 mg.

Dosage form: Injection.

Formulation: The drug product is a liquid formulation and each vial is filled with 25 mg/mL of bevacizumab, an active ingredient.   Based on various investigations, 60 mg/mL trehalose as an isotonizing agent, 51 mmol/L sodium phosphate (pH 6.2) as a buffer, and 0.04 *W/V*% PS20 as a stabilizer have been selected.   The composition of the sodium phosphate buffer is sodium dihydrogen phosphate monohydrate and sodium phosphate dibasic anhydrous.   No overages are used.

Stability: The proposed shelf life for Avastin® is 24 months when stored at 2-8 °C, protected from light, and the proposed temperature during transportation is 2-8 °C, protected from light; The proposed storage time of bevacizumab drug substance is 24 months when stored at -20 ± 5 °C, 45 days at 5 ± 3 °C and up to 5 freeze/thaw cycles.

Amino Acid Sequence[27]

❖ Avastin® contains the antineoplastic agent bevacizumab, a recombinant humanized IgG1 monoclonal antibody (93.0% human, 7.0% murine sequences) that binds with high affinity to human vascular endothelial growth factor (VEGF). Bevacizumab was generated by humanization of the murine parent antibody A4.6.1.

❖ Molecular formula: $C_{6538}H_{10000}O_{2032}N_{1716}S_{44}$

❖ Light chain: $C_{1034}H_{1591}N_{273}O_{338}S_6$

❖ Heavy chain: $C_{2235}H_{3413}N_{585}O_{678}S_{16}$

```
  1  Asp-Ile-Gln-Met-Thr-Gln-Ser-Pro-Ser-Ser-Leu-Ser-Ala-Ser-Val-Gly-Asp-Arg-Val-Thr-Ile-Thr- Cys²³-Ser-Ala-
 26  Ser-Gln-Asp-Ile-Ser-Asn-Tyr-Leu-Asn-Trp-Tyr-Gln-Gln-Lys-Pro-Gly-Lys-Ala-Pro-Lys-Val-Leu-Ile-Tyr-Phe-
 51  Thr-Ser-Ser-Leu-His-Ser-Gly-Val-Pro-Ser-Arg-Phe-Ser-Gly-Ser-Gly-Ser-Gly-Thr-Asp-Phe-Thr-Leu-Thr-Ile-
 76  Ser-Ser-Leu-Gln-Pro-Glu-Asp-Phe-Ala-Thr-Tyr-Tyr-Cys⁸⁸-Gln-Gln-Tyr-Ser-Thr-Val-Pro-Trp-Thr-Phe-Gly-Gln-
101  Gly-Thr-Lys-Val-Glu-Ile-Lys-Arg-Thr-VaL-ALa-ALa-Pro-Ser-Val-Phe-Ile-Phe-Pro-Pro-Ser-Asp-Glu-Gln-Leu-
126  Lys-Ser-Gly-Thr-Ala-Ser-Val-Val- Cys¹³⁴-Leu-Leu-Asn-Asn-Phe-Tyr-Pro-Arg-Glu-Ala-Lys-Val-Gln-Trp-Lys-Val-
151  Asp-Asn-Ala-Leu-Gln-Ser-Gly-Asn-Ser-Gln-Glu-Ser-Val-Thr-Glu-Gln-Asp-Ser-Lys-Asp-Ser-Thr-Tyr-Ser-Leu-
176  Ser-Ser-Thr-Leu-Thr-Leu-Ser-Lys-Ala-Asp-Tyr-Glu-Lys-His-Lys-Val-Tyr-Ala-Cys¹⁹⁴-Glu-Val-Thr-His-Gln-Gly-
201  Leu-Ser-Ser-Pro-Val-Thr-Lys-Ser-Phe-Asn-Arg-Gly-Glu-Cys²¹⁴
```

Light chain

—: Disulfide bond.

The underlined parts: The complementarity-determining regions.

```
  1  Glu-Val-Gln-Leu-Val-Glu-Ser-Gly-Gly-Gly-Leu-Val-Gln-Pro-Gly-Gly-Ser-Leu-Arg-Leu-Ser-Cys²²-Ala-Ala-Ser-
 26  Gly-Tyr-Thr-Phe-Thr-Asn-Tyr-Gly-Met-Asn-Trp-Val-Arg-Gln-Ala-Pro-Gly-Lys-Gly-Leu-Glu-Trp-Val-Gly-Trp-
 51  Ile-Asn-Thr-Tyr-Thr-Gly-Glu-Pro-Thr-Tyr-Ala-Ala-Asp-Phe-Lys-Arg-Arg-Phe-Thr-Phe-Ser-Leu-Asp-Thr-Ser-
 76  Lys-Ser-Thr-Ala-Tyr-Leu-Gln-Met-Asn-Ser-Leu-Arg-Ala-Glu-Asp-Thr-Ala-Val-Tyr-Tyr-Cys⁹⁶-Ala-Lys-Tyr-Pro-
101  His-Tyr-Tyr-Gly-Ser-Ser-His-Trp-Tyr-Phe-Asp-Val-Trp-Gly-Gln-Gly-Thr-Leu-Val-Thr-Val-Ser-Ser-Ala-Ser-
126  Thr-Lys-Gly-Pro-Ser-Val-Phe-Pro-Leu-Ala-Pro-Ser-Ser-Lys-Ser-Thr-Ser-Gly-Gly-Thr-Ala-Ala-Leu-Gly-Cys¹⁵⁰-
151  Leu-Val-Lys-Asp-Tyr-Phe-Pro-Glu-Pro-Val-Thr-Val-Ser-Trp-Asn-Ser-Gly-Ala-Leu-Thr-Ser-Gly-Val-His-Thr-
176  Phe-Pro-Ala-Val-Leu-Gln-Ser-Ser-Gly-Leu-Tyr-Ser-Leu-Ser-Ser-Val-Val-Thr-Val-Pro-Ser-Ser-Ser-Leu-Gly-
201  Thr-Gln-Thr-Tyr-Ile-Cys²⁰⁶ -Asn-Val-Asn-His-Lys-Pro-Ser-Asn-Thr-Lys-Val-Asp-Lys-Lys-Val-Glu-Pro-Lys-Ser-
226  Cys²²⁶-Asp-Lys-Thr-His-Thr-Cys²³²*-Pro-Pro-Cys²³⁵**-Pro-Ala-Pro-Glu-Leu-Leu-Gly-Gly-Pro-Ser-Val-Phe-Leu-Phe-Pro-
251  Pro-Lys-Pro-Lys-Asp-Thr-Leu-Met-Ile-Ser-Arg-Thr-Pro-Glu-Val-Thr-Cys²⁶⁷ -Val-Val-Val-Asp-Val-Ser-His-Glu-
276  Asp-Pro-Glu-Val-Lys-Phe-Asn-Trp-Tyr-Val-Asp-Gly-Val-Glu-Val-His-Asn-Ala-Lys-Thr-Lys-Pro-Arg-Glu-Glu-
301  Gln-Tyr-Asn³⁰³-Ser-Thr-Tyr-Arg-Val-Val-Ser-Val-Leu-Thr-Val-Leu-His-Gln-Asp-Trp-Leu-Asn-Gly-Lys-Glu-Tyr-
326  Lsy-Cys³²⁷-Lys-Val-Ser-Asn-Lys-Ala-Leu-Pro-Ala-Pro-Ile-Glu-Lys-Thr-Ile-Ser-Lys-Ala-Lys-Gly-Gln-Pro-Arg-
351  Glu-Pro-Gln-Val-Tyr-Thr-Leu-Pro-Pro-Ser-Arg-Glu-Glu-Met-Thr-Lys-Asn-Gln-Val-Ser-Leu-Thr-Cys³⁷³-Leu-Val-
376  Lsy-Gly-Phe-Tyr-Pro-Ser-Asp-Ile-Ala-Val-Glu-Trp-Glu-Ser-Asn-Gly-Gln-Pro-Glu-Asn-Asn-Tyr-Lys-Thr-Thr-
401  Pro-Pro-Val-Leu-Asp-Ser-Asp-Gly-Ser-Phe-Phe-Leu-Tyr-Ser-Lys-Leu-Thr-Val-Asp-Lys-Ser-Arg-Trp-Gln-Gln-
426  Gly-Asn-Val-Phe-Ser-Cys⁴³¹-Ser-Val-Met-His-Glu-Ala-Leu-His-Asn-His-Tyr-Thr-Gln-Lys-Ser-Leu-Ser-Leu-Ser-
451  Pro-Gly-Lys
```

Heavy chain

—: Disulfide bond.   *,** : Disulfide bond between the leavy chains. Asn³⁰³: N-linked glycosylation site.

The underlined parts: The complementarity-detemining regions.

Predicted Carbohydrate Structure

Structure	Abbreviation

Manα (1→6) ⟍
          Manα (1→6) ⟍
 Manα (l→3) ⟋   Manβ (1→4) GlcNAcβ (1→4) GlcNAc-
          Manα (l→3) ⟋
	Man5

Fucα (1→6)
            Manα (1→6) ⟍ |
 GlcNAcβ (1→2) {   Manβ (1→4) GlcNAcβ (1→4) GlcNAc-
            Manα (1→3) ⟋
	G-1

GlcNAcβ (1→2) Manα (1→6) ⟍ Manβ (l→4) GlcNAcβ (l→4) GlcNAc- GlcNAcβ (1→2) Manα (1→3) ⟋	G0-F
Manα (1→6) ⟍ Manα (1→6) ⟍ Manα (1→3) ⟋ Manβ (1→4) GlcNAcβ (1→4) GlcNAc- Manα (1→2) Manα (1→3) ⟋	Man 6

Fucα (1→6)
                Manα (1→6) ⟍ |
 Galβ (1→4) GlcNAcβ (1→2) {   Manβ (1→4) GlcNAcβ (1→4) GlcNAc-
                Manα (1→3) ⟋
	G1-1

Fucα (1→6) GlcNAcβ (1→2) Manα (1→6) ⟍ | Manβ (1→4) GlcNAcβ (1→4) GlcNAc- GlcNAcβ (1→2) Manα (1→3) ⟋	G0

Galβ (1→4) GlcNAcβ (1→2) Manα (1→6) ⟍   Fucα (1→6)
                               |
                         Manβ (1→4) GlcNAcβ (1→4) GlcNAc-
 GlcNAcβ (1→2) Manα (1→3) ⟋
	G1 (1-6)

Fucα (1→6) GlcNAcβ (1→2) Manα (1→6) ⟍ | Manβ (1→4) GlcNAcβ (1→4) GlcNAc- Galβ (1→4) GlcNAcβ (1→2) Manα (1→3) ⟋	G1 (1-3)

Galβ (1→4) GlcNAcβ (1→2) Manα (1→6) ⟍   Fucα (1→6)
                               |
                         Manβ (1→4) GlcNAcβ (1→4) GlcNAc-
 Galβ (1→4) GlcNAcβ (1→2) Manα (1→3) ⟋
	G2

Man: Mannose. Fuc: Fucose. Gal: Galactose. GlcNAc: N-acetylglucosamine.

Figure 4   Predicted Carbohydrate Structure of Bevacizumab[27]

Production Process[27]

❖ Production platform: CHO G7 cell line.
❖ Protein yield: NA.
❖ Protein purity: NA.

4 Pre-clinical Pharmacodynamics

Summary

Overview of *in vitro* Activities[27]

❖ Bevacizumab binded to human VEGF$_{165}$ and rabbit VEGF, the K$_d$ was 1.1 ± 0.80 nmol/L and 8.0 ± 5.1 nmol/L, respectively, but bevacizumab did not bind to mouse VEGF.

❖ A4.6.1 recognized all of VEGF$_{121}$, VEGF$_{165}$ and VEGF$_{189}$, but did not bind to PDGF, EGF, acid-FGF, NGF, and HGF.

❖ A4.6.1 inhibited human VEGF-induced proliferation of bovine adrenal cortex vascular endothelial cells.

❖ A4.61 inhibited angiogenesis of chick embryo chorioallantoic membrane induced by VEGF$_{165}$ at a ten-fold molar ratio.

❖ Both bevacizumab and A4.6.1 inhibited proliferation of bovine adrenal cortex vascular endothelial cells induced by VEGF$_{165}$, with an IC$_{50}$ was 50 and 48 ng/mL, respectively.

❖ Both bevacizumab and A4.6.1 inhibited proliferation of umbilical vein endothelial cells induced by VEGF$_{165}$, with an IC$_{50}$ was 0.89 and 0.61 nmol/L, respectively.

❖ Bevacizumab inhibited proliferation of human umbilical vein endothelial cells induced by human VEGF$_{165}$, VEGF$_{121}$ and VEGF$_{110}$, with an IC$_{50}$ was 60, 86 and 32 ng/mL.

Overview of *in vivo* Activities[27]

❖ VEGF-induced vascular permeability in guinea pigs:
  • A4.6.1 inhibited subcutaneous permeability completely by a ten-fold molar ratio.

❖ Human rhabdomyosarcoma A673 cells xenograft nude mice model:
  • Tumor weights were reduced by 90.0% and 95.0% by bevacizumab 0.5 and 5 mg/kg, respectively, compared to the control group.
  • Tumor weights were reduced by 85.0% and 93.0% by A4.6.1 0.5 and 5 mg/kg, respectively, compared to the control group.

❖ Human rhabdomyosarcoma A673 cells xenograft nude mice model:
  • A4.6.1 inhibited tumor growth at doses $\geqslant$10 μg/mouse.
  • Tumor weights were reduced by 96.0% by A4.6.1 100 μg compared to the control group.
  • Vascular density in the tumor tissue was reduced by A4.6.1 compared to the control group.

❖ Human glioblastoma multiforme G55 cells xenograft nude mice model:
  • A4.6.1 inhibited tumor growth at doses $\geqslant$10 μg/mouse.
  • Tumor weights were reduced by 80.0% by A4.6.1 100 μg compared to the control group.

❖ Human leiomyosarcoma SK-LMS-1 cells xenograft nude mice model:
  • Tumor weights were reduced by 70.0% by A4.6.1 100 μg compared to the control group.

❖ Human rhabdomyosarcoma A673 cells xenograft nude mice model:
  • Anti-tumor growth activity was similar between A4.6.1 2.5 mg/kg and 5 mg/kg.
  • The mean plasma concentration of A4.6.1 in the 2.5 mg/kg group was 30.6 μg/mL.

Overview of *in vitro* Activities

Cell-based Activities *in vitro*

Table 5　*In vitro* Activities of Anti-VEGF mAb[21]

Experimental System	Treatment	Concentration	Model Induction	Efficacy
Bovine adrenal cortex-derived capillary endothelial cells	A4.6.1	NA	NA	48 ± 8 ng/mL.
	rhuMab VEGF			50 ± 5 ng/mL.
HUVEC	Bevacizumab	3.9-1,000 ng/mL	rhVEGF$_{165}$, rhVEGF$_{121}$, rhVEGF$_{110}$ 10 ng/mL	Proliferation induced by all splice variants of VEGF was dose-dependently inhibited by bevacizumab, with IC$_{50}$s in the range of 32-86 ng/mL.
HUVEC	Bevacizumab	500 ng/mL	VEGF$_{165}$ 50 ng/mL	Bevacizumab abolished VEGF-induced nitric-coxide production.
HUVEC	Bevacizumab	Bevacizumab:VEGF = 10:1		Bevacizumab abolished VEGF-induced permeability in HUVEC.
HUVEC	Bevacizumab	500 ng/mL	VEGF$_{165}$ 50 ng/mL	Bevacizumab abolished the cell survival activity.

HUVEC: Human umbilical vein endothelial cells.　NA: Not available.　VEGF: Vascular endothelial growth factor.

Overview of *in vivo* Activities

Table 6   Anti-tumor Efficacy of Bevacizumab in Xenograft Mouse Models[27, 31-35]

Xenograft Model				Drug	Dose (mg/kg)	Route & Schedule	Effect	
Cell Line	Type	Implant Method	Animal				ED[a] (µg/injection/ mouse)	Finding
LS174T	Human colon adenocarcinoma	s.c.	Athymic nu/nu mice	A4.6.1	100 µg/injection/ mouse	i.p. & alternate days	100	Inhibited tumor growth, TGD is 12 days; decreased microvessel density by 36.0%; induction of neoplastic cell apoptosis; reduced IFP.
				Combined with radiation	20 Gy (Normal blood flow); 30 Gy (Normal blood flow); 30 Gy (Hypoxic); 40 Gy (Hypoxic)	i.p. & alternate days	100	In comparison with radiation alone, the combination increased the TGD.
U87	Human glioblastoma multiforme	s.c.	Athymic nu/nu mice	A4.6.1	100 µg/injection/ mouse	i.p. & alternate days	100	Inhibited tumor growth, TGD is 22 days; decreased microvessel density by 60.0%; induction of neoplastic cell apoptosis; reduced IFP; increased the median pO$_2$.
				Combined with radiation	20 Gy (Normal blood flow); 30 Gy (Normal blood flow); 30 Gy (Hypoxic); 40 Gy (Hypoxic)	i.p. & alternate days	100	In comparison with radiation alone, the combination increased the TGD.
A673	Human rhabdomyosarcoma cell line	Dorsal skin-fold chamber	Beige nude/ xid mice	A4.6.1	200 µg/injection/ mouse	i.p. & twice weekly	200	Suppressed the tumor growth; inhibited neovascularization of microtumors.
A673	Human rhabdomyosarcoma cell line	s.c.	Beige nude mice	A4.6.1	0.05, 0.1, 0.25, 0.5, 1.0, 2.5, 5.0	i.p. & twice weekly for a total of 8 doses	2.5 mg/kg	Anti-tumor growth activity was similar between A4.6.1 2.5 and 5 mg/kg. The mean plasma concentration of A4.6.1 in the 2.5 mg/kg group was 30.6 µg/mL.
				Anti-gp120 antibody	5.0			
A673	Human rhabdomyosarcoma cell line	s.c.	BALB/c nude mice	A4.6.1	0.5, 5	i.p. & twice weekly for a total of 8 doses	0.5 mg/kg	Tumor growth was suppressed markedly; the decrease in tumor weight were 85.0% and 93.0%, respectively at each dose.
				rhuMAb	0.5, 5			Tumor growth was suppressed markedly; the decrease in tumor weight were 90.0% and 95.0%, respectively at each dose.
				Control murine Mab	5			
A673	Human rhabdomyosarcoma cell line	s.c.	Beige nude/ xid mice	A4.6.1	10, 50, 100, 200, 400 µg/injection/ mouse	i.p. & twice weekly for a total of 8 doses	10	Tumor growth was suppressed markedly; the decrease in tumor weight was 96.0% at 100 µg/mouse.
G55	Human glioblastoma multiforme	s.c.	Beige nude/ xid mice	A4.6.1	10, 50, 100, 200, 400 µg/injection/ mouse	i.p. & twice weekly for a total of 8 doses	10	Tumor growth was suppressed markedly; the decrease in tumor weight was 80.0% at 100 µg/mouse.
SK-LM S-1		s.c.	Beige nude/ xid mice	A4.6.1	10, 50, 100, 200, 400 µg/injection/ mouse	i.p. & twice weekly for a total of 8 doses	100	Tumor growth was suppressed; the decrease in tumor weight was 70.0% at 100 µg/mouse.
SKOV-3	Human ovarian carcinoma cell line	s.c. / i.p.	Balb/c nude mice	A4.6.1	100 µg/injection/ mouse	i.p. & twice weekly for a total of 8 doses	100	Tumor growth was inhibited. Ascites production was inhibited completely; tumor growth was inhibited partially.

Continued

Xenograft Model				Drug	Dose (mg/kg)	Route & Schedule	Effect	
Cell Line	Type	Implant Method	Animal				ED[a] (μg/injection/ mouse)	Finding
LS LiM6	s.c.		Balb/c ncr-nu athymic mice	A4.6.1	10, 50, 100, 200 μg/mouse	i.p. & twice weekly for 3 weeks	10 μg/ mouse	Significant reduction of tumor weight.
HM7	s.c.		Balb/c ncr-nu athymic mice	A4.6.1	10, 50, 100, 200 μg/mouse	i.p. & twice weekly for 2 weeks	10 μg/ mouse	Significant reduction of tumor weight.
HM7		Splenic injection	Balb/c ncr-nu athymic mice	A4.6.1	100 μg/mouse	i.p. & twice weekly for 4 weeks	100 μg/ mouse	Dramatic reduction in the number and size of liver metastases and liver weights, as well as tumor volume per liver.

IFP: Interstitial fluid pressure.   i.p.: Intraperitoneal.   s.c.: Subcutaneous.   TGD: Tumor growth delay.

Table 7   Efficacy of Combination of Anti-VEGF mAb with Chemotherapies in Xenografted Mouse Models[36-40]

Xenograft Model			Drug	Dose (mg/kg)	Route & Schedule	Effect
Cell Line	Implant Method	Animal				
OVCAR3	i.p.	Female athymic nude mice	rhuVEGF mAb	5	i.p. & twice weekly for 6 weeks	Tumor burden in rhuVEGF mAb plus paclitaxel and paclitaxel alone group was reduced 58.5% and 59.5%, respectively. No ascites developed in the combined treatment group or the group treated with VEGF mAb alone. Paclitaxel alone reduced ascites slightly, but not significantly.
			Paclitaxel	20	i.p. & three times weekly for 6 weeks	
MCF-7	Matrigel s.c.	Nude mice	rhuMAb-VEGF	0.25	i.p. & Days 7, 10 or i.p. & Days 7-14 (alone)	Combination of rhuMAb-VEGF and docetacel inhibited angiogenesis effectively, rhuMAb-VEGF overcomed the resistance to docetaxel induced by VEGF.
			Docetaxel	3	i.p. & Days 7, 10	
MCF-7 ZR-75 SK-BR-3	Dorsal skinfold chamber, s.c.	Nude mice	A4.6.1	200 μg/mouse	i.p. & twice weekly for 2 weeks	Significant suppression of angiogenic activity and reduced extensive vascular network was observed.
MCF-7	Dorsal skinfold chamber, s.c.	Nude mice	A4.6.1	200 μg/mouse	i.p. & twice weekly for 2 weeks	Angiogenesis was inhibited and tumor nodules were reduced in A4.6.1 treatment group. Tumor growth was inhibited in doxorubicin treatment group, but without suppression of angiogenesis. In the combination group, angiogenesis was inhibited and tumor was shrinked, and sometimes without viable tumor cells in the tumor, doxorubicin enhanced the anti-angiogenic effect of A4.6.1.
			Doxorubicin	5	i.v. & weekly	
SK-NEP-1	Kidney inoculum	NCR nude mice	A4.6.1	100 μg/dose	i.p. & 2 days per week for 5 weeks	Tumor angiogenesis, tumor weight and tumor lung metastases were inhibited, the effects was stronger in the combination group than the other two treatment groups. Rebound tumor growth was inhibited more significantly in combination group after treatment termination than the other two treatment groups.
			Topotecan	0.36	i.p. & 5 days per week for 2 weeks, followed by a rest week, 2 cycles	
NGP[a]	Kidney inoculum	Female NCR athymic mice	A4.6.1	100 μg/dose	i.p. & twice a week for 5 weeks	Topotecan either with or without anti-VEGF antibody significantly suppresses neuroblastoma xenograft growth in comparison with controls or anti-VEGF antibody alone. Combining topotecan with anti-VEGF antibody significantly inhibited rebound tumor growth in comparison with anti-VEGF antibody alone. Combination therapy may improve durability of antiangiogenic inhibition of neuroblastoma.
			Topotecan	0.36	i.p. & 5 times a week for 5 weeks	

i.p.: Intraperitoneal.   s.c: Subcutaneous.   VEGF: Vascular endothelial growth factor.   [a] NGP: Human neuroblastoma cell line.

5 Toxicology

Summary

Non-clinical Single-Dose Toxicology[21]

❖ Not performed.

Non-clinical Repeated-Dose Toxicology[21]

❖ The 4-week toxicity study in young monkeys treated with vehicle or bevacizumab 2, 10 or 50 mg/kg twice weekly:
  • Physeal dysplasia of the distal femur in the male of 10 and 50 mg/kg group were noted, the physeal dysplasia was slight to moderate at 10 mg/kg and moderate to severe at 50 mg/kg.
  • Physeal dysplasia was present in both males following 4-week recovery, being slight in one animal and severe in the other.
  • Antibodies to bevacizumab were not detected in any animal at any time point.

❖ The 13-week toxicity study in young monkeys treated with vehicle or bevacizumab 2, 10 or 50 mg/kg twice weekly:
  • Ovarian and uterine weights were reduced in females at 10 or 50 mg/kg, coincided with a reduced number or absence of corpora lutea. The effect was partially reversible upon treatment cessation.
  • A dose-dependent increased incidence and severity of physeal dysplasia was noted, and in males it was seen at all dose levels and regarded as moderately severe at 10 and 50 mg/kg, in females it was minimal to slight at 10 or 50 mg/kg.
  • Antibodies to bevacizumab were not detected in any animal at any time point.

❖ The 26-week toxicity study in adult monkeys treated with vehicle or bevacizumab 2, 10 or 50 mg/kg once weekly or twice weekly at 10 mg/kg:
  • Mildly lower albumin and albumin-to-globulin ratio and moderately higher globulin were seen in males at 10 mg/kg (twice weekly) and 50 mg/kg.
  • Body weights, weight gain and food consumption were reduced for males in 10 mg/kg (twice weekly) and 50 mg/kg group.
  • In females, a dose of 10 mg/kg or higher reduced endometrial proliferation, produced lower uterine weights and decreased the incidence of menstrual cycles.
  • At 50 mg/kg and 10 mg/kg (twice weekly), follicular maturation was inhibited at the early Graafian follicle stage in ovaries.
  • Corpora lutea were absent at 10 mg/kg (twice weekly) and at 50 mg/kg.
  • Dose-dependent increase in the incidence and severity of physeal dysplasia was noted in both genders.
  • The toxic effects were reversible or partial reversible following recovery.
  • Only one 50 mg/kg animal at Day 183 were found anti-drug antibody (ADA) positive.

❖ The toxicity study in rabbits treated with vehicle or bevacizumab 50 mg/kg over a 10-day period:
  • Bevacizumab exposure inhibited the function of the corpus luteum at a dose of 50 mg/kg given every 2 days in the rabbit.

❖ The toxicity study in female rabbits treated with vehicle or bevacizumab 2, 10 or 50 mg/kg over a 9-day period:
  • Rabbits given 50 mg/kg of bevacizumab plus hCG had fewer corpora lutea than vehicle-treated animals.

❖ The toxicity study in monkeys treated with bevacizumab in combination with chemotherapeutic regimens (Irinotecan + 5-fluorouracil leucovorin (IFL), or cisplatin + paclitaxel):
  • The co-administration of bevacizumab with IFL did not alter the magnitude of the effects related to treatment with the antineoplastic therapy regimen.

Safety Pharmacology[21]

❖ Not performed.

Genotoxicity study[21]

❖ Not performed.

Carcinogenicity[21]

❖ Not performed.

Reproductive Toxicity[21]

❖ Presumed pregnant NZW rabbits treated i.v. with vehicle or bevacizumab at dose levels of 10, 30 or 100 mg/kg on GDs 6, 9, 12, 15 and 18:
  • A dose-related significant decrease in maternal body weight gain and significant mean body weight loss were observed in the two higher dose groups.
  • Foetal body weights were significantly reduced in all treatment groups.
  • The number of late resorptions was increased in the 100 mg/kg dose group.
  • Dose-related increase in foetal malformations was observed.

- In addition, the number of ossification sites per foetus per litter for metacarpals was reduced or significantly reduced in all treatment groups.
- The maternal NOAEL was 10 mg/kg.
- The foetal NOAEL was less than 10 mg/kg.
- Antibody titers to bevacizumab were detected in maternal serum of 9/73 (12.0%), foetal serum of 9/71 (13.0%), and amniotic fluid from 7/73 (10.0%) of pregnant treated with bevacizumab on GD 29.
- Following the administration of a single-dose or multiple-dose on GDs 6, 9, 12, 15, and 18 of bevacizumab, concentrations in maternal serum and amniotic fluid increased linearly with dose, while concentrations in foetal serum increased less than proportionally.

Other Toxicology[21]

- ❖ Bevacizumab did not cause hemolysis of Cynomolgus monkey or human erythrocytes and was compatible with Cynomolgus monkey and human serum and plasma.
- ❖ No cross-reactivity between bevacizumab and different tissues from rabbit, Cynomolgus monkey, or human was observed with an immunohistochemical method.
- ❖ Bevacizumab interfered with wound healing in the rabbit.
- ❖ Bevacizumab could induce thrombus in rabbit, but no changes in haematology or coagulation parameters were noted.

Anti-product Antibody Profile[21]

- ❖ In rabbits, anti-bevacizumab antibodies could be easily induced.
- ❖ In monkeys, the immunogenicity of bevacizumab was very weak.

Non-clinical Multiple-Dose Toxicology

Table 8   Repeated-Dose Toxicity Studies of Bevacizumab[27]

Species	Duration (Week)	Dose (mg/kg)	NOEL (mg/kg)	Finding
Cynomolgus monkey	4	Male & female: 2, 10 or 50, i.v. twice weekly	<2	Epiphyseal dysplasia of the distal femur was noted in males treated with 10 or 50 mg/kg, the severity of epiphyseal dysplasia was slight to moderate in males treated with 10 mg/kg and moderate to severe in males treated with 50 mg/kg. Epiphyseal abnormalities were not observed in females at any dose level.
	13	Male & female: 2, 10 or 50, i.v. twice weekly	<2	Ovarian and uterine weights were reduced in females in 10 and 50 mg/kg groups, which coincided with a reduction in number or an absence of corpora lutea. The severity and incidence of epiphyseal dysplasia were dose-dependent and an additional finding of linear fissuring of the cartilaginous growth plate was occasionally observed. Epiphyseal dysplasia was noted in all males treated with bevacizumab and the severity was minimal to severe in 2 mg/kg group and slight to severe in 10 and 50 mg/kg groups. Minimal to slight epiphyseal dysplasia was present in all females in 10 and 50 mg/kg group, but none in 2 mg/kg group.
	26	Male & female: 2, 10 or 50, i.v. once weekly	<2	Significantly decreased body weight and food consumption were observed in 50 mg/kg group. Slightly decreased body weight was found in 2 and 10 mg/kg groups. Abnormal menstrual cycles (decreased number of menstrual cycles) and lower uterine weight and reduced endometrial proliferation were observed in females at ≥10 mg/kg. In addition, treatment with 50 mg/kg inhibited follicular maturation at the early Graafian follicle stage and resulted in an absence of corpora lutea. The severity and incidence of epiphyseal dysplasia were increased dose-dependently and additionally, linear fissuring was noted in 1 male in 50 mg/kg group. Epiphyseal dysplasia was not present following the 12-week recovery period.

Continued

Species	Duration (Week)	Dose (mg/kg)	NOEL (mg/kg)	Finding
	26	Male & female: 10, i.v. twice weekly	<2	Decreased body weight and food consumption in males were observed, that could be recovered. Abnormal menstrual cycles (decreased number of menstrual cycles), lower uterine weight, reduced endometrial proliferation, inhibited follicular maturation at the early Graafian follicle stage and absence of corpora lutea were observed. Moderate epiphyseal dysplasia was found and linear fissuring was noted in 1 male. Epiphyseal dysplasia was not present following the 12-week recovery period.
Cynomolgus monkey	2	Bevacizumab 10 mg/kg on Days 1 and 8, i.v.; Irinotecan hydrochloride 100 or 125 mg/m², 5-FU 500 mg/m², and LV 20 mg/m² on Days 1 and 8, i.v.	NA	No death occurred in any group. Co-administration of bevacizumab did not enhance the toxic effects of IFL.
	3	Bevacizumab 10 mg/kg on Days 1, 4, 8, 11, 15 and 18, i.v.; Cisplain (CDDP) 1 mg/kg and PTX 4 mg/kg on Day 18, i.v.	NA	No death occurred in any group. In the CDDP/PTX group and the CDDP/PTX + bevacizumab group, vomiting occurred and decreased body weight and transient decreases in white blood cell and neutrophil counts compared to the control group were also noted. The alterations observed in the CDDP/PTX + bevacizumab group were similar to those in the CDDP/PTX group and the coadministration of bevacizumab did not enhance the toxic effects.

CDDP: cis-Diaminedichloroplatinum.   IFL: Irinotecan + 5-fluorouracil leucovorin.   i.v.: Intravenous.   NA: Not available.   PTX: Paclitaxel.

Reproductive Toxicology

Table 9   Reproductive and Developmental Toxicology Studies of Bevacizumab[27]

Study	Species	Dose [mg/(kg·dose)]	Route & Schedule	Finding
Fertility	Rabbits (female)	10 or 100	i.v., gestation on Day 18	Maternal serum bevacizumab concentrations were increased in a dose-proportional manner. The mean of fetal serum bevacizumab concentrations between the doses was about 3.
		10, 30, 100	i.v., gestation on Days 6, 9, 12, 15, 18	Bevacizumab concentrations in maternal serum and amniotic fluid were largely dose-proportional. The ratio of fetal serum bevacizumab concentrations between the doses was less than the ratio of the doses.

Other Toxicology

Table 10   Special Toxicology Studies of Bevacizumab[27]

Special Toxicology	Species	Bevacizumab	Dose/Concentration (mg/kg)	Finding
Hemolysis and compatibility	Human or monkey whole blood and serum and plasma	Solution	5 mg/mL	No hemolysis.
Tissue specificity	9 normal rabbit tissues, 30 normal Cynomolgus monkey tissues, and 36 normal human tissues	Solution	10-400 µg/mL	No cross-reactivity.
Wound healing	Rabbit	Solution	0.5, 1 or 2 on Days -2, 1, 3, i.v.	Wound healing was interfered.
Wound healing	Rabbit	Solution	50, every other day for 2 weeks, i.v.	Delayed in wound healing.

Continued

Special Toxicology	Species	Bevacizumab	Dose/Concentration (mg/kg)	Finding
Wound healing	Rabbit	Solution	2 or 10 on Days 1, 4, 8, 11, i.v.	Delayed in wound healing.
Wound healing	Cynomolgus monkey	Solution	0.5, 2 on Days -2, 1, 3, 5, i.v.	Delayed in wound healing, but the results were extremely variable.
Thrombosis	Rabbits	Solution	75, i.v., daily for 8 days	No marked changes in hematology and coagulation.
Kidney deposition	NZW rabbits	Solution	2, 10 or 100 on Days 1, 3, i.v.	No deposition.
Renal function	NZW rabbits (CDDP-induced model)	Solution	50 on Days 8, 10, 12, i.v.	No effect was observed.
Renal function	NZW rabbits (BSA-induced model)	Solution	50, i.v., every other day during Week 8 for 4 doses total	No renal disorder was caused by bevacizumab.
Epiphyseal dysplasia	Rabbits	Solution	10, 50, or 75 on Days 1, 4, 7, 10, i.v.	Bevacizumab could lead to a slight thicking of the growth plate cartilage, but did not inhibit vascular invasion or induce subchondral bony plate formation.
Ovarian function	Rabbits	Solution	50 on Days -3, 1, 4, 7, i.v.	Ovarian function was inhibited.
Ovarian function	Rabbits	Solution	2, 10 or 50 on Days -4, 1, 5, i.v.	Ovarian function was inhibited dose-dependently.

BSA: Bovine serum albumin.   CDDP: cis-Diaminedichloroplatinum.   i.v.: Intravenous.

Anti-product Antibody Profile

Table 11   Special Toxicology Studies of Bevacizumab[27]

Special Toxicology	Species	Treatment	Dose (mg/kg)	Finding
Immunogenicity	Cynomolgus monkey	Bevacizumab	Male & female: 2, 10 or 50, twice weekly for 4 weeks	No ADA detected.
			Male & female: 2, 10 or 50, twice weekly for 13 weeks	No ADA detected.
			Male & female: 2, 10 or 50, once weekly for 26 weeks	ADA was positive for 1 animal of the 50 mg/kg group on Day 183.
			Male & female: 10, twice weekly for 26 weeks	No ADA detected.

ADA: Anti-drug antibody.

6   Non-clinical Pharmacokinetic/ADME/Toxicokinetics

Summary

Non-clinical Pharmacokinetics[21]

❖ Absorption-bioavailability
  • Absorption of bevacizumab subsequent to a single intraperitoneal (i.p.) or subcutaneous (s.c.) administration has been examined in mouse, rat, and Cynomolgus monkey.
    ♦ Absorption subsequent to i.p. administration was complete in mouse.
    ♦ s.c. administration resulted in a slower absorption that was complete in mouse (>100%) and Cynomolgus monkey (98.0%), but with a bioavailability of 69.0% in rat.
  • Following i.v. administration of bevacizumab to mice, rats, rabbits, and Cynomolgus monkeys:

- Bevacizumab concentrations decreased with an initial half-life ($t_{1/2\alpha}$) of approximately 1 day followed by a slower phase, with a terminal half-life ($t_{1/2\beta}$) that was between approximately 1 and 2 weeks.
- Nonlinear PK parameters were observed in mice, rats, and rabbits following administration of doses of <1 mg/kg.
- Bevacizumab clearance (CL) was slower following administration of higher doses, the difference was reflected in increased half-time.
- In Cynomolgus monkeys, bevacizumab PK was linear over the range of 2-50 mg/kg. The mean CL was approximately 6 mL/(kg·day), and the $t_{1/2\alpha}$ and $t_{1/2\beta}$ were ≤1 and 10 days, respectively.

❖ Distribution
- Tissue distribution of ^{125}I-labeled bevacizumab was examined in male rabbit following i.v. bolus administration.
  - Trichloracetic acid (TCA)-precipitable radioactivity was localized primarily in plasma (approximately 0-fold higher than in tissues). Radioactivity decreased by nearly 2.5-fold between 2 and 48 hours.
  - The organs that exhibited the highest levels of radioactivity per gram of tissue were, in decreasing order, kidney > testis > spleen > heart > lung > thymus (ranging from 0.069%-0.018% TCA-precipitable dose/g of tissue).
- Bevacizumab was shown to distribute into foetal serum and into the amniotic fluid in two reproduction toxicity studies conducted in rabbit.

❖ Metabolism (*in vitro/in vivo*)
- In the distribution study in rabbit, minimal degradation was noted for as long as 48 hours after ^{125}I-labeled bevacizumab administration.
- The degradation pattern appeared to vary from tissue to tissue.

❖ Excretion
- In the distribution study in rabbit, less than 10.0% of the radioactivity in the urine at 2 and 48 hours post-dose was TCA-precipitable.

❖ Drug-Drug interaction
- The safety and PK of the combination of IFL (irinotecan/5-FU/FA), with or without bevacizumab, were investigated in Cynomolgus monkeys.
  - The PK parameters of irinotecan and 5-FU disposition were unchanged by the concomitant administration of bevacizumab.

Non-clinical Pharmacokinetics

Table 12   *In vivo* Pharmacokinetic Parameters of Bevacizumab in Mice, Rats and Cynomolgus Monkeys after Single Administration[41]

Species	Route	Dose (mg/kg)	T_{max} (min)	C_{max} (μg/mL)	AUC_{0-t} (μg·day/mL)	AUC_{0-inf} (μg·day/mL)	$t_{1/2}$ (Day)	CL or CL/F [mL/(day·kg)]	V_c (mL/kg)	MRT (Day)
Mice (female)	i.v.	9.3	5	174	442	593	6.8	15.7	53.0	9.7
	s.c.	9.3	32 h	74.1	539	682	6.1	13.6	119	8.7
Rats (male)	i.v.	0.66	15	29.7 ± 1.8	69.0 ± 12.0	80.9 ± 14.0	5.4 ± 0.82	8.4 ± 1.4	25.0 ± 0.90	7.1 ± 0.99
	i.v.	10.1	5	341 ± 39.0	1,240 ± 130	2,160 ± 500	12.3 ± 3.2	4.8 ± 1.1	30.8 ± 2.7	17.1 ± 4.7
	s.c.	10.1	7 d	147 ± 13.0	1,260 ± 200	1,480 ± 240	3.0 ± 0.17	7.0 ± 1.1	30.5 ± 5.1	4.4 ± 0.24
Cynomolgus monkeys (female)	i.v.	2.0	18	68.0 ± 6.2	369 ± 68.0	430 ± 72.0	9.9 ± 1.9	4.8 ± 0.88	30.1 ± 2.0	13.4 ± 2.2
	i.v.	10.0	33	290 ± 29.0	1,620 ± 160	1,810 ± 140	8.8 ± 0.84	5.6 ± 0.46	36.3 ± 2.4	12.0 ± 1.0
	i.v.	50.0	5	400 ± 210	7,760 ± 790	8,800 ± 1,400	10.3 ± 3.1	5.8 ± 0.84	36.8 ± 4.9	13.1 ± 3.5
	s.c.	10.0	3 d	120 ± 3.0	1,520 ± 210	1,770 ± 260	9.4 ± 0.46	5.7 ± 0.85	77.6 ± 11.0	13.5 ± 0.66

i.v.: Intravenous.   s.c: Subcutaneous.

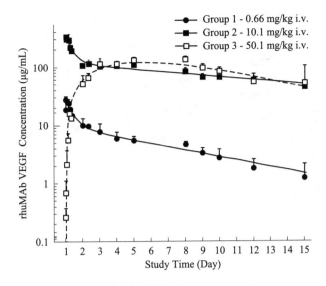

Figure 5　Serum Concentrations vs. Time Profiles of Bevacizumab in Rats after Single Administration[41]

Table 13　*In vivo* Pharmacokinetic Parameters of Bevacizumab after Multiple-Doses in Monkeys[27]

Species	Schedule	Dose [mg/(kg·dose)]	$t_{1/2}$ (Day)	AUC$_{0-inf}$ (µg·day/mL)	MRT (Day)	CL [mL/(h·kg)]	V$_{ss}$ (mL/kg)
Rabbit	i.v., Days 1, 4, 8, 11	10	5.5			8.1	39.9
Cynomolgus monkey	i.v., twice weekly for 4 weeks	2					
		10					
		50	9.9 ± 1.2	9,900 ± 760	13.6 ± 1.6	5.1 ± 0.40	68.4 ± 5.5
Cynomolgus monkey	i.v., twice weekly for 13 weeks	2					
		10					
		50	11.4 ± 3.8	8,070 ± 860	13.6 ± 1.4	6.3 ± 0.71	84.3 ± 2.5
Cynomolgus monkey	i.v., once weekly for 26 weeks	2					
		10					
		50	20.4 ± 8.7	13,000 ± 2,600	16.5 ± 2.6	4.0 ± 0.81	64.7 ± 9.6

i.v.: Intravenous.

Table 14　*In vivo* Tissue Distribution of Bevacizumab in Rabbits[27]

Species	Dose (µg/kg)	Route	Finding
Rabbit	4.8~5.2	i.v.	Total radioactivity in all tissues was similar to TCA-precipitable radioactivity at both 2 and 48 hours post-dose. Total radioactivity was localized primarily in plasma at 2 and 48 hours post-dose. The organs that exhibited the highest levels of TCA-precipitable radioactivity were: kidney > testis > spleen > heart > lung > thymus. The pattern of tissue distribution between bevacizumab and the control IgG1 antibody was similar.

i.v.: Intravenous.　TCA: Trichloracetic acid.

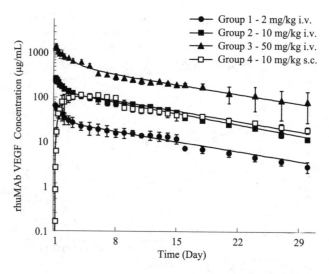

Figure 6   Serum Concentrations vs. Time Profiles of Bevacizumab in Cynomolgus Monkeys after Single Administration[41]

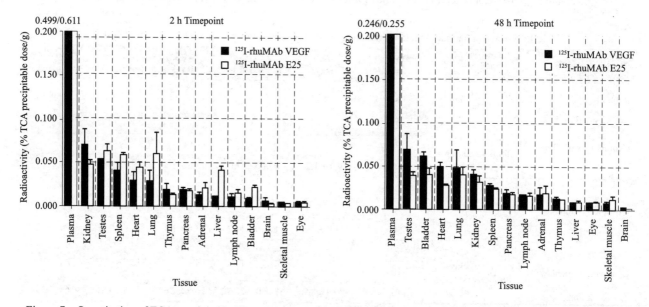

Figure 7   Quantitation of TCA-precipitable Tissue Radioactivity of ^{125}I-rhuMAb VEGF and ^{125}I-rhuMAb E25 at 2 h and 48 h[41]

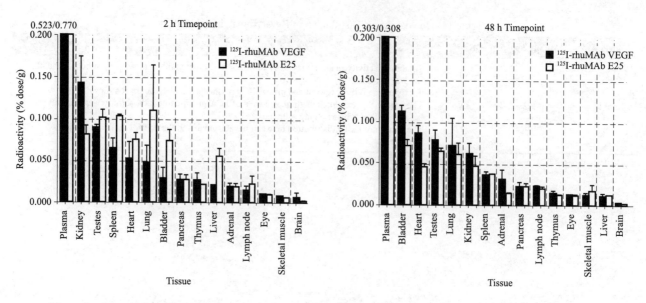

Figure 8   Quantitation of Total Tissue Radioactivity of ^{125}I-rhuMAb VEGF and ^{125}I-rhuMAb E25 at 2 h and 48 h[41]

Table 15　Metabolism/Excretion Profiles of ^{125}I-Bevacizumab in Rabbits after Single-Dose[27]

Species	Dose (µg/kg)	Route	Finding
Rabbit	4.8-5.2	i.v.	Intact ^{125}I-labeled bevacizumab was predominantly detected in plasma at 48 h post-dose with very weak bands for degradation products. Small amounts of low molecular weight degradation products were detected in the tissues of the kidney, testis, spleen, heart, and lung, the degradation pattern varied from tissue to tissue. TCA-precipitable radioactivity in urine represented only 6.0%-9.0% at 2 and 48 h post-dose, unchanged bevacizumab was not detected in the urine at 48 h post-dose. Similar results were obtained for the control IgG1 antibody, omalizumab.

i.v.: Intravenous.

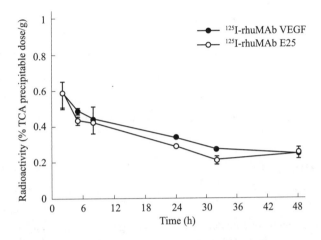

Figure 9　Plasma Concentrations vs. Time Profiles of ^{125}I-rhuMAb VEGF and ^{125}I-rhuMAb E25[41]

Table 16　*In vivo* Pharmacokinetic Parameters of Bevacizumab in Cynomolgus Monkeys after Single or Combination Dose[27]

Bevacizumab (mg/kg)	Route & Schedule	Combination Drug (mg/kg)	Route & Schedule	Result
10	i.v. & Days 1, 4, 8, 11, 15, 18	Cisplatin 1	i.v. & Day 18	Multiple-dose of bevacizumab had no effects on the PK of either CDDP or PTX.
		Paclitaxel 4	i.v. & Day 18	Concurrent CDDP/PTX had no effects on the PK of bevacizumab.
10	i.v. & Days 1, 8	Irinotecan hydrochloride 125 mg/m²	i.v. & Days 1, 8	The PK of irinotecan or 5-FU is not altered by concurrent bevacizumab.
		5-FU 500 mg/m²	i.v. & Days 1, 8	
		LV 20 mg/m²	i.v. & Days 1, 8	

5-FU: 5-fluorouracil.　CDDP: cis-Diaminedichloroplatinum.　i.v.: Intravenous.　LV: Leucovorin.　PK: Pharmacokinetic.　PTX: Paclitaxel.

Table 17　rhuMAb VEGF Pharmacokinetic Parameters[41]

Parameter	Group 2-rhuMAb VEGF	Group 4-rhuMAb VEGF + Cisplatin + Taxol®
T_{max} (median, min)	30.0	30.0
C_{max} (µg/mL)	676 ± 100	744 ± 120
V_c/W (mL/kg)	46.1 ± 10.0	37.1 ± 15.0
V_{ss}/W (mL/kg)	78.0 ± 8.4	72.5 ± 7.0
CL/W [mL/(day·kg)]	4.6 ± 1.3	4.0 ± 0.76
$t_{1/2}\alpha 1$ (h)	28.6 ± 34.0	23.2 ± 14.0
$t_{1/2}\alpha 2$ (Day)	13.5 ± 5.1	14.5 ± 2.7
MRT (Day)	18.0 ± 6.0	18.5 ± 2.7
AUC (µg·day/mL)	2,330 ± 740	2,580 ± 510
AUC1 (%)	7.4 ± 8.0	11.8 ± 9.0
AUC2 (%)	92.6 ± 8.0	88.2 ± 9.0

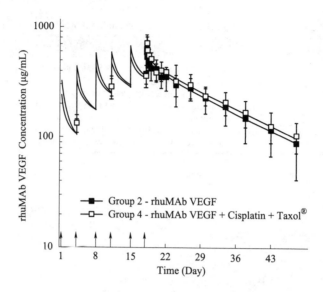

Figure 10   rhuMAb VEGF Serum Concentrations after Multiple Administration[41]

7   Clinical Efficacy and Safety

Overview Profile

❖ Avastin® (Bevacizumab) is a recombinant humanized monoclonal IgG1 antibody which in combination with intravenous 5-fluorouracil-based chemotherapy, is indicated for first- or second-line treatment of patients with metastatic carcinoma of the colon or rectum.   On Feb 26, 2004, FDA approved Avastin® for treatment for metastatic colorectal cancer.

❖ On Oct 11, 2006, FDA approves Avastin® in combination with chemotherapy for first-line treatment of most common type of lung cancer.

❖ On Feb 25, 2008, FDA grants accelerated approval of Avastin® in combination with paclitaxel chemotherapy for first-line treatment of advanced HER2-negative breast cancer.

❖ On May 6, 2009, FDA grants accelerated approval of Avastin® for brain cancer (Glioblastoma) that has progressed following prior therapy.

❖ On Aug 3, 2009, FDA approves Avastin® for the most common type of kidney cancer.

❖ On Nov 18, 2011, FDA revokes breast cancer indication for Avastin® (bevacizumab).

❖ On Aug 14, 2014, FDA approves Avastin® for metastatic cervical cancer.

❖ On Nov 14, 2014, FDA approves Avastin® plus chemotherapy for platinum-resistant recurrent ovarian cancer.

❖ On Dec 6, 2016, FDA approves Avastin® plus chemotherapy for a specific type of advanced ovarian cancer.

Indications 1: Metastatic Colorectal Cancer (mCRC)

Clinical Efficacy

❖ Study AVF2107g: The primary evidence for the efficacy of bevacizumab in the first-line treatment of patients with advanced or recurrent colorectal cancer who are not candidates for curative resection, for filing a NDA for bevacizumab in the US and EU.

❖ Study 16966: The results of this study has demonstrated the add-on effect of bevacizumab in combination with chemotherapy (FOLFOX4 or XELOX), as measured by progression-free survival (PFS), in the first-line treatment of patients with advanced or recurrent colorectal cancer who are not candidates for curative resection.

❖ The efficacy and safety of second-line or subsequent treatment with bevacizumab alone and in combination with FOLFOX4 was evaluated in Study E3200 conducted at 220 centers overseas by the Eastern Cooperative Oncology Group (ECOG) in patients with previously treated (a fluoropyrimidine and an irinotecan hydrochloride-based regimen used either alone or in combination), advanced or metastatic colorectal cancer.

❖ Efficacy data are derived from E4599, a single, multicenter, randomized, open-label, active-controlled trial that enrolled 878 patients receiving initial systemic treatment for unresectable (recurrent, metastatic or locally advanced) non-squamous, non-small cell lung cancer.   Patients were randomized 1:1 to an acceptable, standard chemotherapy regimen (paclitaxel and carboplatin for 6 cycles) or to the same chemotherapy regimen with the addition of bevacizumab at a dose of 15 mg/kg every three weeks.   Bevacizumab was administered until disease progression.

❖ Adverse events (AEs): Adverse events uniquely associated with bevacizumab include gastrointestinal perforation, delayed healing of wound, haemorrhage, thromboembolism, hypertension, reversible posterior leukoencephalopathy syndrome (RPLS), proteinuria, cardiotoxicity (congestive heart failure), and infusion reactions.

Table 18 Summary of Individual Clinical Studies and the Major Efficacy Results[27]

Region	Study No.	Phase	Study Design	Study Population	Dosage Regimen (mg/kg)	No. of Cases	Major Endpoint	Major Result
Overseas	AVF2107g	3	Multicenter, randomized, comparative study	First-line treatment of mCRC	IFL ± Bev. 5, (every 2 weeks up to 96 weeks)	IFL group: 411 cases; IFL + Bev. group: 402	OS, PFS	PFS: 10.6 months, HR: 0.58; Median OS: 20.4 months, HR: 0.71.
Overseas	NO16966	3	Multinational, randomized, comparative study	First-line treatment of mCRC	FOLFOX4 ± Bev. 5, (every 2 weeks); XELOX ± Bev. 7.5, (every 3 weeks)	2,035	PFS	XELOX (with or without Bev.) vs. FOLFOX4 (with or without Bev.): HR: 1.1. Superiority test for PFS: chemotherapy vs. chemotherapy + Bev. HR: 0.83 (97.5% *CI*: 0.72, 0.95), *P* = 0.0023.
Overseas	E3200	3	Randomized, open-label, clinical study	Advanced or mCRC previously treated with a fluoropyrimidine and an irinotecan-based regimen used either alone or in combination	FOLFOX4 ± Bev. 10, (every 2 weeks until disease progression)	FOLFOX4 group: 292 cases; FOLFOX + Bev. group: 293	OS, PFS	FOLFOX4 + Bev. group: Median PFS: 7.5 months, HR: 0.52; Median OS: 13.0 months, HR: 0.75.
Overseas	E4599	3	Randomized, open-label, active-controlled, multicenter study	First treatment of locally advanced, metastatic, or recurrent non-squamouse NSCLC	Paclitaxel + Carboplatin ± Bev. 15	878	OS	Median OS: 12.3 months.
Overseas	Study BO17705	3	Multicenter, randomized, double-blind study	Metastatic renal cell carcinoma	IFN + Bev. 10, (every 2 weeks)	649	OS	Median OS: 23.3 months, HR: 0.91.

Bev.: Bevacizumab. b-IFL: Bolus irinotecan/5-fluorouracil/folinic acid. FOLFOX4: Oxaliplatin + 5-FU continuous i.v. infusion + Leucovorin. HR: Hazard ratio. IFL: Irinotecan + 5-fluorouracil leucovorin. IFN: Interferon. mCRC: Metastatic colorectal cancer. NSCLC: Non-small cell lung cancer. OS: Overall Survival. PFS: Progression-free survival. XELOX: Oxaliplatin.

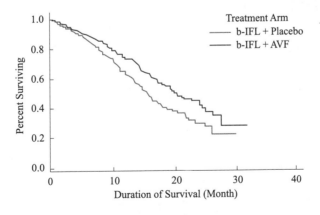

Figure 11 Overall Survival in Study AVF2107g[27]

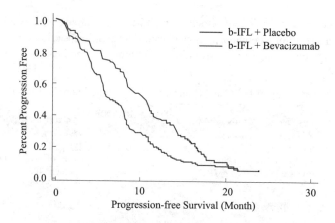

Figure 12   Progression-free Survival in Study AVF2107g[21]

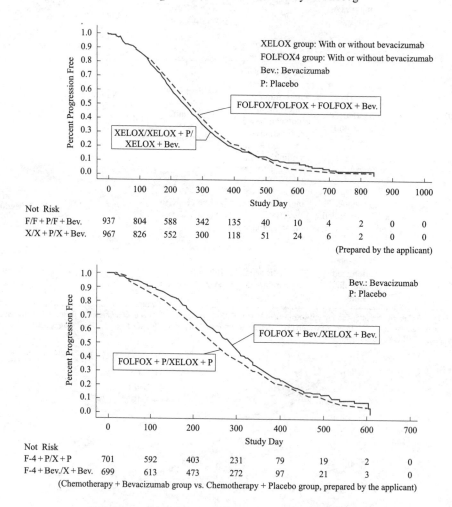

Figure 13   Progression-free Survival in Study NO16966[27]

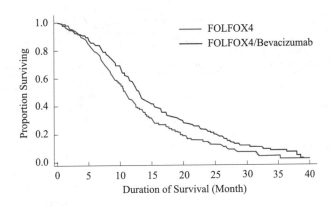

Figure 14　Duration of Survival in Study E3200[27]

Clinical Safety

Table 19　The Incidences of Gastrointestinal Perforation in Major Clinical Studies[27]

Study No.	Treatment Group	No. of Cases with Gastrointestinal Perforation (%)
AVF2107g	IFL + Bevacizumab	8/392 (2.0%)
	IFL + Placebo	0/397 (0.0%)
AVF2192g	5-FU/LV + Bevacizumab	2/100 (2.0%)
	5-FU/LV + Placebo	0/104 (0.0%)
E3200	FOLFOX4 + Bevacizumab	5/287 (1.7%)
	FOLFOX4	0/285 (0.0%)
	Bevacizumab alone	4/234 (1.7%)
NO16966	FOLFOX4 + Bevacizumab	1/341 (0.30%)
	FOLFOX4 + Placebo	0/336 (0.0%)
	XELOX + Bevacizumab	3/353 (0.80%)
	XELOX + Placebo	2/339 (0.60%)

5-FU/LV: 5-Fluorouracil/Leucovorin.　IFL: Irinotecan hydrochloride + 5-FU/LV.　FOLFOX4: Oxaliplatin + 5-FU continuous i.v. infusion + LV.　XELOX: Oxaliplatin.

Table 20　The Incidences of Delayed Healing of Wound in Major Clinical Studies[27]

Study No.	Treatment Group	No. of Cases with Gastrointestinal Perforation (%)
AVF2107g	IFL + Bevacizumab	5/60 (8.3%)
	IFL + Placebo	1/44 (2.3%)
AVF2192g	5-FU/LV + Bevacizumab	5/15 (33.3%)
	5-FU/LV + Placebo	0/3 (0.0%)
E3200[a]	FOLFOX4 + Bevacizumab	-
	FOLFOX4	-
	Bevacizumab alone	-
NO16966[b]	FOLFOX4 + Bevacizumab	9/341 (2.6%)
	FOLFOX4 + Placebo	4/336 (1.2%)
	XELOX + Bevacizumab	3/353 (0.80%)
	XELOX + Placebo	3/339 (0.90%)

5-FU/LV: 5-Fluorouracil/Leucovorin.　IFL: Irinotecan hydrochloride + 5-FU/LV.　FOLFOX4: Oxaliplatin + 5-FU continuous i.v. infusion + LV.　XELOX: Oxaliplatin.　[a] The details are unknow and currently being checked.　[b] Information on the proportion of patients with wound or those who underwent surgery is being saught.

Table 21　The Incidences of Thrombosis in Major Clinical Studies[27]

Study No.	No. of Cases with Arterial Thromboembolism		No. of Cases with Venous Thromboembolism	
	Bevacizumab Group	Control Group	Bevacizumab Group	Control Group
AVF0780g	0/35 (0.0%) (5 mg group)	1/36 (2.8%)	9/35 (25.7%) (5 mg group)	2/36 (5.6%)
	2/33 (6.1%) (10 mg group)		2/33 (6.1%) (10 mg group)	
AVF2107g	14/392 (3.6%)	5/397 (1.3%)	68/392 (17.3%)	62/397 (15.6%)
AVF2192g	10/100 (10.0%)	5/104 (4.8%)	9/100 (9.0%)	14/104 (13.5%)
E3200[a]	3/287 (1.0%) (FOLFOX + bevacizumab group)	1/285 (0.40%)	10/287 (3.5%) (FOLFOX + bevacizumab group)	7/285 (2.5%)
	2/234 (0.90%) (Single agent bevacizumab group)		1/234 (0.40%) (Single agent bevacizumah group)	
NO16966C	17/694 (2.4%)	10/675 (1.5%)	92/694 (13.3%)	64/675 (9.5%)

[a] ≥ Grade 3 for Study E3200.

Table 22　The Incidences of Heamorrhage in Major Clinical Studies[27]

Study No.	Treatment Group	No. of Cases with Gastrointestinal Perforation (%)
AVF2107g	IFL + Bevacizumab	13/392 (3.3%)
	IFL + Placebo	10/397 (2.5%)
AVF2192g	5-FU/LV + Bevacizumab	5/100 (5.0%)
	5-FU/LV + Placebo	3/104 (2.9%)
E3200	FOLFOX4 + Bevacizumab	11/287 (3.8%)
	FOLFOX4	1/285 (0.40%)
	Bevacizumab alone	7/234 (3.0%)
NO16966	FOLFOX4 + Bevacizumab	7/341 (2.1%)
	FOLFOX4 + Placebo	2/336 (0.60%)
	XELOX + Bevacizumab	6/353 (1.7%)
	XELOX + Placebo	6/339 (1.8%)

5-FU/LV: 5-Fluorouracil/Leucovorin.　IFL: Irinotecan hydrochloride + 5-FU/LV.　FOLFOX4: Oxaliplatin + 5-FU continuous i.v. infusion + LV.　XELOX: Oxaliplatin.

Table 23　The Incidences of Hypertension in Major Clinical Studies[27]

Study No.	Treatment Group	No. of Cases with Gastrointestinal Perforation (%)
AVF2107g	IFL + Bevacizumab	96/392 (24.5%)
	IFL + Placebo	34/397 (8.6%)
AVF2192g	5-FU/LV + Bevacizumab	32/100 (32.0%)
	5-FU/LV + Placebo	5/104 (4.8%)
E3200	FOLFOX4 + Bevacizumab	18/287 (6.3%)
	FOLFOX4	5/285 (1.8%)
	Bevacizumab alone	17/234 (7.3%)
NO16966	FOLFOX4 + Bevacizumab	70/341 (20.5%)
	FOLFOX4 + Placebo	27/336 (8.0%)
	XELOX + Bevacizumab	61/353 (17.3%)
	XELOX + Placebo	16/339 (4.7%)

5-FU/LV: 5-Fluorouracil/Leucovorin.　IFL: Irinotecan hydrochloride + 5-FU/LV.　FOLFOX4: Oxaliplatin + 5-FU continuous i.v. infusion + LV.　XELOX: Oxaliplatin.

Table 24   The Incidences of Proteinuria in Major Clinical Studies[27]

Study No.	Treatment Group	No. of Cases with Gastrointestinal Perforation (%)
AVF2107g	IFL + Bevacizumab	113/392 (28.8%)
	IFL + Placebo	89/397 (22.4%)
AVF2192g	5-FU/LV + Bevacizumab	38/100 (38.0%)
	5-FU/LV + Placebo	20/104 (19.2%)
E3200	FOLFOX4 + Bevacizumab	2/287 (0.70%)
	FOLFOX4	0/285 (0.0%)
	Bevacizumab alone	0/234 (0.0%)
NO16966	FOLFOX4 + Bevacizumab	21/341 (6.2%)
	FOLFOX4 + Placebo	19/336 (5.7%)
	XELOX + Bevacizumab	14/353 (4.0%)
	XELOX + Placebo	11/339 (3.2%)

5-FU/LV: 5-Fluorouracil/Leucovorin.   IFL: Irinotecan hydrochloride + 5-FU/LV.   FOLFOX4: Oxaliplatin + 5-FU continuous i.v. infusion + LV.   XELOX: Oxaliplatin.

Indications 2: First-line Non-Squamous Non-Small Cell Lung Cancer (NSCLC)

❖ The safety and efficacy of Avastin® as first-line treatment of patients with locally advanced, metastatic, or recurrent non-squamous NSCLC was studied in a single, large, randomized, active-controlled, open-label, multicenter study [E4599 (NCT00021060)].

- A total of 878 chemotherapy-naïve patients with locally advanced, metastatic or recurrent non-squamous NSCLC were randomized (1:1) to receive six 21-day cycles of paclitaxel (200 mg/m^2) and carboplatin (AUC6) with or without Avastin® 15 mg/kg.   After completing or discontinuing chemotherapy, patients randomized to receive Avastin® continued to receive Avastin® alone until disease progression or until unacceptable toxicity.
- OS was statistically significantly longer for patients receiving Avastin® with paclitaxel and carboplatin compared with those receiving chemotherapy alone.   Median OS was 12.3 months vs. 10.3 months [HR: 0.80 (95% *CI*: 0.68, 0.94), final *P*-value of 0.013, stratified log-rank test].   Based on investigator assessment which was not independently verified, patients were reported to have longer PFS with Avastin® with paclitaxel and carboplatin compared to chemotherapy alone.

❖ The safety and efficacy of Avastin® in patients with locally advanced, metastatic or recurrent non-squamous NSCLC, who had not received prior chemotherapy was studied in another randomized, double-blind, placebo-controlled study [BO17704 (NCT00806923)].

- A total of 1,043 patients were randomized (1:1:1) to receive cisplatin and gemcitabine with placebo, Avastin® 7.5 mg/kg or Avastin® 15 mg/kg.   The main outcome measure was PFS.   Secondary outcome measure was OS.
- PFS was significantly higher in both Avastin®-containing arms compared to the placebo arm HR: 0.75 (95% *CI*: 0.62, 0.91), *P*-value of 0.0026 for Avastin® 7.5 mg/kg and HR: 0.82 (95% *CI*: 0.68, 0.98), *P*-value of 0.030 for Avastin® 15 mg/kg.   The addition of Avastin® to cisplatin and gemcitabine failed to demonstrate an improvement in the duration of OS [HR: 0.93 (95% *CI*: 0.78, 1.1), *P*-value of 0.42 for Avastin® 7.5 mg/kg and HR: 1.0 (95% *CI*: 0.86, 1.2), *P*-value of 0.76 for Avastin® 15 mg/kg].

Clinical Efficacy

Table 25   Survival Outcomes by Histology Type a Overall Survival, by Histology Subtype: Hazard Ratios and Forest Plots[42]

Baseline Characteristic	Total No.	PC		PCB		Hazard Ratio	95% CI
		N	Median (Month)	N	Median (Month)		
All patients	878	444	10.3	434	12.3	0.80	0.69-0.93
Histological type							
Adenocarcinoma	602	302	10.3	300	14.2	0.69	0.58-0.83
Large cell undifferentiated	48	30	8.7	18	10.0	1.2	0.60-2.2
Squamous	3	2	12.3	1	22.4	0.0	0.0-
BAC	23	11	17.7	12	10.0	1.5	0.57-3.9
NSCLC, NOS	165	86	10.0	79	9.5	1.2	0.84-1.6
Other	34	11	12.6	23	8.4	0.92	(0.43-2.0)

BAC: Bronchoalveolar.   CI: Confidence interval.   NOS: Not otherwise specified.   NSCLC: Non-small cell lung cancer.   PC: Paclitaxel/carboplatin.   PCB: Paclitaxel/Carboplatin_bevacizumab.

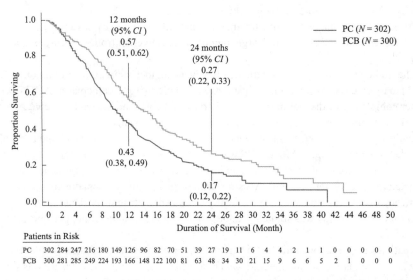

Figure 15   During of Survival for Adenocarcinoma, by Treatment[42]

Table 26   Progression-free Survival: Hazard Ratios[a] and Forest Plots[b, 42]

Baseline Characteristic	Total No.	PC		PCB		Hazard Ratio	95% CI
		N	Median[c] (Month)	N	Median[c] (Month)		
All patients	878	444	4.8	434	6.4	0.66	0.57-0.77
Histological type							
Adenocarcinoma	602	302	5.0	300	6.6	0.65	0.54-0.78
Large cell undifferentiated	48	30	4.3	18	8.5	0.35	0.15-0.79
Squamous	3	2	7.1	1	22.4	0.0	0.0-
BAC	23	11	4.5	12	6.1	1.1	0.43-2.8
NSCLC, NOS	165	86	4.7	79	5.7	0.78	0.55-1.1
Other	34	11	6.0	23	6.6	0.54	0.19-1.5

BAC: Bronchoalveolar.   CI: Confidence interval.   HR: Hazard ratio.   NOS: Not otherwise specified.   NSCLC: Non-small cell lung cancer.   OS: Overall survival. PC: Paclitaxel/carboplatin.   PCB: Paclitaxel/carbiolatin_bevacizumab.   PFS: Progression-free survival.   [a] Median OS and HR with forest plots are shown for PC- or PCB-treated NSCLC patients with different histology types.   HRs are from unstratified models.   [b] Kaplan-Meier curves are shown for OS of patients with adenocarcinoma histology treated with PC or PCB; 12- and 24-month survival rates are indicated.   [c] Median PFS, described as for OS in (A).

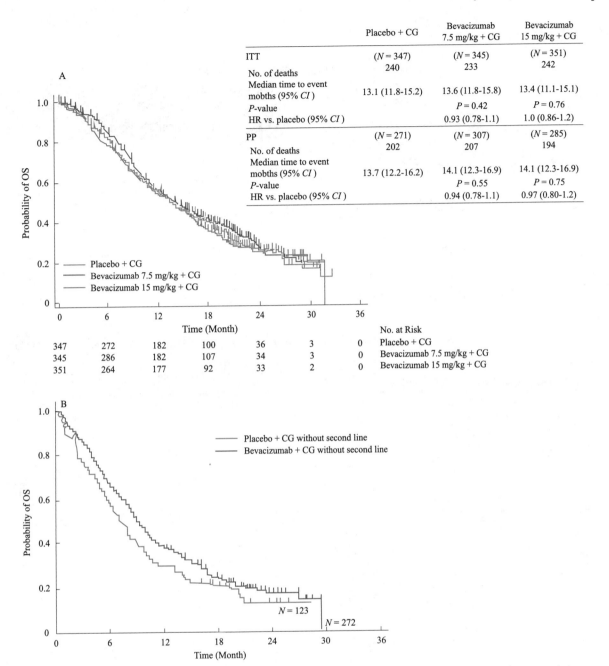

	Placebo + CG	Bevacizumab 7.5 mg/kg + CG	Bevacizumab 15 mg/kg + CG
ITT	(N = 347)	(N = 345)	(N = 351)
No. of deaths	240	233	242
Median time to event mobths (95% CI)	13.1 (11.8-15.2)	13.6 (11.8-15.8)	13.4 (11.1-15.1)
P-value		P = 0.42	P = 0.76
HR vs. placebo (95% CI)		0.93 (0.78-1.1)	1.0 (0.86-1.2)
PP	(N = 271)	(N = 307)	(N = 285)
No. of deaths	202	207	194
Median time to event mobths (95% CI)	13.7 (12.2-16.2)	14.1 (12.3-16.9)	14.1 (12.3-16.9)
P-value		P = 0.55	P = 0.75
HR vs. placebo (95% CI)		0.94 (0.78-1.1)	0.97 (0.80-1.2)

No. at Risk

347	272	182	100	36	3	0	Placebo + CG
345	286	182	107	34	3	0	Bevacizumab 7.5 mg/kg + CG
351	264	177	92	33	2	0	Bevacizumab 15 mg/kg + CG

Plots of Kaplan-Meier estimates for OS (ITT population) for the bevacizumab 7.5 mg/kg group and the bevacizumab 15 mg/kg group relative to placebo, together with time to event data for the OS analysis in the ITT and PP populations (A) and for the subgroup of patients who did not receive poststudy therapy (B).   In panel B, data from the two bevacizumab groups have been pooled.   CG: Cisplatin-gemcitabine.   CI: Confidence interval. HR: Hazard ratio.   ITT: Intent-to-treat.   OS: Overall survival.   PP: Per protocol.

Figure 16   Plots of Kaplan-Meier Estimates for OS[43]

Clinical Safety

Table 27   Adverse Events for Treated Patients[a, 42]

	Adenocarcinoma Histology (N = 596)		NSCLC NOS Histology (N = 164)		Other Histologies[b] (N = 108)	
	PC[c] (N = 299)	PCB[d] (N = 297)	PC[c] (N = 86)	PCB[d] (N = 78)	PC[c] (N = 56)	PCB[d] (N = 52)
Any Bleeding Event[e]						
Grade 3	2 (0.70)	4 (1.3)	0	1 (1.3)	0	2 (3.8)
Grade 4	0	4 (1.3)	0	0	0	1 (1.9)
Grade 5	3 (0.10)	4 (1.3)	0	3 (3.8)	0	1 (1.9)
Pulmonary Hemorrhage[f]						
Grade 3	1 (0.30)	2 (0.70)	0	0	0	0
Grade 4	0	1 (0.30)	0	0	0	0
Grade 5	1 (0.30)	2 (0.70)	0	3 (3.8)	0	1 (1.9)[g]
Hypertension						
Grade 3	0	24 (8.1)	1 (1.2)	4 (5.1)	1 (1.8)	3 (5.8)
Grade 4	1 (0.30)	2 (0.70)	0	0	0	0
Arterial Thromboembolic Event						
Grade 3	0	1 (0.30)	0	1 (1.3)	0	1 (1.9)
Grade 4	5 (1.7)	3 (1.0)	0	1 (1.3)	0	0
Grade 5	1 (0.30)	3 (1.0)	0	1 (1.3)	0	1 (1.9)
Venous Thromboembolic Events						
Grade 3	5 (1.7)	8 (2.7)	2 (2.3)	0	0	1 (1.9)
Grade 4	5 (1.7)	12 (4.0)	2 (2.3)	2 (2.6)	0	0
Grade 5	0	1 (0.30)	0	0	0	0
Gastrointestinal Perforation						
Grade 3	1 (0.30)	4 (1.3)	0	2 (2.6)	1 (1.8)	0
Grade 4	0	3 (1.0)	0	0	0	1 (1.9)
Proteinuria						
Grade 3	0	9 (3.0)	0	1 (1.3)	0	1 (1.9)
Grade 4	0	2 (0.70)	0	0	0	0
Neutropenia[h]						
Grade 4	55 (18.4)	83 (27.9)	12 (14.0)	20 (25.6)	9 (16.1)	10 (19.2)

NCI-CTC: National Cancer Institute Common Terminology Criteria.   NOS: Not otherwise specified.   NSCLC: Non-small cell lung cancer.   PC: Paclitaxel/carboplatin.   PCB: Paclitaxel/carboplatin + bevacizumab.   [a] Events were graded according to NCI-CTC, version 2.0.   Events of maximum severity are reported for each patient.   Rows for Grade 5 events are only included for adverse events categories that included Grade 5 events.   [b] Other histologies include large cell undifferentiated, bronchoalveolar, squamous, and other.   [c] Source data are from the case report form.   [d] Source data are from the case report form and from the NCI Adverse Event Expedited Reporting System.   [e] Any Grade 3 to 5 bleeding events, including pulmonary hemorrhage.   [f] Pulmonary hemorrhage events are a subset of bleeding events described in the row above.   "Hemoptysis" was a preferred term for pulmonary hemorrhage events.   [g] This patient had large cell undifferentiated histology.   [h] Only Grade 4+ hematologic events are reported.

Indications 3: Recurrent Glioblastoma (GBM)[44]

❖ The safety and efficacy of Avastin® were evaluated in a multicenter, randomized (2:1), open-label study in patients with recurrent GBM (EORTC 26101, NCT01290939).

- Patients with first progression following radiotherapy and temozolomide were randomized (2:1) to receive Avastin® (10 mg/kg every 2 weeks) with lomustine (90 mg/m² every 6 weeks) or lomustine (110 mg/m² every 6 weeks) alone until disease progression or unacceptable toxicity. Randomization was stratified by World Health Organization (WHO) performance status (0 vs. >0), steroid use (yes vs. no), largest tumor diameter (≤40 vs. >40 mm), and institution.
- The main outcome measure was OS. Secondary outcome measures were investigator-assessed PFS and ORR per the modified Response Assessment in Neuro-oncology (RANO) criteria, health related quality of life (HRQoL), cognitive function, and corticosteroid use.
- No difference in OS (HR: 0.91, *P*-value of 0.46) was observed between arms; therefore, all secondary outcome measures are descriptive only. PFS was longer in the Avastin® with lomustine arm [HR: 0.52 (95% *CI*: 0.41, 0.64)] with a median PFS of 4.2 months in the Avastin® with lomustine arm and 1.5 months in the lomustine arm. Among the 50.0% of patients receiving corticosteroids at the time of randomization, a higher percentage of patients in the Avastin® with lomustine arm discontinued corticosteroids (23.0% vs. 12.0%).

❖ One single arm single center study (NCI 06-C-0064E) and a randomized noncomparative multicenter study [AVF3708g (NCT00345163)] evaluated the efficacy and safety of Avastin® 10 mg/kg every 2 weeks in patients with previously treated GBM.

- Response rates in both studies were evaluated based on modified WHO criteria that considered corticosteroid use. In AVF3708g, the response rate was 25.9% (95% *CI*: 17.0%, 36.1%) with a median duration of response of 4.2 months (95% *CI*: 3.0, 5.7). In Study NCI 06-C-0064E, the response rate was 19.6% (95% *CI*: 10.9%, 31.3%) with a median duration of response of 3.9 months (95% *CI*: 2.4, 17.4).

Clinical Efficacy

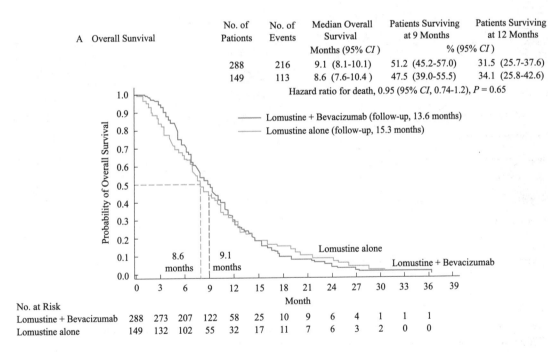

A Overall Survival	No. of Patients	No. of Events	Median Overall Survival	Patients Surviving at 9 Months	Patients Surviving at 12 Months
			Months (95% *CI*)	% (95% *CI*)	
	288	216	9.1 (8.1-10.1)	51.2 (45.2-57.0)	31.5 (25.7-37.6)
	149	113	8.6 (7.6-10.4)	47.5 (39.0-55.5)	34.1 (25.8-42.6)

Hazard ratio for death, 0.95 (95% *CI*, 0.74-1.2), *P* = 0.65

—— Lomustine + Bevacizumab (follow-up, 13.6 months)
—— Lomustine alone (follow-up, 15.3 months)

No. at Risk												
Lomustine + Bevacizumab	288	273	207	122	58	25	10	9	6	4	1	1	1
Lomustine alone	149	132	102	55	32	17	11	7	6	3	2	0	0

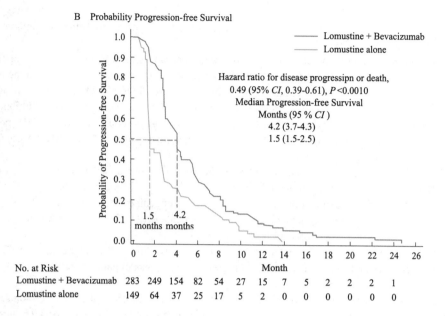

B   Probability Progression-free Survival

Figure 17   Overall Survival and Progression-free Survival in the Intention-to-Treat Population[45]

Clinical Safety

Table 28   Adverse Events for Treated Patients[45]

Event	Lomustine Alone (N = 147)	Lomustine + Bevacizumab (N = 238)
	N (%)	N (%)
Any adverse event	139 (94.6)	278 (98.2)
Treatment-related adverse event	78 (53.1)	241 (85.2)
Grade 3-5 adverse event	56 (38.1)	180 (63.6)
Treatment-related serious adverse event	14 (9.5)	109 (38.5)
Pulmonary embolism	0	14 (4.9)
Arterial hypertension	1 (0.70)	67 (23.7)
Hematologic toxic effects	73 (49.7)	152 (53.7)
Death[a]	1 (0.70)	5 (1.8)

[a] In the monotherapy group, one patient died from a lung infection.   In the combination group, two patients died from myocardial infarction and one each died from large-intestine perforation, sepsis, and intracranial hemorrhage.

Indications 4: Metastatic Renal Cell Carcinoma (mRCC)[44]

❖ Patients with treatment-naïve mRCC were evaluated in a multicenter, randomized, double-blind, international study [BO17705 (NCT00738530)] comparing interferon alfa Avastin® versus placebo.

  • A total of 649 patients who had undergone a nephrectomy were randomized (1:1) to receive either Avastin® (10 mg/kg every 2 weeks; N = 327) or placebo (every 2 weeks; N = 322) with interferon alfa (9 MIU subcutaneously three times weekly for a maximum of 52 weeks).   Patients were treated until disease progression or unacceptable toxicity.   The main outcome measure was investigator-assessed PFS.   Secondary outcome measures were ORR and OS.

  • PFS was statistically significantly prolonged among patients receiving Avastin® compared to placebo; median PFS was 10.2 months vs. 5.4 months [HR: 0.60, (95% CI: 0.49, 0.72), P-value <0.00010, stratified log-rank test].   Among the 595 patients with measurable disease, ORR was also significantly higher (30.0% vs. 12.0%, P-value <0.00010, stratified CMH test).   There was no improvement in OS based on the final analysis conducted after 444 deaths, with a median OS of 23 months in the patients receiving Avastin® with interferon alfa and 21 months in patients receiving interferon alone [HR: 0.86, (95% CI: 0.72, 1.0)].

Clinical Efficacy

Table 29　Efficacy of Bevacizumab plus IFN in Patients with Single or Multiple Metastatic Sites[46]

Metastatic Sites	Placebo + IFN		Bevacizumab + IFN		Hazard Ratio	95% CI for HR
	Patient (N)	Event (N)	Patient (N)	Event (N)		
<1	76	64	76	44	0.57	0.39-0.84
>1	245	214	249	196	0.66	0.54-0.80
<2	198	163	196	130	0.67	0.53-0.84
>3	123	111	129	100	0.54	0.41-0.72
Sum of Baseline Target Lesions						
< median	142	111	156	102	0.65	0.49-0.85
> median	147	136	150	115	0.60	0.47-0.77

CI: Confidence interval.　HR: Hazard radio.　IFN: Interferon.

Clinical Safety

Table 30　Overview of the Adverse Events Experience in Metastatic Renal Cell Carcinoma Trials with Bevacizumab[46]

Parameter	AVOREN		AVF0890s			RACE[a]	
	Placebo + IFN[b]	Bev.[a] + IFN[b]	Placebo	Bev. 3 mg/kg	Bev. 10 mg/kg	Bev.[a] + Placebo	Bev.[a] + Erlotinib[c]
Patients (N)	304	337	40	37	39	53	51
Any AE	287 (94.0%)	328 (97.0%)	NR	NR	NR	NR	NR
Grade 3 AE	129 (42.0%)	192 (57.0%)	NR	NR	NR	31 (59.0%)[d]	33 (65.0%)[d]
Grade 4 AE	12 (4.0%)	21 (6.0%)	0	0	0	31 (59.0%)[d]	33 (65.0%)[d]
Related AE (any grade)	238 (78.0%)	293 (87.0%)	NR	NR	NR	NR	NR
Serious AE	50 (16.0%)	98 (29.0%)	NR	NR	NR	18 (34.0%)	14 (28.0%)
Targeted AE (Grade ≥3)							
Any[e]	6 (2.0%)	58 (17.0%)	NR	NR	NR	24 (45.0%)	26 (51.0%)
Proteinuria	0	22 (7.0%)	0	2 (5.0%)	3 (8.0%)	3 (6.0%)	4 (8.0%)
Hypertension	2 (<1.0%)	13 (4.0%)	0	0	8 (21.0%)	14 (26.0%)	16 (31.0%)
Bleeding	1 (<1.0%)	11 (3.0%)	0	0	0	2 (4.0%)	3 (6.0%)
Arterial TE	1 (<1.0%)	4 (1.0%)	0	0	0	0	1 (2.0%)
Venous TE	2 (<1.0%)	6 (2.0%)	0	0	0	2 (4.0%)	0
Gastrointestinal perforation	0	5 (1.0%)	0	0	0	0	1 (2.0%)
Wound healing complication	0	2 (<1.0%)	0	0	0	2 (4.0%)	0
Congestive heart failure	0	1 (<1.0%)	0	0	0	1 (2.0%)	1 (2.0%)
AE leading to:							
Bev./placebo discontinuation	17 (6.0%)	63 (19.0%)	NR	NR	NR	16 (30.0%)[f]	13 (26.0%)[f]
Bev./placebo modification	57 (19.0%)	109 (32.0%)	NR	NR	NR		
Death not due to PD[g]	7 (2.0%)	8 (2.0%)	0 (0.0%)	0 (0.0%)	0 (0.0%)	0 (0.0%)	1 (2.0%)

AE: Adverse event.　AVF0890s: Deaths possibly related to bevacizumab.　AVOREN: Avastin® and Roferon® in renal cell carcinoma (BO17705).　Bev.: Bevacizumab.　NR: Not reported.　PD: Progression of disease.　TE: Thromboembolic event.　RACE: Randomized, double-blind, Phase 2 trial of bevacizumab with or without erlotinib.　[a]Bevacizumab 10 mg/kg twice weekly.　[b]IFN 9 million IU three-time weekly.　[c]Includes hypertension, proteinuria, wound healing complications, bleeding/hemorrhage, gastrointestinal perforation, TEs, congestive heart failure.　[d]Erlotinib 150 mg/d.　[e]Grade 3 and 4 AEs combined.　[f]AEs leading to change, hold or discontinuation of bevacizumab.　[g]AVOREN: All AEs reported with an outcome of death (related and unrelated, no time limit).

Indications 5: Persistent, Recurrent, or Metastatic Cervical Cancer[44]

❖ Patients with persistent, recurrent, or metastatic cervical cancer were evaluated in a randomized, four-arm, multicenter study comparing Avastin® with chemotherapy vs. chemotherapy alone [GOG-0240 (NCT00803062)].
  • A total of 452 patients were randomized (1:1:1:1) to receive paclitaxel and cisplatin with or without Avastin®, or paclitaxel and topotecan with or without Avastin®.
  • Patients were treated until disease progression or unacceptable adverse reactions. The main outcome measure was OS. Secondary outcome measures included ORR.
  • The ORR was higher in patients who received Avastin® with chemotherapy [45.0% (95% *CI*: 39.0, 52.0)] compared to patients who received chemotherapy alone [34.0% (95% *CI*: 28.0, 40.0)].
  • The HR for OS with Avastin® with cisplatin and paclitaxel as compared to cisplatin and paclitaxel alone was 0.72 (95% *CI*: 0.51, 1.02). The HR for OS with Avastin® with topotecan and paclitaxel as compared to topotecan and paclitaxel alone was 0.76 (95% *CI*: 0.55, 1.06).

Clinical Efficacy

Table 31　Efficacy Results in Study GOG-0204[44]

Efficacy Parameter	Avastin® with Chemotherapy (N = 227)	Chemotherapy (N = 225)
Overall Survival, median (Month)[a]	16.8	12.9
Hazard ratio (95% *CI*)	0.74 (0.58; 0.94) (*P*-value[b] = 0.013)	

[a] Kaplan-Meier estimates.　[b] Log-rank test (stratified).

Table 32　Efficacy Results in Study GOG-0204[44]

Efficacy Parameter	Topotecan and Paclitaxel with or without Avastin® (N = 223)	Cisplatin and Paclitaxel with or without Avastin® (N = 229)
Overall Survival, median (Month)[a]	13.3	15.5
Hazard ratio (95% *CI*)	1.2 (0.91; 1.46) (*P*-value[b] = 0.023)	

[a] Kaplan-Meier estimates.　[b] Log-rank test (stratified).

Indications 6: Recurrent Epithelial Ovarian, Fallopian Tube, or Primary Peritoneal Cancer[44]

❖ Avastin® was evaluated in a multicenter, open-label, randomized study [MO22224 (NCT00976911)] comparing Avastin® with chemotherapy vs. chemotherapy alone in patients with platinum-resistant, recurrent epithelial ovarian, fallopian tube, or primary peritoneal cancer that recurred within <6 months from the most recent platinum-based therapy (N = 361).
  • The main outcome measure was investigator-assessed PFS. Secondary outcome measures were ORR and OS.
  • The addition of Avastin® to chemotherapy demonstrated a statistically significant improvement in investigator-assessed PFS, which was supported by a retrospective independent review analysis.
❖ AVF4095g (NCT00434642) was a randomized, double-blind, placebo-controlled study studying Avastin® with chemotherapy vs. chemotherapy alone in the treatment of patients with platinum-sensitive recurrent epithelial ovarian, fallopian tube, or primary peritoneal cancer who have not received prior chemotherapy in the recurrent setting or prior bevacizumab treatment (N = 484).
  • The main outcome measures were investigator-assessed PFS. Secondary outcome measures were ORR and OS.
  • A statistically significant prolongation in PFS was demonstrated among patients receiving Avastin® with chemotherapy compared to those receiving placebo with chemotherapy. Independent radiology review of PFS was consistent with investigator assessment [HR: 0.45 (95% *CI*: 0.35, 0.58)]. OS was not significantly improved with the addition of Avastin® to chemotherapy [HR: 0.95 (95% *CI*: 0.77, 1.2)].
❖ Study GOG-0213 (NCT00565851) was a randomized, controlled, open-label study of Avastin® with chemotherapy vs. chemotherapy alone in the treatment of patients with platinum-sensitive recurrent epithelial ovarian, fallopian tube, or primary peritoneal cancer, who have not received more than one previous regimen of chemotherapy (N = 673).
  • The main outcome measure was OS. Other outcome measures were investigator-assessed PFS, and ORR.

Clinical Efficacy

Table 33　Efficacy Results in Study MO22224[44]

Efficacy Parameter	Avastin® with Chemotherapy (N = 179)	Chemotherapy (N = 182)
PFS per Investigator		
Median (95% CI), in months	6.8 (5.6, 7.8)	3.4 (2.1, 3.8)
HR (95% CI)[a]	0.38 (0.30, 0.49)	
P-value[b]	<0.00010	
Overall Survival		
Median (95% CI), in months	16.6 (13.7, 19.0)	13.3 (11.9, 16.4)
HR (95% CI)[a]	0.89 (0.70, 1.1)	
Overall Response Rate		
No. of patients with measurable disease at baseline	142	144
Rate, % (95% CI)	28.0% (21.0%, 36.0%)	13.0% (7.0%, 18.0%)
Duration of Response		
Median, in months	9.4	5.4

[a] Per stratified Cox proportional hazards model.　[b] Per stratified log-rank test.

Table 34　Efficacy Results in Study MO22224 by Chemotherapy[44]

Efficacy Parameter	Paclitaxel		Topotecan		Pegylated Liposomal Doxorubicin	
	Avastin® with Chemotherapy (N = 60)	Chemotherapy (N = 55)	Avastin® with Chemotherapy (N = 57)	Chemotherapy (N = 63)	Avastin® with Chemotherapy (N = 62)	Chemotherapy (N = 64)
Progression-free Survival per Investigator						
Median (Month) (95% CI)	9.6 (7.8, 11.5)	3.9 (3.5, 5.5)	6.2 (5.3, 7.6)	2.1 (1.9, 2.3)	5.1 (3.9, 6.3)	3.5 (1.9, 3.9)
Hazard ratio[a] (95% CI)	0.47 (0.31, 0.72)		0.24 (0.15, 0.38)		0.47 (0.32, 0.71)	
Overall Survival						
Median (Month) (95% CI)	22.4 (16.7, 26.7)	13.2 (8.2, 19.7)	13.8 (11.0, 18.3)	13.3 (10.4, 18.3)	13.7 (11.0, 18.3)	14.1 (9.9, 17.8)
Hazard ratio[a] (95% CI)	0.64 (0.41, 1.0)		1.1 (0.73, 1.7)		0.94 (0.63, 1.4)	
Overall Response Rate						
No. of patients with measurable disease at baseline	45	43	46	50	51	51
Rate, % (95% CI)	53.0 (39.0, 68.0)	30.0 (17.0, 44.0)	17.0 (6.0, 28.0)	2.0 (0.0, 6.0)	16.0 (6.0, 26.0)	8.0 (0.0, 15.0)
Duration of Response						
Median (Month)	11.6	6.8	5.2	NE	8.0	4.6

NE: Not estimable.　[a] Per stratified Cox proportional hazards model.

Table 35   Efficacy Results in Study AVF4095[44]

Efficacy Parameter	Avastin® with Gemcitabine and Carboplatin (N = 242)	Placebo with Gemcitabine and Carboplatin (N = 242)
Progression-free Survival		
Median PFS (Month)	12.4	8.4
Hazard ratio (95% CI)	0.46 (0.37, 0.58)	
P-value	<0.00010	
Overall Response Rate		
% patients with overall response	78.0%	57.0%
P-value	<0.00010	

Table 36   Efficacy Results in Study GOG-0213[44]

Efficacy Parameter	Avastin® with Carboplatin and Paclitaxel (N = 337)	Carboplatin and Paclitaxel (N = 336)
Overall Survival		
Median OS (Month)	42.6	37.3
Hazard ratio (95% CI) (IVRS)[a]	0.84 (0.69, 1.0)	
Hazard ratio (95% CI) (eCRF)[b]	0.82 (0.68, 1.0)	
Progression-free Survival		
Median PFS (Month)	13.8	10.4
Hazard ratio (95% CI) (IVRS)[a]	0.61 (0.51, 0.72)	
Overall Response Rate		
No. of patients with measurable disease at baseline	274	286
Rate, %	213 (78.0%)	159 (56.0%)

[a] HR was estimated from Cox proportional hazards models stratified by the duration of treatment free-interval prior to enrolling onto this study per IVRS (interactive voice response system) and secondary surgical debulking status.   [b] HR was estimated from Cox proportional hazards models stratified by the duration of platinum free-interval prior to enrolling onto this study per eCRF (electronic case report form) and secondary surgical debulking status.

Cardiotoxicity (Congestive Heart Failure)

❖ The incidence of heart failure associated with bevacizumab was 2.0% (2/100 patients) in the bevacizumab group of Study AVF2192g and 1.0% (4/392 patients) in Study AVF2107g.

❖ Of the 568 patients in the chemotherapy + bevacizumab groups from clinical studies involving patients with colorectal cancer to date, 7 patients (1.2%) experienced heart failure.

Infusion Reactions

❖ Eight patients experienced "anaphylactic reaction"; 1 patient was untreated with bevacizumab and all of the other 7 patients did not develop anaphylactic reaction after rechallenge.

❖ Two patients had "fatal hypersensitivity" among approximately 67,500 patients exposed to bevacizumab.

Anti-drug Antibody (ADA) Analysis

❖ Four out of the 837 patients who underwent antibody test (Study AVF2107g: 3 patients, Study AVF2119g: 1 patient) had positive results at baseline.

❖ In Study JO18157, 3 out of the 18 patients (5 mg/kg group: 1 patient, 10 mg/kg group: 2 patients) had positive results at baseline.

8　Clinical Pharmacokinetics

Summary

❖ Phase 1 study of single agent bevacizumab (AVF0737g)
  • Serum bevacizumab was eliminated monophasically or biphasically.
  • Serum bevacizumab in 0.1 and 0.3 mg/kg declined rapidly compared with the 1, 3, and 10 mg/kg groups.
  • The mean and standard deviation of the clearance (CL) of bevacizumab were higher in 0.1 and 0.3 mg/kg compared with the 1, 3, and 10 mg/kg groups.
  • The volume of distribution of the central compartment V_c was similar to the serum volume, and the volume of distribution at steady-state (V_{ss}) and V_c were almost constant, being independent of the dose of bevacizumab.
  • There were no changes in CL or V_c at doses of 1 to 10 mg/kg and linearity was observed.
❖ Phase 1/2 study of bevacizumab with 5-FU/LV regimen (JO18157)
  • AUC_{inf} following the administration of bevacizumab alone was increased in a dose-proportional manner and the CL was constant.
  • The ratios of the CL and V_c of bevacizumab for bevacizumab in combination with 5-FU/LV/single agent bevacizumab (estimates) were 0.90 and 1.1, respectively.
  • Combined with 5-FU/LV, the CL of bevacizumab tends to be decreased and the V_c tends to be increased, but the degrees are small and the effects on the PK are small.
❖ Phase 1 study of bevacizumab in combination with chemotherapy (AVF0761g)
  • PK parameters of serum bevacizumab were almost equivalent for all groups and based on a pooled analysis of PK data.
  • PK parameters were similar to the results of Study AVF0737g where single agent bevacizumab was administered.
  • No clear difference in the pharmacokinetics of bevacizumab was observed in combination with DXR, CBDCA/PTX, or 5-FU/LV compared to single agent bevacizumab.
  • PK of these chemotherapy agents was not altered by the administration of bevacizumab.
❖ Phase 2 study of bevacizumab in combination with 5-FU/LV regimen (AVF0780g)
  • The trough concentration of bevacizumab increased after multiple dosing and reached a steady-state by Day 100.
  • Regardless of the dose of bevacizumab, the CL and V_c were constant.
❖ Phase 3 study of bevacizumab in combination with IFL regimen (AVF2107g)
  • The CL and V_c of serum bevacizumab were 3.1 mL/kg/day and 40.3 mL/kg, respectively, which were consistent with the results from Study AVF0780g.
  • The trough serum bevacizumab concentration (mean ± SD) when bevacizumab was combined with IFL or 5-FU/LV was 28.6 ± 10.6 and 32.5 ± 18.8 μg/mL, respectively, on Day 14, and 83.6 ± 31.4 and 77.0 ± 26.9 μg/mL, respectively, on Day 84.
  • Serum bevacizumab concentrations were similar between the IFL + bevacizumab group and the 5-FU/LV + bevacizumab group.

Single-Dose Pharmacokinetics

Table 37　The Pharmacokinetics after Single-Dose of Bevacizumab (Study AVF0737g)[47]

Dose (mg/kg)	N	CL [mL/(day·kg)]	V_c (mL/kg)	V_{ss} (mL/kg)	$t_{1/2, initial}$ (Day)	$t_{1/2, terminal}$ (Day)	MRT (Day)	AUC_{inf} (μg·day/mL)
0.1	5	9.3 ± 7.1	48.0 ± 17.4	50.1 ± 17.0	NA	5.2 ± 2.4	7.4 ± 3.4	18.5 ± 14.3
0.3	5	5.1 ± 2.4	48.6 ± 13.0	60.3 ± 7.3	1.9	10.4 ± 5.3	13.9 ± 6.1	68.7 ± 26.8
1	5	3.3 ± 0.81	37.9 ± 7.8	60.4 ± 18.8	1.3 ± 0.54	14.7 ± 6.9	19.9 ± 9.3	322 ± 84.0
3	4	3.7 ± 2.1	41.4 ± 12.0	53.4 ± 12.0	0.84	12.8 ± 6.6	18.1 ± 9.4	1,073 ± 595
10	5	2.8 ± 0.47	43.5 ± 12.6	53.0 ± 10.9	2.2	14.2 ± 3.4	19.3 ± 3.2	3,730 ± 722

NA: Not available.

Table 38　The Pharmacokinetics of Bevacizumab in Combination with 5-FU/LV (Study JO18157)[47]

Dose (mg/kg)	AUC_{inf} (μg·day/mL)	V_d (mL/kg)	CL [mL/(day·kg)]	$t_{1/2}$ (Day)
3	852 ± 237	62.5 ± 11.1	3.8 ± 1.2	12.3 ± 4.5
5	1,387 ± 427	73.5 ± 18.3	3.9 ± 1.3	13.4 ± 2.8
10	2,811 ± 345	60.3 ± 8.9	3.6 ± 0.48	11.7 ± 1.7

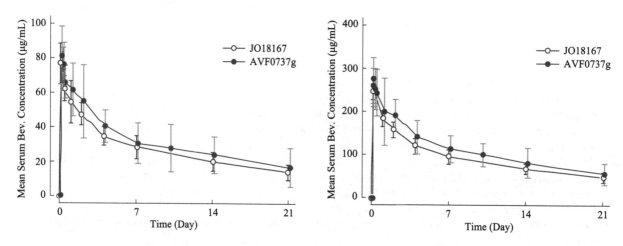

Figure 18   Serum Bevacizumab Concentration over Time following the Administration of Single Agent Bevacizumab in Japanese and Foreign Clinical Studies[27]

Table 39   The Pharmacokinetics of Bevacizumab in Combination with Chemotherapy (Study AVF0761g)[21]

Dose (mg/kg)	N	Chemotherapy	CL [mL/(day·kg)]	V_c (mL/kg)	$t_{1/2, terminal}$ (Day)	MRT (Day)	AUC_{inf} (μg·day/mL)
3	3	Doxorubicin	3.7 ± 0.56	64.8 ± 8.7	12.1 ± 0.60	17.4 ± 0.85	814 ± 122
3	4	Carboplatin/ Paclitaxel	2.5 ± 0.44	51.7 ± 14.0	14.2 ± 1.6	20.6 ± 2.3	1,243 ± 241
3	4	5-FU/FA	3.3 ± 0.86	56.0 ± 12.3	12.5 ± 4.4	18.1 ± 6.4	966 ± 256

5-FU/FA: 5-fluorouracil/folinic acid.

Multiple-Dose Pharmacokinetics

Table 40   The Pharmacokinetics of Bevacizumab in Combination with 5-FU/FA Regimen (Study AVF0780g)[21]

Dose (mg/kg)	N	Chemotherapy	CL [mL/(day·kg)]	V_c (mL/kg)	$t_{1/2, terminal}$ (Day)	MRT (Day)	AUC_{inf} (μg·day/mL)
5	34	5-FU/FA	2.8 ± 0.85	45.4 ± 9.0	12.0 ± 3.2	17.3 ± 4.7	2,009 ± 653
10	28	5-FU/FA	2.8 ± 0.66	46.1 ± 8.8	12.0 ± 3.5	17.4 ± 5.0	3,810 ± 1,002

5-FU/FA: 5-fluorouracil/folinic acid.

Table 41   The Pharmacokinetics of Bevacizumab in Combination with IFL Regimen (Study AVF2107g)[21]

Dose (mg/kg)	N	Chemotherapy	CL [mL/(day·kg)]	V_c (mL/kg)	$t_{1/2, terminal}$ (Day)	MRT (Day)	AUC_{inf} (μg·day/mL)
5	214	Arm 2: IFL Arm 3: 5-FU/FA	3.1	40.3	NA	13.1	1,610

5-FU/FA: 5-fluorouracil/folinic acid.

Anti-drug Antibody (ADA) Analysis

❖ In Study JO18157, 3/18 subjects (5 mg/kg group: 1 subject, 10 mg/kg group: 2 subjects) at baseline and 4/4 subjects (2 subjects each in 3 mg/kg group and 5 mg/kg group) at the end of the study (3 weeks after the last dose of bevacizumab) were tested positive for serum anti-bevacizumab antibodies.

❖ There are no major differences in the PK of bevacizumab between subjects with a positive antibody reaction and those with a negative antibody reaction.

9　Patent

❖ Bevacizumab was approved by the U.S. Food and Drug Administration (FDA) in 2004. It was developed and marketed as Avastin® by Genentech Inc., a subsidiary of Roche.

Summary

❖ The patent applications (WO9845331A2 and WO9845332A2) related to the anti-VEGF antibody (i.e. Bevacizumab). The two applications were filed by Genentech on Apr 3, 1998. The patent families of these applications were granted in the United State, Europe, Japan and China, respectively.

Table 42　Originator's Key Patent of Bevacizumab in Main Countries and/or Region

Country/Region	Publication/Patent No.	Application Date	Granted Date	Estimated Expiry Date
WO	WO9845331A2	04/03/1998	/	/
	WO9845332A2	04/03/1998	/	/
US	US6884879B1	08/06/1997	04/26/2005	08/06/2017
	US7060269B1	08/06/1997	06/13/2006	07/04/2019
	US7169901B2	08/06/1997	01/30/2007	03/23/2019
EP	EP1325932B9	04/03/1998	04/20/2005	04/03/2018
	EP0971959B1	04/03/1998	12/28/2005	04/03/2018
	EP0973804B1	04/03/1998	12/27/2006	04/03/2018
JP	JP3957765B2	04/03/1998	08/15/2007	04/03/2018
	JP4191258B2	04/03/1998	08/09/2017	04/03/2018
CN	CN1191276C	04/03/1998	03/02/2005	04/03/2018
	CN100480269C	04/03/1998	04/22/2009	04/03/2018
	CN101210051B	04/03/1998	12/26/2012	04/03/2018
	CN101665536B	04/03/1998	07/03/2013	04/03/2018

Table 43　Originator's International Patent Protection of Use and/or Method of Bevacizumab

Publication No.	Title	Publication Date
Technical Subjects	TREATMENT METHOD	
WO2006066086A1	Anti-angiogenesis therapy of autoimmune disease in patients who have failed prior therapy	06/22/2006
WO2008077077A2	VEGF-specific antagonists for adjuvant and neoadjuvant therapy and the treatment of early stage tumors	06/26/2008
WO2011015348A2	Responsiveness to angiogenesis inhibitors	02/10/2011
WO2011119656A1	Anti-angiogenesis therapy for treating abdominal aortic aneurysm	09/29/2011
WO2016077227A2	Predicting response to a VEGF antagonist	05/19/2016
Technical Subjects	DIAGNOSTIC METHOD	
WO2009061800A2	Methods and compositions for diagnostic use in cancer patients	05/14/2009
WO2009073540A3	VEGF polymorphisms and anti-angiogenesis therapy	06/11/2009
WO2010010155A1	Monitoring anti-angiogenesis therapy	01/28/2010
WO2010025414A3	Diagnostics and treatments for VEGF-independent tumors	03/04/2010
WO2010075420A1	Methods and compositions for diagnostic use in cancer patients	07/01/2010
WO2011008696A3	Diagnostic methods and compositions for treatment of cancer	01/20/2011
WO2011020049A1	Biological markers for monitoring patient response to VEGF antagonists	02/17/2011
WO2011033006A1	Methods and compositions for diagnostic use in cancer patients	03/24/2011

Continued

Publication No.	Title	Publication Date
WO2011089101A1	Tumor tissue-based biomarkers for bevacizumab combination therapies	07/28/2011
WO2012076582A1	AGTR1 as a marker for bevacizumab combination therapies	06/14/2012
WO2014001232A1	Blood plasma biomarkers for bevacizumab combination therapies for treatment of breast cancer	01/03/2014
WO2016011052A1	Diagnostic methods and compositions for treatment of glioblastoma	01/21/2016
WO2017181111A2	Methods for monitoring and treating cancer	10/19/2017
WO2017181079A2	Methods for monitoring and treating cancer	10/19/2017
Technical Subjects	**COMBINATION METHOD**	
WO2005000900A1	Treatment with anti-VEGF antibodies	01/06/2005
WO2006014729A2	Inhibitors of angiopoietin-like 4 protein, combinations, and their use	02/09/2006
WO2006091693A3	Extending time to disease progression or survival in cancer patients using a HER dimerization inhibitor	08/31/2006
WO2007107329A1	Tumor therapy with an antibody for vascular endothelial growth factor and an antibody for human epithelial growth factor receptor type 2	09/27/2007
WO2008073509A2	Compositions and methods for treating a neoplasm	12/13/2007
WO2008094969A2	Combination therapy with angiogenesis inhibitors	08/07/2008
WO2009039337A2	Inhibition of angiogenesis	03/26/2009
WO2010006232A1	Methods and compositions for diagnostic use for tumor treatment	01/14/2010
WO2010059969A2	Use of anti-VEGF antibody in combination with chemotherapy for treating breast cancer	05/27/2010
WO2011014457A1	Combination treatments	02/03/2011
WO2011143665A1	Treatment methods	11/17/2011
WO2011153243A3	Anti-angiogenesis therapy for treating gastric cancer	12/08/2011
WO2012010546A1	Blood plasma biomarkers for bevacizumab combination therapies for treatment of pancreatic cancer	01/26/2012
WO2012010551A1	Method to identify a patient with an increased likelihood of responding to an anti-cancer therapy	01/26/2012
WO2012010552A1	Blood plasma biomarkers for bevacizumab combination therapies for treatment of pancreatic cancer	01/26/2012
WO2012020123A2	Neuropilin as a biomarker for bevacizumab combination therapies	02/16/2012
WO2012022747A1	Combination therapy of an afucosylated CD20 antibody with an anti-VEGF antibody	02/23/2012
WO2012062653A1	Combination of bevacizumab and 2,2-dimethyl-N-((S)-6-oxo-6,7-dihydro-5H-dibenzo[b,d]azepin-7-yl)-N'-(2,2,3,3,3-pentafluoro-propyl)-malonamide for the treatment of proliferative disorders	05/18/2012
WO2013082511A1	Methods for overcoming tumor resistance to VEGF antagonists	06/06/2013
WO2013135602A2	Combination therapy for the treatment of ovarian cancer	09/19/2013
WO2014025813A1	Combination therapy for the treatment of glioblastoma	02/13/2014
WO2015031782A1	Combination therapy for the treatment of glioblastoma	03/05/2015
Technical Subjects	**PREPERATION**	
WO2005016968A2	Reducing protein a leaching during protein A affinity chromatography	02/24/2005
WO2006012500A2	Crystallization of antibodies or fragments thereof	02/02/2006
WO2009058812A1	Antibody purification by cation exchange chromatography	05/07/2009
WO2009114641A1	Antibodies with enhanced ADCC function	09/17/2009
WO2011019620A1	Antibodies with enhanced ADCC function	02/17/2011
WO2011019622A1	Cell culture methods to make antibodies with enhanced ADCC function	02/17/2011

Continued

Publication No.	Title	Publication Date
Technical Subjects	**FORMULATION**	
WO2008135380A1	Method for stabilizing a protein	11/13/2008
WO2011084750A1	Antibody formulation	07/14/2011
WO2013173687A1	High-concentration monoclonal antibody formulations	11/21/2013
WO2014160490A1	Antibody formulations	10/02/2014
WO2016044334A1	Antibody formulations	03/24/2016

The data was updated until Jan 2018.

10   Reference

[1] Leung D W, Cachianes G, Kuang W J, et al. Vascular endothelial growth factor is a secreted angiogenic mitogen [J]. Science, 1989, 246(4935): 1306-1309.

[2] Keck P J, Hauser S D, Krivi G, et al. Vascular permeability factor, an endothelial cell mitogen related to PDGF [J]. Science, 1989, 246(4935): 1309-1312.

[3] Senger D R, Galli S J, Dvorak A M, et al. Tumor cells secrete a vascular permeability factor that promotes accumulation of ascites fluid [J]. Science, 1983, 219(4587): 983-985.

[4] Ferrara N, Henzel W J. Pituitary follicular cells secrete a novel heparin-binding growth factor specific for vascular endothelial cells [J]. Biochemical and Biophysical Research Communications, 1989, 161(2): 851-858.

[5] Ferrara N. VEGF and the quest for tumor angiogenesis factors [J]. Nature Reviews Cancer, 2002, 2: 795-803.

[6] Ferrara N, Gerber H P, Lecouter J. The biology of VEGF and its receptors [J]. Nature Medicine, 2003, 9(6): 669-676.

[7] Olsson A K, Dimberg A, Kreuger J, et al. VEGF receptor signaling-in control of vascular function [J]. Nature Reviews Molecular Cell Biology, 2006, 7(5): 359-371.

[8] Terman B L, Dougher-vermazen M, Carrion M E, et al. Identification of the KDR tyrosine kinase as a receptor of vascular endothelial cell growth factor [J]. Biochemical and Biophysical Research Communications, 1992, 187(3): 1579-1586.

[9] http://www.ncbi.nlm.nih.gov/protein/AAK95847.1.

[10] http://www.ncbi.nlm.nih.gov/protein/XP_016811082.1.

[11] http://www.ncbi.nlm.nih.gov/protein/AFE64645.1.

[12] http://www.ncbi.nlm.nih.gov/protein/AAL07526.1.

[13] http://www.ncbi.nlm.nih.gov/protein/EDL23467.1.

[14] https://blast.ncbi.nlm.nih.gov.

[15] Herbert S P, Stainier D Y. Molecular control of endothelial cell behavior during blood vessel morphogenesis [J]. Nature Reviews Molecular Cell Biology, 2011, 12(9): 551-564.

[16] Park J E, Chen H H, Winer J, et al. Placenta growth factor. Potentiation of vascular endothelial growth factor bioactivity, *in vitro* and *in vivo*, and high affinity binding to Flt-1 but not to Flk-1/KDR [J]. Journal of Biological Chemistry, 1994, 269(41): 25646-25654.

[17] Gerber H P, Mcmurtrey A, Kowalski J, et al. VEGF regulates endothelial cell survival by the PI3K-kinase/Akt signal transduction pathway. Requirement for Flk-1/KDR activation [J]. Journal of Biological Chemistry, 1998, 273(46): 30366-30343.

[18] Broxmeyer H E, Cooper S, Li Z H, et al. Myeloid progenitor cell regulatory effects of vascular endothelial cell growth factor [J]. International Journal of Hematology, 1995, 62(4): 203-215.

[19] Dvorak H F, Brown L F, Detmar M, et al. Vascular permeability factor/vascular endothelial growth factor, microvascular hyperpermeability, and angiogenesis [J]. The American Journal of Pathology, 1995, 146(5): 1029-1039.

[20] Yang R, Thomas G R, Bunting S, et al. Effects of vascular endothelial growth factor on hemodynamics and cardiac performance [J]. Journal of Cardiovascular Pharmacology, 1996, 27(6): 838-844.

[21] European Medicines Agency (EMA) Database. http://www.ema.europa.eu/docs/en_GB/document_library/EPAR_-_Scientific_Discussion/human/000582/WC500029262.pdf.

[22] Ellis L M. Mechanism of action of bevacizumab as a component of therapy for metastatic colorectal cancer [J]. Seminars in Oncology, 2006, 33(10): S1-S7.

[23] http://pdl.com/royalty-revenue/historical-product-revenue/the financial reports of Genentech.

[24] EMA Database. http://www.ema.europa.eu/ema/index.jsp?curl=pages/medicines/human/medicines/000582/human_med_000663.jsp&mid=WC0b01ac058001d124.

[25] U.S. Food and Drug Administration (FDA) Database. https://www.accessdata.fda.gov/scripts/cder/daf/index.cfm?

event=overview.process&ApplNo=125085.

[26] China Food and Drug Administration (CFDA) Database. http://app1.sfda.gov.cn/datasearch/face3/base.jsp?tableId=36&tableName=TABLE36&title=进口药品&bcId=1243566515641464152144244405468.

[27] Pharmaceuticals and Medical Devices Agency (PMDA) Database. http://www.pmda.go.jp/files/000153070.pdf.

[28] FDA Database. http://101.96.10.43/www.accessdata.fda.gov/drugsatfda_docs/label/2009/125085s0169lbl.pdf.

[29] FDA Database. http://www.accessdata.fda.gov/scripts/cder/drugsatfda/index.cfm?fuseaction=Search.Label_ApprovalHistory#apphist.

[30] PMDA Database. https://ss.pmda.go.jp/en_all/search.x?q=bevacizumab&ie=utf8&cat=0&pagemax=10&imgsize=1&pdf=ok&zoom=1&suggest=1&counsel=1&ref=www.pmda.go.jp&pid=y07Zn6fg4KFKmobOA-dEaQ..&qid=hc7fqUTkppOiei3tq_SINzeTaiojD2eP&d=Drugs%09Prescription+drugs.

[31] Lee C G, Heijn M, Di Tomaso E, et al. Anti-vascular endothelial growth factor treatment augments tumor radiation response under normoxic or hypoxic conditions [J]. Cancer Research, 2000, 60(19): 5565-5570.

[32] Borgstrom P, Hillan K J, Sriramarao P, et al. Complete inhibition of angiogenesis and growth of microtumors by anti-vascular endothelial growth factor neutralizing antibody: novel concepts of angiostatic therapy from intravital videomicroscopy [J]. Cancer Research, 1996, 56(17): 4032-4039.

[33] Kim K J, Li B, Winer J, et al. Inhibition of vascular endothelial growth factor-induced angiogenesis supresses tumor growth *in vivo* [J]. Nature, 1993, 362(6423): 841-844.

[34] Mesiano S, Ferrara N, Jaffe R B. Role of vascular endothelial growth factor in ovarian cancer inhibition of ascites formation by immunoneutralization [J]. The American Journal of Pathology, 1998, 153(4): 1249-1256.

[35] Warren R S, Yuan H, Matli M R, et al. Regulation by vascular endothelial growth factor of human colon cancer tumorigenesis in a mouse model of experimental liver metastasis [J]. The Journal of Clinical Investigation, 1995, 95(4): 1789-1797.

[36] Hu L, Hofmann J, Zaloudek C, et al. Vascular endothelial growth factor immunoneutralization plus paclitaxel markedly reduces tumor burden and ascites in athymic mouse model of ovarian cancer [J]. The American Journal of Pathology, 2002, 161(5): 1917-1924.

[37] Sweeney C J, Miller K D, Sissons S E, et al. The antiangiogenic property of docetaxel is synergistic with a recombinant humanized monoclonal antibody against vascular endothelial growth factor or 2-methoxyestradiol but antagonized by endothelial growth factor [J]. Cancer Research, 2001, 61(8): 3369-3372.

[38] Borgstrom P, Gold D P, Hillan K J, et al. Importance of VEGF for breast cancer angiogenesis *in vivo*: implications from intravital microscopy of combination treatments with an anti-VEGF neutralizing monoclonal antibody and doxorubicin [J]. Anticancer Research, 1999, 19(5B): 4203-4214.

[39] Soffer S Z, Moore J T, Kim E, et al. Combination antiangiogenic therapy: increased efficacy in a murine model of Wilm tumor [J]. Journal of Pediatric Surgery, 2001, 36(8): 1177-1181.

[40] Kim E S, Soffer S Z, Huang J Z, et al. Distinct response of experimental neuroblastoma to combination antiangiogenic strategies [J]. Journal of Pediatric Surgery, 2002, 37(3): 518-522.

[41] FDA Database. https://www.accessdata.fda.gov/drugsatfda_docs/nda/2004/STN-125085_Avastin_Pharmr.pdf.

[42] Sandler A, Yi J, Dahlberg S, et al. Treatment outcomes by tumor histology in Eastern Cooperative Group Study E4599 of bevacizumab with paclitaxel/carboplatin for advanced non-small cell lung cancer [J]. Journal of Thoracic Oncology, 2010, 5(9): 1416-1423.

[43] Reck M, Pawel J V, Zatloukal P. Overall survival with cisplatin-gemcitabine and bevacizumab or placebo as first-line therapy for nonsquamous non-small-cell lung cancer: results from a randomized phase III trial (AVAiL) [J]. Annals of Oncology, 2010, 21(9): 1804-1809.

[44] FDA Database. https://www.accessdata.fda.gov/drugsatfda_docs/label/2017/125085s319lbl.pdf.

[45] Wick W W, Gorlia T, Bendszus M, et al. Lomustine and bevacizumab in progressive glioblastoma [J]. The New England Journal of Medicine, 2017, 377(50): 1954-1963.

[46] Escudier B, Cosaert J, Pisa P. Bevacizumab: direct anti-VEGF therapy in renal cell carcinoma [J]. Expert Review of Anticancer Therapy, 2008, 8(10): 1545-1557.

[47] FDA Database. http://101.96.10.43/www.accessdata.fda.gov/drugsatfda_docs/nda/2004/STN-125085_Avastin_BioPharmr.pdf.

CHAPTER

4

Blinatumomab

Blinatumomab

(Blincyto®)

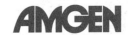

Research code: AMG-103, BiTE-MT-103, bscCD19xCD3, MEDI-538, MT-103

1 Target Biology

The CD19 Receptor

❖ CD19 is present on both healthy and malignant cells of B-lineage origin, and is critically important for B-cell function and tumor survival.

❖ CD19 is expressed on essentially all stages of B-cell lineage acute lymphoblastic leukemia (ALL), with expression levels of ≥95.0% on B-lineage cells.

❖ CD19 is also expressed across all non-Hodgkin's lymphoma (NHL) subtypes and in chronic lymphoblastic leukemia (CLL).

Biology Activity[1-3]

❖ The human CD19 gene is located on the short arm of chromosome 16 at band p11.2 and contains 15 exons and 18 introns, spanning 7.59 kb of DNA.

❖ The CD19 gene encodes for a 95 kDa transmembrane glycoprotein of the immunoglobulin superfamily. CD19 is a type I one-pass transmembrane protein.

❖ The human CD19 is 556 amino acids in length with an extracellular N-terminus and an intracellular C-terminus. It consists of two extracellular immunoglobulin-like domains, a short hydrophobic transmembrane region, and a roughly 242-amino acid-long cytoplasmic tail.

❖ CD19 is an adaptor and activator of PI3 kinase, an important signaling protein in malignant B cells.

❖ Expression of CD19 has also been described for leukemia-initiating cells with self-renewal capacity.

The CD3 Receptor

❖ CD3 is the specific marker of T cells, and is a component of the T-cell receptor (TCR) complex. Crosslinking of TCR complex leads to T cells activation.

Biology Activity[4, 5]

❖ With a protein transiently linking CD3+ polyclonal T cells to target cells, it induces cytotoxic T-lymphocyte (CTL) and T-helper cell activation followed by T-cell-mediated serial target cell lysis and concomitant T-cell proliferation.

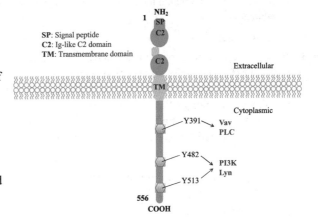

2 General Information

Blincyto®

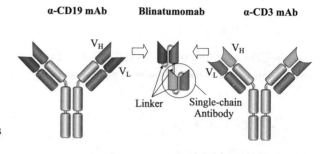

❖ Blincyto® (Blinatumomab) is a bispecific CD19-directed CD3 T-cell engager that binds to CD19 (expressed on cells of B-lineage origin) and CD3 (expressed on T cells).

❖ Blincyto® is a single chain bispecific antibody. The antibody struct was developed by genetic engineering from two distinct murine monoclonal antibodies: HD37, which recognizes the pan-B cell antigen CD19 and L2K-07, which binds the T-cell receptor-associated complex CD3.[3]

❖ The anti-CD19 scFv was generated by PCR with a 15-amino-acid (G4S1) 3 linker between the VH and VL chains. The anti-CD19 scFv was subsequently cloned into the bluescript KS vector containing the bispecific single-chain antibody 17-1AxCD3. The 17-1A scFv was substituted for the CD19 scFv, with an intact (G4S1)1 linker connecting it to the C-terminal of the anti-CD3 scFv. The DNA fragment, VLCD19-VHCD19-VHCD3-VLCD3 was subcloned into the mammalian expression vector pEF-DHFR (dihydrofolate reductase). It is expected to allow the two scFvs a high degree of rotational flexibility as may be needed for simultaneous binding to two epitopes positioned on cell membranes of two separate cells.[3, 6]

❖ Blincyto® is produced in Chinese hamster ovary cells. DHFR-negative Chinese hamster ovary (CHO) cells were electroporated with the plasmid DNA and grown in roller bottles in alpha-minimum essential medium.

❖ A hexahistidine sequence (6X-His) at the C-terminus is used for highly efficient capture from cell culture medium and for affinity purification of blinatumomab using nickel-nitrilotriacetic acid (Ni-NTA) column and eluted with 200 mM imidazole.

❖ The total sales of 115 million US$ for 2016; No sales data as of 2017.

❖ It consists of 504 amino acids and has a molecular weight of approximately 54 kDa.

❖ The CD19 binding N-terminal domain contains 4 cysteine residues that are involved in intramolecular disulfide bonds. The CD3 binding C-terminal domain contains 5 cysteine residues of which 4 are involved in intramolecular disulfide bonds.

❖ Blincyto® does not contain the N-linked glycosylation sequon and is aglycosylated.

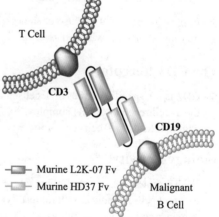

Mechanism of Action

❖ Blincyto® activates endogenous T cells by connecting CD3 in the T-cell receptor (TCR) complex with CD19 on benign and malignant B cells. Blinatumomab mediates the formation of a synapse between the T-cell and the tumor cell, upregulation of cell adhesion molecules, production of cytolytic proteins, release of inflammatory cytokines, and proliferation of T cells, which result in redirected lysis of CD19+ cells.[4, 6, 7]

Sponsor

❖ Blincyto® (Blinatumomab) was developed and marketed by Amgen.

World Sales[8]

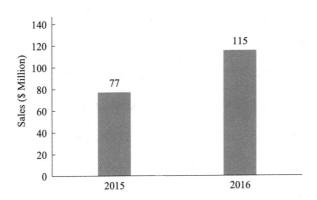

Figure 1   World Sales of Blinatumomab since 2015

Approval and Indications

Table 1   Summary of the Approved Indication[7-9]

Approval (Year)	Agency	Indication
2014	FDA	Philadelphia chromosome-negative (Ph⁻) relapsed or refractory B-cell precursor acute lymphoblastic leukemia (ALL) for use in adults.
2015	EMA	Used in adults with Ph⁻ relapsed or refractory B-cell precursor ALL.
2015	Korea	Used in adults with Ph⁻ relapsed or refractory B-cell precursor ALL.
2016	Canada	Conditionally approved for using in adults with Ph⁻ relapsed or refractory B-cell precursor ALL.
2016	FDA	Treatment of pediatric patients with Ph⁻ relapsed or refractory B-cell precursor ALL.

ALL: Acute lymphoblastic leukemia.

Table 2   Summary of the Approval of Blincyto®[7, 9]

	US (FDA)	EU (EMA)
First approval date	12/03/2014	11/23/2015
Application or approval No.	BLA125557	EMEA/H/C/003731
Brand name	Blincyto®	Blincyto®
Indication	Precursor Cell Lymphoblastic Leukemia-Lymphoma	Precursor Cell Lymphoblastic Leukemia-Lymphoma
Authorization holder	Amgen	Amgen

Till Jan 2018, it had not been approved by PMDA (Japan) and CFDA (China).

Table 3   Administration of Blincyto®[7, 9]

Patient Weight	Cycle 1ª			Cycle 2 and Subsequent Cyclesª	
	Days 1-7	Days 8-28	Days 29-42	Days 1-28	Days 29-42
≥45 kg (fixed dose)	9 mcg/day	28 mcg/day	14 days treatment free interval	28 mcg/day	14 days treatment free interval
<45 kg (BSA-based dose)	5 mcg/m²/day (not to exceed 9 mcg/day)	15 mcg/m²/day (not to exceed 28 mcg/day)		15 mcg/m²/day (not to exceed 28 mcg/day)	

ª A single cycle of treatment of Blincylo® consists of 28 days of continuous intravenous infusion followed by a 14-day treatment-free interval (total 42 days).

3 CMC Profile

Product Profile

Dosage route: IV infusion.

Administration: Administer as a continuous intravenous infusion at a constant flow rate using an infusion pump.

Dosage form and strength: 35 mcg of lyophilized powder in a single-dose vial for reconstitution.

Formulation:

Powder: Citric acid monohydrate (E330); Trehalose dehydrate; Lysine hydrochloride; Polysorbate 80; Sodium hydroxide (for pH-adjustment).

Solution (stabiliser): Citric acid monohydrate (E330); Lysine hydrochloride; Polysorbate 80; Sodium hydroxide (for pH-adjustment); Water for injections.

Dissolution: Reconstitution with 3 mL of preservative-free sterile water for injection, USP, then prepare the infusion bag accordingly based on the dosage requirement.

Stability: Based on the stability data provided, a 36-month expiration dating period is granted for the drug product when stored at 5 ± 3 °C and protected from light.

Amino Acid Sequence

❖ Blincyto® is a single chain bispecific antibody containing scFvs from two different antibodies.

❖ Molecular formula: $C_{2367}H_{3577}N_{649}O_{772}S_{19}$[10]

```
DIQLTQSPAS  LAVSLGQRAT  ISCKASQSVD  YDGDSYLNWY  QQIPGQPPKL  50
LIYDASNLVS  GIPPRFSGSG  SGTDFTLNIH  PVEKVDAATY  HCQQSTEDPW  100
TFGGGTKLEI  KGGGGSGGGG  SGGGGSQVQL  QQSGAELVRP  GSSVKISCKA  150
SGYAFSSYWM  NWVKQRPGQG  LEWIGQIWPG  DGDTNYNGKF  KGKATLTADE  200
SSSTAYMQLS  SLASEDSAVY  FCARRETTTV  GRYYYAMDYW  GQGTTVTVSS  250
GGGGSDIKLQ  QSGAELARPG  ASVKMSCKTS  GYTFTRYTMH  WVKQRPGQGL  300
EWIGYINPSR  GYTNYNQKFK  DKATLTTDKS  SSTAYMQLSS  LTSEDSAVYY  350
CARYYDDHYC  LDYWGQGTTL  TVSSVEGGSG  GSGGSGGSGG  VDDIQLTQSP  400
AIMSASPGEK  VTMTCRASSS  VSYMNWYQQK  SGTSPKRWIY  DTSKVASGVP  450
YRFSGSGSGT  SYSLTISSME  AEDAATYYCQ  QWSSNPLTFG  AGTKLEKLHH  500
HHHH                                                      504
```

Disulfide bridges location/Position des ponts disulfure/Posiciones de los puentes disulfuro
23-92 148-222 277-351 415-479
N-glycosylation sites/Sites de *N*-glycosylation/Posicipnes de *N*-glcosilacion
307 (but Pro in 308)

Production Process

❖ Production platform: CHO cells platform.

❖ Protein yield: NA.

❖ Protein purity: NA.

4 Pre-clinical Pharmacodynamics

Summary

Overview of *in vitro* Activities[11]

❖ Blinatumomab bound to B and T lymphocytes from human and chimpanzee peripheral blood mononuclear cells (PBMC), but it did not bind to PBMC from the mouse, rat, beagle dog, squirrel monkey, African Green monkey, Cynomolgus monkey, rhesus monkey and baboon.

❖ *In vitro*, binding of blinatumomab to CD3+ (CD45RO+CD8+ and CD4+) T cells and CD19+ tumor cell lines resulted in cytokine release (i.e. IL-2 and TNF-alpha), T-cell proliferation, increased expression of granzyme B, and redirected cytotoxicity of CD19+ target cells.

Overview of *in vivo* Activities[12]

❖ Human CD19+ leukemia cell line NALM-6 xenograft mouse models
  • Complete tumor growth inhibition with dose ⩾0.1 μg.

❖ Human CD19+ leukemia cell line Raji xenograft mouse models

• $\geqslant$0.5 µg/kg: Statistically significant inhibition or impairment of tumor formation vs. vehicle-treated control group.

Overview of *in vitro* Activities

Target Binding and Mechanism of Action

❖ AMG-103 had K_d values of 1.5 nM and 25 microM for CD19 and CD3, respectively.

❖ Blinatumomab binds in a dose-dependent manner to malignant B-cell lines NALM-6 and Raji, and could also bind to normal human B cells.

Cell-based Activities *in vitro*

Table 4　The EC_{50} of Blinatumomab toward CD19+ Target Cells[7, 11]

Effector Cell	Target Cell	EC_{50} (pg/mL)
Human PBMC	Human autologous B cells	130 ± 11.0
Chimpanzee PBMC	Chimpanzee autologous B cells	150 ± 15.0
Human PBMC	NALM-6	50.0 ± 3.0
Chimpanzee PBMC	NALM-6	40.0 ± 2.0

❖ The specificity of blinatumomab activity was investigated using target cells not expressing CD19 such as human HT29 colon carcinoma cells. The viability of HT29 cells remained unaffected at blinatumomab concentrations up to 100 ng/mL, i.e. 1,000-fold greater than the EC_{50} values determined in NALM-6 cells.

Overview of *in vivo* Activities

Table 5　Summary of *in vivo* Activities of Blinatumomab[13]

Study	Tumor Model[a]	Treatment[b]	Main Result
103-PCD-0057	s.c. NALM-6 100:1	i.v.; Once daily for 5 days starting on the day of inoculation; 0.001, 0.01, 0.1, 1 µg/day.	$\geqslant$0.1 µg: Complete inhibition of tumor growth.
103-PCD-0059	s.c. NALM-6 80:1	i.v.; Once daily for 5 days starting on the day of inoculation; Blinatumomab: 1 µg/day; MT102: 1 µg/day.	Blinatumomab: Complete inhibition of tumor growth (specific effect did not impact on tumor growth in MT102-treated animals-all died by Day 35).
103-PCD-0058	s.c. NALM-6 78:1	i.v.; Once daily for 5 days starting on either the day of inoculation, or 4, 8, or 12 days following inoculation; 1 µg/day.	Complete inhibition of tumor growth in groups treated from Day 0 or Day 4. Protection no longer observed in groups treated 8 or 12 days after inoculation (due to short half-life of human T cells?).
103-PCD-0099	s.c. SEMc 1:2	i.v.; Once daily for 10 days starting on the day of inoculation; 13, 67, 334 µg/(kg·day).	Significant inhibition or delay of tumor growth in all treatment groups. On Days 40, 6/10, 6/10, and 8/10 animals were tumor-free or with tumor volume <50 mm³ in groups dosed at 13, 67, and 334 µg/kg, respectively (1/10 in vehicle control).
103-PCD-0097	SC Raji 1:2	i.v.; Once daily for 10 days starting on the day of inoculation; 13, 67, 334 µg/(kg·day).	Significant growth delay of tumors. Complete prevention of tumor formation in 4/10, 3/10 and 9/10 animals treated at 13, 67, and 334 µg/kg, respectively (all vehicle-treated animals developed tumors) on Day 26.
R20130026	s.c. Raji 5:1	i.v.; Once daily for 5 days starting on the day of inoculation; 0.5, 5, 50, 500 µg/(kg·day).	$\geqslant$0.5 µg/kg: Statistically significant inhibition or impairment of tumor formation vs. vehicle-treated control group. Tumor-free animals (Day 29): 1/8 and 3/8 at 50 and 500 µg/kg, respectively. Small (encapsulated) tumor tissue remnants (Day 29): 2/8 and 7/8 animals.

[a] Route of injection, tumor cell, E:T ratio.　[b] Route, schedule, doses.

Efficacy Studies

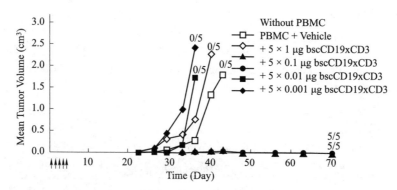

Study: The effect of bscCD19xCD3 on s.c. NALM-6 B lymphoma growth in NOD/SCID mice.

Animal: NOD/SCID mice.

Model: NALM-6 B lymphoma cells were inoculated s.c. into the nude mice.

Administration: The indicated doses of bscCD19xCD3 were administrated i.v. on Days 0, 1, 2, 3 and 4, following tumor cell/PBMC inoculation.

Starting: Upon tumor inoculation.

Test: Measured tumor volumes.

Result: At cumulative doses of 5 or 0.5 μg bscCD19xCD3, none of the animals developed detectable tumors and survived inoculation of NALM-6 cells for the entire observation period of 76 days. Cumulative doses of bscCD19xCD3 of 0.05 and 0.005 μg were not effective in preventing tumor growth.

Figure 2　The Effect of bscCD19xCD3 on s.c. NALM-6 B Lymphoma Growth in NOD/SCID Mice[12]

5　Toxicology

Summary

Non-clinical Single-Dose Toxicology
❖ No single-dose toxicology studies were submitted.

Non-clinical Repeated-Dose Toxicology
❖ The exposure of chimpanzees in term of AUC_{inf} was 2.9 (M) and 5.6 (F) ng·h/mL with C_{max} of 0.90 (M) and 1.4 (F) ng/mL, i.e. higher than C_{ss} reached at the clinical doses of 9 μg/day (211 pg/mL) and 28 μg/day (621 pg/mL) for the treatment of relapsed/refractory ALL.
❖ Since there are very limited possibilities to evaluate the toxicology of blinatumomab in the only non-clinical relevant species for ethical reasons, a surrogate BiTE molecule specific for murine CD3 and murine CD19 from rat monoclonal antibodies were developed. Additional studies were conducted in mice with this surrogate muS103 new.

Cross-reactivity
❖ No unspecific binding was found when following tissues were stained: Adrenal, brain (cerebellum, cortex), blood leuko-cytes, blood vessels (endothelium), bone marrow, mammary gland, eye, fallopian tube, GI tract (colon, oesophagus, small intestine, stomach), heart, kidney, liver, lung, lymph node, ovary, pancreas, parathyroid, peripheral nerve, pituitary, placenta, prostate, salivary gland, skin, spinal cord, spleen, striated muscle, testis, thymus, thyroid, tonsil, ureter, urinary bladder, and uterus (endometrium, cervix).

Reproductive Toxicology
❖ Reproductive toxicity studies have not been conducted with blinatumomab.
❖ In an embryo-foetal developmental toxicity study performed in mice, the murine surrogate crossed the placenta to a limited extent (foetal-to-maternal serum concentration ratio <1.0%) and did not induce embryo-foetal toxicity or teratogenicity.
❖ There were no effects on male or female reproductive organs in toxicity studies with the murine surrogate.

Anti-drug Antibody (ADA)
❖ Development of ADAs in the pivotal toxicity studies did not impact on their validity since neither the kinetics nor the pharmacological effect of muS103new or blinatumomab were affected. The occurrence of ADAs was mainly reported at low dose levels, which may not have completely disrupted humoral immunity.

Other Toxicology
❖ *In vitro* and *in vivo* genotoxicity studies were not performed.
❖ No carcinogenicity studies were performed.
❖ No local irritation was observed when trastuzumab was given by single bolus i.v. injection into the rabbit ear vein.
❖ No effect on sedimentation and thrombin in human and monkey blood *in vitro*.

6 Non-clinical Pharmacokinetic/ADME/Toxicokinetics

Summary

❖ In mice treated with blinatumomab, a dose-proportional increase in exposure was noted in the i.v. groups. The volume of distribution based on the terminal phase ranged from 150 to 350 mL/kg, and the clearance from 70.0 to 105 mL/h·kg. The absolute s.c. bioavailability reached 35.0%. The half-life did not exceed 2.5 hours.
❖ In rats, an over-proportional increase in systemic exposure was noted over the 25.0 to 2,500 µg/kg dose range given by i.v. route. In contrast, s.c. administration of the same dose levels by the s.c. route resulted in a dose-proportional increase in exposure. Absolute s.c. bioavailability ranged from 8.0% to 16.0%. The half-life values were 5-7 hours after i.v. dosing. In the s.c. groups, it reached 8 hours at the high dose level (2,500 µg/kg) and increased with decreasing doses at up to 126 hours.
❖ In Cynomolgus monkeys, the absolute s.c. bioavailability was 21.0%. Upon i.v. administration, the systemic exposure increased in a dose-proportional manner from 10.0 to 500 µg/kg. The half-life ranged from 1 to 2.7 hours at up to 100 µg/kg, and reached 6.3 hours at 500 µg/kg.
❖ In the pharmacologically-relevant species (chimpanzee), blinatumomab was administered i.v. by means of 2-hour infusions once weekly. The half-life ranged from 1.5 to 2.6 hours. C_{max} levels remained constant throughout the dosing period in the 4-week study.
❖ The volume of distribution (V_z) of blinatumomab was estimated from i.v. dosing in various animal species. It reached 268, 55.0, and 68.0-110 mL/kg in mice, dogs, and chimpanzee, respectively.

Non-clinical Pharmacokinetics

Table 6　*In vivo* Pharmacokinetic Parameters of Blinatumomab in Chimpanzees[14]

Dosage (lg/kg)	C_{max} (ng/mL)	AUC_{last} (ng·h/mL)	Half-life (h)
0.06	0.42	1.6	1.9
0.1	0.72	2.4	1.8
0.12	0.75	2.5	1.7

❖ The clearance ranged between 35.3 mL/(h·kg) and 46.1 mL/(h·kg) and the volume of distribution between 94.6 mL/kg and 110 mL/kg.

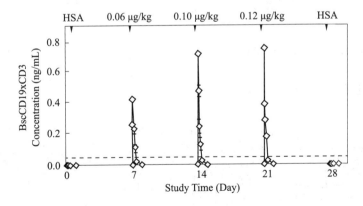

Figure 3　The Pharmacokinetic Profile of Blinatumomab[14]

❖ The pharmacokinetic profile of bscCD19xCD3 paralleled the pharmacodynamic effects induced by bscCD19xCD3 in the dose escalation study. Escalating doses of bscCD19xCD3 induced a marked but transient increase in serum levels of IL-6, IFN-γ and soluble CD25 (sCD25) following each bscCD19xCD3 infusion. Data shown in Figure 4.

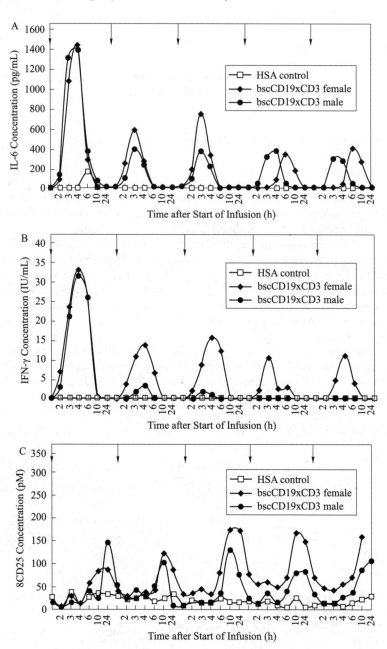

Figure 4　The Pharmacodynamic Effects Induced by bscCD19xCD3 in the Dose Escalation Study[14]

Non-clinical Multiple-Dose Toxicology

Table 7　Repeated-Dose Toxicity Studies of Blinatumomab[13]

Species	Duration	Dose [μg/(kg·day)]	Gender	C_{max} (ng/mL)	AUC_{last} (ng·h/mL)	AUC_{inf} (ng·h/mL)
Chimpanzee	28 days (5 weekly doses) + 4-week recovery period	0.1 μg/kg, on Days 0, 7, 14, 21, 28	Male	17.7	2.9	3.0
			Female	59.0	5.1	5.6

7   Clinical Efficacy and Safety

Overview Profile

❖ In December 2014, blinatumomab was launched in the US for the treatment of adults with Ph-relapsed/refractory B-precursor ALL, based on Phase 2 data.

❖ In November 2015, blinatumomab was granted centralized conditional approval in the EU in all 28-member states plus Iceland, Lichtenstein and Norway for the treatment of adults with Ph-relapsed/refractory B-precursor ALL with full approval upon fulfillment of postmarketing requirements.

❖ In September 2016, the FDA approved blinatumomab for the treatment of pediatric patients with Ph-relapsed or refractory B-cell precursor ALL based on the sBLA data from the Phase 1/2 study (MT103-205).

❖ In July 2017, FDA expanded blinatumomab's indication to include Ph-relapsed or refractory B-cell precursor ALL based on a single arm, multicenter study (ALCANTARA) and approved blinatumomab for the treatment of relapsed or refractory B-cell precursor ALL in adults and children.

Table 8   Summary of the Pivotal Clinical Studies Supporting Blinatumomab's Approval in FDA[15-18]

ID	Phase	N	Population	Design, Objectives	Study Posology
MT 103-211	2	189	Adults with R/R Ph⁻ALL	Open-label, multicenter, single arm study to investigate the efficacy, safety, tolerability, PK and PD.	CTM4 & CTM5 9/28 µg/day cIV for 4 weeks followed by 2 weeks off drug per cycle.
MT 103-205	2	93	Pediatric subjects <18 years with ALL	Multicenter, single arm study preceded by dose evaluation to investigate the efficacy, safety, and tolerability of blinatumomab in pediatric and adolescent subjects with R/R ALL.	Phase 1: 3.75 to 60 µg/(m²·day) cIV for 4 weeks followed by 2 weeks off. Phase 2: Up to 5 cycles with dose of blinatumomab established in Phase 1.
ALCANTARA	2	45	Adults with R/R Ph⁺ ALL	Multicenter, single arm study to evaluate the efficacy and tolerability of blinatumomab in subjects with R/R Ph⁺ ALL.	Blinatumomab was administered 9 µg/day in Week 1 of Cycle 1, followed by 28 µg/day. Each treatment cycle included 4 weeks of cIV followed by a 2-week treatment free interval.
TOWER	3	405	Adults with R/R Ph⁻ ALL	Multicenter, single arm study to investigate the efficacy and safety of blinatumomab in subjects with Ph⁻ B-cell precusor R/R ALL.	Blinatumomab was administered 9 µg/day on Days 1-7 and 28 µg/day on Days 8-28 for Cycle 1 in a 42-day cycle, at 28 µg/day on Days 1-28 for Cycles 2-5 in 42-day cycles, and at 28 µg/day on Days 1-28 for Cycles 6-9 in 84-day cycles.

cIV: Continuous intravenous infusion.   CR: Complete remission.   CRh: Complete remission with partial hematological recovery. C_{ss}: Steady-state concentration. CTM4: Process 4 clinical material.   CTM5: Process 5 clinical material.   MRD: Minimal residual disease.   R/R: Relapsed/refractory.

Clinical Efficacy

Table 9   Efficacy Data of the Pivotal Study (MT103-211) for Blinatumomab's Approval in Adults with R/R Ph⁻ ALL[15]

	Patients	Proportion (95% *CI*)
CR or CRh during the first two cycles	81/189	43.0% (36-50)
Best response during the first two cycles[a]		
CR	63/189	33.0% (27-41)
CRh	18/189	10.0% (6-15)
No response to therapy[b]	90/189	48.0%
Not evaluable[c]	18/189	10.0%
Allogeneic HSCT after CR or CRh	32/81	40.0%
Allogeneic HSCT after CR	28/63	44.0%
Allogeneic HSCT after CRh	4/18	22.0%
MRD response during the first two cycles in patients with CR or CRh[d]	60/73	82.0% (7,290)
100-day mortality from day of HSCT	32	11.0% (0-23)

Data are *n/N*, %, or % (95% *CI*).   ANC: Absolute neutrophil count.   CR: Complete remission.   CRh: CR with partial recovery of peripheral blood counts.   HSCT: Haemopoietic stem-cell transplantation.   MRD: Minimal residual disease.   [a] Three patients with CRh as best response during the first two cycles achieved CR by cycle three or beyond.   One initial nonresponder achieved CR after cycle three, for a total of 82 patients with CR or CRh (the patient continued treatment after a haematological response in cycle two although the presence of extramedullary leukaemia should have prompted discontinuation).   [b] Includes no response to blinatumomab (*n* = 41), progressive disease (*n* = 27), blast-free hypocellular bone marrow (blasts ≤5.0% with either platelets <50,000 cells/μL or ANC <500 cells/μL; *n* = 17), and partial remission (*n* = 5).   [c] Death before the first response assessment (nine patients) or adverse events leading to treatment discontinuation before the first response assessment (nine patients).   [d] Evaluable patients with CR or CRh response in the first two cycles and available MRD data.   Eight patients among the 81 responders in the first two cycles had no MRD assessment due to technical limitations or sample quality.

Table 10   Efficacy Data of the Pivotal Study (MT103-205) for Blinatumomab's Approval in Pediatric R/R Ph⁻ ALL[16]

Efficacy Outcomes and Ability to Proceed to alloHSCT	Patients in Phase 2 (*N* = 44)[a]			All Patients at Recommended Dosage (*N* = 70)[a]			Patients <2 Years at Recommended Dosage (*N* = 10)[a]		
	n	%	95% *CI*	*n*	%	95% *CI*	*n*	%	95% *CI*
Hematologic response									
CR with in the first two cycles	14	32.0	19-48	27	39.0	27-51	6	60.0	26-88
Nonresponders (did not achieve CR)									
Partial remission	3	7.0		4	6.0		0	0.0	
Blast-free hypoplastic or aplastic bone marrow	0	0.0		2	3.0		0	0.0	
Progressive disease	8	18.0		10	14.0		2	20.0	
No response	14	32.0		21	30.0		2	20.0	
No response assessment[b]	5	11.0		6	9.0		NA	NA	
CR within the first two cycles by baseline bone marrow blast count									
<50.0% blasts at baseline	5/12	42.0	15-72	10/18	56.0	31-79	2/2	100	16-100
≥50.0% blasts at baseline	9/32	28.0	14-47	17/52	33.0	20-47	4/8	50.0	16-84
Relapse or death after CR[c]	10/14	71.0		7/27	26.0		4/6	67.0	
MRD response in patients who achieved CR within the first two cycles									
MRD response	8/14	57.0	29-82	14/27	52.0	32-71	3/6	50.0	12-88
Complete MRD response	8/14	57.0	29-82	14/27	52.0	32-71	3/6	50.0	
No MRD response	6/14	43.0		12	44.0		3/6	50.0	
No data available	0	0.0		1	4.0	32-71	0	0.0	
Ability to proceed to HSCT									
Patients who received alloHSCT	13	30.0		24	34.0		4	10.0	

Continued

Efficacy Outcomes and Ability to Proceed to alloHSCT	Patients in Phase 2 (N = 44)[a]			All Patients at Recommended Dosage (N = 70)[a]			Patients <2 Years at Recommended Dosage (N = 10)[a]		
	n	%	95% CI	n	%	95% CI	n	%	95% CI
Patients in blinatumomab-induced CR	5	11.0		13	19.0		4	40.0	
Patients in CR who received only blinatumomab	2	5.0		8	11.0				
100-day mortality rate[d]		NE	NE		25.0	7-69		NE	NE
Nonresponders who received subsequent treatments[e]	8	18.0		11	16.0		NA	NA	

alloHSCT: Allogeneic hematopoietic stem-cell transplantation.   CR: Complete remission.   HSCT: Hematopoietic stem-cell transplantation.   MRD: Minimal residual disease.   NA: Not applicable.   NE: Not evaluated.   [a] All patients treated at 5/15 μA/(m²·day) in Phase 1 or 2.   [b] Patients died (n = 5) or withdrew consent (n = 1) before the first response assessment.   [c] Relapse during the efficacy follow-up (no chemotherapy or alloHSCT between end of blinatumomab treatment and relapse).   [d] Calculated from the date of alloHSCT for all patients who received only blinatumomab at the recommended dose.   Not calculated for the other two patient groups because of limited sample size.   [e] Patients who were refractory to blinatumomab but who received subsequent treatments and then proceeded to alloHSCT.

Table 11   Efficacy Data of the Pivotal Study (ALCANTARA) for Blinatumomab's Approval in Adults R/R Ph⁺ ALL[17]

Outcome	Patients (n/NI)[a]	Proportion (%)	95% CI
Primary endpoint			
CR/CRh during the first two cycles	16/45	36.0	22-51
Philadelphia chromosome and other cytogenetic abnormalities	10/22	45.0	24-68
ABL kinase domain mutations	6/17	35.0	14-62
T315I mutation	4/10	40.0	12-74
P190 BCR/ABL1 isoform[b]	10/26	39.0	20-59
P210 BCR/ABL1 isoform[b]	5/16	31.0	11-59
No. of prior TKI therapies			
1	1/7	14.0	<1-8
2	8/17	33.0	15-57
≥3	8/17	47.0	23-72
Prior ponatinib	8/23	35.0	16-57
Prior alloHSCT	5/20	25.0	9-49
Age 18 to <55 years	8/22	36.0	17-59
Age ≥55 years	8/23	35.0	16-57
Bone marrow blasts <50.0%	7/11	64.0	31-89
Bone marrow blasts ≥50.0%	9/34	27.0	13-44
Secondary endpoint			
Best response during the first two cycles			
CR	14/45	31.0	18-47
CRh	2/45	4.0	1-15
Complete MRD response[c]	14/16	88.0	62-98
alloHSCT after blinatumomab-induced remission[d]	4/16	25.0	7-52
Age 18 to <55 years	2/8	25.0	3-65
Age ≥55 years	2/8	25.0	3-65
100-day post-transplant mortality rate[d]	1/4	25.0	4-87

Complete MRD response was defined as no detectable PCR amplification of BCR-ABL1 genes (sensitivity ≥10⁻⁵) as assessed by a central laboratory.   alloHSCT: Allogeneic hematopoietic stem-cell transplantation.   ABL1: Abelson murine leukemia viral oncogene homolog 1.   BCR: Breakpoint cluster region.   CR: Complete remission.   CRh: CR with partial hematologic recovery.   MRD: Minimal residual disease.   TKI: Tyrosine kinase inhibitor.   [a] n/NI, number of responders/total number of patients with evaluable data under each category.   [b] Isoform designation was determined by MRD status at baseline by using reverse transcription quantitative polymerase chain reaction (PCR) on pretreatment bone marrow aspirates.   A subset of patients (n = 10) had both p190 and p210 transcripts, although in all of these patients, p210 was 2.1- to 3.5-log higher; the transcripts were thus assigned a designation of p210.   Further details are provided in Patients and Methods.   [c] Among CR/CRh responders only; includes all four CR/CRh patients with the T315I mutation.   [d] For patients who received alloHSCT during blinatumomab-induced remission without other antileukemia therapy.

Table 12   Efficacy Data of the Clinical Benefit Confirmed Study (TOWER) for Blinatumomab's Approval in Adults R/R Ph⁻ ALL (Best Hematologic Response within 12 Weeks after Treatment Initiation[a])[18]

	Blinatumomab Group (N = 271)		Chemotherapy Group (N = 134)		Treatment Difference (95% CI)	P-value[b]
	n	% (95% CI)	n	% (95% CI)	Percentage points	
Complete remission with full hematologic recovery	91	33.6 (28.0-39.5)	21	15.7 (10.0-23.0)	17.9 (9.6-26.2)	<0.0010
Complete remission with full, partial, or incomplete hematologic recovery	119	43.9 (37.9-50.0)	33	24.6 (17.6-32.8)	19.3 (9.9-28.7)	<0.0010
Complete remission with partial hematologic recovery	24	8.9 (5.8-12.9)	6	4.5 (1.7-9.5)		
Complete remission with incomplete hematologic recovery	4	1.5 (0.40-3.7)	6	4.5 (1.7-9.5)		

[a] Data are summarized for all patients who underwent randomization (intention-to-treat population).   Complete remission was defined as 5.0% or less bone marrow blasts and no evidence of disease and was further characterized according to the extent of recovery of peripheral blood counts as follows: complete remission with full recovery (platelet count of >100,000 per microliter and absolute neutrophil count of >1,000 per microliter), complete remission with partial recovery (platelet count of >50,000 per microliter and absolute neutrophil count of >500 per microliter), or complete remission with incomplete recovery (platelet count of >100,000 per microliter or absolute neutrophil count of >1,000 per microliter).   [b] Rates were compared with the use of a Cochran-Mantel-Haenszel test, with adjustment for the following stratification factors: age (<35 vs. ≥35 years), previous salvage therapy (yes vs. no), and previous allogeneic stem-cell transplantation (yes vs. no).

Clinical Safety

Table 13   AEs of Blinatumomab's Pivotal Study MT103-211[15]

	Any Grade n (%)	Worst Grade 1-2 n (%)	Worst Grade 3 n (%)	Worst Grade 4 n (%)	Worst Grade 5 n (%)
Patients with adverse events	188 (99.0)	33 (17.0)	71 (38.0)	56 (30.0)	28 (15.0)
Adverse events of worst Grade ≥3 occurring in ≥5.0% of patients					
Febrile neutropenia	53 (28.0)	5 (3.0)	46 (24.0)	2 (1.0)	0 (0.0)
Neutropenia	33 (17.0)	3 (2.0)	9 (5.0)	21 (11.0)	0 (0.0)
Anaemia	38 (20.0)	11 (6.0)	25 (13.0)	2 (1.0)	0 (0.0)
Pneumonia	18 (10.0)	1 (<1.0)	13 (7.0)	2 (1.0)	2 (1.0)
Thrombocytopenia	21 (11.0)	5 (3.0)	2 (1.0)	14 (7.0)	0 (0.0)
Hyperglycaemia	24 (13.0)	9 (5.0)	15 (8.0)	0 (0.0)	0 (0.0)
Leucopenia	19 (10.0)	4 (2.0)	7 (4.0)	8 (4.0)	0 (0.0)
Alanine aminotransferase increased	24 (13.0)	11 (6.0)	12 (6.0)	1 (<1.0)	0 (0.0)
Hypokalaemia	45 (24.0)	32 (17.0)	10 (5.0)	3 (2.0)	0 (0.0)
Pyrexia	113 (60.0)	100 (53.0)	13 (7.0)	0 (0.0)	0 (0.0)
Sepsis	13 (7.0)	2 (1.0)	3 (2.0)	4 (2.0)	4 (2.0)
Hypophosphatemia	13 (7.0)	3 (2.0)	8 (4.0)	2 (1.0)	0 (0.0)
Patients with neurologic events	98 (52.0)	74 (39.0)	20 (11.0)	4 (2.0)	0 (0.0)
All patients with neurologic events of worst Grade ≥3					
Tremor	33 (17.0)	32 (17.0)	1 (<1.0)	0 (0.0)	0 (0.0)
Dizziness	26 (14.0)	25 (13.0)	1 (<1.0)	0 (0.0)	0 (0.0)
Confusional state	14 (7.0)	11 (6.0)	3 (2.0)	0 (0.0)	0 (0.0)
Encephalopathy	10 (5.0)	4 (2.0)	5 (3.0)	1 (<1.0)	0 (0.0)
Ataxia	9 (5.0)	6 (3.0)	2 (1.0)	1 (<1.0)	0 (0.0)
Somnolence	9 (5.0)	8 (4.0)	1 (<1.0)	0 (0.0)	0 (0.0)
Aphasia	7 (4.0)	5 (3.0)	2 (1.0)	0 (0.0)	0 (0.0)
Mental status change	7 (4.0)	5 (3.0)	2 (1.0)	0 (0.0)	0 (0.0)
Dysarthria	6 (3.0)	5 (3.0)	1 (<1.0)	0 (0.0)	0 (0.0)

Continued

	Any Grade n (%)	Worst Grade 1-2 n (%)	Worst Grade 3 n (%)	Worst Grade 4 n (%)	Worst Grade 5 n (%)
Neurotoxicity[a]	5 (3.0)	3 (2.0)	2 (1.0)	0 (0.0)	0 (0.0)
Convulsion	4 (2.0)	3 (2.0)	0 (0.0)	1 (<1.0)	0 (0.0)
Nervous system disorder[a]	3 (2.0)	0 (0.0)	3 (2.0)	0 (0.0)	0 (0.0)
Dysaesthesia	3 (2.0)	2 (1.0)	1 (<1.0)	0 (0.0)	0 (0.0)
Cognitive disorder	3 (2.0)	2 (1.0)	1 (<1.0)	0 (0.0)	0 (0.0)
Bradyphrenia	2 (1.0)	1 (<1.0)	1 (<1.0)	0 (0.0)	0 (0.0)
Hemiparesis	2 (1.0)	1 (<1.0)	1 (<1.0)	0 (0.0)	0 (0.0)
Altered state of consciousness	1 (<1.0)	0 (0.0)	1 (<1.0)	0 (0.0)	0 (0.0)
Febrile delirium	1 (<1.0)	0 (0.0)	0 (0.0)	1 (<1.0)	0 (0.0)
Neurologic symptom[a]	1 (<1.0)	0 (0.0)	1 (<1.0)	0 (0.0)	0 (0.0)
Stupor	1 (<1.0)	0 (0.0)	1 (<1.0)	0 (0.0)	0 (0.0)
Syncope	1 (<1.0)	0 (0.0)	1 (<1.0)	0 (0.0)	0 (0.0)

Data are *n* (%), where *n* is the number of patients. Table shows events for all patients (*n* = 189) during the treatment period and until the end-of-core-study visit (30 days after last treatment or before allogeneic HSCT). [a] Terms provided by study sites without further specification.

Table 14   AEs of Blinatumomab's Pivotal Study MT103-205[16]

Adverse Event	All Patients[a] (*N* = 70)
Patients with adverse events	70 (100)
Adverse events of worst Grade ≥3 occurring in ≥5.0% of patients	61 (87.0)
Anemia	25 (36.0)
Thrombocytopenia	15 (21.0)
Febrile neutropenia	12 (17.0)
Hypokalemia	12 (17.0)
Neutropenia	12 (17.0)
Alanine aminotransferase increased	11 (16.0)
Platelet count decreased	10 (14.0)
Pyrexia	10 (14.0)
Neutrophil count decreased	9 (13.0)
Aspartate aminotransferase increased	8 (11.0)
Leukopenia	7 (10.0)
White blood cell count decreased	7 (10.0)
Cytokine-release syndrome	4 (6.0)
Hypertension	4 (6.0)
Fatal adverse events on study[b]	6 (7.0)
Multiorgan failure[c]	2 (3.0)
Sepsis	1 (1.0)
Fungal infection	1 (1.0)
Respiratory failure[c]	1 (1.0)
Thrombocytopenia	1 (1.0)

Table shows adverse events regardless of relationship to treatment that occurred during the treatment period and until 30 days after the last treatment or before allogeneic hematopoietic stem-cell transplantation or start of chemotherapy. AEs: Adverse events. [a] All patients who received the recommended dose of 5/15 mg/(m²·day) in Phase 1 or 2. [b] Does not include two deaths caused by disease progression, including one patient who died as a result of recurrent leukemia. These deaths were reported by the investigators as adverse events. [c] Patient died after allogeneic hematopoietic stem-cell transplantation after blinatumomab-induced remission (only one of the patients with multiorgan failure).

Table 15 AEs of Blinatumomab's Pivotal Study-ALCANTARA[17]

Event	Any Grade		Grade 1-2		Grade 3		Grade 4	
	n	%	n	%	n	%	n	%
Patients with AEs	45	100	45	100	33	73.0	16	36.0
AEs of Grade ≥3 occurring in ≥5.0% of patients[a]								
Pyrexia	26	58.0	24	53.0	5	11.0	0	0.0
Febrile neutropenia	18	40.0	9	20.0	12	27.0	0	0.0
Headache	14	31.0	13	29.0	3	7.0	0	0.0
Anemia	13	29.0	9	20.0	7	16.0	1	2.0
Thrombocytopenia	10	22.0	4	9.0	5	11.0	7	16.0
Pain	7	16.0	4	9.0	4	9.0	0	0.0
Increased aspartate aminotransferase	6	13.0	3	7.0	3	7.0	2	4.0
Increased alanine aminotransferase	5	11.0	1	2.0	5	11.0	0	0.0
Device-related infection	5	11.0	3	7.0	3	7.0	0	0.0
Neutropenia	3	7.0	0	0.0	0	0.0	3	7.0
Patients with neurologic events	21	47.0	20	44.0	3	7.0	0	0.0
Neurologic events occurring in ≥2 patients								
Paresthesia	6	13.0	6	13.0	0	0.0	0	0.0
Confusional state	5	11.0	5	11.0	0	0.0	0	0.0
Dizziness	4	9.0	4	9.0	0	0.0	0	0.0
Tremor	4	9.0	4	9.0	0	0.0	0	0.0
Aphasia	2	4.0	1	2.0	1	2.0	0	0.0
Cerebellar syndrome	2	4.0	2	4.0	0	0.0	0	0.0
Memory impairment	2	4.0	2	4.0	0	0.0	0	0.0
Nervous system disorder	2	4.0	1	2.0	1	2.0	0	0.0

AEs: Adverse events.   [a] Cutoff based on Grade ≥3 AEs.

Table 16 AEs of Blinatumomab's Clinical Benefit Confirmed Study TOWER[18]

Event	Blinatumomab Group (N = 267)	Chemotherapy Group (N = 109)
	n (%)	n (%)
Any adverse event	263 (98.5)	108 (99.1)
Events leading to premature discontinuation of trial treatment	33 (12.4)	9 (8.3)
Serious adverse events	165 (61.8)	49 (45.0)
Fatal serious adverse events	51 (19.1)	19 (17.4)
Any adverse events of Grade ≥3	231 (86.5)	100 (91.7)
Grade ≥3 adverse event of interest reported in at least 3.0% of patients in either group		
Neutropenia	101 (37.8)	63 (57.8)
Infection	91 (34.1)	57 (52.3)
Elevated liver enzyme	34 (12.7)	16 (14.7)
Neurologic event	25 (9.4)	9 (8.3)
Cytokine release syndrome	13 (4.9)	0
Infusion reaction	9 (3.4)	1 (0.90)

Continued

Event	Blinatumomab Group (N = 267)	Chemotherapy Group (N = 109)
	n (%)	n (%)
Lymphopenia	4 (1.5)	4 (3.7)
Any decrease in platelet count	17 (6.4)	13 (11.9)
Any decrease in white-cell count	14 (5.2)	6 (5.5)

Data were summarized for all patients who received at least one dose of trial treatment.   AEs: Adverse events.

8 Clinical Pharmacokinetics

Summary

❖ To the best of our knowledge, no single-dose studies were conducted to characterize the pharmacokinetic profile of blinatumomab.

❖ Blinatumomab demonstrated linear pharmacokinetics.   Mean steady-state serum concentrations (C_{ss}) values increased approximately dose proportionally from 5 to 90 $\mu g/(m^2 \cdot day)$.

❖ During continuous intravenous over 4 weeks, blinatumomab C_{ss} were achieved within a day and remained stable during the infusion period.

❖ The estimated blinatumomab mean volume of distribution (V_z) was 4.5 L, mean systemic clearance (CL) was 2.9 L/h, and mean elimination half-life ($t_{1/2}$) was 2.1 hours.

❖ The pharmacokinetic profiles of blinatumomab were not affected by body weight, BSA, age, or sex in adult patients.

❖ Limited pharmacokinetic analyses indicate that steady concentrations of blinatumomab were comparable in adults and pediatrics (2 to 17 years old) at a given BSA-based dose.

Blinatumomab's Pharmacokinetic Clinical Trials

Table 17   Summary of Blinatumomab's Clinical Trials with Pharmacokinetic Data[19-21]

Study No.	N	Study Design	Objective	Key Entry Criteria	Test Product, Dosage Regimen
MT103-104	76	Phase 1, non-randomized, non-controlled, open-label, interpatient dose escalation study	Determine the maximal tolerable dose, PK, PD, and antitumor activity	Adults with relapsed NHL	CTM, 0.5, 1.5, 5, 15, 30, 60, 90 $\mu g/(m^2 \cdot day)$ cIV for 4-8 weeks.
MT103-202	21	Phase 2, non-randomized, non-controlled, open-label study	Investigate the efficacy (MRD response rate), safety, tolerability, PK, and PD	Adults with B-precursor ALL in complete hematological remission with MRD	CTM4, 15/30 $\mu g/(m^2 \cdot day)$, cIV for 4 weeks followed by 2 weeks off drug per cycle.
MT103-203	32	Phase 2, a confirmatory multicenter, single arm study	Assess the efficacy, safety, and tolerability of blinatumomab	Adults with MRD of ALL	15 $\mu g/(m^2 \cdot day)$, cIV for 4 weeks followed by 2 weeks off drug per cycle for up to 4 cycles.
MT103-206	36	Phase 2, open-label, multicenter, exploratory study	Evaluate the efficacy, safety, tolerability, PK, and PD	Adults with R/R ALL	CTM4, 5/15/30 $\mu g/(m^2 \cdot day)$, cIV for 4 weeks followed by 2 weeks off drug per cycle.
MT103-208	25	Phase 2, open-label multicenter, single-agent study	Investigate the efficacy, toxicity, and tolerability of blinatumomab	Adults with R/R DLBCL	Cohort 1: 9 $\mu g/day$ first week, 28 $\mu g/day$ second week and 112 $\mu g/day$ thereafter; Cohort 2: A flat dose of blinatumomab 112 $\mu g/day$. Cycle1: cIV for up to 8 weeks, followed by 4 treatment-free weeks; Cycle 2: 4 weeks of consolidation.

Continued

Study No.	N	Study Design	Objective	Key Entry Criteria	Test Product, Dosage Regimen
MT103-211	189	Phase 2, open-label, multicenter, single arm study	Evaluate the efficacy, safety, tolerability, PK, and PD	Adults with R/R ALL	CTM4 & CTM5, 9/28 µg/day cIV for 4 weeks followed by 2 weeks off drug per cycle.
MT103-205	Phase 1: 48 Phase 2: 40	Phase 1/2, multicenter, single arm study preceded by dose evaluation	Evaluate the efficacy, safety, and tolerability of blinatumomab in pediatric and adolescent subjects with R/R ALL	Pediatric subjects <18 years with ALL	Phase 1: 3.75-60 µg/(m²·day) cIV, 4 weeks on followed by 2 weeks off; Phase 2: Up to 5 cycles with dose blinatumomab established in Phase 1.

ALL: Acute lymphoblastic leukemia. DLBCL: Diffuse large B-cell lymphoma. MRD: Minimal residual disease. NHL: Non-Hodgkin's lymphoma. PD: Pharmacodynamics. PK: Pharmacokinetics.

Table 18   Steady-state Concentration (C_{ss}) and PK Parameters of Blinatumomab in Pediatrics and Adults[22]

Daily Dose Adult	C_{ss} (pg/mL, Mean ± SD)					CL (L/h)	V_z (L)	$t_{1/2, z}$ (h)
	5 µg/m² or 9 µg	15 µg/m² or 28 µg	30 µg/m²	60 µg/m² or 112 µg	90 µg/m²			
Adults (≥18 years)								
MT103-104 NHL[a] (n)	210 ± 85.0 (n = 32)	651 ± 307 (n = 36)	1,210 ± 476 (n = 6)	2,730 ± 985 (n = 34)	3,490 ± 904 (n = 4)	2.3 ± 1.2 (n = 66)	4.8 ± 3.2 (n = 32)	2.5 ± 1.6 (n = 32)
MT103-202 MRD⁺ ALL[a] (n)		696 ± 147 (n = 19)				1.8 ± 0.58 (n = 19)	3.9 ± 2.3 (n = 18)	1.5 ± 0.53 (n = 18)
MT103-203 MRD⁺ ALL[a] (n)		771 ± 312 (n = 32)				2.3 ± 3.0 (n = 32)		
MT103-206 R/R ALL[a] (n)	167 ± 66.0 (n = 31)	552 ± 237 (n = 34)	1,180 ± 820 (n = 5)			2.5 ± 1.2 (n = 36)		
MT103-208 DLBCL[b] (n)	277 ± 210 (n = 20)	565 ± 208 (n = 16)		2,800 ± 1,150 (n = 12)		2.0 ± 0.96 (n = 23)		
MT103-211 R/R ALL[b] (n)	211 ± 258 (n = 132)	621 ± 502 (n = 160)				3.4 ± 3.5 (n = 177)		
Combined all studies (n)						2.7 ± 2.7 (n = 366)	4.5 ± 2.9 (n = 50)	2.1 ± 1.4 (n = 50)
Pediatrics (MT103-205) R/R ALL[a]						**CL [L/(h·m²)]**	**CL (L/h)**	**V_z (L/m²)** ... $t_{1/2, z}$ (h)
<2 years	110 ± 42.6 (n = 8)	508 ± 215 (n = 8)				1.6 ± 0.44 (n = 8)	0.68 ± 0.15 (n = 8)	
2-6 years	208 ± 275 (n = 10)	434 ± 353 (n = 15)	2,300[c] (1,090, 3,520) (n = 2)			2.3 ± 2.5 (n = 21)	1.8 ± 2.1 (n = 21)	5.1 ± 4.3 (n = 9) ... 2.4 ± 1.9 (n = 9)
7-17 years	157 ± 109 (n = 9)	686 ± 510 (n = 11)	1,210 ± 635 (n = 5)			1.5 ± 1.4 (n = 16)	1.6 ± 1.1 (n = 16)	3.0 ± 2.2 (n = 11) ... 2.0 ± 1.3 (n = 11)
≤17 years	162 ± 179 (n = 27)	533 ± 392 (n = 34)	1,520 ± 1,020 (n = 7)			1.9 ± 1.9 (n = 45)	1.5 ± 1.6 (n = 45)	3.9 ± 3.4 (n = 20) ... 2.2 ± 1.5 (n = 20)

ALL: Acute lymphoblastic leukemia. CL: Clearance. DLBCL: Diffuse large B-cell lymphoma. MRD: Minimal residual disease. NHL: Non-Hodgkin's lymphoma. R/R: Relapsed/refractor. SD: Standard deviation. $t_{1/2, z}$: Terminal half-life. V_z: Volume of distribution based on terminal phase. [a] BSA-based dosing. [b] Fixed dosing. [c] n = 2, median (range), mean (SD) was only calculated when n ≥3.

Anti-product Antibody (APA) Analysis[9]

❖ In clinical studies, less than 1.0% of patients treated with Blincyto® tested positive for binding anti-blinatumomab antibodies. All patients who tested positive for binding antibodies also tested positive for neutralizing anti-blinatumomab antibodies. Anti-blinatumomab antibody formation may affect pharmacokinetics of Blincyto®.

9 Patent

❖ Blinatumomab was approved by the U.S. Food and Drug Administration (FDA) in 2014. It was developed and marketed as Blincyto® by Amgen.

Summary

❖ The patent application (WO2004106381A1) related to the bispecific antibody targeting both CD3 and CD19 (i.e. Blinatumomab), nucleic acid encoding the same and pharmaceutical compositions thereof was filed by Amgen on May 26, 2004. Accordingly, its PCT counterpart has, among the others, been granted USPTO (US7635472B2), JPO (JP6025502B2) and SIPO (CN100509850C), respectively. Another patent application (WO2005052004A2) related to the composition comprising a polypeptide comprising at least two antigen binding sites was filed on Nov 26, 2004. Accordingly, EP1691833B1 was granted by EPO.

Table 19   Originator's Key Patents of Blinatumomab in Main Countries and/or Region

Country/Region	Publication/Patent No.	Application Date	Granted Date	Estimated Expiry Date
WO	WO2004106381A1	05/26/2004	/	/
US	US7635472B2	05/26/2004	12/22/2009	11/28/2025
EP	EP1629012A1	05/26/2004	/	/
JP	JP6025502B2	05/26/2004	11/16/2016	05/26/2024
	JP2015110628A	05/26/2004	/	/
CN	CN100509850C	05/26/2004	07/08/2009	05/26/2024
WO	WO2005052004A2	11/26/2004	/	/
US	US2007249529A1	11/26/2004	/	/
EP	EP1691833B1	11/26/2004	3/3/2010	11/26/2024

Table 20   Originator's International Patent Protection of Use and/or Method of Blinatumomab

Publication No.	Title	Publication Date
Technical Subjects	**TREATMENT METHOD**	
WO2010052014A1	Treatment of acute lymphoblastic leukemia	05/14/2010
WO2010052013A1	Treatment of pediatric acute lymphoblastic leukemia	05/14/2010
WO2011051307A1	Dosage regimen for administering a CD19xCD3 bispecific antibody	05/05/2011
WO2012055961A1	Means and methods for treating DLBCL	05/03/2012
WO2014122251A2	Anti-leukocyte adhesion for the mitigation of potential adverse events caused by CD3-specific binding domains	08/14/2014
WO2015181683A1	Risk-stratification of B-precursor acute lymphoblastic leukemia patients	12/03/2015
Technical Subjects	**COMBINATOIN METHOD**	
WO2012062596A1	Prevention of adverse effects caused by CD3 specific binding domains	05/18/2012
Technical Subjects	**FORMULATION**	
WO2017129585A1	Pharmaceutical composition comprising bispecific antibody constructs	08/03/2017

The data was updated until Jan 2018.

10 Reference

[1] Fujimoto M, Fujimoto Y, poe J C, et al. CD19 regulates Src family protein tyrosine kinase activation in B lymphocytes through processive amplification [J]. Immunity, 2000, 13(1): 47-57.

[2] Wang K, Wei G, Liu D. CD19: a biomarker for B cell development, lymphoma diagnosis and therapy [J]. Experimental Hematology & Oncology, 2012, 1(1): 36-42.

[3] Loffler A, Kufer P, Lutterbuse R, et al. A recombinant bispecific single-chain antibody, CD19xCD3, induces rapid and high lymphoma-directed cytotoxicity by unstimulated T lymphocytes [J]. Blood, 2000, 95(6): 2098-2103.

[4] Zimmerman Z, Maniar T, Nagorsen D. Unleashing the clinical power of T cells: CD19/CD3 bi-specific T cell engager (BiTE(R)) antibody construct blinatumomab as a potential therapy [J]. International Immunology, 2015, 27(1): 31-37.

[5] Stieglmaier J, Benjamin J, Nagorsen D. Utilizing the BiTE (bispecific T-cell engager) platform for immunotherapy of cancer [J]. Expert Opinion on Biological Therapy, 2015, 15(8): 1093-1099.

[6] Nagorsen D, Kufer P, Baeuerle P A, et al. Blinatumomab: a historical perspective [J]. Pharmacology & Therapeutics, 2012, 136(3): 334-342.

[7] European Medicines Agency (EMA) Database. http://www.ema.europa.eu/docs/en_GB/document_library/EPAR_-_Product_Information/human/003731/WC500198228.pdf.

[8] The financial reports of AmGen; http://data.pharmacodia.com/web/homePage/index.

[9] U. S. Food and Drug Administration (FDA) Database. http://www.accessdata.fda.gov/drugsatfda_docs/label/2014/125557lbl.pdf.

[10] International nonproprietary names for pharmaceutical substances (INN). WHO Drug Information, 2009, 23: 240-241.

[11] FDA Database. http://www.accessdata.fda.gov/drugsatfda_docs/nda/2014/125557Orig1s000PharmR.pdf.

[12] Dreier T, Baeuerle P A, Fichtner I, et al. T cell costimulus-independent and very efficacious inhibition of tumor growth in mice bearing subcutaneous or leukemic human B cell lymphoma xenografts by a CD19-/CD3- bispecific single-chain antibody construct [J]. The Journal of Immunology, 2003, 170(8): 4397-4402.

[13] EMA Datebase. http://www.ema.europa.eu/docs/en_GB/document_library/EPAR_-_Public_assessment_report/human/003731/WC500198227.pdf.

[14] Schlereth B, Quadt C, Dreier T, et al. T-cell activation and B-cell depletion in chimpanzees treated with a bispecific anti-CD19/anti-CD3 single-chain antibody construct [J]. Cancer Immunology, Immunotherapy, 2006, 55(5): 503-514.

[15] Topp M S, Gokbuget N, Stein A S, et al. Safety and activity of blinatumomab for adult patients with relapsed or refractory B-precursor acute lymphoblastic leukaemia: a multicenter, single arm, phase 2 study [J]. Lancet Oncology, 2015, 16(1): 57-66.

[16] Von Stackelberq A, Locatelli F, Zuqmaier G, et al. Phase I/Phase II Study of blinatumomab in pediatric patients with relapsed/refractory acute lymphoblastic leukemia [J]. Journal of Clinical Oncology, 2016, 34(36): 4381- 4389.

[17] Martinelli G, Boissel N, Chevallier P, et al. Complete hematologic and molecular response in adult patients with relapsed/refractory philadelphia chromosome-positive B-precursor acute lymphoblastic leukemia following treatment with blinatumomab: results from a Phase II, single-arm, multicenter study [J]. Journal of Clinical Oncology, 2017, 35(16): 1795-1802.

[18] Hagop Kantarjian M D, Anthony Stein M D, Nicola Gökbuget M D, et al. Blinatumomab versus chemotherapy for advanced acute lymphoblastic leukemia [J]. The New England Journal of Medicine, 2017, 376(9): 836-847.

[19] FDA Database. http://www.accessdata.fda.gov/drugsatfda_docs/nda/2014/125557Orig1s000 ClinPharmRedt.pdf.

[20] Viardot A, Goebeler M E, Hess G, et al. Phase 2 study of the bispecific T-cell engager (BiTE) antibody blinatumomab in relapsed/refractory diffuse large B-cell lymphoma [J]. Blood, 2016, 127(11): 1410-1416.

[21] https://clinicaltrials.gov/ct2/show/study/NCT01207388?term=MT103-203&rank=1.

[22] FDA Database. https://www.accessdata.fda.gov/drugsatfda_docs/nda/2016/125557Orig1s005ClinPharmRedt.pdf.

CHAPTER

5

Cetuximab

Cetuximab

(Erbitux®)

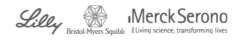

Research code: BMS-564717, C-225, ch-225, EMD-271786, GT-MAB-5.2, IMC-C225, LY-2939777, NSC-714692

---

1 Target Biology

Biology Activity

❖ Epidermal growth factor receptor (EGFR), also known as human epidermal growth factor receptor 1 (HER1), or ErbB1, is a trans-membrane receptor encoded by the c-ErbB1 proto-oncogene with a molecular weight of approximately 170 kDa. EGFR belongs to subclass I family of receptor tyrosine kinases (RTKs) and is the receptor to at least six distinct ligands including epidermal growth factor (EGF), transforming growth factor α (TGF-α), heparin-binding EGF, amphiregulin, betacellulin, and epiregulin.[1, 2]

❖ EGFR subclass I family of RTKs includes HER1 (ErbB-1), HER2/neu (ErbB-2); HER3 (ErbB-3), and HER4 (ErbB-4). These receptors function in various homodimeric and heterodimeric pairs, depending on their density on cell surface, the concentrations of a particular ligand, and intrinsic dimerization preference between the receptors.[3, 4]

❖ Binding of a ligand to the extracellular domain of EGFR induces a conformational change of receptor, which in turn results in a) increased binding affinity for the other receptors and b) tyrosine autophosphorylation.[5, 6] These phosphorylated residues within the receptor's cytoplasmic domain serve as docking sites for other molecules involved in the regulation of intracellular signaling cascades. The major signaling cascades activated by EGFR include the Ras/MAP kinase, PLC-gamma, PI-3 kinase/Akt and STAT3 pathways. The integrated biological responses to EGFR signaling are pleiotropic, including mitogenesis or apoptosis, enhanced cell motility, protein secretion, cell adhesion, invasion, differentiation or dedifferentiation, and increased neovascularization.[7, 8]

❖ EGFR is normally expressed in a wide variety of epithelial tissues as well as in the central nervous system. Expression of EGFR is upregulated in a variety of human solid tumors, including head and neck squamous cell cancer and carcinomas of cervix, renal cell, lung, prostate, bladder, colorectal, pancreatic, and breast, as well as melanoma, glioblastoma, and meningioma. Several tumor types, including colorectal cancers, have been demonstrated to co-express EGFR and its ligands, leading to an autocrine activation of the receptor and poor outcome in the clinic.[7-11] Mutants of EGFR, because of gene rearrangement that results in in-frame deletion of portions of the extracellular domain of the receptor, have been found in a significant fraction of EGFR-expressing tumors. For example, the most common mutation (EGFRvIII)-with a deletion of exons 2-7 of EGFR gene-that is frequently found in brain tumors, such as glioblastoma, results in a protein with defective ligand binding capacity but is constitutively activated and its tumorigenicity *in vivo* is enhanced.[12, 13]

❖ Expression of EGFR in human cancers has a significant effect on their biological behavior, thus providing the rationale for the development of EGFR antagonists as potentially useful therapeutic strategies for the treatment of EGFR-expressing cancers. In this regard, a number of EGFR targeted therapeutics, including monoclonal antibodies (mAb) such as cetuximab and panitumumab, and small-molecule tyrosine kinase inhibitors (TKI) such as gefitinib, erlotinib, vandetanib and lapatinib, have been developed for the treatment of several human cancers.[14-20]

Sequence of Human EGFR Proteins[21]

Length: 1210 aa.   Accession: CAA25240.

```
   1 MRPSGTAGAA LLALLAALCP ASRALEEKKV CQGTSNKLTQ LGTFEDHFLS LQRMFNNCEV
  61 VLGNLEITYV QRNYDLSFLK TIQEVAGYVL IALNTVERIP LENLQIIRGN MYYENSYALA
 121 VLSNYDANKT GLKELPMRNL QEILHGAVRF SNNPALCNVE SIQWRDIVSS DFLSNMSMDF
 181 QNHLGSCQKC DPSCPNGSCW GAGEENCQKL TKIICAQQCS GRCRGKSPSD CCHNQCAAGC
 241 TGPRESDCLV CRKFRDEATC KDTCPPLMLY NPTTYQMDVN PEGKYSFGAT CVKKCPRNYV
 301 VTDHGSCVRA CGADSYEMEE DGVRKCKKCE GPCRKVCNGI GIGEFKDSLS INATNIKHFK
 361 NCTSISGDLH ILPVAFRGDS FTHTPPLDPQ ELDILKTVKE ITGFLLIQAW PENRTDLHAF
 421 ENLEIIRGRT KQHGQFSLAV VSLNITSLGL RSLKEISDGD VIISGNKNLC YANTINWKKL
 481 FGTSGQKTKI ISNRGENSCK ATGQVCHALC SPEGCWGPEP RDCVSCRNVS RGRECVDKCK
 541 LLEGEPREFV ENSECIQCHP ECLPQAMNIT CTGRGPDNCI QCAHYIDGPH CVKTCPAGVM
 601 GENNTLVWKY ADAGHVCHLC HPNCTYGCTG PGLEGCPTNG PKIPSIATGM VGALLLLLVV
 661 ALGIGLFMRR RHIVRKRTLR RLLQERELVE PLTPSGEAPN QALLRILKET EFKKIKVLGS
 721 GAFGTVYKGL WIPEGEKVKI PVAIKELREA TSPKANKEIL DEAYVMASVD NPHVCRLLGI
 781 CLTSTVQLIT QLMPFGCLLD YVREHKDNIG SQYLLNWCVQ IAKGMNYLED RRLVHRDLAA
 841 RNVLVKTPQH VKITDFGLAK LLGAEEKEYH AEGGKVPIKW MALESILHRI YTHQSDVWSY
 901 GVTVWELMTF FRELIIEFSK GSKPYDGIPA SEISSILEKG ERLPQPPICT IDVYMIMVKC
 961 FRELIIEFSK GSKPYDGIPA SEISSILEKG ERLPQPPICT IDVYMIMVKC WMIDADSRPK
1021 QGFFSSPSTS MARDPQRYLV IQGDERMHLP SPTDSNFYRA LMDEEDMDDV VDADEYLIPQ
1081 SIDDTFLPVP RTPLLSSLSA TSNNSTVACI DRNGLQSCPI KEDSFLQRYS SDPTGALTED
1141 TVQPTCVNST EYINQSVPKR PAGSVQNPVY HNQPLNPAPS RDPHYQDPHS TAVGNPEYLN
1201 APQSSEFIGA FDSPAHWAQK GSHQISLDNP DYQQDFFPKE AKPNGIFKGS TAENAEYLRV
```

❖ The homology analysis data of different species are listed in Table 1 and amino acid sequence alignments of different species are summarized in Table 2.   The amino acids which are different from the human EGFR are listed in the table.   The point mutations among the same species are highlight with yellow.

Table 1   Summary of EGFR Proteins from Different Species[22]

Species	Accession	Length	Max Score	Total Score	Query Cover (%)	Identity %, (n/N)	Positive %, (n/N)	Gap (%)
Human	CAA25240.1	1,210	2,522	2,522	100	100 (1,210/1,210)	100 (1,210/1,210)	0.0 (0/1,210)
	NP005219.2	1,210	2,521	2,521	100	99.9 (1,209/1,210)	99.9 (1,209/1,210)	0.0 (0/1,210)
	AA266620.1	1,210	2,518	2,518	100	99.8 (1,208/1,210)	99.8 (1,208/1,210)	0.0 (0/1,210)
	AAT52212.1	1,210	2,516	2,516	100	99.8 (1,208/1,210)	99.8 (1,208/1,210)	0.0 (0/1,210)
	BAF83041.1	1,210	2,513	2,513	100	99.8 (1,207/1,210)	99.8 (1,208/1,210)	0.0 (0/1,210)
Chimpanzee	XP_519102.3	1,210	2,516	2,516	100	99.6 (1,205/1,210)	99.6 (1,205/1,210)	0.0 (0/1,210)
	XP_8967087.1	1,157	2,410	2,410	95.0	99.5 (1,151/1,157)	99.8 (1,155/1,157)	0.0 (0/1,157)
Rhesus monkey	XP-014988922.1	1,210	2,506	2,506	100	99.3 (1,201/1,210)	99.6 (1,205/1,210)	0.0 (0/1,210)
	XP-014988923.1	1,157	2,401	2,401	95.0	99.2 (1,148/1,157)	99.6 (1,152/1,157)	0.0 (0/1,157)
	EHH17303.1	1,181	2,452	2,452	97.0	99.2 (1,172/1,181)	99.6 (1,176/1,181)	0.0 (0/1,181)
Norway rat	NP_113695.1	1,209	2,236	2,236	100	90.3 (1,093/1,211)	94.1 (1,139/1,211)	0.25 (3/1,211)
	ADT91284.1	1,209	2,242	2,242	100	91.5 (1,096/1,211)	94.1 (1,141/1,211)	0.25 (3/1,211)
	ADT91285.1	1,209	2,242	2,242	100	90.4 (1,095/1,211)	94.1 (1,141/1,211)	0.25 (3/1,211)
	EDL97896.1	1,209	2,240	2,240	100	90.4 (1,095/1,211)	94.1 (1,140/1,211)	0.25 (3/1,211)
House mouse	AAA17899.1	1,210	2,269	2,269	100	90.2 (1,093/1,212)	94.7 (1,148/1,212)	0.0033 (4/1,212)
	AAG24388.1	1,210	2,268	2,268	100	90.2 (1,093/1,212)	94.7 (1,148/1,212)	0.0033 (4/1,212)
	NP_997538.1	1,210	2,269	2,269	100	90.3 (1,094/1,212)	94.7 (1,148/1,212)	0.0033 (4/1,212)

Table 2　Alignment of EGFR Proteins from Different Species[21]

Amino acid sequence (positions 1–112)

Species	Accession #	Sequence
Human	CAA25240.1	MRPSGTAGAALLALLAALCPASRALEEKKVCQGTSNKLTQLGTFEDHFLSLQRMFNNCEVVLGNLEITYVQRNYDLSFLKTIQEVAGYVLIALNTVERIPLE
Human	NP005219.2	
Human	AA266620.1	...C...
Human	AAT52212.1	
Human	BAF83041.1	
Chimpanzee	XP 519102.3	
Chimpanzee	XP 008967087.1	sequence missing
Rhesus Monkey	XP-014988922.1	sequence missing
Rhesus Monkey	XP-014988923.1	
Rhesus Monkey	EHH17303.1	sequence missing
Norway rat	NP 113695.1	R T K . L . . . A . G G . . . R
Norway rat	ADT91284.1	R T K . L . . . A . G G . . . R
Norway rat	ADT91285.1	R T K . L . . . A . G G . . . R
Norway rat	EDL97896.1	R T K . L . . . A . G G . . . R
House mouse	AAA17899.1	R T T . V T . A . G G . . . R . Y
House mouse	AAG24388.1	R T T . V T . A . G G . . . R . Y
House mouse	NP 997538.1	R T T . V T . A . G G . . . R . Y

Amino acid sequence (positions 103–234)

Species	Accession #	Sequence
Human	CAA25240.1	NLQIIRGNMYYENSYALAVLSNYDANKTGLKELPMRNLQEILHGAVRFSNNPALCNVESIQWRDIVSSDFLSNMSMDFQNHLGSCQKCDPSCPNGSCWGAGE
Rhesus Monkey	XP-014988922.1	...E...
Rhesus Monkey	XP-014988923.1	...E...
Rhesus Monkey	EHH17303.1	...E...
Norway rat	NP 113695.1	A L . T . G T . R . I . I . M T . Q D V . V R . T G P . R
Norway rat	ADT91284.1	A L . T . G T . R . I . I . M T . Q D V . V R . T G P . R
Norway rat	ADT91285.1	A L . T . G T . R . I . I . M T . Q D V . V R . T G P . R
Norway rat	EDL97896.1	A L . T . G T . R . I . I . M T . Q D V . V R . T G P . R
House mouse	AAA17899.1	A L . T . I . G T R . R . I . I . M D T . Q N V M . L S . P S P . G
House mouse	AAG24388.1	A L . T . I . G T R . R . I . I . M D T . Q N V M . L S . P S P . G
House mouse	NP 997538.1	A L . T . I . G T R . R . I . I . M D T . Q N V M . L S . P S P . G

Amino acid sequence (positions 205–306)

Species	Accession #	Sequence
Human	CAA25240.1	ENCQKLTKIICAQQCSGRCRGKSPSDCCHNQCAAGCTGPRESDCLVCRKFRDEATCKDTCPPLMLYNPTTYQMDVNPEGKYSFGATCVKKCPRNYVVTDHGS
Norway rat	NP 113695.1	R . R . H R
Norway rat	ADT91284.1	R . R . H R
Norway rat	ADT91285.1	R . R . H R
Norway rat	EDL97896.1	R . R . H R
House mouse	AAA17899.1	H . R . Q K Q
House mouse	AAG24388.1	H . R . Q K Q
House mouse	NP 997538.1	H . R . Q K Q

Amino acid sequence (positions 307–408)

Species	Accession #	Sequence
Human	CAA25240.1	CVRACGADSYEMEEDGVRKCKKCEGPCRKVCNGIGIGEFKDSLSINATNIKHFKNCTSISGDLHILPVAFRGDSFTHTPPLDPQELDILKTVKEITGFLLIQ
Chimpanzee	XP 519102.3	...T...
Chimpanzee	XP 008967087.1	...T...
Rhesus Monkey	XP-014988922.1	...T...
Rhesus Monkey	XP-014988923.1	...T...
Rhesus Monkey	EHH17303.1	...T...
Norway rat	NP 113695.1	P Y V . S . D . T . Y A . K . R . R E
Norway rat	ADT91284.1	P Y V . S . D . T . Y A . K . R . R E
Norway rat	ADT91285.1	P Y V . S . D . T . Y A . K . R . R E
Norway rat	EDL97896.1	P Y V . S . D . T . Y A . K . R . R E
House mouse	AAA17899.1	P Y V . I . D . T . Y A . K . R . R E
House mouse	AAG24388.1	P Y V . I . D . T . Y A . K . R . R E
House mouse	NP 997538.1	P Y V . I . D . T . Y A . K . R . R E

Amino acid sequence (positions 409–510)

Species	Accession #	Sequence
Human	CAA25240.1	AWPENRTDLHAFENLEIIRGRTKQHGQFSLAVVSLNITSLGLRSLKEISDGDVIISGNKNLCYANTINWKKLFGTSGQKTIISNRGENSCKATGQVCHALC
Rhesus Monkey	XP-014988922.1	...S...
Rhesus Monkey	XP-014988923.1	...S...
Rhesus Monkey	EHH17303.1	...S... . P N . M N . A K D . N H . N P
Norway rat	NP_113695.1	W . G . R . P N . M N . A K D . N H . N P
Norway rat	ADT91284.1	W . G . R . P N . M N . A K D . N H . N P
Norway rat	ADT91285.1	W . G . R . P N . M N . A K D . N H . N P
Norway rat	EDL97896.1	W . G . R . P N . M N . A K D . N H . N P
House mouse	AAA17899.1	D W . G . R . P N . M N . A K D . V N H . N P
House mouse	AAG24388.1	D W . G . R . P N . M N . A K D . V N H . N P
House mouse	NP_997538.1	D W . G . R . P N . M N . A K D . V N H . N P

Amino acid sequence (positions 511–612)

Species	Accession #	Sequence
Human	CAA25240.1	SPEGCWGPEPRDCVSCRNVSRGRECVDKGKLLEGEPREFVENSECIQCHPECLPQAMNITCTGRGPDNCIQCAHYIDGPHCVKTCPAGVMGENNTLVWKYAD
Human	NP005219.2	...N...
Human	AA266620.1	...N...
Human	AAT52212.1	...N...
Human	BAF83041.1	...N...
Chimpanzee	XP 519102.3	...N I...
Chimpanzee	XP 008967087.1	...N I... I
Rhesus Monkey	XP-014988922.1	Q . N V . V
Rhesus Monkey	XP-014988923.1	Q . N V . V
Rhesus Monkey	EHH17303.1	Q . N I . V
Norway rat	NP_113695.1	S . T . Q . N I . T . K . V . S I . F
Norway rat	ADT91284.1	S . T . Q . N I . T . K . V . S I . F
Norway rat	ADT91285.1	S . T . Q . N I . T . K . V . S I . F
Norway rat	EDL97896.1	S . T . Q . N I . T . K . V . S I . F
House mouse	AAA17899.1	S . Q . E . N I . I
House mouse	AAG24388.1	S . Q . E . N I . I
House mouse	NP 997538.1	S . Q . E . N I . I

Amino acid sequence (positions ~613–734)

Species	Accession #	Sequence
Human	CAA25240.1	AGHVCHLCHPNCTYGCTGPGLEGCPTN--GPKIPSIATGMVGALLLLLVVALGIGLFMRRRHIVRKRTLRRLLQERELVEPLTPSGEAPNQALLRILKETEF
Human	NP005219.2	
Human	AA266620.1	
Human	AAT52212.1	
Human	BAF83041.1	
Chimpanzee	XP_519102.3	
Chimpanzee	XP_008967087.1	
Rhesus Monkey	XP-014988922.1	A R
Rhesus Monkey	XP-014988923.1	A R
Rhesus Monkey	EHH17303.1	A R
Norway rat	NP_113695.1	N N A A K QQP E I G F I V Q L H
Norway rat	ADT91284.1	N N A A K QQP E I G F I I H
Norway rat	ADT91285.1	N N A A K QQP E I G F I I H
Norway rat	EDL97896.1	N N A A K QQP E I G F I V H K
House mouse	AAA17899.1	N N A A Q E V W P S I G F I V H
House mouse	AAG24388.1	N N A A Q E V W P S I G F I V H
House mouse	NP_997538.1	N N A A Q E V W P S I G F I V H

Amino acid sequence (positions ~715–836)

Species	Accession #	Sequence
Human	CAA25240.1	KKIKVLGSGAFGTVYKGLWIPEGEKVKIPVAIKELREATSPKANKEILDEAYVMASVDNPHVCRLLGICLTSTVQLITQLMPFGCLLDYVREHKDNIGSQYL
Human	NP005219.2	
Human	AA266620.1	
Human	AAT52212.1	
Human	BAF83041.1	
Chimpanzee	XP_519102.3	
Chimpanzee	XP_008967087.1	
Rhesus Monkey	XP-014988922.1	
Rhesus Monkey	XP-014988923.1	
Rhesus Monkey	EHH17303.1	
Norway rat	NP_113695.1	Y
Norway rat	ADT91284.1	Y
Norway rat	ADT91285.1	Y
Norway rat	EDL97896.1	Y
House mouse	AAA17899.1	Y
House mouse	AAG24388.1	Y
House mouse	NP_997538.1	Y

Amino acid sequence (positions ~817–938)

Species	Accession #	Sequence
Human	CAA25240.1	LNWCVQIAKGMNYLEDRRLVHRDLAARNVLVKTPQHVKITDFGLAKLLGAEEKEYHAEGGKVPIKWMALESILHRIYTHQSDVWSYGVTVWELMTFGSKPYD
Human	NP005219.2	
Human	AA266620.1	
Human	AAT52212.1	
Human	BAF83041.1	H C
Chimpanzee	XP_519102.3	
Chimpanzee	XP_008967087.1	
Rhesus Monkey	XP-014988922.1	
Rhesus Monkey	XP-014988923.1	
Rhesus Monkey	EHH17303.1	
Norway rat	NP_113695.1	
Norway rat	ADT91284.1	
Norway rat	ADT91285.1	
Norway rat	EDL97896.1	
House mouse	AAA17899.1	
House mouse	AAG24388.1	
House mouse	NP_997538.1	

Amino acid sequence (positions ~912–1090)

Species	Accession #	Sequence
Human	CAA25240.1	GIPASEISSILEKGERLPQPPICTIDVYMIMVKCWMIDADSRPKFRELIIEFSKMARDPQRYLVIQGDERMHLPSPTDSNFYRALMDEEDMDDVVDADEYLI
Human	NP005219.2	
Human	AA266620.1	
Human	AAT52212.1	
Human	BAF83041.1	
Chimpanzee	XP_519102.3	
Chimpanzee	XP_008967087.1	
Rhesus Monkey	XP-014988922.1	
Rhesus Monkey	XP-014988923.1	
Rhesus Monkey	EHH17303.1	
Norway rat	NP_113695.1	L E E
Norway rat	ADT91284.1	L E E
Norway rat	ADT91285.1	L E E
Norway rat	EDL97896.1	L E E
House mouse	AAA17899.1	D L F E
House mouse	AAG24388.1	D L E
House mouse	NP_997538.1	D L E T

Amino acid sequence (positions ~1029–1152)

Species	Accession #	Sequence
Human	CAA25240.1	PQQGFFSSPSTSRTPLLSSLSATSNNSTVACIDRNGLQSCPIKEDSFLQRYSSDPTGALTEDSIDDTFLPVPEYINQSVPKRPAGSVQNPVYHNQPLNPAPS
Human	NP005219.2	
Human	AA266620.1	
Human	AAT52212.1	P
Human	BAF83041.1	
Chimpanzee	XP_519102.3	M T
Chimpanzee	XP_008967087.1	M T
Rhesus Monkey	XP-014988922.1	
Rhesus Monkey	XP-014988923.1	
Rhesus Monkey	EHH17303.1	
Norway rat	NP_113695.1	N N S N - - G R V A S V N H G
Norway rat	ADT91284.1	N N S N - - G R V A S V N H G
Norway rat	ADT91285.1	N N S N - - G R V A S V N H G
Norway rat	EDL97896.1	N N S A N - - G R V A S V N H G
House mouse	AAA17899.1	N T N - - G R V A V N A V H G
House mouse	AAG24388.1	N T N - - G R V A V N A V H G
House mouse	NP_997538.1	N T N - - G R V A V N A V H G

Amino acid sequence (positions ~1124–1242)

Species	Accession #	Sequence
Human	CAA25240.1	RDPHYQDPHSTAVGNPEYLNTVQPTCVNSTFDSPAHWAQKGSHQISLDNPDYQQDFFPKEAKPNGIFKGSTAENAEYLRVAPQSSEFIGA
Human	NP005219.2	
Human	AA266620.1	
Human	AAT52212.1	
Human	BAF83041.1	
Chimpanzee	XP_519102.3	
Chimpanzee	XP_008967087.1	
Rhesus Monkey	XP-014988922.1	
Rhesus Monkey	XP-014988923.1	
Rhesus Monkey	EHH17303.1	
Norway rat	NP_113695.1	L N N S A L S G S L I M P P S
Norway rat	ADT91284.1	L N N S A L S G S L I M P P
Norway rat	ADT91285.1	L N N S A L S G S L I M P P
Norway rat	EDL97896.1	L N N S A L S G S L I M P P
House mouse	AAA17899.1	L N N A L S G N L I M T P P
House mouse	AAG24388.1	L N N A L S G N L M T P P
House mouse	NP_997538.1	L N N A L S G N L I M T P P

2   General Information

Erbitux®

❖ Erbitux® (Cetuximab) is a human/mouse chimeric monoclonal IgG1
antibody produced in a stably transfected murine myeloma cell line (Sp2/0)
by recombinant DNA technology.

❖ Erbitux® was engineered by fusing the variable domains of the parental
murine antibody (M225) into the constant domain of a human IgG1 and
targets the extracellular domain of the ErbB-1/EGFR.

❖ The total sales of 1,664 million US$ for 2016; No sales data as of 2017.

❖ Chimeric IgG1κ monoclonal antibody: $C_{6484}H_{10042}N_{1732}O_{2023}S_{36}$, ~146 kDa
(calculated molecular mass) (Table 3).

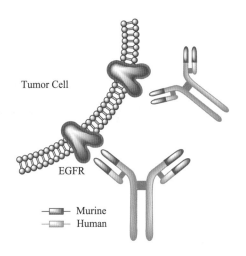

Table 3   Summary of Erbitux®[23]

Generic Name	Cetuximab
CAS registry No.	205923-56-4
Chemical name	Chimerical anti-EGFR IgG1κ monoclonal antibody
Molecular formula	$C_{6484}H_{10042}N_{1732}O_{2023}S_{36}$
Molecular weight[a]	145.8
Pharmacological class	EGFR neutralized antibody

[a] Peptide chains only.

Mechanism of Action[15, 20]

❖ Erbitux® is a chimeric monoclonal IgG1 antibody that is specifically directed against EGFR, not the other members
belonging to the HER family.   EGFR signaling pathways are involved in the control of cell survival, cell cycle progression,
angiogenesis, cell migration and cellular invasion/metastasis.

❖ Erbitux® binds to EGFR with an affinity that is approximately 5- to 10-fold higher than that of the endogenous ligands and
blocks binding of the endogenous ligands, resulting in inhibition of the function of the receptor.   It further induces the
internalization of EGFR, which can lead to downregulation of EGFR.

❖ Erbitux® also targets cytotoxic immune effector cells towards EGFR expressing tumor cells, resulting in antibody dependent
cell-mediated cytotoxicity (ADCC).

❖ Erbitux® can inhibit cell-cycle progression, DNA repair and angiogenesis; there is evident to demonstrate that Erbitux®
can increase apoptosis in tumor cell lines by upregulating pro-apoptosis regulator Bax, decreasing expression of the antiapoptotic molecule Bcl-2.

❖ The protein product of the proto-oncogene RAS (rat sarcoma) is a central down-stream signal transducer of EGFR.   In
tumors, activation of RAS by EGFR contributes to EGFR-mediated increased proliferation, survival and the production of
pro-angiogenic factors.   RAS is one of the most frequently activated families of oncogenes in human cancers.   Mutations
of RAS genes at certain hot-spots on exons 2, 3 and 4 result in constitutive activation of RAS proteins independently of
EGFR signaling.

Sponsor

❖ Erbitux® (Cetuximab) was initially developed by ImClone Systems (acquired by Eli Lilly in November 2008) and Merck
Serono, and co-marketed by Eli Lilly, Bristol-Myer Squibb and Merck Serono.

World Sales[24]

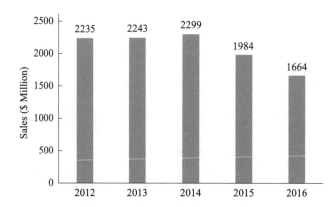

Figure 1   World Sales of Cetuximab since 2012

Approval and Indication

❖ Erbitux® is an EGFR antagonist indicated for treatment of squamous cell carcinoma of the head and neck (SCCHN) and colorectal cancer as approved by FDA (US), EMA (EU), PMDA (Japan) and CFDA (China) (Table 4).   The detail indications and administration are listed in Table 5.

Table 4   Summary of the Approval of Erbitux®[25-28]

	US (FDA)	EU (EMA)	Japan (PMDA)	China (CFDA)
First approval date	02/12/2004	06/29/2004	07/16/2008	01/25/2011
Application or approval No.	BLA125084	EMEA/H/C/000558	22000AMX01771000	国药准字 S20110009
Brand name	Erbitux®	Erbitux®	Erbitux®	Erbitux®
Indication	CC, H&N	CRC, H&N	CC, H&N	CC, H&N
Strength	100 mg/50 mL; 200 mg/100 mL	100 mg/20 mL; 500 mg/100 mL	100 mg/20 mL	100 mg/20 mL
Authorization holder	LLY/BMY	Merck KGaA	Merck KGaA	Merck KGaA

BMS: Bristol-Myers Squibb.   CC: Colorectal cancer.   CRC: Metastatic colorectal cancer.   H&N: Head and neck cancer.   LLY: Eli Lilly.

Table 5   Indication and Administration[28]

Administration	Indication
Combination with radiation therapy or with platinum-based therapy with 5-FU: • The recommended initial dose is 400 mg/m² administered one week prior to initiation of a course of radiation therapy or on the day of initiation of platinum-based therapy with 5-FU as a 120 min intravenous infusion (maximum infusion rate 10 mg/min). Complete cetuximab administration 1 h prior to platinum-based therapy with 5-FU. • The recommended subsequent weekly dose (all other infusions) is 250 mg/m² infused over 60 min (maximum infusion rate 10 mg/min) for the duration of radiation therapy (6-7 weeks) or until disease progression or unacceptable toxicity when administered in combination with platinum-based therapy with 5-FU. Complete cetuximab administration 1 h prior to radiation therapy or platinum-based therapy with 5-FU. Monotherapy: • The recommended initial dose is 400 mg/m² administered as a 120 min intravenous infusion (maximum infusion rate 10 mg/min). • The recommended subsequent weekly dose (all other infusions) is 250 mg/m² infused over 60 min (maximum infusion rate 10 mg/min) until disease progression or unacceptable toxicity.	SCCHN • Single agent for the treatment of patients with recurrent or metastatic squamous cell carcinoma of the head and neck for whom prior platinum-based therapy has failed. • Combination with radiation therapy for the initial treatment of locally or regionally advanced SCCHN. • Combination with platinum-based therapy with 5-FU for the first line treatment of patients with recurrent locoregional disease or metastatic SCCHN.

Continued

Administration	Indication
• The recommended initial dose, either as monotherapy or in combination with irinotecan, is 400 mg/m² administered as a 120 min intravenous infusion (maximum infusion rate 10 mg/min). • The recommended subsequent weekly dose, either as monotherapy or in combination with irinotecan, is 250 mg/m² infused over 60 min (maximum infusion rate 10 mg/min) until disease progression or unacceptable toxicity.	Colorectal Cancer • Single agent for the treatment of EGFR-expressing metastatic colorectal cancer after failure of both irinotecan- and oxaliplatin-based regimens. • Single agent for the treatment of EGFR-expressing metastatic colorectal cancer in patients who are intolerant to irinotecan-based regimens. • Combination with irinotecan for the treatment of EGFR-expressing metastatic colorectal carcinoma in patients who are refractory to irinotecan-based chemotherapy.

Sourced from US FDA drug label information.   5-FU: 5-Fluorouracil.   EGFR: Epidermal growth factor receptor.   SCCHN: Squamous cell carcinoma of the head and neck.

Recommended Premedication[28]

❖ Premedicate with an H1 antagonist (eg, 50 mg of diphenhydramine) intravenously 30-60 min prior to the first dose; Premedication should be administered for subsequent cetuximab doses based upon clinical judgment and presence/severity of prior infusion reactions.

Does Modification[28]

❖ Infusion reactions: Reduce the infusion rate by 50.0% for NCI CTC Grade 1 or 2 and non-serious NCI CTC Grade 3 infusion reactions.   Immediately and permanently discontinue cetuximab for serious infusion reactions, requiring medical intervention and/or hospitalization.

Dermatologic Toxicity

❖ Recommended dose modifications for severe (NCI CTC Grade 3 or 4) acneiform rash are specified in Table 6.

Table 6   Dose Modification Guideline for Rash[28]

Severe Acneiform	Cetuximab	Outcome	Cetuximab Dose Modification
1st occurrence	Delay infusion 1 to 2 weeks	Improvement No improvement	Continue at 250 mg/m² Discontinue Erbitux®
2nd occurrence	Delay infusion 1 to 2 weeks	Improvement No improvement	Reduce dose to 200 mg/m² Discontinue Erbitux®
3rd occurrence	Delay infusion 1 to 2 weeks	Improvement No improvement	Reduce dose to 150 mg/m² Discontinue Erbitux®
4th occurrence	Discontinue Erbitux®	-	-

-: Not available.

Other EGFR Antagonists

Table 7   Other Marketed EGFR-targeting Drugs[25-29]

Drug	Trade	Sponsor	Type	Approval	Indication
Nimotuzumab	BIOMab-EGFR®	CIM/BIOTECH PHARMA/Biocon	EGFR antagonist mAb	07/2006-IN 01/2008-CFDA	H&N
Panitumumab	Vectibix®	AMGN/Takeda	EGFR antagonist mAb	09/2006-FDA 12/2007-EMA 04/2010-PMDA 06/2011-PMDA	CRC
Necitumumab	Portrazza®	Eli Lilly	EGFR antagonist mAb	11/2015-FDA 02/2016-EMA	NSCLC
Gefitinib	Iressa®	AstraZeneca	EGFR tyrosine kinase inhibitor (TKI)	03/2003-FDA 07/2015-FDA 07/2002-PMDA 06/2009-EMA 06/2014-CFDA	Metastatic NSCLC NSCLC Metastatic NSCLC NSCLC Metastatic NSCLC

Continued

Drug	Trade	Sponsor	Type	Approval	Indication
Erlotinib hydrochloride	Tarceva®	ROCHE (Genentech)/ Astellas	EGFR TKI	11/2004-FDA 09/2005-EMA 10/2007-PMDA 11/2004-FDA 09/2005-EMA 10/2012-CFDA	Metastatic NSCLC and PC Metastatic NSCLC Metastatic NSCLC and PC Metastatic NSCLC-25mg
Lapatinib ditosylate hydrate	Tykerb® Tyverb® Tykerb® Tykerb®	GlaxoSmithKline	Dual HER2/ EGFR TKI	03/2007-FDA 06/2008-EMA 04/2009-PMDA 11/2013-CFDA	Breast Cancer
Vandetanib	Caprelsa®	AstraZeneca	Multi-targeted receptor TKI	04/2011-FDA 02/2012-EMA 09/2015-PMDA	MTC
Icotinib hydrochloride	Conmana®	Beta pharmaceutical	EGFR TKI	06/2011-CFDA	NSCLC
Afatinib dimaleate	Gilotrif® Giotrif® Giotrif®	Boehringer Ingelheim	Pan EGFR TKI	07/2013-FDA 09/2013-EMA 01/2014-PMDA	NSCLC
Osimertinib mesylate	Tagrisso®	GENZYME	EGFR TKI	11/2015-FDA 02/2016-EMA 03/2016-PMDA	NSCLC
Olmutinib	Olita®	Hanmi/Boehringer Ingelheim/Zai Lab	EGFR mutant selective inhibitor	05/2016-KR	NSCLC

EGFR: Epidermal growth factor receptor.   H&N: Head and neck cancer.   mAb: Monoclonal antibody.   MTC: Medullary thyroid cancer.   NSCLC: Non-small cell lung cancer.   PC: Pancreatic cancer.   TKI: Tyrosine kinase inhibitor.

3   CMC Profile

Product Profile[28, 30]

Dosage route: IV infusion.
Dosage form and Strength: US: 100 mg/50 mL and 200 mg/100 mL; EU: 100 mg/20 mL and 500 mg/100 mL; JP: 100 mg/20 mL; CN: 100 mg/20 mL.
Formulation: 100 mg/50 mL (final concentration 2 mg/mL): Cetuximab is formulated in a solution with no preservatives, which contains 8.48 mg/mL sodium chloride, 1.88 mg/mL sodium phosphate dibasic heptahydrate, 0.41 mg/mL sodium phosphate monobasic monohydrate, and water for injection, USP.
Stability: Shelf-life: 4 years.
Storage: Store vials under refrigeration at 2-8 °C (36-46 °F).   Do not freeze.   Increased particulate formation may occur at temperatures at or below 0 °C.   This product contains no preservatives.   Preparations of cetuximab in infusion containers are chemically and physically stable for up to 12 h at 2-8 °C (36-46 °F) and up to 8 h at controlled room temperature (20-25 °C; 68-77 °F).   Discard any remaining solution in the infusion container after 8 h at controlled room temperature or after 12 h at 2-8 °C.   Discard any unused portion of the vial.

Amino Acid Sequence

❖ Cetuximab is a recombinant mouse/human chimerical monoclonal antibody, an IgG1 that contains human constant domain regions (66.0%) with the variable region of a murine antibody (34.0%) that binds to EGFR.
❖ Molecular formula:[31]
Amino acid sequence of light chain:

```
DILLTQSPVI  LSVSPGERVS  FSCRASQSIG  TNIHWYQQRT  NGSPRLLIKY  ASESISGIPS
RFSGSGSGTD  FTLSINSVES  EDIADYYCQQ  NNNWPTTFGA  GTKLELKRTV  AAPSVFIFPP
SDEQLKSGTA  SVVCLLNNFY  PREAKVQWKV  DNALQSGNSQ  ESVTEQDSKD  STYSLSSTLT
LSKADYEKHK  VYACEVTHQG  LSSPVTKSFN  RGEC
```

Amino acid sequence of heavy chain:

```
QVQLKQSGPG  LVQPSQSLSI  TCTVSGFSLT  NYGVHWVRQS  PGKGLEWLGV  IWSGGNTDYN
TPFTSRLSIN  KDNSKSQVFF  KMNSLQSNDT  AIYYCARALT  YYDYEFAYWG  QGTLVTVSAA
STKGPSVFPL  APSSKSTSGG  TAALGCLVKD  YFPEPVTVSA  LTSGVHTFPA  VLQSSGLYSL
SSVVTVPSSS  LGTQYICNVN  HKPSNTKVDK  KVEPKSCDKT  HTCPPCPAPE  LLGGPSVFLF
PPKPKDTLMI  SRTPEVTCVV  VDVSHEDPEV  KFNWYVDGVE  VHNAKTKPRE  EQYNSTYRVV
SVLTVLHQDW  LNGKEYKCKV  SNKALPAPIE  KTISKAKGQP  REPQVYTLPP  SRDELTKNQV
SLTCLVKGFY  PSDIAVEWES  NGQPENNYKT  TPPVLDSDGS  FFLYSKLTVD  KSRWQQGNVF
SCSVMHEALH  NHYTQKSLSL  SPGK
```

4　Pre-clinical Pharmacodynamics

Summary

Overview of *in vitro* and *in vivo* Activities
- ❖ M225, the parental murine antibody of cetuximab, efficiently competes with EGF and TGF-β for binding to the receptor, inhibits both ligand stimulated activation of the receptor and downstream signaling molecules, and inhibits tumor cell mitogenesis and proliferation.　Binding of M225 to EGFR induces rapid receptor internalization, hence effectively stripping the receptor from tumor cell surface.　M225 also induces apoptosis in some EGFR-overexpressing tumor cell lines and inhibits tumor growth in numerous human tumor cell lines *in vivo*.
- ❖ Cetuximab (also called IMC-C225), the engineered chimeric form of M225 to minimize immunogenicity in human, has a higher binding affinity to EGFR than the paternal M225.　Cetuximab can also compete with ligands binding to the receptor, therefore, block the activation and phosphorylation of receptor and downstream molecules such Akt and MAPK.
- ❖ Cetuximab can generate antibody-dependent cellular cytotoxicity (ADCC) in tumor cells expressing wild-type or mutant EGFR.　The activity of ADCC is correlated to the EGFR expression level.
- ❖ Cetuximab inhibits EGFR/HER2 heterodimerization and phosphorylation/activation stimulated by EGF in EGFR and HER2 coexpressing cell line CAL27, NCI-H226 and NCI-N87.　Cetuximab can also block the phosphorylation of downstream molecules such as Akt, MAPK and STAT-3 in these cells and tumor growth in the xenograft model.
- ❖ Cetuximab can effectively inhibit the growth of almost all EGFR-positive tumor cell lines *in vitro* and *in vivo* in various animal models.　The sensitivity to the treatment is varied.　The combination treatment with other anti-cancer agents or irradiation markedly enhanced tumor inhibition over treatment with either agent alone, in some models, led to tumor regression and eradication of established tumors.

Overview of *in vitro* Activities

Target Binding and Mechanism of Action
- ❖ The binding affinity (K_d) of cetuximab and M225 to EGFR is 0.15 nM and 1.2 nM, respectively, as measured by ELISA for binding to fixed A431 cells.　When analyzed by surface plasmon resonance (SPR), the K_d of cetuximab and M225 for binding to soluble EGFR is 0.2 nM and 0.87 nM, respectively.[20]
- ❖ Cetuximab binds to EGFR with 2-log higher affinity than the endogenous ligands (EGF and TGF-α).[15, 20, 32]
- ❖ Competition experiments showed that cetuximab displaced FITC-labeled EGF bound to human epidermal vulva cancer derived cell line A431 cells with a avidity 6-fold higher than that of unlabeled EGF.[15, 20]
- ❖ Cetuximab induces ADCC against tumor cells with wild-type or mutant EGFR (Table 8)[33] in most EGFR positive cell lines.　The ADCC activity was correlative to the EGFR expression level.
- ❖ Cetuximab inhibited the formation of EGFR-EGFR homodimers and EGFR-HER2 heterodimers and blocked the phosphorylation of receptor and downstream molecules (Figure 2, 3).[34]

Table 8   Correlation between EGFR Expression Level and ADCC Activity[33]

Cell Line	EGFR Expression (R-1)	EGFR Expression (Cetuximab)	ADCC (%)
A431	286 ± 13.7	319 ± 98.2	30.7
PC-9	9.7 ± 6.2	20.1 ± 10.2	20.1
PC-14	17.6 ± 1.5	42.2 ± 8.6	26.8
A549	9.1 ± 1.9	19.1 ± 6.2	24.2
Ma-1	13.8 ± 1.4	27.5 ± 2.9	22.3
11_18	6.1 ± 0.60	12.6 ± 1.1	15.5
K562	1.1 ± 0.40	2.8 ± 1.6	7.0
293M	3.7 ± 1.6	8.6 ± 3.2	8.2
293W	40.2 ± 6.2	39.7 ± 6.2	16.3
293D	55.2 ± 21.9	53.0 ± 8.2	18.9

The mean of expression values from three different experiments and standard deviations are shown.   A431: Vulva squamous carcinoma.   A541: Ma-1 and 11_18: Human non-small cell lung cancer (NSCLC).   K562: Human chronic myelogenous leukemia (CML).   PC-9 and PC-14: Prostatic carcinoma cell lines.   PC-9 and Ma-1 are known to contain E746_A750del, and 11_18 is known to contain L858R in tyrosine kinase domains of EGFR.   The other cell lines are known to have wild-type EGFR. 293M, 293W and 293D: HEK293 stably transfected cell lines with an empty vector only, vector containing the wild type EGFR or E746-A750 deletion as that observed in PC-9 cells.   EGFR values were measured by FACS with the anti-EGFR antibody R-1 from Santa Cruz and cetuximab.   In ADCC assay, PBMC was used in a ratio 10:1 to the target cells.

Overview of *in vivo* Activities

Human Colorectal Cancer Cell DLD-1 and HT-29 Xenograft Mouse Models[35]

❖ Cetuximab (0.5 or 1 mg, q3d) with or without irinotecan CPT-11 (100 mg/kg, q7d): (Figure 2, A and B)
  • Cetuximab alone: No significant inhibition was observed for DLD-1 or HT-29 tumors ($P > 0.050$) in two different dosages (1 or 0.5 mg, q3d).
  • CPT-11 alone [100 mg/(kg·week)]: Was active against DLD-1 ($P < 0.020$) tumors, and no significant inhibition for HT-29 tumors ($P > 0.050$).
  • Combination of cetuximab and CPT-11: Enhanced antitumor activity was observed in both DLD-1 and HT-29 tumors compared with the two controls, cetuximab or CPT-11 alone.
❖ Cetuximab (1 mg, q3d) with MDT dosage of CPT-11 (150 mg/kg, q7d): (Figure 3, C & D)
  • DLD-1: Combination resulted in a significant inhibition of tumor growth compared with single-agent cetuximab ($P < 0.0020$) or CPT-11 ($P < 0.030$).   Complete inhibition of tumor growth was observed in the majority of animals. In addition, regression of established DLD-1 tumors was observed in 60.0% of animals.
  • HT-29 model: Regression of established HT-29 tumors was observed in 100% of the animals treated with cetuximab and CPT-11 combination therapy.

Human Squamous Cell Carcinoma of the Head and Neck[36]

❖ *In vitro*
  • Cetuximab induced G1 cell cycle arrest with an associated decrease in the S-phase fraction.
  • Cetuximab inhibited squamous cell carcinoma (SCC) tumor cell proliferation and alternated the expression of key regulators of the G1-S cell cycle phase transition.
  • Exposure of SCCs to cetuximab in culture enhances radiosensitivity following single-dose radiation exposure.
❖ *In vivo* (SCC tumor xenografts in athymic mice)
  • Profound augmentation of the radiation response of SCC tumor xenografts in athymic mice.   Potential underlying mechanisms of action for the combination of cetuximab and radiation may include: (a) proliferative growth inhibition, (b) enhancement of radiation-induced apoptosis, (c) inhibition of damage repair, and (d) downregulation of tumor angiogenic response.

Human Pancreatic Carcinoma Xenograft Models[37]

❖ *In vitro*
  • Cetuximab inhibited exogenous ligand-stimulated tyrosine phosphorylation of the EGF receptor on BxPC-3 tumor cells.
  • Cetuximab inhibited DNA synthesis (23.8%) and colony formation in soft agar (45.6%).
❖ *In vivo* (BxPC-3 tumor xenografts in athymic mice) (Figure 4)
  • Cetuximab alone significantly suppressed the growth of BxPC-3 tumors compared with treatment with vehicle alone ($P < 0.0030$).
  • Combination of cetuximab the chemotherapeutic agent 5-fluorouracil enhanced the antitumor effects compared with either agent alone and resulted in regression of pancreatic tumors in several animals.

- Histologic examination of pancreatic tumors from mice treated with cetuximab showed extensive tumor necrosis that coincided with a substantial decrease in tumor cell proliferation and an increase in tumor cell apoptosis.

Summary of Some *in vivo* and *in vitro* Studies[15, 20]

❖ Extensive preclinical studies using a variety of assays, including ligand competition, receptor phosphorylation, cell proliferation, and anchorage-independent growth in soft agar, demonstrated that cetuximab inhibits EGFR activation and the growth of several different EGFR-expressing human tumor cell lines *in vitro*, including those carcinomas of the bladder, breast, colon, epidermoid carcinoma, kidney, ovary, pancreas, brain, and prostate (Table 9). The extent of cell growth inhibition varies among different tumor cell lines used in each study, and is dependent on the type of assay utilized, EGFR expression levels, the presence of autocrine stimulatory pathways and the intrinsic biology of the tumor cell lines. Cetuximab treatment under optimal *in vitro* culture conditions results in suppression of tumor cell growth ranging from 10.0% to 90.0%.

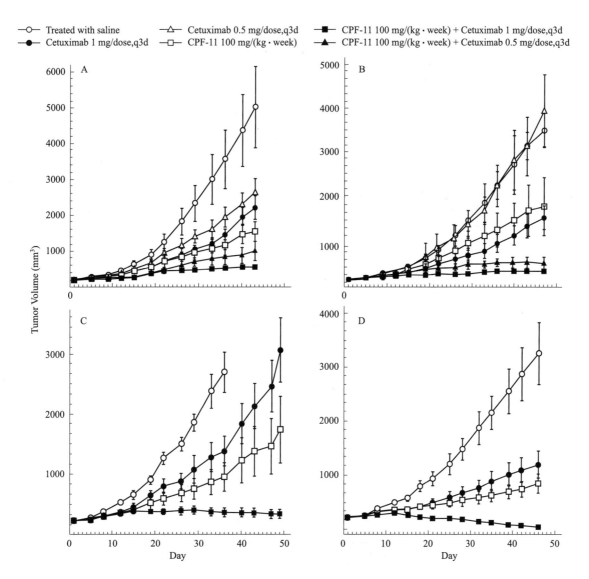

Figure 2   Growth Inhibitions of DLD-1 and HT-29 Colorectal Tumor Xenografts in Nude Mice[35]

Study: A and B: Dose-dependent effects are shown for treatment of established DLD-1 (A) and HT-29 (B) tumors treated with saline (open cycle). C and D: Combination therapy on established DLD-1 (C) and HT-29 (D) tumors treated with saline (open cycle).

Animal: Nude Mice.

Administration: A and B: Cetuximab: 1 mg (solid cycle) or 0.5 mg (open triangle) per dose/q3d; CPT-11: 100 mg/(kg·week) (open square); CPT-11 [100 mg/(kg·week)] plus cetuximab at 1 mg/dose/q3d (solid square); CPT-11 [100 mg/(kg·week)] plus cetuximab at 0.5 mg/dose/q3d (solid triangle). Bars, ± SE.   C and D: Cetuximab: 1 mg (solid cycle); CPT-11 at 150 mg/(kg·week) (open square); CPT-11 [150 mg/(kg·week)] plus IMC-C225 at 1 mg/dose/q3d (solid square).   Bars, ± SE.

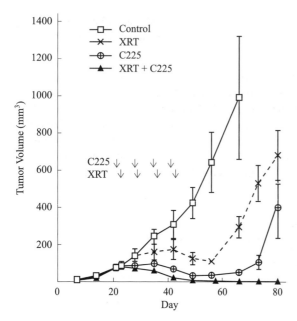

Study: Human SCC-1 xenografts were raised s.c. in the dorsal flank of athymic mice.

Administration: i.p. 0.2 mg of cetuximab, once a week, for a total of four injections. The radiation (XRT)-treated groups received a single 8-Gy treatment at 24 h following each injection of cetuximab.

Starting: Tumors reached a size of ~100 mm³ at 23 days.

Test: Measured tumor volumes. Values represent mean tumor size (mm³) ± SE (n = 8 per group).

Figure 3   SCC Xenograft Response[36]

❖ Dose-dependent effects of cetuximab therapy alone on BxPC-3 tumors are shown. Open circles: Saline control; triangles: cetuximab at 17 mg/kg; filled circles: 33 mg/kg. (B) Effects of cetuximab combined with 5-fluorouracil (5-FU) on BxPC-3 xenografts. Open circles: Saline control; filled circles: cetuximab; open squares: 5-FU; filled squares: combined cetuximab and 5-FU therapy. Error bars indicate standard error.

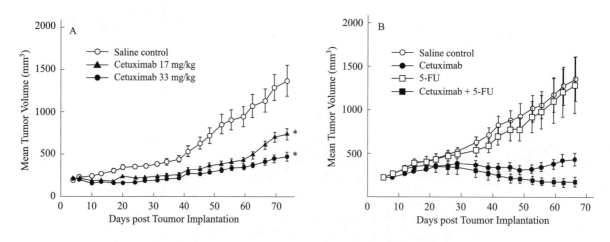

Figure 4   Growth Inhibition of BxPC-3 Xenografts in Nude Mice by Cetuximab[37]

Table 9   Summary of Cell-based and Animal Studies Performed Prior to Year 1999[15, 20]

Treatment	Cell Line/Model	Finding
Cetuximab	Human epidermoid carcinoma (A431) xenografts	Effectively inhibited tumor growth and resulted in complete remission in many cases.
Cetuximab	Human epidermoid carcinoma (A431)	Down-regulation of the expression of vascular endothelial growth factor (VEGF) *in vitro* and *in vivo*. Significant reduction in tumor blood vessels and regression of established tumors.
Cetuximab + Doxorubicin	Human epidermoid carcinoma (A431) cell lines	Combined therapy enhanced the cell cycle arrest induced by doxorubicin alone in a manner suggestive of apoptosis, augmented the inhibition of proliferation, and further decreased receptor activation.
Cetuximab + Doxil®	Human epidermoid carcinoma (A431) xenografts	Combined therapy resulted in significant tumor regression and many complete remissions.

Continued

Treatment	Cell Line/Model	Finding
Cetuximab + Cisplatin	Human epidermoid carcinoma (KB) xenografts	Neither agent alone affected tumor growth, but combined therapy significantly inhibited tumor growth and EGFR activation-related phosphorylation.
Cetuximab	Prostatic carcinoma (LNCaP, PC-3, DuI45) cell lines and (Du145) xenografts	Inhibition of cell proliferation *in vitro* and tumor regression *in vivo*.
Cetuximab + Doxorubicin	Prostatic carcinoma cell lines and (PC-3, Du145) xenografts	Cetuximab blocked EGF-induced receptor activation and induced receptor internalization. Tumor progression of well-established xenografts was inhibited by cetuximab alone or combined with doxorubicin.
Cetuximab + Hydroxyflutamide	Prostatic carcinoma cell line MDA PCa2b	Combined treatment augmented inhibition of tumor cell growth *in vitro*.
Cetuximab	Human renal cell carcinoma (A498, Caki-1, SK-RC-4, SK-RC-29, SW839) cell lines and (Caki-1 ascites, SK-RC-29 subcutaneous) xenografts	Decreased DNA synthesis and inhibition of tumor cell growth *in vitro*. Dose-dependent inhibition of tumor growth and increased survival time *in vivo*.
Cetuximab + Protein kinase A antisense	Human renal cell carcinoma (769-D, ACHN, A498, SW839)	Combined treatment inhibited tumor cell growth *in vitro* and caused regression of tumor xenografts *in vivo*.
Cetuximab + Protein kinase A antisense	Human colon carcinoma (GEO) xenografts	Combined therapy inhibited tumor growth and cell production of autocrine growth factors and angiogenic factors.
Cetuximab + Topotecan	Human colon carcinoma (GEO) xenografts	Combined therapy resulted in a supra-additive inhibition of tumor growth *in vitro* and tumor regression of established xenografts *in vivo*.
Cetuximab + anti-HER2 mAb 4D5	Human ovarian carcinoma (OVCA 420)	Combined treatment augmented anti-proliferative effect on tumor cells that was accompanied by enhanced G1 cell distribution, increased levels of p27Kip1, and decreased activity of CDK kinases.
Cetuximab	Human transitional cell carcinoma (TCC) cultures and xenografts	Blocked EGF-induced cell invasion of a Matrigel matrix and metallo-proteinase-9 (MMP-9) production. Inhibited tumor growth and metastasis.
Cetuximab	Human TCC (253J B-V) cultures and orthotopic tumors	Inhibited *in vitro* production of angiogenic peptides VEGF, interleukin 8 (IL-8) and basic fibroblast growth factor (bFGF) in a dose-dependent manner. Resulted in significant tumor regression, inhibition of metastasis, and decreased production of VEGF, IL-8, and bFGF.
Cetuximab + Taxol®, cisplatin	Human TCC cultures	Cetuximab + Taxol®, but not cisplatin, exerted an additive cytotoxic effect.
Cetuximab + Irradiation	Human SCCHN	Exposure of tumor cells to cetuximab in culture inhibited cell proliferation and induced accumulation of cells in G1 phase. Cetuximab exposure also induced apoptosis and enhanced radio sensitivity of tumor cells.
Cetuximab + Irradiation	Human glioblastoma xenografts (U251)	Mice bearing established intracranial tumors had increased survival when treated with cetuximab band irradiation.
Cetuximab + 5-FU	Human pancreatic carcinoma xenografts (BXPC-3)	Inhibited tumor cell growth *in vitro* and inhibited established tumor xenografts *in vivo*. Combined therapy with 5-FU resulted in regression of established tumors.
Cetuximab + Gemcitabine	Human pancreatic carcinoma xenografts (L3.6p1)	Combination treatment inhibited growth and metastasis of established orthotopic tumors.

5-FU: 5-Fluorouracil. OVCA: Ovarian carcinoma. SCCHN: Squamous cell carcinoma of the head and neck. TCC: Transitional cell carcinoma. VEGF: Vascular endothelial growth factor.

5 Toxicology[38, 39]

Summary

Non-clinical Single-Dose Toxicology
- ❖ No single-dose toxicity studies were performed in relevant species.
- ❖ Doses of 300 mg/kg in mice and 200 mg/kg in rats revealed no significant signs of toxicity in all parameters analyzed, including body weight, food consumption, clinical hematology, serum biochemistry and gross necropsy.

Non-clinical Repeated-Dose Toxicology
- ❖ Repeated-dose toxicity study in Cynomolgus monkeys for 39 weeks study

- Six animals were included in each group and two additions animal were added to the high dose group. The initial doses and subsequent weekly doses were 12 and 7.5 mg/kg for the low dose group, 38 and 24 mg/kg for the intermediate dose group, and 120 and 75 mg/kg for the high dose group.
- Severe toxicity was observed with cetuximab. Dose-related skin lesions were observed in all animals. Occasionally other epithelial effects e.g. conjunctivitis, reddened and swollen eyes were noted, as were signs of intestinal disturbances. Half of the animals in the high dose group died as a result of the treatment, which caused lesions of the skin, tongue, nasal cavity, and oesophagus.
- Pathogenically the skin lesions were considered to be related to a cetuximab induced maturation defect of the epidermis. This defect accounts for parakeratosis, acanthosis, and acanthosis with clefts, pustules, and vesicle formation, summarized as dermatosis. Secondary bacterial superinfections, especially in high dose animals caused an erosive to ulcerative dermatitis with subsequent involvement of inner organs due to septicemia, especially in liver, spleen, bone marrow, and kidney.

❖ Repeated-dose toxicity study in Sprague-Dawley rat for 4 weeks
- 0, 2.5, 10 and 40 mg/kg cetuximab were administered to groups of 30 rats (15F + 15M) for 4 weeks.
- Parameters for the study: Food consumption/body weight; hematology, clinical chemistry and urinalysis.
- No significant change was observed by the administration of cetuximab.

Reproductive Toxicology

❖ No reproductive and developmental toxicity studies were performed.

❖ In the 39-week repeated-dose toxicity study in Cynomolgus monkeys, examination of individual sexual cycle length from Week 25 onwards, including the treatment-free period, revealed an impairment of menstrual cyclicity in cetuximab treated females such as increased incidences of irregular cyclicity or absence of cyclicity when compared to controls. However, since pre-treatment cycles were not evaluated in any of the females in any group, this result cannot be confirmed. Evaluation of testosterone data and sperm analysis did not show any toxicologically significant differences among the treated groups when compared to controls. Histological examinations of organs of the reproductive system in the males and females treated with cetuximab revealed no abnormalities attributable to cetuximab.

Carcinogenicity and Genotoxicity

❖ Carcinogenicity: No studies were performed.

❖ Genotoxicity: *Salmonella typhimurium* and *Escherichia coli* were used as test systems with and without addition of liver S9 mix as external metabolic system yielded no indications of a mutagenic potential of cetuximab. Furthermore, in an *in vivo* cytogenetic assay performed as a micronucleus test in male Wistar rats, cetuximab was not genotoxic. The results of the micronucleus test are considered of limited value due to the lack of immunoreactivity of cetuximab with tissues from rats.

Local Tolerance

❖ Local tolerance testing has been performed in New Zealand white rabbits with material originating from three different production processes. Cetuximab drug product and the vehicle were administered to female rabbits (6 females received intravenous (i.v.), intramuscular (i.m.), and subcutaneous (s.c.) injections and 6 females received intra-arterial (i.a.) and paravenous (p.v.) injections) as a single injection of each type of administration on Day 1. Afterwards animals were observed for 48 hours (3 females that received i.v., i.m., and s.c.; 3 females that received i.a. and p.v.) or 96 h (the remaining 3 females of each group) before their scheduled necropsy.

❖ No signs of systemic toxicity were observed. Gross pathological and histological examinations revealed no toxicologically relevant alterations.

Other Toxicity Studies

❖ Immunogenicity
- Antigenicity was demonstrated in rats as expected for chimeric proteinaceous product. Antibody responses were observed in 3/22 (13.6%) Cynomolgus monkeys. An effect on cetuximab serum concentrations was observed for one of these animals only. The assay for anti-cetuximab response was a non-species specific double antigen radiometric assay.

❖ Immunotoxicity
- No separate studies were performed.

❖ Dependence
- No studies were performed.

❖ Metabolites
- No studies were performed.

❖ Studies on Impurities
- No studies were performed.

❖ Ecotoxicity/Environmental Risk Assessment
  • No environmental risk assessment was submitted.

Table 10   Non-clinical Repeated-Dose Toxicology Studies of Cetuximab[38, 39]

Species	Duration (Week)	Dose	Finding
Cynomolgus monkey	39	The initial doses and subsequent weekly doses were 12 and 7.5 mg/kg for the low dose group, 38 and 24 mg/kg for the intermediate dose group, and 120 and 75 mg/kg for the high dose group	Severe toxicity was observed with cetuximab. Dose-related skin lesions were observed in all animals. Occasionally other epithelial effects e.g. conjunctivitis, reddened and swollen eyes were noted, as were signs of intestinal disturbances. Half of the animals in the high dose group died as a result of the treatment, which caused lesions of the skin, tongue, nasal cavity and oesophagus. Pathogenically the skin lesions were considered to be related to a cetuximab induced maturation defect of the epidermis. This defect accounts for parakeratosis, acanthosis, and acanthosis with clefts, pustules, and vesicle formation, summarized as dermatosis. Secondary bacterial superinfections, especially in high dose animals caused an erosive to ulcerative dermatitis with subsequent involvement of inner organs due to septicemia, especially in liver, spleen, bone marrow, and kidney.
Sprague-Dawley rat	4	Male & female: 0, 2.5, 10, 40 mg/kg	Parameters for the study: Food consumption/body weight, hematology, clinical chemistry and urinalysis. No significant change was observed by the administration of cetuximab.

6   Non-clinical Pharmacokinetic/ADME/Toxicokinetics

Summary

Non-clinical Pharmacokinetics[38, 39]
❖ Single-dose pharmacokinetics in Cynomolgus monkey (Table 11)
  • C_{max} and AUC increased with increasing dose.
  • Non-linear pharmacokinetics in Cynomolgus monkeys, with a pattern of supra-proportional increases in AUC in the dose of 7.5, 24, 75 mg/kg.
  • Clearance decreased and terminal half-life increased with increasing dose.
  • Half-life ranging between 2.7-6.8 days (Table 11 and Figure 5).
❖ Multiple-dose pharmacokinetics in Cynomolgus monkey
  • Repeated-dose (0, 12, 38 and 120 mg/kg at Week 1, subsequent weekly doses 0, 7.5, 24, and 75 mg/kg).
  • No accumulation after daily dosing beyond Week 4 was observed.
  • AUC_{last} and C_{max} at the 4, 13, 26, and 39 weeks were comparable.
❖ Absorption-Bioavailability
  • Cetuximab is administered intravenously and the bioavailability is therefore 100%.
  • No studies have been performed to address absorption of cetuximab.
❖ Distribution
  • No studies in a relevant species have been performed to address the distribution of cetuximab.   [111]Indium-labeled mouse monoclonal M225 was studied in mouse xenograft models of human tumors, showing specific uptake into the tumors.
❖ Metabolism and excretion
  • No studies addressing the metabolism and excretion of cetuximab were performed.
❖ Pharmacokinetic drug interactions
  • No pharmacokinetic drug interaction studies in non-clinical models of disease were performed.

Table 11 Summary of Mean Pharmacokinetic Parameters after a Single Infusion[38]

Dose (mg/kg)	7.5		24		75	
Gender (No. of Animals)	**M (3)**	**F (3)**	**M (3)**	**F (3)**	**M (3)**	**F (3)**
$C_{max}{}^a$ (µg/mL)	166	175	949	936	2,300	2,460
C_{max} (nM)	1,100	1,150	6,200	6,100	15,000	16,000
C_{max}/Dose [(µg/mL)/(mg/kg)]	22.0	23.0	40.0	39.0	31.0	33.0
$t_{1/2}$ (Day)	2.7	3.1	4.0	4.7	6.8	6.7
AUC_{last} (µg·h/mL)	10,933	8,854	61,113	65,523	200,753	213,637
AUC_{inf}/Dose [(µg·h/mL)/(mg/kg)]	1,619	1,354	2,623	2,777	3,149	3,187
CL [mL/(h·kg)]	0.60	0.80	0.40	0.30	0.30	0.30
V_{ss} (mL/kg)	61.0	76.0	50.0	48.0	67.0	64.0

F: Female.   M: Male.   ª AUC at the last measurement taken.

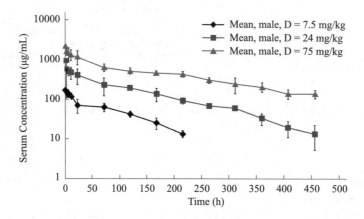

Figure 5   Serum Concentrations of Cetuximab after a Single Infusion in Cynomolgus Monkeys (N = 3)[40]

7   Clinical Efficacy and Safety

Overview Profile

Clinical Efficacy

❖ On February 12, 2004, the FDA approved cetuximab, in combination with irinotecan for the treatment of EGFR-expressing, recurrent metastatic colorectal carcinoma in patients who are refractory to irinotecan-based chemotherapy, and as a single agent in patients who have failed oxaliplatin- and irinotecan-based chemotherapy or who are intolerant to irinotecan, based on the results from three Phase 2 trials, EMR 62202-007 (BOND study), supplemental by IMCL-CP02-9923 and IMCL-CP02-0141.[35]

❖ On March 1, 2006, the FDA granted approval to cetuximab for use in combination with radiation therapy (RT) for the treatment of locally or regionally advanced SCCHN or as a single agent for the treatment of patients with recurrent or metastatic SCCHN for whom prior platinum-based therapy has failed.   This approval is based on a statistically significant improvement in overall survival and duration of locoregional disease control for RT plus cetuximab when compared to RT alone (EMR62 202-006 or NCT00865098).[35]

❖ On November 7, 2011, the FDA approved cetuximab in combination with platinum-based therapy plus 5-FU for the first-line treatment of patients with recurrent and/or metastatic SCCHN.   The approval was based primarily on the results of a multicenter clinical study conducted outside the United States in 442 patients with metastatic or locally recurrent head and neck cancer who were not suitable for potentially curative treatment with surgery or radiation (EMR62 202-002).[35]

❖ On July 6, 2012, the FDA granted approval to cetuximab for use in combination with FOLFIRI (irinotecan, 5-fluorouracil, and leucovorin) for first-line treatment of patients with KRAS mutation-negative (wild-type), EGFR-expressing metastatic colorectal cancer (mCRC) as determined by FDA-approved tests.   FDA also approved the Thrascreen® KRAS RGQ PCR Kit (QIAGEN Manchester, Ltd) concurrent with this cetuximab approval.   This approval was based on retrospective analyses of tumor samples from patients enrolled in the CRYSTAL trial and in two supportive studies, CA225025 and EMR 62 202-047 (OPUS), according to KRAS mutation status.[36]

❖ Two open labeled, randomized clinical trials (FIRE-3 and CALGB 80405) were performed to compare cetuximab plus FOLFIRI or FOLFOX (leucovorin, 5-fluorouracil and oxaliplatin) and bevacizumab plus FOLFIRI or FOLFOX head-to-head to treat patients with KRAS-wild type metastatic colorectal cancer. FIRE-3 trial result was presented in 2013 ASCO (American Society of Clinical Oncology) annual meeting, and 2013 European Cancer Congress; CALGB 80405 results were presented in 2014 ESMO (European Society of Medical Oncology). The FIRE-3 trial demonstrated a 7.5 to 12 months survival advantage with the use cetuximab; but CALGB 8045 showed no difference between cetuximab and bevacizumab treatment.[37]

Combination and Monotherapy of Cetuximab for Advanced Metastatic Colorectal Cancer[41]

❖ Three Phase 2 trials were designed to study the efficacy of cetuximab alone or in combination with irinotecan in patients with metastatic colorectal adenocarcinoma expressing the epidermal growth factor receptor (EGFR) and progressing on a defined irinotecan based regimen. EMR 62 202-007 was a multicenter, randomized, controlled clinical trial conducted in 329 patients (218 patients for cetuximab plus Irinotecan) or cetuximab monotherapy (111 patients). IMCL-CP02-9923 was an open-label, single arm trial (138 patients) of cetuximab plus irinotecan. IMCL-CP02-0141 was an open-label single arm trial (57 patients) of cetuximab as a single reagent.

❖ The recommended dose of cetuximab, in combination with irinotecan or as monotherapy, is 400 mg/m^2 as an initial loading dose (first infusion only) administered as a 120 min i.v. infusion. The recommended weekly maintenance dose is 250 mg/m^2 infused over 60 min.

❖ The overall objective response rate (ORR) of EMR 62 202-007 was 23.0% with a median duration of response of 5.7 months in the cetuximab plus irinotecan arm. The overall response rate was 12.0% with a median duration of response of 4.1 months in the cetuximab monotherapy arm. The median time to progression was significantly longer for patients receiving combination therapy (4.1 vs. 1.5 months). Comparable results were observed in the single arm studies of cetuximab plus irinotecan (15.0% ORR, 6.5 months median response duration) and cetuximab monotherapy (9.0% ORR, 1.4 months median response duration).

Combination Treatment of Cetuximab plus Radiation for Advanced Squamous Cell Cancer of the Head and Neck[30]

❖ EMR 62 202-006 was a randomized study compared the combination of cetuximab and radiation therapy (208 patients) with radiation therapy alone (212 patients) in patients with locally advanced SCCHN.

❖ Cetuximab was administered as a 400 mg/m^2 initial dose, followed by 250 mg/m^2 weekly for the duration of RT (6-7 weeks), starting one week before RT. RT was administered for 6-7 weeks as once daily, twice daily or concomitant boost.

❖ The median overall survival (OS) time was 49 months on the cetuximab plus RT versus 29.3 months observed in patients receiving RT alone [$P = 0.030$, stratified log-rank test; HR: 0.74, (95% CI: 0.56, 0.97)]. The median duration of loco-regional control was 24.4 months in patients receiving cetuximab plus RT versus 14.9 months for those receiving RT alone [$P = 0.0050$, stratified log-rank test; HR: 0.68, (95% CI: 0.52, 0.89)].

Combination Treatment of Cetuximab plus Cisplatin in the First-line Therapy for Squamous Cell Cancer of the Head and Neck[42]

❖ EMR 62 202-002 was a randomized study in patients with recurrent and/or metastatic squamous cell cancer of the head and neck who had not received prior chemotherapy for this disease compared the combination of cetuximab and cisplatin or carboplatin plus infusional 5-fluorouracil (219 patients) to the same chemotherapy alone (215 patients).

❖ Either cisplatin (100 mg/m^2 intravenously Day 1) or carboplatin (5 mg/(mL·min) intravenously Day 1) with 5-FU [1,000 mg/(m^2·day) continuous intravenous infusion Days 1-4] were administered every three weeks (one cycle). A maximum of six cycles was administered in the absence of disease progression or unacceptable toxicity. For patients randomly assigned to the cetuximab group, cetuximab was administered as an initial dose of 400 mg/m^2 intravenously, followed by a weekly dose of 250 mg/m^2 intravenously. After completion of six planned courses, patients demonstrating at least stable disease on cetuximab in combination with chemotherapy continued cetuximab monotherapy [250 mg/(m^2·week)] in the absence of disease progression or unacceptable toxicity.

❖ The major efficacy outcome measure of the trial was OS. Other outcome measures included ORR and progression-free survival (PFS). OS was significantly improved in patients receiving cetuximab plus chemotherapy compared with those receiving chemotherapy alone [HR: 0.80; (95% CI: 0.64, 0.98); $P = 0.034$, stratified log-rank test]. The median survival for patients receiving cetuximab plus chemotherapy was 10.1 months, compared with 7.4 months for those receiving chemotherapy alone. PFS was also significantly improved in patients receiving cetuximab plus chemotherapy [HR: 0.57; (95% CI: 0.46, 0.72); $P < 0.00010$, stratified log-rank test]. The median PFS times were 5.5 months in the patients receiving cetuximab plus chemotherapy and 3.3 months in the patients receiving chemotherapy alone. The ORRs were 35.6% in the patients receiving cetuximab plus chemotherapy and 19.5% in the patients receiving chemotherapy alone [Odds Ratio (OR): 2.3; (95% CI: 1.5, 3.6); $P = 0.00010$, Cochran-Mantel-Haenszel test].

Single Arm Treatment of Cetuximab for Squamous Cell Cancer of the Head and Neck[42]

❖ This study was a single arm, multicenter clinical trial in 103 patients with recurrent or metastatic SCCHN. All patients had documented disease progression within 30 days of a platinum-based chemotherapy regimen. Eighty percent had metastatic disease.

❖ Patients received a 20-mg test dose of Erbitux® on Day 1, followed by a 400 mg/m² initial dose, and 250 mg/m² weekly until disease progression or unacceptable toxicity.

❖ The ORR was 12.6% (95% *CI*: 7.0, 21.0). Median duration of response was 5.8 months [range 1.2-5.8 months, (95% *CI*: 2.9, 5.8)].

Cetuximab as Single Agent in Comparison to the Best Support Care in Advanced Chemo-refractory CRC Patients[43]

❖ CA225025: A total of 242 advanced CRC patients who had received prior oxaliplatin-, irinotecan- and fluoropyri-midine-based treatment were randomly assigned (1:1) to receive either cetuximab plus best supportive care (BSC) or BSC alone treatment. Tumor tissue was evaluable for retrospective KRAS mutation status analysis in 79.0% patients (453 patients).

❖ The recommended initial dose is 400 mg/m² administered as a 120 min intravenous infusion (maximum infusion rate 10 mg/min). The recommended subsequent weekly dose is 250 mg/m² infused over 60 min (maximum infusion rate 10 mg/min) until disease progression or unacceptable toxicity.

❖ CA225025 efficacy results:

- KRAS wild-type subgroup (245/453, 54.0%): Cetuximab plus BSC resulted in an improvement in OS compared with BSC alone [HR: 0.63 (95% *CI*: 0.47, 0.84)]. The median OS was 8.6 versus 5.0 months in the cetuximab plus BSC and BSC groups, respectively. The median PFS was 3.8 and 1.9 months in the cetuximab plus BSC and the BSC groups, respectively [HR: 0.42 (95% *CI*: 0.32, 0.56)].

- KRAS mutant subgroup (208/453, 46.0%): No improvements in OS, PFS or ORR were observed with the addition of cetuximab to BSC compared with BSC alone.

Cetuximab Combined with Irinotecan in First-line Therapy for Metastatic Colorectal Cancer[44]

❖ Two open-label randomized controlled trials were designed to treat patients with EGFR-expressing mCRC in first-line. KRAS mutation was analyzed partially to check mutants located in codons 12 and 13 (exon 2): G12A, G12D, G12R, G12C, G12S, G12V, 574 G13D.

- CRYSTAL: Total 667 mCRC patients who had not received prior chemotherapy were randomly assigned (1:1) to receive either cetuximab in combination with FOLFIRI or FOLFIRI alone. Tumor tissue was evaluable for retrospective KRAS mutation status analysis in 89.0% patients.

- OPUS: A total of 337 mCRC patients who had not received prior chemotherapy were randomly assigned (2:1) to receive either cetuximab in combination with FOLFOX-4 (5-flourouracil, folinic acid, and oxaliplatin) or FOLFOX-4 alone. Tumor tissue was evaluable for retrospective KRAS mutation status analysis in 93.0% patients (315 patients).

❖ The recommended initial dose, either as monotherapy or in combination with irinotecan or FOLFIRI (irinotecan, 5-fluorour-acil, leucovorin), is 400 mg/m² administered as a 120 min intravenous infusion (maximum infusion rate 10 mg/min). Complete Erbitux® administration 1 hour prior to FOLFIRI. The recommended subsequent weekly dose either as mono-therapy or in combination with irinotecan or FOLFIRI, is 250 mg/m² infused over 60 min (maximum infusion rate 10 mg/min) until disease progression or unacceptable toxicity. Complete Erbitux® administration 1 hour prior to FOLFIRI.

❖ CRYSTAL efficacy result:

- All patients (1,217): A statistically significant improvement in PFS was observed in patients treated with cetuximab plus FOLFIRI compared with patients treated with FOLFIRI alone [median PFS: 8.9 vs. 8.1 months; HR: 0.85; (95% *CI*: 0.74, 0.99); *P* = 0.036]. There was not a statistically significant improvement in the planned OS analysis [HR: 0.93; (95% *CI*: 0.82, 1.1); *P* = 0.33, 838 events]. In an updated analysis with an additional 162 events, the median OS was 19.6 months for patients treated with cetuximab plus FOLFIRI compared with 18.5 months for patients treated with FOLFIRI alone [HR: 0.88, (95% *CI*: 0.78, 1.0)].

- KRAS wild-type patients (673/1079, 63.0%): The addition of cetuximab to FOLFIRI resulted in a favorable effect on OS, PFS, and ORR in patients with KRAS wild-type tumors. The median OS was 23.5 months for patients treated with cetuximab plus FOLFIRI, compared with 19.5 months for patients treated with FOLFIRI alone [HR: 0.80; (95% *CI*: 0.67, 0.94)]. The median PFS for patients treated with cetuximab plus FOLFIRI was 9.5 compared with 8.1 months for patients treated with FOLFIRI alone [HR: 0.70; (95% *CI*: 0.57, 0.86)]. ORR was 57.0% in patients treated with cetuximab plus FOLFIRI compared with 39.0% in patients treated with FOLFIRI alone.

- KRAS mutant patients (406/1,079, 37.0%): Improvements in OS, PFS or ORR were not observed with the addition of cetuximab to FOLFIRI compared to FOLFIRI alone.

❖ OPUS efficacy results:

- KRAS wild type (179 patients, 57.0%): The primary endpoint ORR was 57.0% (95% *CI*: 46.0, 68.0) in patients treated with cetuximab plus FOLFOX-4 compared with 34.0% (95% *CI*: 25.0, 44.0) in patients treated with FOLFOX-4. The median PFS was 8.3 months in patients treated with cetuximab plus FOLFOX-4, compared with 7.2 months in patients treated with FOLFOX-4 [HR: 0.57; (95% *CI*: 0.38, 0.86)]; The median OS for patients treated with cetuximab plus FOLFOX-4 was 22.8 months, vs. 18.5 months for patients treated with FOLFOX-4. OS improvement was also observed [HR: 0.86; (95% *CI*: 0.60, 1.22)].

- KRAS mutant subgroup (136 patients, 43.0%): No improvements in OS, PFS, or ORR were observed in patients treated with cetuximab plus FOLFOX-4 compared with patients treated with FOLFOX-4 alone.

Combination Study of Cetuximab with Bevacizumab Plus Capecitabine or Oxaliplatin[45]

- ❖ NCT 00208546 was a multicenter randomized Phase 3 study investing head-to-head capecitabine, oxaliplatin, and bevacizumab with or without cetuximab. A total of 755 patients with previously untreated metastatic colorectal cancer were randomly assigned to capecitabine, oxaliplatin, and bevacizumab (CB regimen, 378 patients) or the same regimen plus weekly cetuximab (CBC regimen, 377 patients).
- ❖ The primary endpoint was PFS. The mutation status of the KRAS gene was evaluated as a predictor of outcome. PFS was shorter in the CBC group than that of the CB group [median PFS was 10.7 months in CB group vs. 9.4 months in the CBC group (*P* = 0.010)]. The OS and ORR were not different significantly in two groups. Quality-of-life scores were lower in the CBC group. Treated patients in CBC group had more Grade 3 or 4 adverse events, which were attributed to cetuximab-related adverse cutaneous effects.

Head-to-head Comparison of Cetuximab plus FOLFIRI to Bevacizumab plus FOLFIRI in First-line mCRC[46]

- ❖ The FIRE-3 study was a multicenter randomized Phase 3 study investigating head-to-head FOLFIRI combined with either cetuximab or bevacizumab in patients with KRAS exon 2 wild-type mCRC. RAS status was evaluable in tumor samples of 407 out of the total of 592 (69.0%) KRAS exon 2 wild-type patients. Of these, 342 patients had RAS wild-type tumors while RAS mutations were identified in the other 65 patients. The RAS mutant population (178 patients) comprises these 65 patients together with 113 patients with KRAS exon 2 mutant tumors treated before study enrolment was stratified to patients with KRAS exon 2 wild-type mCRC.
- ❖ The efficacy data generated in this study are summarized in the Table 23. In the KRAS wild-type patients, the primary endpoint, ORR, was not significantly different between the cetuximab and bevacizumab group (65.5% in the cetuximab group vs. 59.6% in the bevacizumab group). Median PFS was almost identical in the two groups. A significant OS advantage, however, was observed for patients treated with first-line FOLFIRI plus cetuximab, with an increase of 7.5 months (33.1 months for cetuximab vs. 25.6 for bevacizumab). No significant difference in ORR, PFS and OS between the two groups in patients with KRAS mutations.

Head-to-head Comparison of Cetuximab and Bevacizumab when Combined with either FOLFOX or FOLFIRI in First-line mCRC[47]

- ❖ The CALGB study was a multicenter randomized Phase 3 study investigating head-to-head FOLFIRI or FOLFOX combined with either cetuximab or bevacizumab in patients with KRAS exon 2 wild-type mCRC. Results of CALGB have been presented at the ASCO and ESMO. A total of 1,137 KRAS wild-type patients were enrolled in this study. This study failed to confirm an advantage for cetuximab in OS or PFS over bevacizumab, as observed in the FIRE-3 study; the median PFS was about 11 months (HR: 1.1; *P* = 0.31) with a median OS of 31-32 months (HR: 0.90; *P* = 0.40) for both treatment arms.

Table 12   Three Phase 2 Studies of Cetuximab Led to FDA Approval for the Treatment of Advanced CRC[48]

Study No.	Study Design	Objective	Population	No. of Patients
EMR 62202-007 (BOND study)	Phase 2, randomized (2:1) cetuximab and irinotecan or cetuximab monotherapy	ORR (primary) Time to progression (secondary)	EGFR positive metastatic CRC who progressive after an irinotecan containing regimen	329 (218/111)
IMCL-CP02-9923	Phase 2, non-randomized, single arm, cetuximab in combination with irinotecan	ORR (primary)	EGFR positive advanced CRC, refractory to treatment with an irinotecan containing regimen	139
IMCL-CP02-0141	Phase 2, single arm cetuximab monotherapy	ORR (primary)	EGFR positive advanced CRC, refractory to treatment with an irinotecan containing regimen	57

CRC: Colorectal cancer.   EGFR: Epidermal growth factor receptor.   ORR: Objective response rate.

Table 13   FDA Analysis of ORR for EMR 62202-007 (BOND) in the Treatment of CRC[48]

Population	Cetuximab + Irinotecan		Cetuximab Monotherapy		Difference	P-value
	N	n (%)	N	n (%)	(95% CI)	
ITT	218	50 (22.9)	111	12 (10.8)	12.1 (4.1-20.2)	0.0074
IRC-PD	132	34 (25.8)	69	10 (14.5)	11.3 (0.10-22.4)	0.074
IRC-PD oxaliplatin failure	80	19 (23.8)	44	5 (11.4)	12.4 (-0.80, 25.6)	0.10

CI: Confidence interval.   CRC: Colorectal cancer.   IRC-PD: All randomized patients who have received two cycles of irinotican-based chemotherapy treatment prior to cetuximab treatment.   ITT: Intent-to-treat.

Table 14   FDA Analysis of Time to Progression for EMR 62202-007 (BOND) in the Treatment of CRC[48]

Population	Cetuximab + Irinotecan (Median, month)	Cetuximba Monotherapy (Median, month)	Hazard Ratio (95% CI)	Log-rank P-value
ITT	4.1	1.5	0.54 (0.42-0.71)	<0.00010
IRC-PD	4.0	1.5	0.52 (0.37-0.73)	0.00010
IRC-PD oxaliplatin failure	2.9	1.5	0.48 (0.31-0.72)	0.00040

CI: Confidence interval.   CRC: Colorectal cancer.   IRC-PD: All randomized patients who have received two cycles of irinotican-based chemotherapy treatment prior to cetuximab treatment.   ITT: Intent-to-treat.

Table 15   Results of the Supportive Studies in the Treatment of CRC (IMCL CP02-9923 and 0141)[41]

		IMCL CP02-9923 (Combination Therapy)		IMCL CP02-0141 (Monotherapy)	
		All treated	IRC-PD	All treated	IRC-PD
		(N = 138)	(N = 83)	(N = 57)	(N = 28)
Primary endpoint	Objective response rate (CR + PR)	15.2%	13.3%	8.8%	14.3%
	(95% CI)	(9.7, 22.3)	(6.8, 22.5)	(2.9, 19.3)	(4.0, 32.7)
Secondary endpoint	Disease control rate (CR + PR + SD)	60.9%	53.0%	45.6%	39.3%
	(95% CI)	(52.2, 69.1)	(41.7, 64.1)	(32.4, 59.3)	(21.5, 59.4)
	Duration of response, median (Month)	6.5	5.7	4.2	4.2
	Time to response, median (Month)	2.6	1.3	1.2	1.9
	Duration of disease control, median (Month)	5.5	5.4	5.3	5.3
	Time to progression (TTP)	2.9	2.6	1.4	1.3
	Median (Month)	(2.6, 4.1)	(17.3, 3.1)	(1.3, 2.8)	(1.3, 3.2)
	Survival time (n/N die)	8.4	7.7	6.4	8.8
	Median (Month)	(7.2, 10.3)	(6.2, 9.8)	(4.1, 10.8)	(4.1, 12.9)
	1-year survival rate	32.0%	25.0%	33.0%	36.0%

Disease control rate (patients with complete response, partial response, or stable disease for at least 6 weeks).   CI: Confidence interval.   CR: Complete response. CRC: Colorectal cancer.   PR: Partial response.   SD: Stable disease.   TTP: Time to progression.

Table 16　Clinical Efficacy in Locoregionally Advanced SCCHN (EMR 62 202-006)[49]

Variable Statistic	Radiation Therapy + Cetuximab (N = 211)	Radiation Therapy Alone (N = 213)
Locoregional Control		
Median, months (95% CI)	24.4 (15.7, 45.1)	14.9 (11.8, 19.9)
Hazard ratio (95% CI)	0.68 (0.52, 0.89)	
Stratified log-rank P-value	0.0050	
Overall Survival Time (OS)		
Median, months (95% CI)	49.0 (32.8, 69.5+)	29.3 (20.6, 41.4)
Hazard ratio (95% CI)	0.73 (0.56, 0.95)	
Stratified log-rank P-value	0.018	
Median Follow-up, months	60.0	60.1
1-year OS rate, % (95% CI)	77.6 (71.4, 82.7)	73.8 (67.3, 79.2)
2-year OS rate, % (95% CI)	62.2 (55.2, 68.4)	55.2 (48.2, 61.7)
3-year OS rate, % (95% CI)	54.7 (47.7, 61.2)	45.2 (38.3, 51.9)
5-year OS rate, % (95% CI)	45.6 (38.5, 52.4)	36.4 (29.7, 43.1)

A '+' denotes that the upper bound limit had not been reached at cut-off.　CI: Confidence interval.　OS: Overall survival.　SCCHN: Squamous cell carcinoma of the head and neck.

Table 17　Clinical Efficacy in Recurrent Locoregional Disease or Metastatic SCCHN (EMR 62 202-002)[49]

Variable Statistic	EU-approved Cetuximab + CTX (N = 222)	CTX (N = 220)
OS		
Median, months (95% CI)	10.1 (8.6, 11.2)	7.4 (6.4, 8.3)
Hazard ratio (95% CI)	0.80 (0.64, 0.99)	
Stratified log-rank P-value	0.036	
PFS		
Median, months (95% CI)	5.6 (5.0, 6.0)	3.3 (2.9, 4.3)
Hazard ratio (95% CI)	0.54 (0.43, 0.67)	
Stratified log-rank P-value	<0.00010	
ORR		
% (95% CI)	35.6 (29.3, 42.3)	19.5 (14.5, 25.4)
Stratified log-rank P-value	0.00010	

CI: Confidence interval.　CTX: Platinum-based chemotherapy.　ORR: Objection response rate.　OS: Overall survival.　PFS: Progression-free survival time.
SCCHN: Squamous cell carcinoma of the head and neck.

Table 18　Three Studies of Cetuximab Led to FDA Approved for the Treatment of mCRC in First-line[50]

Study No.	Study Design	Objective	Population	Total/KRAS Analysis/ KRAS Wild-type
CRYSTAL	Phase 3, open-label randomized (1:1), Cetuximab + FOLFIRI or FOLFIRI alone	ORR, PFS (primary) and OS; KRAS mutation analysis	EGFR positive metastatic CRC patients who had not received prior treatment	1,217/1,079 (89.0%)/ 673 (63.0%)
CA225025	Phase 2/3, open-label randomized (1:1), Cetuximab + BSC or BSC alone	OS; KRAS mutation analysis; OS comparision of two arms	EGFR positive advanced CRC, patients who had received prior oxaliplatin-, irinotecan- and fluoropyrimidine-based treatment	572/453 (79.0%)/ 245 (54.0%)
EMR 62 202-047 (OPUS)	Phase 2, open-label randomized (2:1), Cetuximab + FOLFOX4 or FOLFOX4 alone	ORR (primary), OS and PFS; KRAS mutation analysis	EGFR positive advanced CRC patients who had not received prior treatment	337/315 (93.0%)/ 179 (57.0%)

EGFR: Epidermal growth factor receptor.　FOLFIRI: Irinotecan, 5-fluorouracil, and leucovorin.　FOLFOX4: Oxaliplatin plus continuous infusional 5-FU/FA.
KRAS: Kirsen rat sarcoma viral oncogene homolog.　mCRC: Metastatic colorectal cancer.　ORR: Objective response rate.　OS: Overall survival.

Table 19   Overall Survival in Previously Treated EGFR-expressing mCRC
(All Randomized or Based on KRAS Status) (CA225025)[51]

	All Randomized		KRAS Mutation Negative		KRAS Mutation Positive	
	Cetuximab + BSC (N = 287)	BSC (N = 285)	Cetuximab + BSC (N = 117)	BSC (N = 128)	Cetuximab + BSC (N = 108)	BSC (N = 100)
Median (Month) (95% CI)	6.1 (5.4, 6.7)	4.6 (4.2, 4.9)	8.6 (7.0, 10.3)	5.0 (4.3, 5.7)	4.8 (3.9, 5.6)	4.6 (3.6, 4.9)
Hazard ratio (95% CI)	0.77 (0.64, 0.92)		0.63 (0.47, 0.84)		0.91 (0.67, 1.2)	
P-value	0.0046					

BSC: Best supportive care.   CI: Confidence interval.   mCRC: Metastatic colorectal cancer.

Table 20   Clinical Efficacy in First-line EGFR-expressing mCRC (All Randomized or Based on KRAS Status) (CRYSTAL)[51]

	All Randomized		KRAS Wild-type Population		KRAS Mutant Positive	
	Cetuximab[a] + FOLFIRI	FOLFIRI	Cetuximab[a] + FOLFIRI	FOLFIRI	Cetuximab[a] + FOLFIRI	FOLFIRI
	(N = 608)	(N = 609)	(N = 320)	(N = 356)	(N = 216)	(N = 187)
PFS						
No. of events (%)	343 (56.0)	371 (61.0)	165 (52.0)	214 (60.0)	138 (64.0)	112 (60.0)
Median (Month)	8.9	8.1	9.5	8.1	7.5	8.2
(95% CI)	(8.0, 9.4)	(7.6, 8.8)	(8.9, 11.1)	(7.4, 9.2)	(6.7, 8.7)	(7.4, 9.2)
Hazard ratio (95% CI)	0.85 (0.74, 0.99)		0.70 (0.57, 0.86)		1.1 (0.88, 1.5)	
Stratified log-rank P-value	0.036					
OS[b]						
No. of events (%)	491 (81.0)	509 (84.0)	244 (76.0)	292 (82.0)	189 (88.0)	159 (85.0)
Median (Month)	19.6	18.5	23.5	19.5	16.0	16.7
(95% CI)	(18.0, 21.0)	(17.0, 20.0)	(21.0, 26.0)	(17.0, 21.0)	(15.0, 18.0)	(15.0, 19.0)
Hazard ratio (95% CI)	0.88 (0.78, 1.0)		0.80 (0.67, 0.94)		1.0 (0.84, 1.3)	
ORR						
ORR (95% CI)	46.0% (42.0, 50.0)	38.0% (34.0, 42.0)	57.0% (51.0, 62.0)	39.0% (34.0, 44.0)	31.0% (25.0, 38.0)	35.0% (28.0, 43.0)

CI: Confidence interval.   FOLFIRI: Irinotecan plus infusional 5-FU/FA.   mCRC: Metastatic colorectal cancer.   ORR: Objective response rate.   OS: Overall survival.   PFS: Progression-free survival time.   [a] Europe-approved.   [b] Post-hoc updated OS analysis, results based on an additional 162 events.

Table 21   Clinical Efficacy in First-line EGFR-expressing mCRC (OPUS)[52]

	RAS Wild-type Population (179/315)		RAS Mutant Population (136/315)	
Variable/Statistic	Cetuximab + FOLFOX4 (N = 82)	FOLFOX4 (N = 97)	Cetuximab + FOLFOX4 (N = 77)	FOLFOX4 (N = 59)
Overall Survival Rate				
No. of events, n (%)	55 (67.1)	71 (73.2)	61 (79.2)	45 (76.3)
Median, months (95% CI)	22.8 (19.3, 25.9)	18.5 (6.4, 44.3)	13.4 (10.5, 17.7)	17.5 (14.7, 24.8)
Hazard ratio (95% CI)	0.86 (0.60, 1.2)		1.3 (0.87, 1.9)	
P-value	0.39		0.20	
PFS				
No. of events, n (%)	34 (46.3)	62 (63.8)	56 (72.7)	34 (57.6)
Median, months (95% CI)	8.3 (7.2, 12.0)	7.2 (5.6, 7.6)	5.5 (4.0, 7.3)	8.6 (6.5, 9.4)
Hazard ratio (95% CI)	0.57 (0.38, 0.86)		1.7 (1.1, 2.7)	
P-value	0.0064		0.015	
ORR				
ORR% (95% CI)	57.3 (45.9, 68.2)	34.0 (24.7, 44.3)	33.6 (23.4, 44.5)	52.5 (39.1, 65.7)
Odds ratio (95% CI)	2.5 (1.4, 4.7)		0.46 (0.23, 0.92)	
P-value	0.0027		0.029	

CI: Confidence interval.   FOLFOX4: Oxaliplatin plus continuous infusional 5-FU/FA.   mCRC: Metastatic colorectal cancer.   NE: Not estimable.   ORR: Objective response rate.   PFS: Progression-free survival.

Table 22   Clinical Efficacy of Cetuximab plus Chemotherapy and Bevacizumab in First-line mCRC (NCT00208546)[53]

Outcome	CB Group (N = 368)	CBC Group (N = 368)	P-value
PFS			0.010
Median, months (95% *CI*)	10.7 (9.7, 12.3)	9.4 (8.4, 10.5)	
OS			0.16
Median, months (95% *CI*)	20.3 (17.8, 24.7)	19.4 (17.5, 21.4)	
Response Rate (%)[a]	50.0	52.7	0.49
Disease control rate (%)[a]	94.0	94.6	0.72
Duration of Treatment			<0.0010
Median, months	7	6	
Range	1-31	1-33	
Primary Reason for Treatment Discontinuation (%)			
Disease progression	54.0	48.5	0.16
Adverse events	25.9	29.6	0.28
Other	20.1	21.9	0.59
60-day mortality (%)	1.9	2.7	0.46

CB group: Capecitabine, oxaliplatin and bevacizumab.   CBC group: Capecitabine, oxaliplatin bevacizumab, and cetuximab.   *CI*: Confidence interval.   mCRC: Metastatic colorectal cancer.   [a] A total of 649 patients (332 in the CB group and 317 in the CBC group) were evaluated for response.

Table 23   Clinical Efficacy of Cetuximab plus FOLFIRI in First-line mCRC, Head-to-head Comparison to Bevacizumab plus FOLFIRI (FIRE-3)[43]

Variable/Statistic	RAS Wild-type Population		RAS Mutant Population	
	Cetuximab + FOLFIRI (N = 171)	Bevacizumab + FOLFIRI (N = 171)	Cetuximab + FOLFIRI (N = 92)	Bevacizumab + FOLFIRI (N = 86)
Overall Response Rate				
Median, months (95% *CI*)	33.1 (24.5, 39.4)	25.6 (22.7, 28.6)	20.3 (16.4, 23.4)	20.6 (17.0, 26.7)
Hazard ratio (95% *CI*)	0.70 (0.53, 0.92)		1.1 (0.78, 1.5)	
P-value	0.011		0.60	
PFS				
Median, months	10.4 (9.5, 12.2)	10.2 (9.3, 11.5)	7.5 (6.1, 9.0)	10.1 (8.9, 12.2)
Hazard ratio (95% *CI*)	0.93 (0.74, 1.2)		1.3 (0.96, 1.8)	
P-value	0.54		0.085	
ORR				
ORR, %	65.5 (57.9, 72.6)	59.6 (51.9, 67.1)	38.0 (28.1, 48.8)	51.2 (40.1, 62.1)
Odds ratio (95% *CI*)	1.3 (0.83, 2.0)		0.59 (0.32, 1.1)	
P-value	0.32		0.097	

CI: Confidence interval.   FOLFIRI: Irinotecan plus infusional 5-FU/FA.   mCRC: Metastatic colorectal cancer.   ORR: Objective response rate.   PFS: Progression-free survival.

Clinical Safety

Cetuximab Alone or Combined with Irinotecan for mCRC

❖ Table 24 contains selected adverse reactions in 667 patients with KRAS mutation-negative (wild-type), EGFR-expressing, metastatic colorectal cancer receiving EU-approved cetuximab plus FOLFIRI or FOLFIRI alone in this study.   Cetuximab was administered at the recommended dose and schedule (400 mg/m^2 initial dose, followed by 250 mg/m^2 weekly). Patients received a median of 26 infusions (range 1-224).

❖ The frequency and nature of adverse events, including adverse events associated with cetuximab (acne-like rash, infusion reactions, cardiac events, and hypomagnesemia), observed in CRYSTAL, CA225025, and OPUS in the KRAS wild-type population were consistent with the known adverse drug reaction profiles of cetuximab, chemotherapy agents, and the underlying disease. No significant differences between the wild-type, mutant, and the overall safety populations have been noted.

- The most serious adverse reactions observed in clinical trials of cetuximab, alone or in combination with irinotecan, were infusion reactions (3.0%), dermatologic toxicity (1.0%), interstitial lung disease (0.50%), fever (5.0%), sepsis (3.0%), renal dysfunction (2.0%), pulmonary embolism (1.0%), dehydration (5.0% in patients receiving cetuximab plus irinotecan; 2.0% in patients receiving cetuximab monotherapy), and diarrhea (6.0% in patients receiving cetuximab plus irinotecan, 0.0% in patients receiving cetuximab monotherapy).
- The most common adverse events seen in 354 patients receiving cetuximab plus irinotecan were acneform rash (88.0%), asthenia/malaise (73.0%), diarrhea (72.0%), nausea (55.0%), abdominal pain (45.0%), and vomiting (41.0%). The most common Grades 3-4 adverse reactions included 307 diarrhea (22.0%), leukopenia (17.0%), asthenia/malaise (16.0%), and acneiform rash (14.0%). Thirty-seven (10.0%) patients receiving cetuximab plus irinotecan and 14 (5.0%) patients receiving cetuximab monotherapy discontinued treatment primarily because of adverse events.
- The most common adverse events seen in 279 patients receiving cetuximab monotherapy were acneform rash (90.0%), asthenia/malaise (49.0%), fever (33.0%), nausea (29.0%), constipation (28.0%), and diarrhea (28.0%).

❖ Table 25 contains selected adverse reactions in 242 patients with KRAS mutation-negative (wild-type), EGFR-expressing, metastatic colorectal cancer who received best supportive care (BSC) alone or with Erbitux® in Study CA225025. Cetuximab was administered at the recommended dose and schedule (400 mg/m² initial dose, followed by 250 mg/m² weekly). Patients received a median of 17 infusions (range 1-51).

Cetuximab in Combination with RT or Platinum-based Therapy and 5-FU in Metastatic SCCHN

❖ Cetuximab alone or combined with radiation therapy for advanced SCCHN

- Table 26 contains selected adverse reactions in 420 patients receiving radiation therapy either alone or with cetuximab for locally or regionally advanced SCCHN. Erbitux® was administered at the recommended dose and schedule (400 mg/m² initial dose, followed by 250 mg/m² weekly). Patients received a median of 8 infusions (range 1-11).
- The most common adverse events reported for both treatment arms were mucositis and radiation dermatitis. The incidence of serious mucositis, radiation dermatitis and allergic/anaphylatoid reaction were >2.0% higher in the RT + cetuximab arm when compared with RT alone. The following serious adverse reactions, some with fatal outcome were observed in the cetuximab plus RT arm: Infusion reactions, cardiopulmonary arrest and/or sudden death and acneform rash.
- The overall incidence of late radiation toxicities (any grade) was higher in cetuximab in combination with radiation therapy compared with radiation therapy alone. The following sites were affected: salivary glands (65.0% vs. 56.0%), larynx (52.0% vs. 36.0%), subcutaneous tissue (49.0% vs. 45.0%), mucous membrane (48.0% vs. 39.0%), esophagus (44.0% vs. 35.0%), and skin (42.0% vs. 33.0%). However, the incidence of Grade 3 or 4 late radiation toxicities was similar between the radiation therapy alone and the Erbitux® plus radiation treatment groups.

❖ Cetuximab in combination with platinum-based therapy with 5-FU

- Table 27 summarizes selected adverse reactions in 434 patients with recurrent loco-regional disease or metastatic SCCHN receiving cetuximab in combination with platinum-based therapy with 5-FU or platinum-based therapy with 5-FU alone. Cetuximab was administered at 400 mg/m² for the initial dose, followed by 250 mg/m² weekly. Patients received a median of 17 infusions (range 1-89).
- The most common adverse reactions (at least 25.0%) in patients treated with cetuximab were nausea, anemia, vomiting, neutropenia, rash, asthenia, diarrhea, and anorexia. Conjunctivitis occurred in 10.0% of the patients receiving cetuximab. Other adverse reactions, sometimes severe, caused by cetuximab included infusion reactions, hypomagnesemia, hypocalcemia and hypokalemia.
- For cardiac disorders, approximately 9.0% of subjects in the cetuximab plus chemotherapy and chemotherapy-only treatment arms experienced a cardiac event. The majority of these events occurred in patients who received cisplatin/5-FU, with or without cetuximab as follows: 11.0% and 12.0% in patients who received cisplatin/5-FU with or without cetuximab, respectively, and 6.0% or 4.0% in patients who received carboplatin/5-FU with or without cetuximab, respectively. In both arms, the incidence of cardiovascular events was higher in the cisplatin with 5-FU containing subgroup. Death attributed to cardiovascular event or sudden death was reported in 3.0% of the patients in the cetuximab plus platinum-based therapy with 5-FU arm and 2.0% in the platinum-based chemotherapy with 5-FU alone arm. Health care providers should closely monitor serum electrolytes, including serum magnesium, potassium, and calcium, during and after cetuximab administration.

Table 24   Incidence of Selected Adverse Reactions (≥10.0%) in Patients with KRAS Wild-type and EGFR-expressing, Metastatic Colorectal Cancer[a, 28]

Body System Preferred Term	EU-approved Cetuximab + FOLFIRI (N = 317)		FOLFIRI Alone (N = 350)	
	Grade 1-4[b]	Grade 3 & 4	Grade 1-4	Grade 3 & 4
	% of Patients			
Blood and Lymphatic System Disorders				
Neutropenia	49.0	31.0	42.0	24.0
Eye Disorders				
Conjunctivitis	18.0	<1.0	3.0	0.0
Gastrointestinal Disorders				
Diarrhea	66.0	16.0	60.0	10.0
Stomatitis	31.0	3.0	19.0	1.0
Dyspepsia	16.0	0.0	9.0	0.0
General Disorders and Administration Site Conditions				
Infusion-related reaction[c]	14.0	2.0	<1.0	0.0
Pyrexia	26.0	1.0	14.0	1.0
Infections and Infestations				
Paronychia	20.0	4.0	<1.0	0.0
Investigations				
Weight decreased	15.0	1.0	9.0	1.0
Skin and Subcutaneous Tissue Disorders				
Acne-like rash[d]	86.0	18.0	13.0	<1.0
Rash	44.0	9.0	4.0	0.0
Dermatitis acneiform	26.0	5.0	<1.0	0.0
Dry skin	22.0	0.0	4.0	0.0
Acne	14.0	2.0	0.0	0.0
Pruritus	14.0	0.0	3.0	0.0
Palmar-plantar erythrodysesthesia syndrome	19.0	4.0	4.0	<1.0
Skin fissures	19.0	2.0	1.0	0.0

EU: Europe.   FOLFIRI: Irinotecan plus infusional 5-FU/FA.   [a] Adverse reactions occurring in at least 10.0% of Erbitux® combination arm with a frequency at least 5.0% greater than that seen in the FOLFIRI arm.   [b] Adverse reactions were graded using the NCI CTC, V 2.0.   [c] Infusion related reaction is defined as any event meeting the medical concepts of allergy/anaphylaxis at any time during the clinical study or any event occurring on the first day of dosing and meeting the medical concepts of dyspnea and fever or by the following events using MedDRA preferred terms: "acute myocardial infarction", "angina pectoris", "angioedema", "autonomic seizure", "blood pressure abnormal", "blood pressure decreased", "blood pressure increased", "cardiac failure", "cardiopulmonary failure", "cardiovascular insufficiency", "clonus", "convulsion", "coronary no-reflow phenomenon", "epilepsy", "hypertension", "hypertensive crisis", "hypertensive emergency", "hypotension", "infusion related reaction", "loss of consciousness", "myocardial infarction", "myocardial ischaemia", "prinzmetal angina", "shock", "sudden death", "syncope", or "systolic hypertension".   [d] Acne-like rash is defined by the events using MedDRA preferred terms and included "acne", "acne pustular", "butterfly rash", "dermatitis acneiform", "drug rash with eosinophilia and systemic symptoms", "dry skin", "erythema", "exfoliative rash", "folliculitis", "genital rash", "mucocutaneous rash", "pruritus", "rash", "rash erythematous", "rash follicular", "rash generalized", "rash macular", "rash maculopapular", "rash maculovesicular", "rash morbilliform", "rash papular", "rash papulosquamous", "rash pruritic", "rash pustular", "rash rubelliform", "rash scarlatiniform", "rash vesicular", "skin exfoliation", "skin hyperpigmentation", "skin plaque", "telangiectasia", or "xerosis".

Table 25   Incidence of Selected Adverse Reactions Occurring in ≥10.0% of Patients with KRAS Wild-type and EGFR-expressing, Metastatic Colorectal Cancer Treated with Cetuximab Monotherapy[a, 28]

Body System Preferred Term	Erbitux® + BSC (N = 118)		BSC Alone (N = 124)	
	Grade 1-4[b]	Grade 3 & 4	Grade 1-4	Grade 3 & 4
	% of Patients			
Dermatology/Skin				
Rash/Desquamation	95.0	16.0	21.0	1.0
Dry skin	57.0	0.0	15.0	0.0
Pruritus	47.0	2.0	11.0	0.0
Other dermatology	35.0	0.0	7.0	2.0
Nail changes	31.0	0.0	4.0	0.0
Constitutional Symptoms				
Fatigue	91.0	31.0	79.0	29.0
Fever	25.0	3.0	16.0	0.0
Infusion reactions[c]	18.0	3.0	0.0	0.0
Rigors, Chills	16.0	1.0	3.0	0.0
Pain				
Pain-other	59.0	18.0	37.0	10.0
Headache	38.0	2.0	11.0	0.0
Bone pain	15.0	4.0	8.0	2.0
Pulmonary				
Dyspnea	49.0	16.0	44.0	13.0
Cough	30.0	2.0	19.0	2.0
Gastrointestinal				
Nausea	64.0	6.0	50.0	6.0
Constipation	53.0	3.0	38.0	3.0
Diarrhea	42.0	2.0	23.0	2.0
Vomiting	40.0	5.0	26.0	5.0
Stomatitis	32.0	1.0	10.0	0.0
Other gastrointestinal	22.0	12.0	16.0	5.0
Dehydration	13.0	5.0	3.0	0.0
Month dryness	12.0	0.0	6.0	0.0
Taste disturbance	10.0	0.0	5.0	0.0
Infection				
Infection without neutropenia	38.0	11.0	19.0	5.0
Musculoskeletal				
Arthralgia	14.0	3.0	6.0	0.0
Neurology				
Neuropathy-sensory	45.0	1.0	38.0	2.0
Insomnia	27.0	0.0	13.0	0.0
Confusion	18.0	6.0	10.0	2.0
Anxiety	14.0	1.0	5.0	1.0
Depression	14.0	0.0	5.0	0.0

BSC: Best supportive care.   [a] Adverse reactions occurring in at least 10.0% of cetuximab plus BSC arm with a frequency at least 5.0% greater than that seen in the BSC alone arm.   [b] Adverse reactions were graded using the NCI CTC, V 2.0.   [c] Infusion reaction is defined as any event (chills, rigors, dyspnea, tachycardia, bronchospasm, chest tightness, swelling, urticaria, hypotension, flushing, rash, hypertension, nausea, angioedema, pain, sweating, tremors, shaking, drug fever, or other hypersensitivity reaction) recorded by the investigator as infusion-related.

Table 26   Incidence of Selected Adverse Reactions (≥10.0%) in Patients with Locoregionally Advanced SCCHN[28]

Body System Preferred Term	Erbitux® + Radiation (N = 208)		Radiation Therapy Alone (N = 212)	
	Grade 1-4	Grade 3 & 4	Grade 1-4	Grade 3 & 4
	% of Patients			
Body as a Whole				
Asthenia	56.0	4.0	49.0	5.0
Fever[a]	29.0	1.0	13.0	1.0
Headache	19.0	<1.0	8.0	<1.0
Infusion reaction[b]	15.0	3.0	2.0	0.0
Infection	13.0	1.0	9.0	1.0
Chills[a]	16.0	0.0	5.0	0.0
Digestive				
Nausea	49.0	2.0	37.0	2.0
Emesis	29.0	2.0	23.0	4.0
Diarrhea	19.0	2.0	13.0	1.0
Dyspepsia	14.0	0.0	9.0	1.0
Metabolic/Nutritional				
Weight loss	84.0	11.0	72.0	7.0
Dehydration	25.0	6.0	19.0	8.0
Alanine tansaminase, high[c]	43.0	2.0	21.0	1.0
Aspartate transaminase, high[c]	38.0	1.0	24.0	1.0
Alkaline phosphatase, high[c]	33.0	<1.0	24.0	0.0
Respiratory				
Pharyngitis	26.0	3.0	19.0	4.0
Skin/Appendages				
Acneiform rash[d]	87.0	17.0	10.0	1.0
Radiation dermatitis	86.0	23.0	90.0	18.0
Application site reaction	18.0	0.0	12.0	1.0
Pruritus	16.0	0.0	4.0	0.0

SCCHN: Squamous cell carcinoma of the head and neck.   [a] Includes cases also reported as infusion reaction.   [b] Infusion reaction is defined as any event described at any time during the clinical study as "allergic reaction" or "anaphylactoid reaction", or any event occurring on the first day of dosing described as "allergic reaction", "anaphylactoid reaction", "fever", "chills", "chills and fever", or "dyspnea".   [c] Based on laboratory measurements, not on reported adverse reactions, the number of subjects with tested samples varied from 205-206 for Erbitux® plus Radiation arm; 209-210 for Radiation alone.   [d] Acneiform rash is defined as any event described as "acne", "rash", "maculopapular rash", "pustular rash", "dry skin", or "exfoliative dermatitis".

Table 27   Incidence of Selected Adverse Reactions (≥10.0%) in Patients with Recurrent Locoregionally Disease or Metastatic[28]

Body System Preferred Term	EU-approved Cetuximab + Platinum-based Therapy (N = 219)		Platinum-based Therapy with 5-FU Alone (N = 215)	
	Grade 1-4	Grade 3 & 4	Grade 1-4	Grade 3 & 4
	% of Patients			
Eye Disorders				
Conjunctivitis	10.0	0.0	0.0	0.0
Gastrointestinal Disorders				
Nausea	54.0	4.0	47.0	4.0
Diarrhea	26.0	5.0	16.0	1.0
General Disorders and Administration Site Conditions				
Pyrexia	22.0	0.0	13.0	1.0
Infusion reaction[a]	10.0	2.0	<1.0	0.0
Infections and Infestations				
Infection[b]	44.0	11.0	27.0	8.0
Metabolism and Nutrition Disorders				
Anorexia	25.0	5.0	14.0	1.0
Hypocalcemia	12.0	4.0	5.0	1.0
Hypokalemia	12.0	7.0	7.0	5.0
Hypomagnesemia	11.0	5.0	5.0	1.0
Skin and Subcutaneous Tissue Disorders				
Acne-like rash[c]	70.0	9.0	2.0	0.0
Rash	28.0	5.0	2.0	0.0
Acne	22.0	2.0	0.0	0.0
Dermatitis acneiform	15.0	2.0	0.0	0.0
Dry Skin	14.0	0.0	<1.0	0.0
Alopecia	12.0	0.0	7.0	0.0

5-FU: 5-Fluorourac.   Chemotherapy: Cisplatin + 5-fluorouracil or carboplatin + 5-fluorourac.   EU: Europe.   [a] Infusion reaction defined as any event of "anaphylactic reaction", "hypersensitivity", "fever and/or chills", "dyspnea", or "pyrexia" on the first day of dosing.   [b] Infection: This term excludes sepsis-related events which are presented separately.   [c] Acneiform rash defined as any event described as "acne", "dermatitis acneiform", "dry skin", "exfoliative rash", "rash", "rash erythematous", "rash macular", "rash papular", or "rash pustular".

8   Clinical Pharmacokinetics

Summary[25, 26]

Single-Dose Studies

❖ Phase 1 studies IMCL CP02_9401 (single-dose), IMCL CP02_ 9502, 9503, 9605, 9607, 9608, 9609, CP02_9710, BMS CA 225004, and EMR 62 202-012 (multiple-does) were performed for dose-escalation studies.   The pharmacokinetics of cetuximab after single-dose ranging from 5 to 500 mg/m^2 have been characterized in a broad range of studies and tumor types and the results were summarized in Table 28.

❖ Cetuximab exhibits nonlinear pharmacokinetics. $AUC_{0-\infty}$ increased in a greater extent than dose proportional manner; Clearance decreased and half-life increased with increasing of doses.

❖ As the dose of cetuximab increased from 20 to 200 mg/m^2, the clearance decreased from 0.080 to 0.020 L/h/m^2 at doses greater than 200 mg/m^2, CL appeared to become constant.   This plateau may be suggestive of a second, linear elimination pathway that becomes pronounced at doses above 200 mg/m^2.

Multiple-Dose Studies

❖ After administration of the target dose of 400 kg/m^2 initial and 250 mg/m^2 weekly, peak and trough concentration of cetuximab were comparable across studies (Table 29).

❖ Reasonably constant cetuximab peak and trough concentrations were generally reached within 3 to 5 weeks after the initiation of treatment and were maintained during later stages of the treatment without any accumulation.

❖ Available data indicate that the PK of cetuximab appears to remain unchanged for up to 4 weeks.

General Pharmacokinetics Data for Cetuximab

❖ Long elimination life: 70-100 hours.

❖ Serum concentration reached stable level: 3 weeks.

❖ Mean peak concentration: 155.8 mg/mL (Week 3) and 151.6 mg/mL (Week 8).

❖ Mean through concentration: 41.3 mg/mL (Week 3) and 55.4 mg/mL (Week 8).

❖ Mean through concentration for the combination of cetuximab and irinotecan: 50 mg/mL (Week 12) and 49.4 mg/mL (Week 36).

Distribution

❖ The mean volume of distribution at steady-state, V_{ss} was about 2.0-3.0 L/m² at the target dose (absolute values about 4.0-6.5 L), suggesting distribution only within the vascular space.

❖ The volume of distribution was independent of dose.

❖ In the population pharmacokinetic analysis, the estimated volumes of the central and peripheral compartments were 4.49 and 4.54 L, respectively, with a 27.0% reduction in the typical value of the central volume in females.

❖ Total V_{ss} from the population analysis was, thus, about 9.0 L.

❖ Plasma protein binding studies were not performed.

Table 28　Single-Dose PK Parameters for Cetuximab Cross all Studies[54]

Dose (mg/m²)	N (Cases)	C_{max} (µg/mL)	$AUC_{0-\infty}$ (µg·h/mL)	$t_{1/2}$ (h)	CL [L/(h·M²)]	V_{ss} (L/m²)
20	13	8.7 ± 4.2	343 ± 228	33.3 ± 29.2	0.079 ± 0.039	2.8 ± 1.1
50	23	22.2 ± 4.7	1,031 ± 440	32.3 ± 9.8	0.059 ± 0.028	2.5 ± 0.70
100	52	46.8 ± 11.6	2,910 ± 1,060	44.8 ± 12.8	0.039 ± 0.015	2.5 ± 0.91
200	14	102 ± 29.4	9,923 ± 3,226	79.8 ± 19.6	0.020 ± 0.010	2.3 ± 1.1
250	8	140 ± 19.6	1,241 ± 3,332	65.9 ± 18.8	0.021 ± 0.0050	2.2 ± 0.16
300	4	133 ± 47.7	16,311 ± 3,786	90.4 ± 13.8	0.019 ± 0.0050	2.5 ± 0.49
400	56	185 ± 54.6	21,142 ± 8,657	97.2 ± 37.4	0.022 ± 0.0090	2.9 ± 0.90
500	20	284 ± 84.1	32,448 ± 12,880	119 ± 76.9	0.018 ± 0.0080	2.6 ± 0.66

Mean ± SD.

Table 29　Combined Pharmacokinetic Parameters of Cetuximab from Different Studies at the Target Dose 400/250 mg/m², Once Weekly Dosing (Modified from Clinical Summary)[41]

Week	Study	Statistic	CL (L/h)	AUC_{last} (µg·h/mL)	$t_{1/2}$ (h)	V_{ss} (L)
1	IMCL CP02-9503, 9504, 9607, 9608, 9709, 9710; CA225004, 005	N (cases)	53	53	53	53
		Mean	0.022	21,142	97.2	2.9
		SD	0.0090	8,657	37.4	0.93
3	IMCL CP02-9709 and EMR 62 202-012	N (cases)	8	8	8	8
		Mean	0.020	22,723	123	2.3
		SD	0.0060	10,313	41.4	0.83
4	IMCL CP02-9607, 9608 and EMR 62 202-012	N (cases)	13	11	11	11
		Mean	0.017	24,329	108	2.0
		SD	0.0060	11,202	29.3	0.59

SD: Standard deviation.

Elimination

❖ The elimination pathways of cetuximab have not been specifically studied.

Dose Proportionality

❖ Single-dose pharmacokinetics of cetuximab as monotherapy at different doses was evaluated in three studies.   Doses from 5 to 500 mg/m^2 were administered as single infusion, and plasma sampling was performed during 3 or 4 weeks after dosing.

❖ In all three studies, C_{max} increased in a dose-related manner, while AUC increased more than dose proportionally.   Mean CL values decreased from 0.079 L/(h·m^2) after a single-dose of 20 mg/m^2 to 0.018-0.022 L/(h·m^2) after a single-dose of 200-500 mg/m^2.   These observations were supported by the population PK, indicating that following single infusions in the range of 250 to 500 mg/m^2 the clearance tends to become constant.

❖ A dose-dependent relationship was also observed for the elimination half-life ($t_{1/2}$).   The mean $t_{1/2}$ values increased with dose from 33.9 h to 119.4 h after single-dose of 20 mg/m^2 to 500 mg/m^2.   At the target dose, 400/250 mg/m^2, $t_{1/2}$ values were about 80-120 h.

Time Dependency

❖ Peak and trough concentrations of cetuximab were determined after up to eight weekly doses.   No apparent changes in pharmacokinetics of cetuximab over time at repeated dosing were observed.   In general, the peak and trough concentration appeared to be stable from dose three or four and onwards, which is consistent with a half-life of about 100 hours.

Antibody Formation

❖ Human anti-chimeric antibody (HACA) data were available from a total of 534 patients.

❖ The incidence of positive antibody response in individual studies was variable and did not follow a clear trend.   In total, only 20 patients (3.7%) displayed positive HACA responses.

❖ Data from two patients indicated that anti-cetuximab antibody response leads to lower cetuximab exposure.

❖ There was no clear relationship between response incidence and cetuximab dose.

Special Populations

❖ There are no formal studies in special patient sub-populations, but a population pharmacokinetic analysis was performed. The database included data from all cetuximab studies with pharmacokinetic sampling.   The final dataset contained 8,388 observations from 906 patients, and from 19 studies.   Approximately 45.0% of the observations came from three studies (CP02-9504, CP02-9710 and EMR202-007).   A two-compartment model with a single saturable elimination pathway was finally selected.   Adding a linear elimination pathway to the model only marginally improved the model, and the linear pathway was estimated to be more than 30 times slower than the saturable pathway.

❖ Impaired renal function
  • Only 49 and 4 patients (of total 906) had moderate and severe impairment, respectively.
  • Renal function (based on CLcr) was not identified as an important factor for cetuximab pharmacokinetics.

❖ Impaired hepatic function
  • More than 90.0% of the patients had normal hepatic function, as assessed by AST and total bilirubin levels.
  • Influence of hepatic function on cetuximab pharmacokinetics could not be adequately estimated.

❖ Gender
  • Male 578 (63.8%); Female 328 (36.2%).
  • Gender was identified as a significant co-variate for volume of the central compartment (absolute volume) and for CL (V_{max} and K_m).   However, the effect did not necessitate dose adjustments based on gender.

❖ Race
  • The majority of patients included in the integrated pharmacokinetic database were Caucasian (815 patients, representing 90.0%).   An evaluation of impact on race could not be made.

❖ Weight
  • The median weight was 73.5 kg, range from 36.8 to 167 kg.
  • Weight and BSA were identified as significant co-variates for volume of the central compartment.

❖ Elderly
  • The median age was 60 and 57 years for males and females, respectively.   The age range was 22 to 88 years.   Age did not seem to have an impact on volume of distribution (absolute volume) or CL.

❖ Children
  • There are no pharmacokinetic data for children.

Interaction Studies

❖ Interaction study with irinotecan (Study EMR 62 202-012): Cetuximab and irinotecan were administered at the therapeutic dosages.   Effects of cetuximab on pharmacokinetics of irinotecan and its active metabolite SN-38 were assessed in patients who received irinotecan on Days 1 and 22, and cetuximab on Days 8, 15 and 22. Effects of irinotecan on cetuximab were evaluated in another group, receiving cetuximab on Days 1, 8, 15 and 22 and irinotecan on Day 22.

❖ Statistical analysis of the data was not performed, but there were no apparent changes in pharmacokinetics of either irinotecan or cetuximab, when administered together with the other drug. For SN-38 the variability was large and since only samples around T_{max} had SN-38 levels above LLQ, a meaningful analysis of data could not be made for the metabolite.

❖ A possible impact of co-administered chemotherapies and radiation therapy on the PK of cetuximab was evaluated in the population pharmacokinetic analysis (data not shown).

9 Patent

❖ Cetuximab was first approved by the U.S. Food and Drug Administration (FDA) on Feb 19, 2004. Cetuximab in the US and Canada by the drug company Bristol-Myers Squibb and outside the US and Canada by the drug company Merck KGaA. In Japan, Merck KGaA, Bristol-Myers Squibb and Eli Lilly have a co-distribution.

Summary

❖ EP0359282B1 and US6217866B1 related to the antibody of cetuximab were granted in 1996 and 2001, separately.

Table 30   Originator's Key Patent of Cetuximab in Main Countries and/or Region

Country/Region	Publication/Patent No.	Application Date	Granted Date	Estimated Expiry Date
US	US6217866B1	06/07/1995	04/17/2001	02/12/2018
EP	EP0359282B1	09/15/1989	05/15/1996	09/15/2009

Table 31   Originator's International Patent Protection of Use and/or Method of Cetuximab

Publication No.	Title	Publication Date
Technical Subjects	DIAGNOSTIC METHOD	
WO2010009794A1	Method of determination of receptor binding saturation effected by monoclonal antibodies	01/28/2010
WO2010145796A2	Biomarkers and methods for determining efficacy of anti-EGFR antibodies in cancer therapy	12/23/2010
Technical Subjects	COMBINATION METHOD	
WO2004032961A1	Bispecific anti-ErbB antibodies and their use in tumor therapy	04/22/2004
WO2009010290A2	Engineered anti-alpha V-integrin hybrid antibodies	01/22/2009
Technical Subjects	FORMULATION	
WO03053465A2	Lyophilized preparation containing antibodies to the EGF receptor	07/03/2003
WO2005051355A1	Solid forms of anti-EGFR-antibodies	06/09/2005
WO2005058365A1	Pharmaceutical preparation containing an antibody for the EGF receptor	06/30/2005
WO2005077414A1	Highly concentrated liquid formulations of anti-EGFR antibodies	08/25/2005
WO2007076923A1	Combination therapy using anti-EGFR and anti-HER2 antibodies	07/12/2007

The data was updated until Jan 2018.

10   Reference

[1] Normanno N, Bianco C. The Erb receptors and their ligands in cancer: an overview [J]. Current Drug Targets, 2005, 6(3): 243-257.

[2] Yarden Y. The EGFR family and its ligands in human cancer signaling mechanisms and therapeutic opportunities [J]. European Journal of Cancer, 2001, 37(Suppl 4): S3-S8.

[3] Carpenter G. The EGF receptor: a nexus for trafficking and signaling [J]. Bioassays, 2000, 22(8): 697-707.

[4] Gulick W J. Type I growth factor receptors: current status and future work [J]. Biochemical Society Symposium, 1998, 63: 193-198.

[5] Yarden Y, Sliwkowski M X. Untangling the ErbB signaling network [J]. Nature Reviews Molecular Cell Biology, 2001, 2(2): 127-137.

[6] Martinelli E, De Palma R. Anti-epidermal growth factor receptor monoclonal antibodies in cancer therapy [J]. Clinical & Experimental Immunology, 2009, 158(1): 1-9.

[7] Brandt R, Eisenbrandt R. Mammary gland specific hEGF receptor transgene expression induces neoplasia and inhibits differentiation [J]. Oncogene, 2000, 19(17): 2129-2137.

[8] Dassonville O, Formento J L. Expression of epidermal growth factor receptor and survival in upper aerodigestive tract cancer [J]. Journal of Clinical Oncology, 1993, 11(10): 1873-1878.

[9] Humphreys R C, Hennighausen L. Transforming growth factor and mouse models of human breast cancer [J]. Oncogene, 2000, 19(8): 1085-1091.

[10] Klijn J G M, Berns P M J J, Schmitz P I M, et al. The clinical significance of epidermal growth factor receptor (EGF-R) in human breast cancer: a review on 5232 patients [J]. Endocrine Reviews, 1992, 13(1): 3-17.

[11] Nicholson R I, GEE J M, HARPER M E. EGFR and cancer prognosis [J]. European Journal of Cancer, 2001, 37(14): S9-S15.

[12] Pedersen M W, Meltorn M, Damstrup L, et al. The type III epidermal growth factor receptor mutation: biological significance and potential target for anti-cancer therapy [J]. Annals of Oncology, 2001, 12(6): 745-760.

[13] Gan H K, Cvrljevc A N, Johns T G. The epidermal growth factor receptor variant III (EGFRvIII): where wild things are altered [J]. FEBS Journal, 2013, 280(21): 5350-5370.

[14] Goldstein N I, Prewett M. Biological efficacy of a chimeric antibody to the epidermal growth factor receptor in a human tumor xenograft model [J]. Clinical Cancer Research, 1995, 1(11): 1311-1318.

[15] Waskal H W. Role of an anti-epidermal growth factor receptor in treating cancer [J]. Cancer and Metastasis Reviews, 1999, 18(4): 427-436.

[16] Arteage C. ErbB-targeted therapeutic approaches in human cancer [J]. Experimental Cell Research, 2003a, 284(1): 122-130.

[17] Arteage C. Targeting HER1/EGFR: A molecular approach to cancer therapy [J]. Seminars in Oncology, 2003b, 30(3): 3-14.

[18] Bianco R, Daniele G. Monoclonal antibodies targeting the epidermal growth factor receptor [J]. Current Drug Targets, 2005, 6(3): 275-287.

[19] Krause D S, Van Etten R A. Tyrosine kinases as targets for cancer therapy [J]. The New England Journal of Medicine, 2005, 353(2): 172-187.

[20] Zhu Z. Cetuximab (ERBITUX®), an anti-epidermal growth factor receptor antibody for the treatment of metastatic colorectal cancer [J]. Target Validation in Drug Discovery, 2007, II: 43-67.

[21] http://www.ncbi.nlm.nih.gov/protein./CAA25240.

[22] https://blast.ncbi.nlm.nih.gov/Blast.cgi.

[23] Yazdi M H, Faramazi M A A. Comprehensive review of clinical trials on EGFR inhibitors such as cetuximab and panitumumab as monotherapy and in combination for treatment of metastatic colorectal cancer [J]. Avicenna Journal of Medical Biotechnology, 2015, 7(4): 134-144.

[24] The financial reports of Eli Lilly, Merck Serono and Bristol-Myers Squibb; http://data.pharmacodia.com/web/homePage/index.

[25] U.S. Food and Drug Administration (FDA) Database. https://www.accessdata.fda.gov/scripts/cder/daf/index.cfm?event=overview.process&ApplNo=125084.

[26] European Medicines Agency (EMA) Database. http://www.ema.europa.eu/ema/index.jsp?curl=pages/medicines/human/medicines/000558/human_med_000769.jsp&mid=WC0b01ac058001d124.

[27] China Food and Drug Administration (CFDA) Database. http://qy1.sfda.gov.cn/datasearch/face3/base.jsp?tableId=36&tableName=TABLE36&title=%E8%BF%9B%E5%8F%A3%E8%8D%AF%E5%93%81&bcId=124356651564146415214424405468.

[28] FDA Database. https://www.accessdata.fda.gov/drugsatfda_docs/label/2015/125084s262lbl.pdf.

[29] Pharmaceuticals and Medical Devices Agency (PMDA) Database. http://www.pmda.go.jp/english/review-services/reviews/approved-information/drugs/0001.html#select22.

[30] EMA Database. http://www.ema.europa.eu/docs/en_GB/document_library/EPAR_-_Product_Information/human/000558/WC500029116.pdf.

[31] FDA Database. https://www.accessdata.fda.gov/drugsatfda_docs/bla/2004/125084_ERBITUX_PHARMR_P1.PDF.

[32] De bono J S, Rowinsky E K. The ErbB receptor family: a therapeutic target for cancer [J]. Trends in Molecular Medicine, 2002, 8(4): S19-S26.

[33] Kimura H, Sakai K, Arao T, et al. Antibody-dependent cellular cytotoxicity of cetuximab against tumor cells with wild-type or mutant epidermal growth factor receptor [J]. Cancer Science, 2007, 98(8): 1275-1280.

[34] Patel D, Bassi R, Hooper A, et al. Anti-epidermal growth factor receptor monoclonal antibody cetuximab inhibits EGFR/HER-2 heterodimerization and activation [J]. International Journal of Oncology, 2009, 34(1): 25-32.

[35] Prewett M, Hooper A T, Prewett M, et al. Enhanced antitumor activity of anti-epidermal growth factor receptor monoclonal antibody IMC-C225 in combination with irinotecan (CPT-11) against human colorectal tumor xenografts [J]. Clinical Cancer Research, 2002, 8(5): 994-1003.

[36] Harari P, Huang S. Head and neck cancer as a clinical model for molecular targeting of therapy: combining EGFR blockade with radiation [J]. International Journal of Radiation Oncology Biology·Physics, 2001, 49(2): 427-433.

[37] Overholser J, Prewett M. Epidermal growth factor receptor blockade by antibody IMC-C225 inhibits growth of a human pancreatic carcinoma xenograft in nude mice [J]. Cancer, 2000, 89(1): 74-82.

[38] FDA Database. https://www.accessdata.fda.gov/drugsatfda_docs/bla/2004/125084_ERBITUX_PHARMR_P2.PDF.

[39] FDA Database. https://www.accessdata.fda.gov/drugsatfda_docs/bla/2004/125084_ERBITUX_PHARMR_P3.PDF.

[40] PMDA Database. http://www.pmda.go.jp/drugs/2008/P200800039/index.html.

[41] EMA Database. http://www.ema.europa.eu/docs/en_GB/document_library/EPAR_-_Scientific_Discussion/human/000558/WC500029113.pdf.

[42] EMA Database. http://www.ema.europa.eu/docs/en_GB/document_library/EPAR_-_Assessment_Report_-_Variation/human/000558/WC500029118.pdf.

[43] EMA Database. http://www.ema.europa.eu/docs/en_GB/document_library/EPAR_-_Assessment_Report_-_Variation/human/000558/WC500029119.pdf.

[44] EMA Database. http://www.ema.europa.eu/docs/en_GB/document_library/EPAR_-_Assessment_Report_-_Variation/human/000558/WC500109161.pdf.

[45] https://clinicaltrials.gov/ct2/show/NCT00208546?term=00208546&rank=1.

[46] https://clinicaltrials.gov/ct2/show/NCT00433927?term=FIRE-3&rank=1.

[47] https://clinicaltrials.gov/ct2/show/NCT01243372?term=calgb%2Fswog+80405&rank=1.

[48] FDA Database. https://www.accessdata.fda.gov/drugsatfda_docs/bla/2004/125084_ERBITUX_MEDR_P1.PDF.

[49] EMA Database. http://www.ema.europa.eu/docs/en_GB/document_library/EPAR_-_Product_Information/human/000558/WC500029119.pdf.

[50] FDA Database. https://www.cancer.gov/about-cancer/treatment/drugs/fda-cetuximab#Anchor-Recur-11711.

[51] https://www.drugs.com/pro/erbitux.html#Section_14.1.

[52] Bokemeyer C, Bondarenko I, Hartmann J T. Efficacy according to biomarker status of cetuximab plus FOLFOX-4 as first-line treatment for metastatic colorectal cancer: the OPUS study [J]. Annals of Oncology, 2011, 22(7): 1535-1546.

[53] Tol J, Koopman M. Chemotherapy, bevacizumab, and cetuximab in metastatic colorectal cancer [J]. The New England Journal of Medicine, 2009, 360(6): 563-572.

[54] FDA Database. https://www.accessdata.fda.gov/drugsatfda_docs/bla/2004/125084_ERBITUX_BIOPHARMR.PDF.

CHAPTER
6

Ipilimumab

Ipilimumab

(Yervoy®)

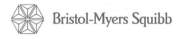
Bristol-Myers Squibb

Research code: Anti-CTLA-4 Mab, BMS-734016, Mab-10D14, MDX010, MDX-101, MDX-CTLA-4, 10D1

---

1 Target Biology

The CTLA-4 Receptor

❖ Cytotoxic T-lymphocyte-associated protein 4, also known as CD152 (cluster of differentiation152), is a protein receptor that functioning as an immune checkpoint, downregulates immune responses.

❖ CTLA-4 is a receptor expressed by activated T lymphocytes. It is expressed by T helper, T-cytotoxic and T-regulatory cells. Engagement of CTLA-4 by its ligands, CD80 (B7.1) and CD86 (B7.2), induces a negative regulatory signal which results in the down modulation of T-cell activation on T-helper and T-cytotoxic cells. Its role in T-regulatory cell activity is not well understood.

❖ CTLA-4 and CD28, the primary co-stimulatory receptor for T cells, bind to the same ligands. CTLA-4, however, has a high affinity for the ligands compared to CD28 and is able to out-compete CD28 for binding to CD80/86. CTLA-4's ability to compete with CD28 for binding to CD80/86 also plays a role in CTLA-4's ability to down modulate T-cell immune response.

Sequence Homology of CLTA-4 Proteins[1, 2]

Human: 223 aa. Accession: NP_005205.2.

```
  1  MACLGFQRHK  AQLNLATRTW  PCTLLFFLLF  IPVFCKAMHV  AQPAVVLASS  RGIASFVCEY
 61  ASPGKATEVR  VTVLRQADSQ  VTEVCAATYM  MGNELTFLDD  SICTGTSSGN  QVNLTIQGLR
121  AMDTGLYICK  VELMYPPPYY  LGIGNGTQIY  VIDPEPCPDS  DFLLWILAAV  SSGLFFYSFL
181  LTAVSLSKML  KKRSPLTTGV  YVKMPPTEPE  CEKQFQPYFI  PIN
```

Chimpanzee: 223 aa. Accession: XP_526000.1.

❖ BLAST:
Max score: 462; Total score: 462; Query cover: 100%.
Identities: 100% (223/223); Positives: 100% (223/223); Gaps: 0.0% (0/223).

```
  1  MACLGFQRHK  AQLNLATRTW  PCTLLFFLLF  IPVFCKAMHV  AQPAVVLASS  RGIASFVCEY
 61  ASPGKATEVR  VTVLRQADSQ  VTEVCAATYM  MGNELTFLDD  SICTGTSSGN  QVNLTIQGLR
121  AMDTGLYICK  VELMYPPPYY  LGIGNGTQIY  VIDPEPCPDS  DFLLWILAAV  SSGLFFYSFL
181  LTAVSLSKML  KKRSPLTTGV  YVKMPPTEPE  CEKQFQPYFI  PIN
```

Rhesus Monkey: 223 aa. Accession: NP_001038204.1.

❖ BLAST:
Max score: 445; Total score: 445; Query cover: 100%.
Identities: 97.0% (216/223); Positives: 98.0% (219/223); Gaps: 0.0% (0/223).

```
  1  MACLGFQRHK  ARLNLATRTR  PMTLLFSLLF  IPVFSKAMHV  AQPAVVLANS  RGIASFVCEY
 61  ASPGKATEVR  VTVLRQADSQ  VTEVCAATYM  MGNELTFLDD  SICTGTSSGN  QVNLTIQGLR
121  AMDTGLYICK  VELMYPPPYY  MGIGNGTQIY  VIDPEPCPDS  DFLLWILAAV  SSGLFFYSFL
181  LTAVSLSKML  KKRSPLTTGV  YVKMPPTEPE  CEKQFQPYFI  PIN
```

Norway Rat: 223 aa. Accession: NP_113862.1.

❖ BLAST:
Max score: 356; Total score: 356; Query cover: 100%.
Identities: 76.0% (169/223); Positives: 85.0% (190/223); Gaps: 0.0% (0/223).

```
  1  MACLGⅢQRⅢK  ⅢⅢLⅢLPⅢRTW  PⅢGⅢLⅢSLLF  IPⅢFSⅢAⅢQV  ⅢQPⅢVVLASS  ⅢGⅢASFⅢCEY
 61  ASⅢⅢⅢⅢⅢEVR  VTVLRQⅢⅢⅢQ  VTEVCAⅢTⅢⅢ  ⅢKNⅢLⅢFLDD  ⅢⅢCⅢGTⅢⅢⅢS  ⅢVNLTIQGLR
121  AⅢDTGLYⅢCK  VELMYPPPYⅢ  ⅢGⅢGNGTQIY  VIDPEPCPDS  DFLLWILAAV  SSGLFFYSFL
181  ⅢTAVSLⅢRⅢL  KKRSPLTTGV  YVKMPPTEPE  CEKQFQPYFI  PIN
```

House Mouse: 223aa.   Accession: NP_033973.2.

❖ BLAST:

Max score: 349; Total score: 349; Query cover: 100%.

Identities: 75.0% (167/223); Positives: 84.0% (189/223); Gaps: 0.0% (0/223).

```
  1  MACLGⅢRRⅢK  AⅢLQLPⅢRTW  PⅢVALⅢⅢLLF  IPVFSⅢAⅢQV  ⅢQPⅢVVLASS  ⅢGⅢASFⅢCEY
 61  ⅢPⅢHNⅢⅢⅢEVR  VTVLRQⅢⅢⅢQ  ⅢTEVCAⅢTⅢⅢ  ⅢKNⅢVGFLDⅢ  ⅢⅢCⅢGⅢⅢNⅢS  ⅢVNLTIQGLR
121  AⅢDTGLYⅢCK  VELMYPPPYⅢ  ⅢGⅢGNGTQIY  VIDPEPCPDS  DFLLWILⅢAV  SⅢGLFFYSFL
181  ⅢTAVSLSKML  KKRSPLTTGV  YVKMPPTEPE  CEKQFQPYFI  PIN
```

Biology Activity

❖ CTLA4 is a member of the immunoglobulin superfamily that is expressed by activated T cells and transmits an inhibitory signal to T cells.

❖ CTLA4 is homologous to the T-cell co-stimulatory protein, CD28, and both molecules bind to CD80 and CD86, also called B7-1 and B7-2, respectively, on antigen-presenting cells.   CTLA-4 binds CD80 and CD86 with greater affinity and avidity than CD28 thus enabling it to out-compete CD28 for its ligands.

❖ CTLA4 transmits an inhibitory signal to T cells, whereas CD28 transmits a stimulatory signal.

❖ CTLA4 is also found in regulatory T cells and contributes to its inhibitory function.   T-cell activation through the T-cell receptor and CD28 leads to increased expression of CTLA-4.

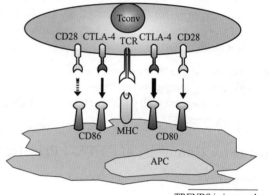

TRENDS in immunology

2   General Information

Yervoy®[3-5]

❖ Yervoy® (Ipilimumab) is a fully human IgG1 kappa monoclonal antibody that is directed against the human cytotoxic lymphocyte antigen-4 (CTLA-4) present on activated T cells.

❖ Yervoy® has been produced from CHO cells maintained in cell culture systems at Bristol-Myers Squibb.

❖ Human IgG1κ monoclonal antibody: ~148 KD.

❖ The total sales of 1,053 million US$ for 2016; No sales data as of 2017.

Mechanism of Action: A Dual Mechanisms of Action *in vitro*[3]

❖ The mechanism of action is believed to be through prevention of the inhibition of the interaction between antigen present-ing cells (APCs) and T cells.   The CTLA-4 antigen on T cells out-competes CD28 for binding to CD80/86 on APCs and induces a negative or inhibitory signal which acts to down-regulate T-cell activity.   Ipilimumab binds to CTLA-4, thus preventing its interaction with CD80/86.   This results in potentiation or up-regulation of T-cell activity.   It is believed that ipilimumab acts by permitting development of an immune response to tumor (self) antigens presented by APCs. This is also thought to be the primary mechanism of ipilimumab toxicity, an unintended pharmacologic effect of enhanced immune response to self-antigens presented by APCs.   As noted by the patent applicant, "blocking CTLA-4 function may permit the emergence of immune-mediated adverse events that result in clinical syndromes resembling autoimmunity".

Sponsor

❖ Yervoy® (Ipilimumab) was developed and marketed by Bristol-Myers Squibb.

World Sales[6]

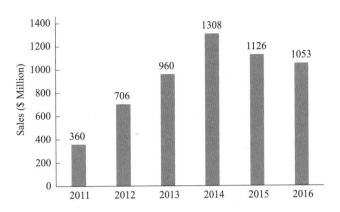

Figure 1   World Sales of Ipilimumab since 2011

Approval and Indication

Table 1   Summary of the Approved Indication[7]

Approval (Year)	Agency	Indication
2011	FDA	The treatment of unresectable or metastatic melanoma.
2011	EMA	Treat advanced melanoma (a type of skin cancer) in adults.
2015	PMDA	Unresectable melanoma.
2015	FDA	Adjuvant treatment of patients with cutaneous melanoma with pathologic involvement of regional lymph nodes of more than 1 mm who have undergone complete resection, including total lymphadenectomy.

Table 2   Summary of the Approval of Yervoy®[6]

	US (FDA)	EU (EMA)	Japan (PMDA)
First approval date	03/25/2011	07/13/2011	07/03/2015
Application or approval No.	BLA125377	EMEA/H/C/002213	22700AMX00069600
Brand name	Yervoy®	Yervoy®	Yervoy®
Indication	Unresectable or metastatic melanoma, cutaneous melanoma	Advanced melanoma	Unresectable melanoma
Authorization holder	BMS	BMS	BMS

Till Jan 2018, it had not been approved by CFDA (China).

Table 3   Indication and Administration[7]

No.	Administration	Indication
1	3 mg/kg administered intravenously over 90 minutes every 3 weeks for a total of 4 doses.	Unresectable or metastatic melanoma
2	10 mg/kg administered intravenously over 90 minutes every 3 weeks for 4 doses, followed by 10 mg/kg every 12 weeks for up to 3 years or until documented disease recurrence or unacceptable toxicity.	Adjuvant melanoma

Sourced from US FDA drug label information.

CTLA-4 Blocker

❖ Yervoy® is the only approved CTLA-4 blocking antibody on the market.

3   CMC Profile

Product Profile[4, 5, 7]

Dosage route: IV infusion.
Strength: US & EU: 50 mg/10 mL, 200 mg/40 mL; JP: 50 mg/10 mL.
Dosage form: Infusion solution.
Formulation: Diethylene triamine pentaacetic acid (DTPA), mannitol, polysorbate 80, sodium chloride, tris-hydrochloride, and water for injection, USP.
Stability: The proposed shelf life of 36 months at 2-8 °C and protected from light Vialed product should not be frozen.

Amino Acid Sequence[5]

❖ Ipilimumab is a fully human monoclonal antibody produced by recombinant DNA technology in a CHO mammalian cell expression system.

❖ Ipilimumab consists of four polypeptide chains with two identical heavy chains of 448 amino acids each and two identical kappa light chains of 215 amino acids each.   Each heavy and light chain pair is linked through an interchain disulfide bond.

❖ Molecular formula: $C_{6472}H_{9972}N_{1732}O_{2004}S_{40}$ (Protein part).

```
EIVLTQSPGT  LSLSPGERAT  LSCRASQSVG  SSYLAWYQQK  PGQAPRLLIY
GAFSRATGIP  DRFSGSGSGT  DFTLTISRLE  PEDFAVYYCQ  QYGSSPWTFG
QGTKVEIKRT  VAAPSVFIFP  PSDEQLKSGT  ASVVCLLNNF  YPREAKVQWK
VDNALQSGNS  QESVTEQDSK  DSTYSLSSTL  TLSKADYEKH  KVYACEVTHQ
GLSSPVTKSF  NRGEC
```

Light Chain

```
QVQLVESGGG  VVQPGRSLRL  SCAASGFTFS  SYTMHWVRQA  PGKGLEWVTF
ISYDGNNKYY  ADSVKGRFTI  SRDNSKNTLY  LQMNSLRAED  TAIYYCARTG
WLGPFDYWGQ  GTLVTVSSAS  TKGPSVFPLA  PSSKSTSGGT  AALGCLVKDY
FPEPVTVSWN  SGALTSGVHT  FPAVLQSSGL  YSLSSVVTVP  SSSLGTQTYI
CNVNHKPSNT  KVDKRVEPKS  CDKTHTCPPC  PAPELLGGPS  VFLFPPKPKD
TLMISRTPEV  TCVVVDVSHE  DPEVKFNWYV  DGVEVHNAKT  KPREEQYNST
YRVVSVLTVL  HQDWLNGKEY  KCKVSNKALP  APIEKTISKA  KGQPREPQVY
TLPPSRDELT  KNQVSLTCLV  KGFYPSDIAV  EWESNGQPEN  NYKTTPPVLD
SDGSFFLYSK  LTVDKSRWQQ  GNVFSCSVMH  EALHNHYTQK  SLSLSPGK
```

Heavy Chain

Production Process

❖ Production platform: CHO cells platform.
❖ Protein yield: NA.
❖ Protein purity: NA.

Analytical Profile

❖ Main structure an disulfide profile:[8]

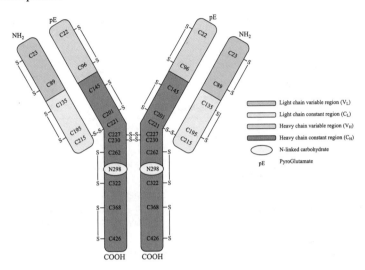

❖ Glycosylation:[5]

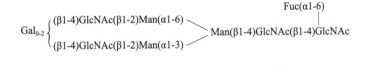

Figure 2   Glycosylation of Ipilimumab[5]

4   Pre-clinical Pharmacodynamics

Summary

Overview of *in vitro* Activities[4]
❖ Ipilimumab binds to CTLA-4 with high affinity ($K_d = 5.3 \pm 3.6$ nM).
❖ Blocks *in vitro* binding of B7.1 (CD80) and B7.2 (CD86) to human CTLA-4 at EC_{50} values of approximately 0.2 μg/mL with maximal blockade between 6-20 μg/mL and 1-3 μg/mL, respectively.
❖ Induced ADCC against resting human T cells; ADCC was enhanced against T cells simulated to express CTLA-4.

Overview of *in vivo* Activities[4, 9]
❖ Unstaged MC38 tumors in hCTLA-4 transgenic mice
  • Ipilimumab exhibited clear antitumor activity, slowing growth of human implanted MC38 tumors and prolonging survival in transgenic mice, genetically engineered to express human CTLA-4, but not mouse CTLA-4.
  • In combination studies:
    ♦ Statistically superior antitumor efficacy in combination with doxorubicin, paclitaxel, cyclophosphamide, methotrexate, etoposide and vinblastine.
    ♦ Antagonistic effect of 5-fluorouracil.
❖ In monkeys, ipilimumab increased the antibody response to HBsAg and SK-mel cells.
❖ In monkeys, Ipilimumab increased the antibody response to KLH.

Overview of *in vitro* Activities

Target Binding and Mechanism of Action

❖ Ipilimumab bound to CTLA-4: $K_d = 5.3 \pm 3.6$ nM.[4]

Table 4   Ipilimumab Reference Standard Binding Affinity Parameters[8]

	k_a (1/M·s)	k_d (1/M·s)	K_A (1/M)	K_D (nM)
Experiment 1	2.6×10^5	7.1×10^{-4}	3.6×10^8	2.8
Experiment 2	1.8×10^5	4.9×10^{-4}	3.7×10^8	2.7
Experiment 3	1.7×10^5	8.8×10^{-4}	1.9×10^8	5.2
Experiment 4	1.9×10^5	2.0×10^{-3}	9.6×10^7	10.4
Average	2.0×10^5	1.0×10^{-3}	2.6×10^8	5.3
SD	4.0×10^4	6.5×10^{-4}	1.3×10^8	3.6

SD: Standard deviation.

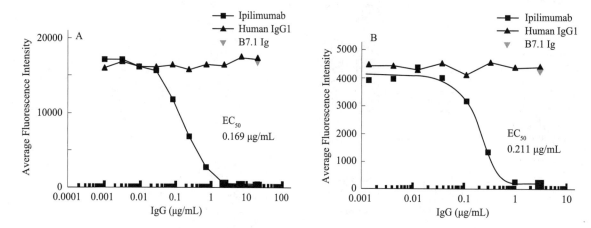

Figure 3   Ipilimumab Inhibited CTLA-4 to Binding B7.1 or B7.2[8]

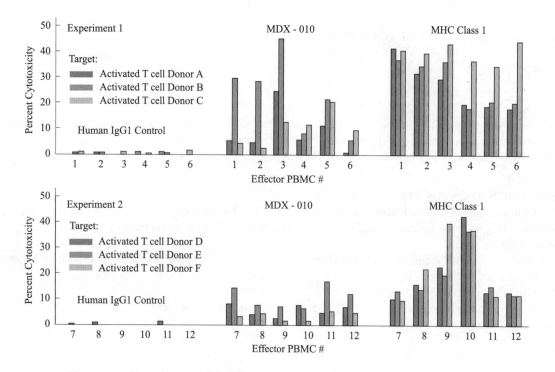

Figure 4   Ipilimumab Induced ADCC in Human T Cells Stimulated to Express CTLA-4[9]

Overview of *in vivo* Activities

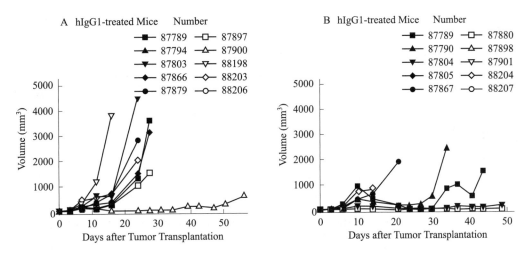

Study: Effects of human anti-CTLA-4 administration on unstaged MC38 tumors in hCTLA-4 transgenic mice.

Animal: Mice.

Model: MC-38 colon carcinoma tumor line was implanted into the human CTLA-4 transgenic mice.

Administration: i.p., Ipilimumab 10 mg/(kg·day).   Control: 10 mg/kg human IgG1 on study Days 0, 3, 6, and 10.

Figure 5   Ipilimumab Inhibits Growth of Human Implanted MC38 Tumors in Transgenic Mice Expressing Human CTLA-4[8]

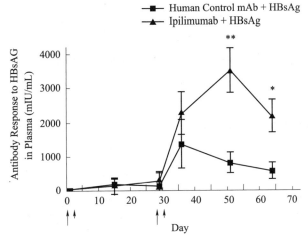

Study: An immunogenic study following combined intravenous/intramuscular administration of MAb10/D1/HBsAg respectively, to Cynomolgus monkeys.

Animal: Cynomolgus monkey.

Dosing: All animal received HBsAg i.m. on Day 2 and Day 30.   Group 1 and group 3 received 10 mg/kg of MAbRSV i.v. on Day 1 and Day 29. Group 2 and group 4 received 10 mg/kg of ipilimumab i.v. on Day 1 and Day 29; Group 3 and group 4 received oligo-CpG i.m. on Day 2 only.

Figure 6   Ipilimumab Increased the Antibody Response to HBsAg in Cynomolgus Monkeys[8]

Table 5   Ipilimumab Increased Monkeys' Antibody Response to HBsAg Vaccine[9]

Treatment	Group 1	Group 2	Group 3	Group 4
D1	0.0	0.0	0.0	0.0
D15	200 ± 170	110 ± 90.0	1,940 ± 1,380	2,270 ± 1,670
D29	110 ± 70.0	310 ± 250	310 ± 190	950 ± 620
D36	1,670 ± 700	2,260 ± 620	6,140 ± 2,130	3,870 ± 1,630
D51	820 ± 290	3,520 ± 630	4,240 ± 1,350	1,530 ± 640
D64	580 ± 240	2,180 ± 480	2,820 ± 920	1,120 ± 690

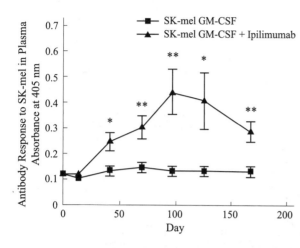

Study: DMX-CTLA-4: A 6-month intravenous toxicity.

Animal: Cynomolgus monkey.

Dosing: Saline i.v., 10 mg/kg ipilimumab i.v., 5×10^6 SK-mel cells s.c., 10 mg/kg ipilimumab and SK-mel, on Days 0, 28, 56, 84 and 140 for all four dose groups.

Figure 7   Ipilimumab Increased the Antibody Response to SK-mel in Cynomolgus Monkeys[8]

Table 6   Ipilimumab Increased Monkeys' Antibody Response to SK-mel Vaccine[9]

Day	Antibody to SK-mel (Flow Cytometry Assay, Mean Fluorescence Intensity)		Antibody to SK-mel (ELISA Assay, Mean Optical Density)	
	SK-mel	Ipilimumab + SK-mel	SK-mel	Ipilimumab + SK-mel
Pre-dose	61.0	67.0	0.12	0.12
D13	80.0	169	0.11	0.13
D41	325	1,280	0.14	0.25
D69	337	798	0.15	0.31
D97	220	1,029	0.13	0.45
D125	281	630	0.14	0.41
D167/168	148	454	0.13	0.29

❖ Ipilimumab increased the antibody response to KLH in Cynomolgus monkeys.

Table 7   Ipilimumab Induced Monkeys' Antibody Response to KLH[9]

Titer (/1,000) Day	Male			Female		
	0	Ipilimumab & BMS-663513	Ipilimumab	0	Ipilimumab & BMS-663513	Ipilimumab
D15	0.40	0.80	0.30	0.80	1.0	0.50
D23	15.0	102	57.0	22.0	137	102
D29	14.0	236	113	46.0	172	224
D36	14.0	240	124	65.0	172	239

PK/PD Studies in Cynomolgus Monkeys[9]

❖ Elimination half-life ($t_{1/2}$):
- $t_{1/2} = 203 \pm 63$ h (following a single 10 mg/kg i.v. dose, data collected for 28 days).
- $t_{1/2} = 339 \pm 112$ h (data collected for 9 weeks after the final dose).

❖ Steady-state volume of distribution (V_{ss}) was variable, but indicates that ipilimumab was confined to the plasma space (approximately 40 to 70 mL/kg):
- $V_{ss} = 44 \pm 6$ mL/kg.
- $V_{ss} = 81 \pm 14$ mL/kg.

❖ Generally, exposure was dose-proportional or greater than dose-proportional.

❖ Accumulation was observed with frequent dosing (e.g. weekly or more often than weekly dosing).

❖ ELISA was used to detect circulating levels of ipilimumab.

5 Toxicology

Non-clinical Single-Dose Toxicology[4]

❖ Pivotal single-dose studies with ipilimumab were not conducted.   No acute toxicity was noted in monkeys following ipilimumab doses up to 30 mg/kg in the repeated-dose toxicology studies.   Further, no adverse toxicities were observed in a single-dose exploratory comparative pharmacokinetics study in monkeys of ipilimumab at 10 mg/kg.

Non-clinical Repeated-Dose Toxicology[4]

❖ A series of i.v. repeated-dose toxicology studies were conducted with ipilimumab in Cynomolgus monkeys (up to 6 months).
   • At 30 mg/kg ipilimumab dosed for 2 weeks, haematological effects were noted.   10 mg/kg was selected as the highest dose tested.
   • Three out of 100 Cynomolgus monkeys presented severe adverse effects.   Fatal colitis and persistent dermatitis/rash observed in two animals along the toxicology program were considered as immune-related adverse event (irAEs) linked with the intended pharmacologic basis of CTLA-4 blockade.
   • Apart from these cases of severe adverse events, ipilimumab generally did not result in adverse toxicities in any other monkeys when administered i.v. at doses up to 30 mg/kg for 1 week, or 10 mg/kg monthly for up to 6 months.

Safety Pharmacology[9]

❖ The results did not raise concerns for effects of ipilimumab on safety pharmacology parameters (i.e. neuromotor, cardiac, or respiratory function).

Reproductive Toxicology[4]

❖ Despite specific binding of ipilimumab to Cynomolgus monkey ovarian tissue, no gross or microscopic ovarian findings were observed in ipilimumab toxicity studies conducted in monkeys and therefore is not expected to have any biological or toxicological relevance, especially since similar binding was not observed with human ovaries.

Other Toxicology[4]

❖ Antigenicity: Ipilimumab generally was not immunogenic in monkeys.
❖ Immunotoxicity: In addition to standard immune hematologic and clinical chemistry assessments and gross and histopathologic examinations of lymphoid tissues included in the repeated-dose studies, specialized immune parameters were incorporated into several of the studies including peripheral blood lymphocyte phenotyping (including activated T-cell and regulatory T-cell subsets), lymphocyte phenotyping in spleen, inguinal lymph node, and colon epithelium, anti-nuclear antibody assessments, T cell-dependent antibody response assessments, DTH assessments, and intracellular staining of *ex vivo* stimulated cytokine (IL-2, TNF-α and/or IFN-γ) production by monkey peripheral blood T cells.   The T-cell dependent response as elicited by KLH administration clearly showed the effect of ipilimumab.

Non-clinical Repeated-Dose Toxicology

Table 8   Repeated-Dose Toxicity Studies[4]

No./Sex	Dose (mg/kg)	Day of Dosing	Antigen	NOEL [mg/(kg·day)]	Major Finding
2/F	3	1, 4, 7	-	3.0	-
2/M	3	1, 4, 7	-	10.0	Small increase CD3+ cells.
2/Sex	10	1, 4, 7	-		
2/M	3	1, 4, 7	-	3.0	30: > leukocyte, WBC, lymph, neutr, mono.
2/Sex	30	1, 4, 7	-		
5/Sex	10	1, 8, 15, 22	KLH	10.0	-
5/Sex	10[a]	1, 8, 15, 22	KLH		
2/Sex	10	1, 29	HBsAg		>10+ CpG: Lymphocyte count.
2/Sex	10[b]	1, 29	HBsAg		
3/Sex	1	1, 29, 57	HBsAg, SK-mel	10.0	-
3/Sex	1	10 × weekly	HBsAg, SK-mel		
3/Sex	10	1, 29, 57	HBsAg, SK-mel		
3/Sex	10[c]	1, 29, 57	HBsAg, SK-mel		
2/Sex	10[c]	0, 28, 56, 84, 140	-		↓ Organ weight (testes, thyroid).
3/Sex	10[c]	0, 28, 56, 84, 140	SK-mel		

[a] Ipilimumab was given together with BMS-663513.   [b] Ipilimumab was administered together with CpG.   [c] Process A material.

6 Pre-clinical Pharmacokinetics/ADME/Toxicokinetics

Summary

Non-clinical Pharmacokinetics[4]

❖ All studies were performed in Cynomolgus monkey and ipilimumab was administered intravenously.
❖ In single-dose kinetics:
  • The half-life time of ipilimumab is 8 to 15 days depending on the study, as was the mean residence time. Consistent with the long $t_{1/2}$, the CLT was low [0.17-0.21 mL/(h·kg)]. The V_{ss} is similar to the plasma volume of monkeys.
❖ Studies with every 3rd day dosing:
  • Serum concentrations increased in males in a manner proportional or greater than dose proportional to the dose increment between 3 and 10 mg/kg.
  • Consistent with the long half-life pre-dose concentrations doubled in these studies between Day 4 and Day 7, indicative of accumulation of ipilimumab when dosed every 3 days.
❖ Studies with weekly dosing:
  • Data from 8 animals followed up after the last administration revealed a long half-life, approximately 12 days.
❖ Studies with monthly dosing:
  • Plasma concentrations of ipilimumab tended to increase with repeated dosing.
❖ In all studies serum/plasma concentrations of ipilimumab were similar between males and females and between animals receiving ipilimumab only or ipilimumab in combination with another substance.
❖ Two non-clinical bridging studies were performed comparing processes. There were no differences in pharmacokinetics (PK) parameters.
❖ Ipilimumab generally was not immunogenic in monkeys.
❖ Distribution
  • Following a single 10 mg/kg i.v. dose of ipilimumab to male and female Cynomolgus monkeys, the V_{ss} was similar to the plasma volume of monkeys, suggesting that ipilimumab does not distribute out of the plasma compartment.
❖ Drug-Drug interaction
  • Ipilimumab is not expected to have interactions with molecules that are metabolized by cytochrome P450 enzymes.
  • In an intermittent-dose study conducted to determine the potential toxicity of ipilimumab administered alone or in combination with BMS-663513, there was no difference between the C_{max} or AUC$_{(0-48 h)}$ values for monkeys receiving ipilimumab alone and monkeys receiving ipilimumab in combination with BMS-663513. These results do not provide any evidence of a PK drug-drug interaction between ipilimumab and BMS-663513 in monkeys.

Non-clinical Pharmacokinetics

Table 9   Mean PK Parameters in the Single-Dose Comparability Study in Monkeys[9]

Process Material	C_{max} (µg/mL)	AUC$_{0-1008 h}$ (µg·h/mL)	AUC$_{inf}$ (µg·h/mL)	$t_{1/2}$ (h)	MRT (h)	CLT [mL/(h·kg)]	V_{ss} (L/kg)
B	252	521,000	57,500	307	410	0.18	0.072
C	234	467,000	55,200	370	507	0.19	0.090

CLT: Clearance rate.   MRT: Mean residence time.

Table 10　PK Parameters following 4 Weekly Injections[a] in Monkeys[9]

Parameter	Day	Animals Measured	Ipilimumab
C_{max} (µg/mL)	1	20	220 ± 26.0
	22	19	339 ± 47.0
$AUC_{0-48\,h}$ (µg·h/mL)	1	20	7,160 ± 1,080
	22	19	17,500 ± 2,830
$AUC_{0-168\,h}$ (µg·h/mL)	1	20	18,000 ± 3,900
$AUC_{0-1512\,h}$ (µg·h/mL)	22	7	90,600 ± 25,300
MRT (h)	22-85	7	432 ± 72.0
$t_{1/2}$ (h)	29-85	7	302 ± 90.0

MRT: Mean residence time.　[a] Study BMS-663513 and BMS-734016, one-month intravenous combination toxicity study in monkeys.

❖ TK data for 10 mg/kg of ipilimumab, i.v. dosing on Days 0, 28, 56, 84 and 140.

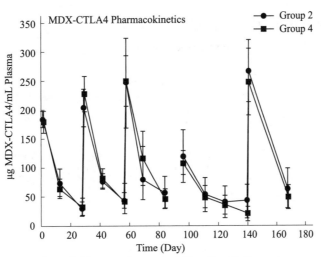

Group 2: The group that received 10 mg/kg of ipilimumab.
Group 4: The group that received 10 mg/kg of ipilimumab + SK-mel.

Figure 8　TK Data for 10 mg/kg of Ipilimumab (i.v.)[9]

7　Clinical Efficacy and Safety

Overview Profile

❖ Ipilimumab is a monoclonal antibody which targets CTLA-4.　The proposed indication for the first approval is for treatment of advanced melanoma in patients who received prior therapy.

❖ Ipilimumab started clinical trials in the US in 2003.

❖ Ipilimumab was approved for the treatment of unresectable or metastatic melanoma in 2011 by US FDA, based on the results from MDX010-20.

❖ Treatment for advanced melanoma (a type of skin cancer) in adults with ipilimumab was approved by EMA in 2011 based on the results from one Phase 3 pivotal study MDX010-20 and seven supportive Phase 1/2 studies.

❖ Ipilimumab was approved for unresectable malignant melanoma by Japan PMDA in 2011.

❖ Ipilimumab was approved for adjuvant treatment of patients with cutaneous melanoma with pathologic involvement of regional lymph nodes of more than 1 mm who have undergone complete resection, including total lymphadenectomy with by US FDA in 2015.

Indications 1: Unresectable or Metastatic Melanoma

Phase 1 Trial

Table 11　The Profile of Phase 1 Clinical Trials of Ipilimumab[4]

ID	Phase	Type of Study	Patient and Treatment Regimen	Aim	Endpoint
MDX010-15 Group B	1/2	Open-label study; In 5 sites in the US	Unresectable Stage 3 or 4 melanoma. 10 mg/kg, q3wk × 4 (induction).	Determine the safety and pharmacokinetic profile of single and multiple-dose of ipilimumab derived from a transfectoma or a hybridoma cell line.	Safety/PK; Secondary endpoints: BORR, DCR, TTR, and DOR.

BORR: Best overall response rate.　DCR: Disease control rate.　DOR: Duration of response.　TTR: Time to response.

Phase 2 Trials

Table 12　The Profile of Phase 2 Clinical Trials of Ipilimumab[4]

ID	Type of Study	Patient and Treatment Regimen	Aim	Endpoint
CA184022	Randomized, double-blind, dose-ranging, 3 group multicenter study; In 66 sites in 13 countries.	Previously treated unrespectable Stage 3 and 4 melanoma, 0.3, 3, or10mg/kgq3wk×4(induction)followed by maintenance dosing q12wk.	Estimate BORR in patients receiving ipilimumab doses 0.3, 3 and 10 mg/kg.	BORR; Secondary endpoints: OS, DCR, PRS, TTR, and DOR.
CA184004	Randomized, double-blind, 2-group, biomarker study; In 14 sites in 7 countries.	Unrespectable Stage 3 or 4 melanoma, 3 or 10 mg/kg q3wk × 4 (induction) followed by maintenance dosing q12wk.	Analyze pre-treatment characteristic of patients and/or tumor with clinical tumor response, in order to identify candidate markers predictive of response and/or serious toxicity to ipilimumab dosed at 3 or 10 mg/kg, q3wk.	Biomarker; Secondary endpoints: BORR, OS, DCR, PFS, TTR, and DOR.
MDX010-08	Randomized, double-blind, 2 group study; In 12 sites in the US.	Chemotherapy naïve metastatic melanoma, 3 mg/kg, q4wk × 4 +/-DTIC (induction).	To determine the safety and activity profile of multiple-dose of ipilimumab and to determine whether the addition of cytotoxic chemotherapy would augment the effects of ipilimumab.	ORR; Secondary endpoints: OS, DCR, PFS, DOR, and TTR.
CA184008	Open-label, single-group study; In 50 sites in Europe and North America.	Previously treated, unrespectable Stage 3 or 4 melanoma, 10 mg/kg q3wk × 4 (induction) followed by maintenance dosing q12wk.	To evaluate the BORR.	BORR; Secondary endpoints; OS, DCR, PFS, TTR, and DOR.
CA184007	Randomized, double-blind, 2 group study; In 11 sites in 6 countries in Europe, North America, and South America.	Unresectable Stage 3 or 4 melanoma, 10 mg/kg, q3wk × 4 +/-budesonide (induction) followed by maintenance dosing q12wk.	To estimate the rate of Grade ≥2 diarrhoea in patients treated ipilimumab at 10 mg/kg given with either prophylactic oral budesonide or placebo.	Safety; Secondary endpoints: BORR, OS, DCR, PFS, TTR, and DOR.
CA184042 Stage 1	Open-label study; In 8 sites in the US.	Stage 4 melanoma with brain metastases, 10 mg/kg q3wk × 4 (induction) followed by maintenance dosing q12wk.	To assess the disease control rate determined after Week 12 using the modified WHO (mWHO) tumor assessment criteria.	DCR; Secondary endpoints: BORR, PFS, and DOR.
MDX010-28 Survival Follow-up Study	Multicenter, Long-term	Patients alive who received any dose of ipilimumab (MDX-010) in MDX010-02, MDX010-08, and MDX010-15	Collect disease status and survival information on patients alive after completing studies MDX010-02, MDX010-08 or MDX010-15.	Disease status and OS.

BORR: Best overall response rate.　DCR: Disease control rate.　DOR: Duration of response.　OS: Overall survival.　PFS: Progression-free survival.　TTR: Time to response.

Table 13   Overall Survival in CA184-004 (Phase 2 Study)[10]

	3 mg/kg Ipilimumab (N = 40)	10 mg/kg Ipilimumab (N = 42)
Survival rate at 1 year, % (95% *CI*)	52.0 (36.6, 67.3)	45.2 (31.0, 59.5)
Survival rate at 18 months, % (95% *CI*)	33.8 (19.8, 49.1)	35.2 (21.2, 49.9)
Overall survival (Month), median, 95% *CI*	12.8 (9.5, 17.6)	11.2 (6.1, 16.9)

CI: Confidence interval.

Table 14   Overall Survival in CA184-007 (Phase 2 Study)[10]

	10 mg/kg Ipilimumab + Budesonide (N = 58)	10 mg/kg Ipilimumab + Placebo (N = 57)
Survival rate at 1 year, % (95% *CI*)	55.9 (42.7, 68.8)	62.4 (49.4, 75.1)
Survival rate at 18 months, % (95% *CI*)	47.9 (34.7, 61.2)	50.9 (37.5, 64.1)
Survival rate at 2 years, % (95% *CI*)	40.6 (27.1, 54.4)	41.8 (28.3, 55.5)
OS (Month), median, 95% *CI*	17.7 (6.3, -)	19.3 (12.0, -)

CI: Confidence interval.   OS: Overall survival.   -: Not reached.

Table 15   Overall Survival in CA184-008 (Phase 2 Study)[10]

	10 mg/kg Ipilimumab (N = 155)
Survival rate at 1 year, % (95% *CI*)	47.2 (39.5, 55.1)
Survival rate at 18 months, % (95% *CI*)	39.4 (31.7, 47.2)
Survival rate at 2 years, % (95% *CI*)	32.8 (25.4, 40.5)
OS (Month), median, 95% *CI*	10.2 (7.6, 16.3)

CI: Confidence interval.   OS: Overall survival.

Table 16   Overall Survival in CA184-022 (Phase 2 Study)[10]

	0.3 mg/kg Ipilimumab (N = 73)	3 mg/kg Ipilimumab (N = 72)	10 mg/kg Ipilimumab (N = 72)
Survival rate at 1 year, % (95% *CI*)	39.6 (28.2, 51.2)	39.3 (28.0, 50.9)	48.6 (36.8, 60.4)
Survival rate at 18 months, % (95% *CI*)	23.0 (13.4, 33.6)	30.2 (19.8, 41.4)	34.5 (23.4, 46.2)
Survival rate at 2 years, % (95% *CI*)	18.4 (9.6, 28.2)	24.2 (14.4, 34.8)	29.8 (19.1, 41.1)
OS (Month), median, 95% *CI*	8.6 (7.7, 12.7)	8.7 (6.7, 12.1)	11.4 (6.9, 16.1)

CI: Confidence interval.   OS: Overall survival.

Phase 3 Trials

Table 17   The Profile of Phase 3 Clinical Trials of Ipilimumab[4]

ID	Type of Study	Patient and Treatment Regimen	Aim	Endpoint
MDX010-20 Pivotal study	Randomized, double-blind, 3 groups multicenter study; In 125 sites in Europe, North America, South America and Africa.	HLA-A2*0201-positive, previously treated, unresectable Stage 3 or 4 melanoma, 3 mg/kg q3wk × 4 +/-gp100 or gp100 alone (induction) followed by re-induction.	Compare OS of patients administered ipilimumab in combination with gp100 vs. those administered ipilimumab placebo in combination with gp100.	OS; Secondary endpoints: BORR, major durable response rate, DOR, PFS, TTP.
CA184024	Randomized, double-blind, 2 groups multicenter study.	Previously untreated patients with unresectable Stage 3 or 4 melanoma, 10 mg/kg q3wk × 4 +/-dacarbazine (induction) followed by maintenance.	To compare overall survival in patients receiving dacarbazine plus 10 mg/kg ipilimumab vs. dacarbazine with placebo.	OS; Secondary endpoints: BORR, PFS, DCR.

BORR: Best overall response rate.   DCR: Disease control rate.   DOR: Duration of response.   OS: Overall survival.   PFS: Progression-free survival.   TTP: Time to progression.

Clinical Efficacy

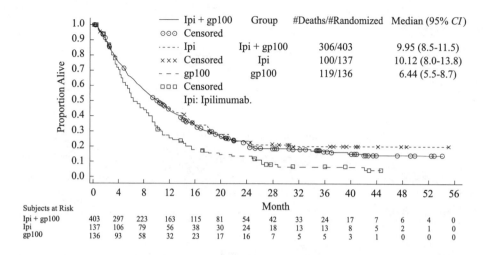

Figure 9   Overall Survival by Treatment (ITT Population) in Trial MDX010-20[10]

Table 18   Overall Survival Analyses in Trial MDX101-20[10]

OS	Primary Comparison	Ipilimumab + gp100 (N = 403)	gp100 (N = 136)
	No. of deaths	306	119
	No. censored	97	17
P-value = 0.00040	Hazard ratio (95% CI)	0.68 (0.55, 0.85)	
	Median OS (Month) (95% CI)	10.0 (8.5, 11.5)	6.4 (5.5, 8.7)
OS	**Secondary Comparison**	**Ipilimumab (N = 137)**	**gp100 (N = 136)**
	No. of deaths	100	119
	No. censored	37	17
P-value = 0.0026	Hazard ratio (95% CI)	0.66 (0.51, 0.87)	
	Median OS (Month) (95% CI)	10.1 (8.0, 13.8)	6.4 (5.5, 8.7)
OS		**Ipilimumab + gp100 (N = 403)**	**Ipilimumab (N = 137)**
	No. of deaths	306	100
	No. censored	97	37
P-value = 0.76	Hazard ratio (95% CI)	1.0 (0.83, 1.3)	
	Median OS (Month) (95% CI)	10.0 (8.5, 11.5)	10.1 (8.0, 13.8)

CI: Confidence interval.   OS: Overall survival.

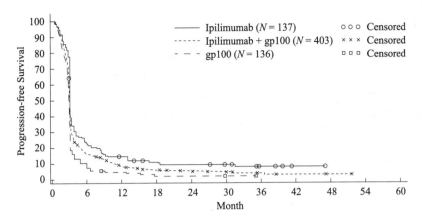

Figure 10   Progression-free Survival by Treatment (MDX010-20 Study-ITT Population)[4]

Table 19   Best Overall Response Based on Modified WHO Criteria by Treatment (MDX010-20 Study, ITT Population)[4]

	Ipilimumab + gp100 (N = 403)	Ipilimumab (N = 137)	gp100 (N = 136)	Total (N = 676)
Best Overall Response	n (%)	n (%)	n (%)	n (%)
CR	1 (0.20)	2 (1.5)	0	3 (0.40)
PR	22 (5.5)	13 (9.5)	2 (1.5)	37 (5.5)
SD	58 (14.4)	24 (17.5)	13 (9.6)	95 (14.1)
PD	239 (59.3)	70 (51.1)	89 (65.4)	398 (58.9)
NE	83 (20.6)	28 (20.4)	32 (23.5)	143 (21.2)
BORR	23 (5.7)	15 (10.9)	2 (1.5)	40 (5.9)
95% CI	(3.7, 8.4)	(6.3, 17.4)	(0.20, 5.2)	(4.3, 8.0)
P-value vs. gp100	0.043	0.0012		
P-value vs. ipilimumab	0.040			

BORR: Best overall response rate.   CI: Confidence interval.   CR: Complete remission.   NE: Not evaluated.   PD: Disease progression.   PR: Partial remission.   SD: Stable disease.

Clinical Safety

Table 20   irAE during the Induction Phase[10]

	% of Subjects				
	Phase 3 Study (MDX010-20)			Phase 2 Study	
	3 mg/kg Ipilimumab (N = 131)	3 mg/kg Ipilimumab + gp100 (N = 380)	gp100 (N = 132)	Pooled 3 mg/kg (N = 111)	Pooled 10 mg/kg (N = 325)
Any irAE	59.5	56.8	31.8	61.3	72.0
Grade 3-4	13.0	10.0	3.0	6.3	24.3
Grade 5	0.80	1.1	0.0	0.90	0.90

irAE: Immune-related adverse events.

Table 21   Incidence of Common ($\geq 5.0\%$) Adverse Reactions and of Severe (Grades 3-5) Adverse Reactions in Patients Receiving a Single Course of Treatment in MDX101-20[3]

System Organ Class Preferred Term	% of Patients					
	3 mg/kg Ipilimumab (N = 131)		3 mg/kg Ipilimumab + gp100[a] (N = 380)		gp100[a] (N = 132)	
	Any Grade	Grade 3-5	Any Grade	Grade 3-5	Any Grade	Grade 3-5
Gastrointestinal Disorders						
Diarrhea	32.0	5.0	37.0	4.0	20.0	1.0
Colitis	8.0	5.0	5.0	3.0	2.0	0.0
Skin and Subcutaneous Tissue Disorders						
Pruritus[a]	31.0	0.0	21.0	0.30	11.0	0.0
Rash[a]	29.0	1.0	25.0	2.0	8.0	0.0
General Disorders and Administration Site Conditions						
Fatigue	41.0	7.0	34.0	5.0	31.0	3.0

[a] Included appropriate combining/remapping of the preferred terms by the applicant.

❖ Treatment-related adverse events were common, leading to discontinuation in 9.9% of patients and to death in 3.1% in MDX010-20.

❖ Most serious adverse events (SAEs) were immune related, as can be expected based on the mechanism of action.

❖ The majority of immune-related AEs could be treated successfully.

Indications 2: Adjuvant Melanoma

❖ The safety and efficacy of Yervoy® for the adjuvant treatment of melanoma were investigated in EORTC 18071, a randomized (1:1), double-blind, placebo-controlled trial in patients with resected Stage 3A (>1 mm nodal involvement), 3B, and 3C (with no in-transit metastases) histologically confirmed cutaneous melanoma.   Patients were randomized to receive Yervoy® 10 mg/kg or placebo as an intravenous infusion every 3 weeks for 4 doses, followed by Yervoy® 10 mg/kg or placebo every 12 weeks from Week 24 to Week 156 (3 years) or until documented disease recurrence or unacceptable toxicity.   Enrollment required complete resection of melanoma with full lymphadenectomy within 12 weeks prior to randomization.   Patients with prior therapy for melanoma, autoimmune disease, and prior or concomitant use of immunosuppressive agents were ineligible.   Randomization was stratified by stage according to American Joint Committee on Cancer (AJCC) 2002 classification (Stage 3A >1 mm nodal involvement, Stage 3B, Stage 3C with 1 to 3 involved lymph nodes, and Stage 3C with ≥ 4 involved lymph nodes) and by region (North America, Europe, and Australia).   The major efficacy outcome measures were independent review committee (IRC)-assessed recurrence-free survival (RFS), defined as the time between the date of randomization and the earliest date of first recurrence (local, regional, or distant metastasis) or death, and overall survival.   Tumor assessment was conducted every 12 weeks for the first 3 years then every 24 weeks until distant recurrence.

❖ Among 951 patients enrolled, 475 were randomized to receive Yervoy® and 476 to placebo.   Median age was 51 years old (range: 18 to 84), 62.0% were male, 99.0% were white, 94.0% had ECOG performance status of 0.   With regard to disease stage, 20.0% had Stage 3A with lymph nodes >1 mm, 44.0% had Stage 3B, and 36.0% had Stage 3C (with no in-transit metastases).   Other disease characteristics of the trial population were: Clinically palpable lymph nodes (58.0%), 2 or more positive lymph nodes (54.0%), and ulcerated primary lesions (42.0%).

Clinical Efficacy

Table 22   Recurrence-free Survival and Overall Survival in EORTC 18071[11]

	Ipilimumab (N = 475)	Placebo (N = 476)
Recurrence-free Survival		
No. of Events, *n* (%)	234 (49.0)	294 (62.0)
Recurrence	220	289
Death	14	5
Median (Month), (95% *CI*)	26 (19.0, 39.0)	17 (13.0, 22.0)
Hazard ratio (95% *CI*)	0.75 (0.64, 0.90)	
P-value (stratified log-rank[a])	*P* <0.0020	
Overall Survival		
Death, *n* (%)	162 (34.0)	214 (45.0)
Hazard ratio (95% *CI*)	0.72 (0.58, 0.88)	
P-value (stratified log-rank[a])	*P* <0.0020	

[a] Stratified by disease stage.

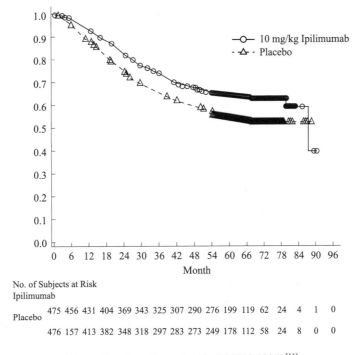

Figure 11   Overall Survival in EORTC 18071[11]

Clinical Safety
❖ Table 23 presents selected adverse reactions from EORTC 18071 which occurred in at least 5.0% of ipilimumab-treated patients and with at least 5.0% increased incidence over the placebo group for all-grade events.

Table 23   Selected Adverse Reactions in EORTC 18071[11]

System Organ Class/Preferred Term	% of Patients[a]			
	Ipilimumab 10 mg/kg (N = 471)		Placebo (N = 474)	
	Any Grade	Grade 3-5	Any Grade	Grade 3-5
Skin and Subcutaneous Tissue Disorders				
Rash	50.0	2.1	20.0	0.0
Pruritus	45.0	2.3	15.0	0.0
Gastrointestinal Disorders				
Diarrhea	49.0	10.0	30.0	2.1
Nausea	25.0	0.20	18.0	0.0
Colitis[b]	16.0	8.0	1.5	0.40
Vomiting	13.0	0.40	6.0	0.20
Investigations				
Weight decreased	32.0	0.20	9.0	0.40
General Disorders and Administration Site Conditions				
Fatigue	46.0	2.3	38.0	1.5
Pyrexia	18.0	1.1	4.9	0.20
Nervous System Disorders				
Headache	33.0	0.80	18.0	0.20
Metabolism and Nutrition Disorders				
Decreased appetite	14.0	0.20	3.4	0.20
Psychiatric Disorders				
Insomnia	10.0	0.0	4.4	0.0

[a] Incidences presented in this table are based on reports of adverse events regardless of causality.   [b] Includes 1 death.

❖ Table 24 presents selected laboratory abnormalities from EORTC 18071 which occurred in at least 10.0% of ipilimumab-treated patients at a higher incidence compared to placebo.

Table 24   Laboratory Abnormalities Worsening from Baseline Occurring in ≥10.0% of Ipilimumab-treated Patients (EORTC 18071)[a, 11]

Test	% of Patients with Worsening Laboratory Test from Baseline[a]			
	Ipilimumab		Placebo	
	Any Grade	Grade 3-4	Any Grade	Grade 3-4
Chemistry				
Increased ALT	46.0	10.0	16.0	0.0
Increased AST	38.0	9.0	14.0	0.20
Increased lipase[b]	26.0	9.0	17.0	4.5
Increased amylase[b]	17.0	2.0	7.0	0.60
Increased alkaline phosphatase	17.0	0.60	6.0	0.20
Increased bilirubin	11.0	1.5	9.0	0.0
Increased creatinine	10.0	0.20	6.0	0.0
Hematology				
Decreased hemoglobin	25.0	0.20	14.0	0.0

[a] Each test incidence is based on the number of patients who had both baseline and at least one on-study laboratory measurement available.   Excluding lipase and amylase, ipilimumab group (range: 466-470 patients) and placebo group (range: 472-474 patients).   [b] For lipase and amylase, ipilimumab group (range: 447-448 patients) and placebo group (range: 462-464 patients).

❖ Table 25 presents the per-patient incidence of severe, life-threatening, or fatal immune-mediated adverse reactions from EORTC 18071.

Table 25   Severe to Fatal Immune-mediated Adverse Reactions in EORTC 18071[11]

	% of Patients[a]
	Ipilimumab 10 mg/kg (*N* = 471)
Any Immune-mediated Adverse Reaction	41.0
Enterocolitis[a, b]	16.0
Hepatitis	11.0
Dermatitis	4.0
Neuropathy[a]	1.7
Endocrinopathy	8.0
Hypopituitarism	7.0
Primary hypothyroidism	0.20
Hyperthyroidism	0.60
Other	
Myocarditis[a]	0.20
Meningitis	0.40
Pericarditis[c]	0.20
Pneumonitis	0.20
Uveitis	0.20

[a] Including fatal outcome.   [b] Including intestinal perforation.   [c] Underlying etiology not established.

Other Clinical Experience[11]

❖ Across clinical studies that utilized ipilimumab doses ranging from 0.3 to 10 mg/kg, the following adverse reactions were also reported (incidence less than 1.0% unless otherwise noted): Urticaria (2.0%), large intestinal ulcer, esophagitis, acute respiratory distress syndrome, renal failure, and infusion reaction.

8   Clinical Pharmacokinetics

Summary[10]

❖ Rich pharmacokinetic (PK) data is available from 84 patients enrolled into 3 clinical trials and sparse PK data is available from 499 patients across 4 clinical trials.
❖ Ipilimumab exhibited linear PK over a dose range of 0.3 to 10 mg/kg with a mean elimination half-life of 15 days.
❖ The inter-individual variability for clearance was approximately 35.0%.

Single-Dose Pharmacokinetics

Table 26   Summary Statistics for Signle-Dose PK Parameters of Ipilimumab in MDX010-15[a, [10]]

PK	Day 1 of Multiple-Dose			Single-Dose			
	2.8 mg/kg (N = 13)	3.0[b] mg/kg (N = 12)	5.0 mg/kg (N = 10)	7.5 mg/kg (N = 6)	10 mg/kg (N = 7)	15 mg/kg (N = 6)	20 mg/kg (N = 11)
C_{max} (μg/mL)	79.9 (24.0%)	84.5 (38.0%)	162 (28.0%)	292 (23.0%)	300 (24.0%)	400 (7.5%)	533 (33.0%)
T_{max} (h)	2.5 (1.5, 5.5)	1.8 (1.5, 4.0)	3.5 (1.5, 5.5)	2.0 (1.5, 2.5)	2.0 (1.5, 7.0)	3.3 (1.5, 22.0)	3.0 (1.4, 5.5)
$AUC_{0-21 d}$ (μg·h/mL)	12,081 (44.0%)	12,383 (32.0%)	26,875 (23.0%)	44,853 (22.0%)	37,706 (24.0%)	67,107 (11.0%)	64,808 (23.0%)
AUC_{inf} (μg·h/mL)	19,583 (74.0%)	19,596 (68.0%)	42,337 (32.0%)	70,847 (19.0%)	60,099 (43.0%)	98,325 (23.0%)	78,258 (46.0%)
Terminal $t_{1/2}$ (Day)	16.0 (9.5)	17.3 (11.0)	16.0 (10.9)	16.1 (6.7)	15.3 (8.3)	16.5 (6.0)	12.4 (8.3)
CL (mL/h)	12.8 (6.8)	13.8 (8.1)	11.6 (5.2)	8.9 (2.1)	15.7 (6.2)	13.6 (2.2)	21.9 (11.5)
V_{ss} (L)	5.5 (2.1)	5.9 (1.6)	5.4 (1.9)	4.7 (1.1)	6.7 (2.3)	6.2 (1.9)	6.1 (1.8)

[a] AUC and C_{max} are expressed as geometric mean (CV%), T_{max} as in media (min, max), all the other parameters are expressed as arithmetic mean (SD).   [b] Response patients who received process A (hybridoma-derived) ipilimumab.

Multiple-Dose Pharmacokinetics

Table 27   Summary Statistics for Multiple-Dose PK Parameters of Ipilimumab in MDX010-15[a, [10]]

Time and Dose No. of Sampling	Group A			Group B
	Day 57 (Dose 2)	Day 57 (Dose 2)	Day 58 (Dose 3)	Day 64 (Dose 4)
PK parameters	2.8 mg/kg (N = 7)	3 mg/kg (N = 5)	5 mg/kg (N = 3)	10 mg/kg (N = 13)
C_{max} (μg/mL)	108 (38.0%)	103 (68.0%)	237 (32.0%)	441 (36.0%)
T_{max} (h)	2.5 (1.3, 4.0)	3 (1.5, 24)	2.5 (1.6, 5.5)	2.5 (1.3, 48)
$AUC_{0-21 d}$ (μg·h/mL)	15,206 (30.0%)	18,396 (33.0%)	37,670 (30.0%)	55,433 (35.0%)
Terminal $t_{1/2}$ (Day)	11 (3.0)	13 (9.0)	NA	15 (9.0)

NA: Not available.   [a] AUC and C_{max} are expressed as geometric mean (CV%), T_{max} as in median (min, max), all the other parameters are expressed as mean (SD).   All the dates are when the last available data is collected.

Anti-product Antibody (APA) Analysis[10]

❖ The incidence of anti-product (ipilimumab) antibody (APA) formation is approximately 1.1% (11 out of 1,024 patients) across 7 clinical studies in patients with advanced melanoma.   None of the binding antibodies were found to have neutralizing capacity.

9   Patent

❖ Ipilimumab was approved by the U.S. Food and Drug Administration (FDA) in 2011.   It was developed and marketed as Yervoy® by Bristol-Myers Squibb.

Summary

❖ The patent application (WO200114424A2) related to the anti-CTLA-4 antibody (i.e. Ipilimumab), nucleic acid encoding the same and therapeutic compositions thereof was filed by Bristol-Myers Squibb on Oct 24, 2000.   Accordingly, its PCT counterpart has, among the others, been granted before USPTO (US6984720B1 and US7605238B2), EPO (EP1212422B1), JPO (JP4093757B2 and JP5599158B2) and SIPO (CN1371416B), respectively.

Table 28   Originator's Key Patent of Ipilimumab in Main Countries and/or Region

Country/Region	Publication/Patent No.	Application Date	Granted Date	Estimated Expiry Date
WO	WO200114424A2	08/24/2000	/	/
US	US6984720B1	08/24/2000	01/10/2006	08/02/2022
	US7605238B2	08/24/2000	10/20/2009	09/07/2021
	US2016257753A1	08/24/2000	/	/
EP	EP1212422B1	08/24/2000	02/21/2007	08/24/2020
	EP3214175A1	08/24/2000	/	/
JP	JP4093757B2	08/24/2000	06/04/2008	08/24/2020
	JP5599158B2	08/24/2000	10/01/2014	08/24/2020
	CN1371416B	08/24/2000	10/10/2012	08/24/2020

Table 29   Originator's International Patent Protection of Use and/or Method of Ipilimumab

Publication No.	Title	Publication Date
Technical Subjects	**TREATMENT METHOD**	
WO03086459A1	Methods of treatment using CTLA-4 antibodies	10/23/2003
WO2007067959A2	CTLA-4 antibody dosage escalation regimens	06/14/2007
WO2013142796A2	Methods of treatments using CTLA4 antibodies	09/26/2013
Technical Subjects	**DIAGNOSTIC METHOD**	
WO2013169971A1	Anti-tumor antibodies as predictive or prognostic biomarkers of efficacy and survival in ipilimumab-treated patients	11/14/2013
Technical Subjects	**COMBINATION METHOD**	
WO2007056540A2	TNF-alpha blocker treatment for enterocolitis associated with immunostimulatory therapeutic antibody therapy	05/18/2007
WO2007056539A2	Prophylaxis and treatment of enterocolitis associated with anti-CTLA-4 antibody therapy	05/18/2007
WO2009089260A2	Combination of anti-CTLA4 antibody with tubulin modulating agents for the treatment of proliferative diseases	07/16/2009
WO2010014784A2	Combination of anti-CTLA4 antibody with diverse therapeutic regimens for the synergistic treatment of proliferative diseases	02/04/2010
WO2010042433A1	Combination of CD137 antibody and CTLA-4 antibody for the treatment of proliferative diseases	04/15/2010
WO2011011027A1	Combination of anti-CTLA4 antibody with diverse therapeutic regimens for the synergistic treatment of proliferative diseases	01/27/2011
WO2011146382A1	Improved immunotherapeutic dosing regimens and combinations thereof	11/24/2011
WO2012027536A1	Combination of anti-CTLA4 antibody with BRAF inhibitors for the synergistic treatment of proliferative diseases	03/01/2012
WO2013173223A1	Cancer immunotherapy by disrupting PD-1/PD-L1 signaling	11/21/2013
WO2014066532A1	Combination of anti-KIR and anti-CTLA-4 antibodies to treat cancer	05/01/2014
WO2015134605A1	Treatment of renal cancer using a combination of an anti-PD-1 antibody and another anti-cancer agent	09/11/2015
WO2015176033A1	Treatment of lung cancer using a combination of an anti-PD-1 antibody and another anti-cancer agent	11/19/2015
WO2016100561A2	Use of immune checkpoint inhibitors in central nervous systems neoplasms	06/23/2016
WO2016176503A1	Treatment of PD-L1-negative melanoma using an anti-PD-1 antibody and an anti-CTLA-4 antibody	11/03/2016

The data was updated until Jan 2018.

10 Reference

[1] http://www.ncbi.nlm.nih.gov/homologene/3820.

[2] https://blast.ncbi.nlm.nih.gov.

[3] U.S. Food and Drug Administration (FDA) Database. http://www.accessdata.fda.gov/drugsatfda_docs/nda/2011/125377 Orig1s000SumR.pdf.

[4] European Medicines Agency (EMA) Database. http://www.ema.europa.eu/docs/en_GB/document_library/EPAR_-_Public_assessment_report/human/002213/WC500109302.pdf.

[5] Pharmaceuticals and Medical Devices Agency (PMDA) Database. http://www.pmda.go.jp/PmdaSearch/iyakuDetail/ResultDataSetPDF/670605_4291430A1026_1_07.

[6] The financial reports of Bristol-Myers Squibb; http://data.pharmacodia.com/web/homePage/index.

[7] FDA Database. http://www.accessdata.fda.gov/drugsatfda_docs/label/2015/125377s073lbl.pdf.

[8] PMDA Database. http://www.pmda.go.jp/drugs/2015/P20150722002/index.html.

[9] FDA Database. http://www.accessdata.fda.gov/drugsatfda_docs/nda/2011/125377Orig1s000PharmR.pdf.

[10] FDA database. http://www.accessdata.fda.gov/drugsatfda_docs/nda/2011/125377Orig1s000ClinPharmR.pdf.

[11] FDA Database. https://www.accessdata.fda.gov/drugsatfda_docs/label/2017/125377s091lbl.pdf.

CHAPTER

7

Ranibizumab

Ranibizumab

(Lucentis®)

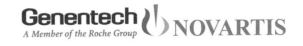

Research code: AMD-Fab, AMD-rhuFab-V2, RFB-002, RG 3645, rhuFab-V2, rhuFab-VEG, Y-0317

1 Target Biology

The VEGF

❖ Vascular endothelial growth factor A (VEGFA, previously known as vascular permeability factor (VPF) identified by Senger and colleagues in 1983) was isolated and sequenced by Ferrara and colleagues in 1989.[1-4]

❖ VEGFA is the prototype member of a family of proteins that includes VEGFB, VEGFC, VEGFD, VEGFE (a virally encoded protein) and placental growth factor (PlGF, also known as PGF).[5]

❖ Multiple isoforms of VEGFA are derived from alternative splicing of exons 6 and 7, including $VEGFA_{121}$, $VEGFA_{165}$, $VEGFA_{189}$ and $VEGF_{206}$. $VEGFA_{165}$ is the most frequently expressed isoform in normal tissues and tumors. $VEGFA_{165}$ has an intermediary behavior between the highly diffusible $VEGFA_{121}$ and the extracellular matrix-bound $VEGFA_{189}$, and is thought to be the most physiologically relevant VEGFA isoform.[6]

❖ VEGFA can bind VEGFR1 and VEGFR2 on endothelial cells *in vivo*. VEGFR2 is the main mediator of the roles of VEGFA in cell proliferation, angiogenesis and vessel permeabilization. VEGFR2 binds to VEGF with a K_d of approximately 75-125 pM and lead to receptor dimerization and autophosphorylation.[7-8]

Sequence Homology of VEGF Proteins[9-14]

Human: 191aa. Accession: AAK95847.1.

```
  1 MNFLLSWVHW  SLALLLYLHH  AKWSQAAPMA  EGGGQNHHEV  VKFMDVYQRS  YCHPIETLVD
 61 IFQEYPDEIE  YIFKPSCVPL  MRCGGCCNDE  GLECVPTEES  NITMQIMRIK  PHQGQHIGEM
121 SFLQHNKCEC  RPKKDRARQE  NPCGPCSERR  KHLFVQDPQT  CKCSCKNTDS  RCKARQLELN
181 ERTCRCDKPR  R
```

Pan troglodytes: 191aa. Accession: XP_016811082.1.

❖ BLAST:
  • Max score: 401; Total score: 401; Query cover: 100%; Identities: 100%.

```
  1 MNFLLSWVHW  SLALLLYLHH  AKWSQAAPMA  EGGGQNHHEV  VKFMDVYQRS  YCHPIETLVD
 61 IFQEYPDEIE  YIFKPSCVPL  MRCGGCCNDE  GLECVPTEES  NITMQIMRIK  PHQGQHIGEM
121 SFLQHNKCEC  RPKKDRARQE  NPCGPCSERR  KHLFVQDPQT  CKCSCKNTDS  RCKARQLELN
181 ERTCRCDKPR  R
```

Macaca mulatta: 191aa. Accession: AFE64645.1.

❖ BLAST:
  • Max score: 401; Total score: 401; Query cover: 100%; Identities: 100%.

```
  1 MNFLLSWVHW  SLALLLYLHH  AKWSQAAPMA  EGGGQNHHEV  VKFMDVYQRS  YCHPIETLVD
 61 IFQEYPDEIE  YIFKPSCVPL  MRCGGCCNDE  GLECVPTEES  NITMQIMRIK  PHQGQHIGEM
121 SFLQHNKCEC  RPKKDRARQE  NPCGPCSERR  KHLFVQDPQT  CKCSCKNTDS  RCKARQLELN
181 ERTCRCDKPR  R
```

Rattus norvegicus: 190aa.   Accession: AAL07526.1.

❖ BLAST:

   • Max score: 334; Total score: 334; Query cover: 100%; Identities: 90.0%.

```
  1  MNFLLSWVHW  ▮LALLLYLHH  AKWSQAAP▮▮  EG▮QK▮HEV▮  KFMDVYQRSY  C▮PIETLVDI
 61  FQEYPDEIEY  IFKPSCVPLM  RC▮GCCNDE▮  LECVPT▮ESN  VTMQIMRIKP  HQ▮QHIGEMS
121  FLQHS▮CECR  PKKDR▮KPEN  ▮C▮PCSERRK  HLFVQDPQTC  KCSCKNTDSR  CKARQLELNE
181  RTCRCDKPRR
```

Mus musculus: 190aa.   Accession: EDL23467.1.

❖ BLAST:

   • Max score: 334; Total score: 334; Query cover: 100%; Identities: 90.0%.

```
  1  MNFLLSWVHW  ▮LALLLYLHH  AKWSQAAP▮▮  EG▮QK▮HEV▮  KFMDVYQRSY  C▮PIETLVDI
 61  FQEYPDEIEY  IFKPSCVPLM  RC▮GCCNDE▮  LECVPT▮ESN  ITMQIMRIKP  HQ▮QHIGEMS
121  FLQHS▮CECR  PKKDR▮KPEN  ▮C▮PCSERRK  HLFVQDPQTC  KCSCKNTDSR  CKARQLELNE
181  RTCRCDKPRR
```

Biology Activity

❖ VEGFA is the master regulator of angiogenesis, binding to VEGFR2 to stimulate the proliferation of endothelial cells via the RAS-RAF-MAPK-ERK signaling pathway.   VEGFA triggers endothelial cell migration, which is an integral component of angiogenesis.[15]

❖ More recent studies have shown that phosphorylation of VEGFR2 Tyr1175 (in humans; Tyr1173 in mice) has a crucial role in regulating VEGFA-dependent angiogenesis.[16]

❖ Binding of VEGFA to VEGFR1 is lack of mitogenic effects following VEGFR1 activation, suggest that VEGFR1 may act at least in some circumstances as a decoy receptor, sequestering VEGFA and regulating VEGFR2 activity.[7]

❖ VEGF is a survival factor for endothelial cells both *in vitro* and *in vivo*.   *In vivo*, the prosurvival effects of VEGF are developmentally regulated.[17]

❖ VEGF promotes monocyte chemotaxis and induces colony formation by mature subsets of granulocyte-macrophage progenitor cells.[18]

❖ VEGF has the ability to induce vascular leakage, which underlies significant roles of this molecule in inflammation and other pathological circumstances.[19]

❖ VEGF induces vasodilatation *in vitro* in a dose-dependent fashion as a result of endothelial cell-derived nitric oxide, and produces transient tachycardia, hypotension and decrease in cardiac output when injected intravenously in conscious, instrumented rats.[20]

❖ VEGF has been implicated in pathological angiogenesis associated with tumors, intraocular neovascular disorders and other conditions.[6]

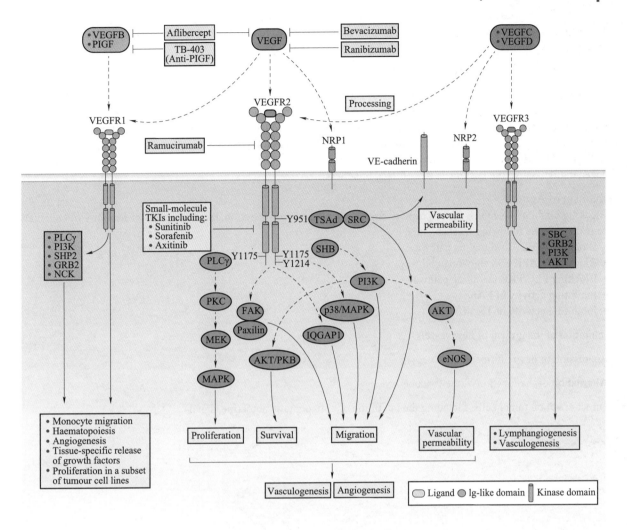

Figure 1   VEGF-VEGFR Signaling[15]

2   General Information

Lucentis®[21]

❖ Lucentis® (Ranibizumab) results from the insertion of murine anti-VEGFA complementary-determining regions (CDRs) into a consensus human IgG1 framework.

❖ Ranibizumab was originally derived from a murine monoclonal antibody (muMAb A4.6.1).

❖ The cDNAs encoding the muMAb A.4.6.1 variable light (V_L) and variable heavy (V_H) chains were isolated using reverse transcriptase-polymerase chain reaction (RT-PCR) from hybridoma cells producing muMAb A.4.6.1.

❖ Ranibizumab is the Fab moiety of a recombinant humanized monoclonal antibody rhuMAb accomplished by site directed mutagenesis of a human IgG1 framework (95.0%) with murine complementarity-determining regions (5.0%).   As a Fab fragment, ranibizumab does not contain the Fc region that is involved in antibody-mediated effector functions.

❖ The 214-residue light-chain of ranibizumab linked by a disulfide bond at its C-terminus extremity to the 231-residue N-terminal segment of the heavy chain.   The molecular weight of ranibizumab is approximately 48 kDa (23 kDa and 25 kDa for the light and heavy chain, respectively).

❖ Ranibizumab contains 10 cysteine residues forming 4 intra-chain and 1 inter-chain disulfide bonds.

❖ To generate a ranibizumab-producing cell line, E. coli 60E4 cells were transformed with pY0317 xaptet and selected for tetracycline resistance.

❖ The total sales of 3,255 million US$ for 2016; No sales data as of 2017.

❖ Ranibizumab binds with high affinity to VEGFA isoforms generated by alternative mRNA splicing, e.g. $VEGF_{121}$, $VEGF_{165}$, and their biologically active proteolytic cleavage product $VEGF_{110}$. The binding of ranibizumab to VEGFA prevents the interaction of VEGFA with its receptors VEGFR-1 and VEGFR-2 on the surface of endothelial cells. Binding of VEGFA to its receptors leads to endothelial cell proliferation and neovascularisation, as well as vascular leakage, all of which are thought to contribute to the progression of the neovascular (wet) form of age-related macular degeneration, one of the leading causes of legal blindness.

Mechanism of Action[22]

❖ Blocking binding of VEGFA to its receptors, inhibiting survival, proliferation, migration and permeability of endothelial cells through the following mechanism:
  • Blocking PI3K/Akt signaling pathway.
  • Blocking MAPK/P38 signaling pathway.
  • Blocking PLC/PKC signaling pathway.
  • Inhibiting activity of FAK.
  • Inhibiting activity of TSAd-Src.

❖ Inhibition of the growth of new vessels.

❖ Regression of newly formed tumor vessels.

❖ Alternation of the function of the vascular bed.

❖ Direct effect on tumor cells, including the inhibition of antiapoptotic autocrine signals.

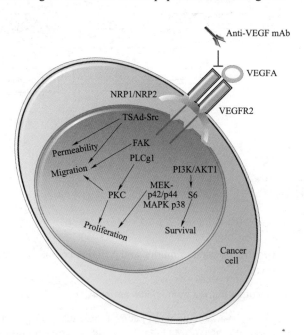

Figure 2   Mechanism of Anti-VEGF mAb[22]

Sponsor
❖ Lucentis® was developed and market by Genentech (a subsidiary of Roche) and Novartis.

World Sales[23]

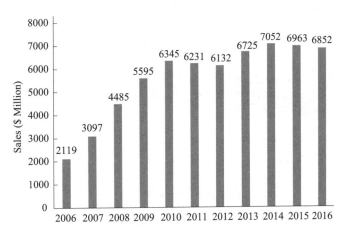

Figure 3   World Sales of Ranibizumab since 2006

Approval and Indication

Table 1   Summary of the Approved Indication[24, 25]

Approval (Year)	Agency	Indications
2006	FDA	Neovascular (wet) age-related macular degeneration.
2007	EMEA	Neovascular (wet) age-related macular degeneration (AMD).
2010	FDA	Macular edema following retinal vein occlusion (RVO).
	EMEA	Visual impairment due to diabetic macular edema (DME).
2011	EMEA	Visual impairment due to retinal vein occlusion (RVO).
2012	FDA	Diabetic macular edema.
2013	EMEA	Visual impairment due to choroidal neovascularization (CNV) to pathologic myopia (PM).

AMD: Age-related macular degeneration.   CNV: Choroidal neovascularization.   DME: Diabetic macular edema.   PM: Pathologic myopia.   RVO: Retinal vein occlusion.

Table 2   Summary of the Approval of Lucentis®[25-29]

	US (FDA)	EU (EMA)	Japan (PMDA)	China (CFDA)
First approval date	30/06/2006	22/01/2007	21/01/2009	31/12/2011
Application or approval No.	BLA125156	EMEA/H/C/000715	22100AMX00399000	S20110085
Brand name	Lucentis®	Lucentis®	Lucentis®	Lucentis®/诺适得®
Indication	wAMD, Macular edema following RVO, DME, DR	wAMD, Macular edema following RVO, DME, CNV caused by PM	wAMD, Macular edema following RVO, myopic CNV, DME	Macular degeneration
Authorization holder	Genentech (Roche)	Novartis	Novartis	Novartis

CNV: Choroidal neovascularisation.   DME: Diabetic macular edema.   DR: Diabetic retinopathy.   RVO: Retinal vein occlusion.   wAMD: Wet age-related macular degeneration.

Table 3   Indication and Administration[26]

No.	Administration	Indication
1	0.5 mg in 0.05 mL by intravitreal injection once a month	Neovascular (wet) age-related macular degeneration.
2	0.5 mg in 0.05 mL by intravitreal injection once a month	Macular edema following RVO.
3	0.3 mg in 0.05 mL by intravitreal injection once a month	Diabetic macular edema and diabetic retinopathy in patients with DME.

Sourced from US FDA drug label information.

Table 4　Marketing VEGF-targeting Drugs[28, 30-38]

Drug	Trade	Sponsor	Type	Approval	Indication
Bevacizumab	Avstin®	Genentech	rhuMab	02/2004-FDA 01/2005-EMA 04/2007-PMDA 07/2015-CFDA	mCRC, MBC, NSNSCLC, Glioblastoma, mRCC, prmCC, prrEOFTPPC
Aflibercept	Zaltrap®	Sanofi-Aventis	Fusion protein	08/2012-FDA 02/2013-EMA 03/2017-PMDA	mCRC
Aflibercept	Eylea®	Bayer Pharma	Fusion protein	11/2011-FDA 11/2012-EMA 09/2012-PMDA	wAMD, macular edema due to BRVO or CRVO, DME, myopic CNV
Conbercept	Langum®/朗沐®	Chengdu Kanghong Biotechnologies Co. Ltd	Fusion protein	11/2013-CFDA	Wet age-related macular degeneration, Choroidal neovascularization of pathological myopia

CNV: Choroidal neovascularisation.　DME: Diabetic macular edema.　DR: Diabetic retinopathy.　mCRC: Metastatic colorectal cancer.　mRCC: Metastatic renal cell cancer.　NSNSCLC: Non-squamous non-small cell lung cancer.　prmCC: Persistent, recurrent, or metastatic carcinoma of the cervix.　prrEOFTPPC: Platinum-resistant recurrent epithelial ovarian, fallopian tube or primary peritoneal cancer.　RVO: Retinal vein occlusion.　wAMD: Wet age-related macular degeneration.

3　CMC Profile

Product Profile[21, 26-29]

Dosage route:　　　Intravitreal injection.

Strength:　　　US: 10 mg/mL solution (Lucentis® 0.5 mg), 6 mg/mL solution (Lucentis® 0.3 mg); EU: 1 mL contains 10 mg ranibizumab.　Each vial contains 2.3 mg of ranibizumab in 0.23 mL solution; JP: 1 mL contains 10 mg ranibizumab. Each vial contains 2.3 mg of ranibizumab in 0.23 mL solution; CN: 10 mg/mL, 0.20 mL/vial.

Dosage form:　　　Injection.

Formulation:　　　A liquid formulation with ranibizumab concentrations of 6 mg/mL and 10 mg/mL with pH 5.5 was used. α,α-trehalose dihydrate (tonicity agent), a histidine buffer, polysorbate 20 (surfactant to minimize the risk of agitation-induced aggregation) are used in the commercial formulation of Lucentis®.　Water for injection is also used as solvent in the formulation.

The proposed container for Lucentis® is a single-use type I glass vial, with an overfill of 0.25 mL.　Lucentis® is supplied with a filter needle for withdrawal of the vial content, a 1 mL syringe and an injection needle.

Stability:　　　36 months at $\leqslant$ -20 °C; 90 days at 5 °C including three freeze/thaw cycles; 18 months at 2-8 °C; Protected from light.

Amino Acid Sequence

❖ Ranibizumab is a humanized monoclonal antibody fragment produced in Escherichia coli cells by standard recombinant DNA technology.　The 214-residue light-chain linked by a disulfide bond at its C-terminus extremity to the 231-residue N-terminal segment of the heavy chain.

❖ The molecular weight of ranibizumab is approximately 48 kDa (23 kDa and 25 kDa for the light and heavy chain, respectively).

❖ Ranibizumab contains 10 cysteine residues forming 4 intra-chain and 1 inter-chain disulfide bonds.　As a Fab fragment, ranibizumab does not contain the Fc region that is involved in antibody-mediated effector functions.

Production Process

❖ Production platform: *E. coli* expression vector.

❖ Protein yield: NA.

❖ Protein purity: NA.

Sequence Strand[39]

```
  1  EVQLVESGGG  LVQPGGSLRL  SCAASGYDFT  HYGMNWVRQA  PGKGLEWVGW
 51  INTYTGEPTY  AADFKRRFTF  SLDTSKSTAY  LQMNSLRAED  TAVYYCAKYP
101  YYYGTSHWYF  DVWGQGTLVT  VSSASTKGPS  VFPLAPSSKS  TSGGTAALGC
151  LVKDYFPEPV  TVSWNSGALT  SGVHTFPAVL  LSKADYEKHK  VVTVPSSSLG
201  TQTYICNVNH  KPSNTKVDKK  VEPKSCDKTH  L
```

```
  1  DIQLTQSPSS  LSASVGDRVT  ITCSASQDIS  NYLNWYQQKP  GKAPKVLIYF
 51  TSSLHSGVPS  RFSGSGSGTD  FTLTISSLQP  EDFATYYCQQ  YSTVPWTFGQ
101  GTKVEIKRTV  AAPSVFIFPP  SDEQLKSGTA  SVVCLLNNFY  PREAKVQWKV
151  DNALQSGNSQ  ESVTEQDSKD  STYSLSSTLT  LSKADYEKHK  VYACEVTHQG
201  LSSPVTKSFN  RGEC
```

Table 5   Sequence Notes[39]

Type	Location	Description	Type	Location	Description
Bridge	CYS-96 CYS-22	Disulfide bridge	Bridge	CYS-194' CYS-134'	Disulfide bridge
Bridge	CYS-206 CYS-150	Disulfide bridge	Bridge	CYS-226 CYS-214'	Disulfide bridge
Bridge	CYS-88' CYS-23'	Disulfide bridge			

4   Pre-clinical Pharmacodynamics

Summary

Overview of *in vitro* Activities[21, 40]

❖ Ranibizumab binds with high affinity to the three biologically active isoforms of VEGF: $VEGF_{165}$ (predominant form), $VEGF_{121}$ and $VEGF_{110}$.

❖ Ranibizumab dose-dependently inhibited VEGF-induced proliferation in human umbilical vein endothelial cell (HUVEC), which are cells that express the VEGF-receptors, with IC_{50} values below 1 nM.   This is 10-20 folds over clinical C_{max}.

❖ Ranibizumab inhibited $rhVEGF_{165}$-induced tissue factor up-regulation in a dose-dependent manner, with an IC_{50} of 0.31 nM.

❖ Ranibizumab has a high, but 40 folds reduced, affinity towards rabbit VEGF ($K_d \pm SD = 8.8 \pm 8.1$ nM) in comparison with human VEGF.

Overview of *in vivo* Activities[21, 40]

❖ Intravitreal/intravitreous (IVT) injected ranibizumab blocks VEGF-induced vascular permeability in a modified Miles assay.

❖ Ranibizumab inhibited angiogenesis and vascular leakage in laser-induced CNV of monkeys.

❖ Combined with verteporfin with PDT, ranibizumab produced an additional effect on the inhibition of vascular leakage without any apparent increase in side effects.

❖ No complement dependent cytotoxicity (CDC) or antibody dependent cell-mediated cytotoxicity (ADCC) effect of ranibizumab was found.

Overview of *in vitro* Activities

Target Binding and Mechanism of Action[21]
❖ VEGF binding.

Table 6   Affinity of Ranibizumab for Three Recombinant Human VEGF Isoforms by SPR Analysis[40]

Parameter	$VEGF_{165}$	$VEGF_{121}$	$VEGF_{110}$
K_a (M^{-1} sec^{-1})	$(5.6 \pm 0.28) \times 10^4$	$(10.1 \pm 2.3) \times 10^4$	$(5.2 \pm 0.020) \times 10^4$
K_d (sec^{-1})	$\leqslant 10^{-5}$	$\leqslant 10^{-5}$	$\leqslant 10^{-5}$
K_A (M^{-1})	$\geqslant 5.6 \times 10^9$	$\geqslant 10.1 \times 10^9$	$\geqslant 5.2 \times 10^9$
K_D (pM)	$\leqslant 179$	$\leqslant 99.0$	$\leqslant 192$

VEGF: Vascular endothelial growth factor.

Cell-based Activities *in vitro*

Table 7   *In vitro* Activities of Anti-VEGF mAb[41, 42]

Experimental System	Treatment	Concentration	Model Induction	Efficacy
VEGFR1 expressing HEK293 cells	Ranibizumab	8.5 pM-500 nM	$VEGFA_{165}$, $VEGFA_{121}$ or hPlGF-2 20 pM induced VEGFR1 activation	IC_{50} is 675 and 1,140 pM for $VEGFA_{121}$ and $VEGFA_{165}$, respectively.
VEGFR2 expressing HEK293 cells	Ranibizumab	8.5 pM-500 nM	$VEGFA_{165}$, $VEGFA_{121}$ or hPlGF-2 20 pM induced VEGFR2 activation	IC_{50} is 576 and 845 pM for $VEGFA_{121}$ and $VEGFA_{165}$, respectively.
HUVEC	Ranibizumab	8.5 pM-500 nM	$VEGFA_{165}$ 20 pM induced Ca^{2+} mobilization	IC_{50} is 335 pM.
HUVEC	Ranibizumab	0.013-13 nM	130 pM human VEGF-A_{165}, 7.1 nM human PLGF-2, or 3.5 nM mouse PLGF-2 induced cell migration	Ranibizumab inhibited $VEGFA_{165}$ induced HUVEC migration dose-dependently.
HUVEC	Ranibizumab	0.02-5.2 nM	$rhVEGF_{165}$ (0.26 nM), $rhVEGF_{121}$ (0.36 nM), or $rhVEGF_{110}$ (0.39 nM) induced cell proliferation	IC_{50} is 0.44 ± 0.070, 0.56 ± 0.14 and 0.23 ± 0.030 nM for $VEGFA_{165}$, $VEGFA_{121}$ and $VEGFA_{110}$, respectively.

hPIGF 2: Human placental growth factor.   HUVEC: Human umbilical vein endothelial cells.   VEGFA: Vascular endothelial growth factor A.

Overview of *in vivo* Activities

Table 8　*In vivo* Activities of Ranibizumab[40]

Model		Drug	Dose	Route & Schedule	Effect
Animal	Model Induction				
Male hairless guinea pigs	Intracardiac injection of 1 mL of 1.0% Evans blue dye	Ranibizumab + VEGF$_{165}$ 100 ng/mL	1-6,000 ng/mL	Intradermal	Ranibizumab inhibited VEGF-induced permeability in a concentration-dependent manner with a mean IC$_{50}$ of 56.7 ± 17.0 ng/mL.　The mean IC$_{90}$ was 113 ± 29.4 ng/mL.
Male hairless guinea pigs	Intracardiac injection of 1 mL of 1.0% Evans blue dye	Ranibizumab + VEGF$_{121}$ 205 ng/mL	1-1,000 ng/mL	Intradermal	Ranibizumab significantly inhibited VEGF-induced permeability in a concentration-dependent manner with a mean IC$_{50}$ of 35.6 ng/mL.
Male hairless guinea pigs	Intracardiac injection of 1 mL of 1.0% Evans blue dye	Ranibizumab + VEGF$_{110}$ 189 ng/mL	1-1,000 ng/mL	Intradermal	Ranibizumab significantly inhibited VEGF-induced permeability in a concentration-dependent manner with a mean IC$_{50}$ of 20.6 ng/mL.
Cynomolgus monkey	Laser-induced CNV	Ranibizumab followed by PDT (on Days 21, 35, 49)	500, 2,000 µg/eye ($\times$ 3) on Days 14, 28, 42, 56.	ITV	ITV ranibizumab administration in combination with verteporfin PDT reduced angiographic leakage relative to PDT alone. No difference was found between ranibizumab combined with PDT group and ranibizumab alone group.
		PDT (on Days 14, 28 and 42) followed by ranibizumab	500, 2,000 µg/eye ($\times$ 2) on Days 21, 35, 49.	ITV	
		PDT (on Days 14, 28, 42) concomitant with ranibizumab	500, 2,000 µg/eye ($\times$ 2) on Days 14, 28, 42.	ITV	
Cynomolgus monkey	Laser-induced CNV	Ranibizumab	500 µg/eye, every other two weeks for 5 doses totally.	ITV	Ranibizumab inhibited the vascular leakage.

CNV: Choroidal neovascularization.　ITV: Intravitreous injection.　PDT: Photon dynamic treatment.　VEGF: Vascular endothelial growth factor.

5　Toxicology

Summary

Non-clinical Single-Dose Toxicology
❖ Not performed.

Non-clinical Repeated-Dose Toxicology
❖ The 4-week intravitreous toxicity study in Cynomolgus monkeys treated with ranibizumab at 450 and 1,800 µg/eye once every other two weeks with 4-week recovery:
  • Administration of ranibizumab at dose levels of 450 and 1,800 µg/eye was associated with dose-related inflammation of the eye, the effect was reversible.
  • The inflammation was evidenced by the presence of cells, fibrin, and flare in the anterior chamber and accumulation of cells in the anterior vitreous.
  • The inflammation was transient in nature and only anterior vitreal cells persisted beyond 7 days post-dose.
  • No systemic toxicity was found.
❖ The 13-week intravitreous toxicity study in Cynomolgus monkeys treated with ranibizumab at 250, 750 and 2,000 µg/eye once every other two weeks with 4-week recovery:
  • Administration of ranibizumab at dose levels of 750 and 2,000 µg/eye was associated with dose-related inflammation, the effect was reversible.
  • The inflammation reaction was the most intense after the first treatment and diminished with subsequent injections, even at the same or greater doses.

- Anterior chamber inflammation was generally transient with either no or mild anterior chamber cell persisting beyond 7 days after each administration in most animals.
- Vitreal cell scores were dose-dependent and the vitreal cells tended to persist, or slowly increase in number throughout the study.
- No drug-related systemic toxicity was found.   Drug-related retinal perivascular infiltrates and subsequently developed varying degrees of white exudates over the surface of the optic disk were observed.
- Inflammatory cell infiltration was noted in many ocular tissues with a higher incidence in mid-dose and high-dose group.
- At the terminal sacrifice, there was a dose-dependent increase in plasma cell infitrates among females in mid-dose and high-dose group.
- Perivascular inflammatory infiltrates were occurred in mid-dose and high-dose group.

❖ The 16-week intravitreous toxicity study in Cynomolgus monkeys treated with ranibizumab at 250 to 2,000 µg/eye once every 2 or 4 weeks with 8-week recovery:
- Intravitreous treatment of Cynomolgus monkeys with ranibizumab 250 to 2,000 µg/eye once every 2 or 4 weeks was associated with inflammation, the effect was reversible.
- Inflammatory cells in the anterior chamber were generally transient in nature with peak scores at 48 h after dosing and spontaneously diminishing to no or mild anterior chamber cell beyond 7 days after dosing in most animals.
- Vitreal cell scores tended to demonstrate a dose-response manner.
- Inflammatory cells in the vitreous were slower to appear and were slower to clear than in the more fluid aqueous humor.
- Two forms of posterior segment inflammation of the eye evidenced by changes around the peripheral retinal venules were noted.   The first form was an acute response characterized by focal or multifocal, perivenous retinal hemorrhages with white centers in the far peripheral retina.   The second form of posterior segment inflammation was characterized as focal or multifocal white, perivascular sheathing around peripheral retinal venules.
- Inflammatory cell infiltrates were noted in various ocular structures among all groups by histopathology examination.

❖ The 26-week intravitreous toxicity study in Cynomolgus monkeys treated with ranibizumab at 500, 1,000, and 2,000 µg/eye once every 2 weeks with 8-week recovery:
- Intravitreous administration of ranibizumab produced a dose-dependent anterior and posterior segment inflammation in monkeys, the inflammatory response was reversible.
- Dose-related increase in aqueous cells that persisted through the end of the treatment period.
- Vitreal cell scores showed a dose- and time-effect.   Inflammatory cells in the vitreous body were slower to appear and to disappear from the vitreous body than the aqueous humor.
- Two forms of posterior segment inflammation of the eye evidenced by changes around the peripheral retinal venules were noted.   The first form was an acute response characterized by focal or multifocal, perivenous retinal hemorrhages with white centers in the far peripheral retina.   The second form of posterior segment inflammation was characterized as focal or multifocal white, perivascular sheathing around peripheral retinal venules.
- A cataractogenic effect was noted that correlated with the intensity and duration of the inflammatory response.
- Inflammation associated venous dilatation and tortuosity, venous beading, possible peripapillary retinal thickening, possible papillary tuft was observed.
- No drug-related systemic toxicity was found.

Genotoxicity
❖ Not performed.

Carcinogenicity
❖ Not performed.

Reproductive Toxicology
❖ Not performed.

Special Toxicology Studies
❖ Cross-reactivity of ranibizumab with normal human tissue:
- No cross-reactive binding of ranibizumab was observed to any human tissues.
❖ Hemolytic potential, blood compatibility, and vitreal fluid compatibility testing with ranibizumab:
- Ranibizumab at concentrations of 20, 7.5, or 2.5 mg/mL did not cause hemolysis of human erythrocytes, and were compatible with Cynomolgus monkey, human serum and plasma, and with human vitreal fluid.
❖ Assessment of the safety of intravitreal injections of ranibizumab in combination with intravenous verteporfin photodynamic therapy in normal Cynomolgus monkeys or monkeys following laser-induced CNV:
- Ranibizumab ITV injection in combination with verteporfin PDT induced no significant increase in toxicity over that

observed following administration of PDT alone.
- The toxicity of ranibizumab in combination with PDT was similar to that of ranibizumab alone.
- Ocular inflammation was observed, characterized by anterior chamber flare along with increased vitreal inflammatory cells.   The greatest amount of anterior chamber inflammation was seen following the initial dose of ranibizumab. Treatment with PDT did not alter the anterior chamber inflammatory response induced by ranibizumab.
- The combined treatment of ranibizumab and PDT did not alter the inflammatory response either in normal eyes or eyes with CNV lesions induced by laser.
- Twenty-four hours after ITV administration at 500 µg/eye and 2,000 µg/eye, mean serum concentrations ranged from 0.045-0.084 µg/mL and 0.16-0.21 µg/mL, respectively.   Serum concentrations were similar across all groups.
❖ Assessment of the safety and efficacy of ITV injections of ranibizumab in a laser-induced CNV model in Cynomolgus monkeys:
- The mitigative effect of ranibizumab on Grade 4 CNV vascular leakage was noted.
- Mild perivenous sheathing and peripapillary swelling were observed in only 2/6 of the ranibizumab-treated eyes.
- Median serum ranibizumab concentration one day after each dose ranged from 43.1 to 80.4 ng/mL, two days after each dose ranged from 31.6 to 87.4 ng/mL.   At necropsy, the median serum ranibizumab concentration was 17.4 ng/mL. The median concentration of ranibizumab in the vitreous humor 8 days after the final ITV dose was 25,650 ng/mL.

Anti-product Antibody Profile
❖ In rabbits, anti-ranibizumab antibody was detected in the vitreous body and serum after ITV administration.

Local Tolerance
❖ Intravitreal local tolerance study with ranibizumab in rabbits:
- Administration of ranibizumab as a single intravitreal injection to male NZW rabbits produced a slight inflammatory response by 7 days post-dose.
- Lower intraocular pressure in some drug-treated eyes might be associated with mild, transient cyclitis.

Safety Pharmacology
❖ No formal *in vivo* safety pharmacology studies were conducted with ranibizumab.
❖ Safety pharmacology endpoints were incorporated into repeated-dose toxicity studies.   No treatment-related effects on physical examination parameters, including respiratory rate, heart rate, and body temperature, were observed in Cynomolgus monkeys administrated up to 2.0 mg/eye of ranibizumab ITV every 2 weeks for up to 26 weeks.

Non-clinical Multiple-Dose Toxicology

Table 9   Repeated-Dose Toxicity Studies of Ranibizumab[21, 40]

Species	Duration (Week)	Dose [mg/(kg·day)]	Finding
	4	450, 1,800 µg/eye, ITV, once every other two weeks	Administration of ranibizumab at dose levels of 450 and 1,800 µg/eye was associated with dose-related inflammation of the eye, the effect was reversible. The inflammation was evidenced by the presence of cells, fibrin, and flare in the anterior chamber and accumulation of cells in the anterior vitreous. The inflammation was transient in nature and only anterior vitreal cells persisted beyond 7 days post-dose. No systemic toxicity was found.
Cynomolgus monkey (Male & Female)	13	250, 750, 2,000 µg/eye, ITV, once every other two weeks	Administration of ranibizumab at dose levels of 750 and 2,000 µg/eye was associated with dose-related inflammation, the effect was reversible. The inflammation reaction was the most intense after the first treatment and diminished with subsequent injections, even at the same or greater doses. Anterior chamber inflammation was generally transient with either no or mild anterior chamber cell persisting beyond 7 days after each administration in most animals. Vitreal cell scores were dose-dependent and the vitreal cells tended to persist, or slowly increase in number throughout the study. Drug-related retinal perivascular infiltrates and subsequently developed varying degrees of white exudates over the surface of the optic disk were observed. Inflammatory cell infiltration was noted in many ocular tissues with a higher incidence in mid-dose and high-dose group. At the terminal sacrifice, there was a dose-dependent increase in plasma cell infiltrates among females in mid-dose and high-dose group. Perivascular inflammatory infiltrates were occurred in mid-dose and high-dose group. No drug-related systemic toxicity was found.

Continued

Species	Duration (Week)	Dose [mg/(kg·day)]	Finding
Cynomolgus monkey (Male & female)	16	250-2,000 µg/eye, ITV, once every 2 or 4 weeks	Intravitreous treatment of Cynomolgus monkeys with ranibizumab 250 to 2,000 µg/eye once every 2 or 4 weeks was associated with inflammation, the effect was reversible. Inflammatory cells in the anterior chamber were generally transient in nature with peak scores at 48 h after dosing and spontaneously diminishing to no or mild anterior chamber cell beyond 7 days after dosing in most animals. Vitreal cell scores tended to demonstrate a dose-response manner. Inflammatory cells in the vitreous were slower to appear and were slower to clear than in the more fluid aqueous humor. Two forms of posterior segment inflammation of the eye evidenced by changes around the peripheral retinal venules were noted. The first form was an acute response characterized by focal or multifocal, perivenous retinal hemorrhages with white centers in the far peripheral retina. The second form of posterior segment inflammation was characterized as focal or multifocal white, perivascular sheathing around peripheral retinal venules. Inflammatory cell infiltrates were noted in various ocular structures among all groups by histopathology examination.
	26	500, 1,000, 2,000 µg/eye, ITV, once every 2 weeks	Intravitreous administration of ranibizumab produced a dose-dependent anterior and posterior segment inflammation in monkeys, the inflammatory response was reversible. Dose-related increase in aqueous cells that persisted through the end of the treatment period. Vitreal cell scores showed a dose- and time-effect. Inflammatory cells in the vitreous body were slower to appear and to disappear from the vitreous body than the aqueous humor. Two forms of posterior segment inflammation of the eye evidenced by changes around the peripheral retinal venules were noted. The first form was an acute response characterized by focal or multifocal, perivenous retinal hemorrhages with white centers in the far peripheral retina. The second form of posterior segment inflammation was characterized as focal or multifocal white, perivascular sheathing around peripheral retinal venules. A cataractogenic effect was noted that correlated with the intensity and duration of the inflammatory response. Inflammation associated venous dilatation and tortuosity, venous beading, possible peripapillary retinal thickening, possible papillary tuft was observed. No drug-related systemic toxicity was found.

Table 10   TK of Ranibizumab in the 4-week Intravitreous Toxicity Study in Cynomolgus Monkeys[40]

Parameter	Serum				Vitreous Humor	
	450 µg/eye (N = 2/sex)	1,800 µg/eye (N = 4/sex)	450 µg/eye (N = 1/sex)	1,800 µg/eye (N = 1/sex)	450 µg/eye (N = 1/sex)	1,800 µg/eye (N = 1/sex)
$AUC_{0-Day\ 29/30}$ (µg·day/mL)	2.6 ± 0.56	9.8 ± 2.7	0.89	2.7		
C_{max} (µg/mL)			0.058	0.19	215	601
$t_{1/2}$ (Day)					2.2	2.5
AUC_{0-last} (µg·day/mL)			1.6	4.3	1,630	5,640

Table 11   TK of Ranibizumab in the 13-week Intravitreous Toxicity Study in Cynomolgus Monkeys[40]

Parameter	Serum			Vitreous Humor		
	250 µg/eye (N = 4/sex)	750 µg/eye (N = 4/sex)	2,000 µg/eye (N = 6/sex)	250 µg/eye (N = 4/sex)	750 µg/eye (N = 4/sex)	2,000 µg/eye (N = 6/sex)
$AUC_{0-Day\ 101}$ (µg·day/mL)	4.3 ± 1.8	16.6 ± 8.8	30.1 ± 21.5	Mean concentration (µg/mL)		
C_{max} (ng/mL)	132 ± 102	624 ± 266	899 ± 774	53.5 ± 7.2	186 ± 24.1	545 ± 87.6
T_{max} (Day)	75.0 ± 34.0	93.0 ± 11.0	75.0 ± 26.0			

Table 12   TK of Ranibizumab in the 26-week Intravitreous Toxicity Study in Cynomolgus Monkeys[40]

Parameter	Serum			Vitreous Humor		
	500 μg/eye (N = 4/sex)	500/1,000 μg/eye (N = 4/sex)	500/1,000/ 2,000 μg/eye (N = 6/sex)	500 μg/eye (N = 4/sex)	500/1,000 μg/eye (N = 4/sex)	500/1,000/ 2,000 μg/eye (N = 6/sex)
$AUC_{0\text{-Day }184}$ (μg·day/mL)	20.5 ± 14.1	23.1 ± 6.5	88.7 ± 54.3	Vitreous concentration		
AUC in ADA positive animals	29.8 ± 14.9					
AUC in ADA negative animals	11.1 ± 2.4					
Mean concentration 48 h after last dose (Day 184, μg/mL)	0.17 ± 0.13	0.27 ± 0.20	1.2 ± 1.1	127 ± 38.9	276 ± 57.5	569 ± 53.5
C_{max} (μg/mL)	0.36 ± 0.30	0.35 ± 0.22	2.1 ± 1.2			
T_{max} (Day)	83.5 ± 51.2	113 ± 54.4	93.3 ± 43.2			

ADA: Anti-drug antibody.

Anti-product Antibody Profile

Table 13   Special Toxicology Studies of Ranibizumab[21, 40]

Special Toxicology	Species	N	Dose	Finding
Immunogenicity	Cynomolgus monkey (male & female)	16	500, 2,000 μg/eye: ITV; Every other 2 weeks for 4 weeks	Four animals developed low to moderate antibody titers to ranibizumab in the serum. No antibodies were detected in the vitreous.
	Cynomolgus monkey (male & female)	28	250, 750, 2,000 μg/eye: ITV; Every other 2 weeks for 8 doses totally	Fifteen out of 28 treated monkeys developed antibodies to ranibizumab in the serum as early as Day 29. Antibodies were also detected in the vitreal fluid in one mid-dose and two high-dose males.
	Cynomolgus monkey (male & female)	28	250-2,000 μg/eye: ITV; Once every 2 or 4 weeks	Eleven of 28 treated monkeys developed low to moderate antibody titers to ranibizumab in the serum. Antibodies were not detected in the vitreal fluid.
	Cynomolgus monkey (male & female)	28	500, 1,000, 2,000 μg/eye: ITV; Every other 2 weeks for 14 doses totally	No ADA was detected in control and mid-dose group. Serum ADA was found in low-dose and high-dose group.
	Cynomolgus monkey	21	500, 2,000 μg/eye: ITV; Every other 2 weeks for 2-3 doses totally	Serum ADA was detected in 2/21 animals. No ADA was detected in the vitreous.
	Cynomolgus monkey	6	500 μg/eye: ITV; Every other 2 weeks for 5 doses totally	Antibodies to ranibizumab were detected in 3/6 animals.

ADA: Anti-drug antibody.   ITV: Intravitreous injection.

6   Non-clinical Pharmacokinetic/ADME/Toxicokinetics

Summary[21, 40]

Non-clinical Pharmacokinetics

❖ PK studies of ranibizumab in both rabbit and monkey after ITV administration
- Ranibizumab was present in vitreous humor, aqueous humor, all layers of the retina, ciliary body, iris, corneal endothelium and serum.
- The terminal $t_{1/2}$ was approximately 2-3 days in all ocular tissues in both species.
- Concentrations in serum following ITV injection were more than 1,000-fold lower than concentrations in vitreous humor and declined in parallel with the concentrations in the ocular compartments.
- Ranibizumab levels in aqueous humor and retina were 2.5-4 folds lower than the vitreous levels.

- Drug clearance from the vitreous is reported to be dependent on molecular size.
- ❖ PK study of ranibizumab following subconjunctival, intracameral and intravitreal injections in rabbits
  - The highest ranibizumab concentrations in retinal tissue and the lowest serum concentrations were measured after ITV administration.
  - Subconjunctival administration slowed delivery of ranibizumab to the retinal tissue.
  - Anti-ranibizumab antibodies were detected in serum in all groups.
- ❖ PK study of ranibizumab following intravenous administration in rabbits
  - The PK appeared to be dose-dependent.
  - No anti-ranibizumab antibodies were detected in serum at pre-dose or 24 h post-dose.
- ❖ PK study of ranibizumab in Cynomolgus monkeys after a single intravitreous administration
  - PK appeared to be dose-linear in vitreous humor, aqueous humor, retinal tissues, and serum.
  - The terminal $t_{1/2}$ was approximately 2-3 days in all ocular matrices and rapid penetration into retinal tissues was observed.
  - Concentrations in serum following ITV injection were more than 1,000-fold lower than concentrations in vitreous humor and declined in parallel with the concentrations in the ocular compartments.
  - The bioavailability was 60.0% and 50.0% after ITV administration of 500 and 2,000 µg/eye.
  - Ranibizumab concentrations were measurable in the vitreous humor, aqueous humor, neural retina layer, RPE/Bruch's layer, and serum after a single intravitreous administration of 2,000 µg/eye.
- ❖ Distribution
  - Tissue distribution of ranibizumab following ITV administration in normal rabbits:
    - ◆ The ocular distribution of human Fab was determined by immunohistochemical method.
    - ◆ rhuFab V1 at 625 µg/eye was present on Day 1 and 7 in the vitreous, all retinal layers, ciliary body epithelium and stroma of the pars plana, iris stroma posterior epithelium, Schlemm's canal, limbal blood vessels and corneal endothelial cell. The staining intensity decreased on Days 14 and 15. Pathy and/or weak retinal staining of specific components persisted up to Day 40.
    - ◆ For rhuFab V2, positive staining in similar tissues was only seen on Day 7. The staining was seen last time in the vitreous, ciliary body epithelium and iris on Day 21.
    - ◆ In microautoradiographic distribution assay with ^{125}I-labeled rhuFab V2, a microautoradiographic signal was present in all retinal layers, perivascularly in the optic nerve head with iris, and corneal endothelium at Days 1, 2, and 4. No signal was seen in choroidal and scleral tissues.
    - ◆ In electron microscopy examinations, radioactive Fab fragments injected into the vitreous of rabbit eyes penetrated into the retina and diffused intercellularly through the various inner layers.
    - ◆ Fab fragment appeared to be internalized by different cell types, including the bipolar cells and the RPE cells. After crossing the Bruch's membrane, radioactive Fab reached the blood vessel in the choroid.
- ❖ Metabolism
  - Ocular degradation is suggested to be limited, since the systemic bioavailability was 50.0-60.0% at 2 days post ITV injections to monkeys.
  - No studies on the metabolism of ranibizumab have been performed, but as with other proteins, once reaching the systemic circulation, if not excreted, ranibizumab is most likely degraded in the liver or kidney.
- ❖ Excretion
  - No studies were performed.
- ❖ Drug-Drug interaction
  - No drug interaction studies were conducted.

Non-clinical Pharmacokinetics

Table 14   Pharmacokinetic Parameters of rhuFab V1 and rhuFab V2 following Single Intravitreal Injection in Rabbits[40]

Tissue	Parameter	rhuFab V1 625 µg/eye (N = 24)	rhuFab V2 25 µg/eye (N = 10)	rhuFab V2 625 µg/eye (N = 24)
Vitreous humor	C_{max} (µg/mL)	743 ± 389	24.2	1,280 ± 308
	$AUC_{0\text{-}inf}$ (µg·day/mL)	2,640	97.1	4,850
	$t_{1/2}$ (Day)	2.4	2.4	2.9
	T_{max} (h)	1.0	24.0	1.0

Continued

Tissue	Parameter	rhuFab V1 625 µg/eye (N = 24)	rhuFab V2 25 µg/eye (N = 10)	rhuFab V2 625 µg/eye (N = 24)
Aqueous humor	C_{max} (µg/mL)	17.7 ± 7.7		57.1 ± 23.4
	$AUC_{0\text{-}inf}$ (µg·day/mL)	131		286
	$t_{1/2}$ (Day)	2.1		3.0
	T_{max} (h)	48.0		48.0
Serum	C_{max} (ng/mL)	30.0		55.0
	$AUC_{0\text{-}inf}$ (µg·day/mL)	0.11		0.27
	$t_{1/2}$ (Day)			
	T_{max} (h)	24.0		24.0

Table15　Pharmacokinetic Parameters of Ranibizumab following Subconjunctival, Intracameral and Intravitreal Injections in Rabbits[40]

Tissue	Parameter	Ranibizumab 500 µg/eye, SCJ (N = 18)	500 µg/eye, IC (N = 18)	500 µg/eye, IVT (N = 15)	4,000 µg/eye, SCJ (N = 21)
Vitreous Humor	C_{max} (µg/mL)			NA	
	$AUC_{0\text{-}inf}$ (µg·day/mL)			1,710	
	$t_{1/2}$ (Day)			5.4	
	T_{max} (h)			NA	
	$AUC_{0\text{-}t}$ (µg·day/mL)	0.22, t = 48 h	0.059, t = 24 h	1,360, t = 264 h	1.3, t = 264 h
Aqueous Humor	C_{max} (µg/mL)			37.2	
	$AUC_{0\text{-}inf}$ (µg·day/mL)			305	
	$t_{1/2}$ (Day)			3.5	
	T_{max} (h)			12.0	
	$AUC_{0\text{-}t}$ (µg·day/mL)	0.12, t = 96 h	21.3, t = 96 h	259, t = 264 h	0.66, t = 96 h
Serum	C_{max} (µg/mL)			0.026	
	$AUC_{0\text{-}inf}$ (µg·day/mL)			0.046	
	$t_{1/2}$ (Day)			1.0	
	T_{max} (h)			12.0	
	$AUC_{0\text{-}t}$ (µg·day/mL)	0.25, t = 48 h	0.12, t = 24 h	0.019, t = 24 h	1.6, t = 48 h
Retina	C_{max} (µg/mL)			112	
	$AUC_{0\text{-}inf}$ (µg·day/mL)			589	
	$t_{1/2}$ (Day)			4.3	
	T_{max} (h)			4.0	
	$AUC_{0\text{-}t}$ (µg·day/mL)	2.9, t = 48 h	0.33, t = 24 h	490, t = 264 h	28.7, t = 264 h

IC: Intracameral.　ITV: Intravitreous injection.　NA: Not applicable.　SCJ: Subconjunctival.

Table 16　Pharmacokinetic Parameters of Ranibizumab following a Single Intravitreous Administration in Cynomolgus Monkeys[40]

Dose (µg)	N	C_{max} (µg/mL)	$AUC_{0\text{-}inf}$ (µg·day/mL)	T_{max} (min)	$t_{1/2}$ (h)
625	5	5.2 ± 0.75	4.9 ± 0.61	5	3.1 ± 1.2
2,500	5	31.5 ± 5.2	29.5 ± 4.3	5	5.3 ± 0.67

Table 17　PK Parameters of Ranibizumab following a Single Intravitreous/Intravenous Administration in Cynomolgus Monkeys[40]

Tissue	Parameter	Ranibizumab			
		500 µg/eye, ITV (N = 3/sex)	2,000 µg/eye, ITV (N = 3/sex)	1,000 µg/animal, IV (N = 2/sex)	4,000 µg/animal, IV (N = 2/sex)
Vitreous Humor	C_{max} (µg/mL)	169	612		
	$AUC_{0\text{-}inf}$ (µg·day/mL)	687	3,230		
	$t_{1/2}$ (Day)	2.3	2.4		
	T_{max} (Day)	0.25	1.0		
	$AUC_{0\text{-}2\,h}$ (µg·day/mL)				
Aqueous Humor	C_{max} (µg/mL)	116	478		
	$AUC_{0\text{-}inf}$ (µg·day/mL)	221	1,550		
	$t_{1/2}$ (Day)	2.4	2.1		
	T_{max} (Day)	0.25	1.0		
	$AUC_{0\text{-}t}$ (µg·day/mL)				
Serum	C_{max} (µg/mL)	0.15	0.62		
	$AUC_{0\text{-}inf}$ (µg·day/mL)	0.46	1.6		
	$t_{1/2}$ (Day)	4.5	3.9	0.65 ± 0.48	0.59 ± 0.23
	T_{max} (Day)	0.25	0.25		
	$AUC_{0\text{-}t}$ (µg·day/mL)			0.25 ± 0.0090	1.2 ± 0.28
Retina	C_{max} (ng/mL)	78.6	227		
	$AUC_{0\text{-}inf}$ (µg·day/mL)	223	909		
	$t_{1/2}$ (Day)	2.5	2.3		
	T_{max} (Day)	0.25	1.0		
	$AUC_{0\text{-}t}$ (µg·day/mL)				

ITV: Intravitreous injection.　IV: Intravenous.

7　Clinical Efficacy and Safety

Overview Profile[43]

❖ FDA has approved Lucentis® (ranibizumab) for the treatment of neovascular (wet) age-related macular degeneration (AMD) on Jun 30, 2006.

❖ On Jun 23, 2010, FDA Approves Lucentis® for the treatment of macular edema following retinal vein occlusion.

❖ On Aug 10, 2012, Lucentis® was approved by the U.S. Food and Drug Administration (FDA) for treatment of diabetic macular edema (DME), an eye condition in people with diabetes that causes blurred vision, severe vision loss and sometimes blindness.

❖ On Feb 6, 2015, FDA today expanded the approved use for Lucentis® 0.3 mg to treat diabetic retinopathy (DR) in patients with diabetic macular edema (DME).

❖ On Oct 14, 2016, FDA Approves Genentech's Lucentis® prefilled syringe.

Table 18 Summary of Individual Clinical Studies and the Major Efficacy Results[44]

Region	Study No.	Phase	Study Design	Study Population	Control	Dosage Regimen	No. of Cases	Major Result
US	FVF3192g, PIER	3b	Sham-controlled study	Sujects with all lesion types of neovascular AMD in the active state	Sham	0.3 or 0.5 mg, IVT every month trough Month 3, and then quarterly	184	Visual acuity was improved following dosing monthly, but returned to baseline after dosing quarterly.
US, EU, Australia	FVF2587g, ANCHOR	3	Randomized, double-masked, double-sham, active treatment-controlled study	Subjects with predominantly classic subfoveal neovascular AMD	Verteporfin PDT (+ sham injection)	0.3 or 0.5 mg, IVT every month, maximum of 24 total injections over 2 years or verteporfin PDT every 3 months as needed	423	Visual acuity was improved; CNV lesions was stablized and CNV leakage was reduced; foveal retinal thickness was reduced.
US	FVF2598g, MARINA	3	Randomized, double-masked, sham-controlled study	Subjects with minimally classic or occult subfoveal neovascular AMD	Sham injection	0.3 or 0.5 mg, IVT every month, maximum of 24 total injections over 2 years	716	Visual acuity was improved; CNV lesions was stablized and CNV leakage was reduced; foveal retinal thickness was reduced.

AMD: Age-related macular degeneration.   CNV: Choroidal neovascularization.   IVT: Intravitral.   PDT: Photon dynamic treatment.

Clinical Efficacy

❖ The primary objective for Studies FVF2598 and FVF2587 was to evaluate the efficacy of intravitreal injections of ranibizumab in preventing vision loss, as measured by the proportion of subjects who lost fewer than 15 letters in visual acuity at 12 months compared with baseline and to evaluate the safety and tolerability of intravitreal injections of ranibizumab administered monthly.

❖ Study FVF2587g also evaluated the non-inferiority of ranibizumab to verteporfin PDT; if non-inferiority was demonstrated, then the treatment differences between ranibizumab and verteporfin PDT were also to be evaluated for superiority.

❖ The primary objective for Study FVF3192 was to evaluate the efficacy and safety of IVT injections of ranibizumab when administered with a reduced dosing frequency.

❖ The safety dossier includes data from seven clinical studies in neovascular AMD: the three pivotal Phase 3 studies (FVF2598g, FVF2587g and FVF3192g) and the four Phase 1 and Phase 1/2 studies (FVF2428g, FVF2128g, FVF2425g, and FVF1770g).

❖ The safety assessments focused on ocular adverse events and visual function effects as well as on systemic adverse events.

Table 19 One-year Data from Studies from FVF2598g (MARINA) and FVF2587g (ANCHOR)[21]

Visual Acuity at 12 Months	Study FVF2598g			Study FVF2587g		
	Sham (N = 238)	Ranibizumab		Verteporfin PDT (N = 143)	Ranibizumab	
		0.3 mg (N = 238)	0.5 mg (N = 240)		0.3 mg (N = 140)	0.5 mg (N = 140)
At a Starting Test Distance of 2 Meters						
n	238	238	240	143	140	139
Loss of <15 letters P-value (vs. control)	148 (62.2%)	225 (94.5%) <0.00010	227 (94.6%) <0.00010	92 (64.3%)	132 (94.3%) <0.00010	134 (96.4%) <0.00010
Gain of ≥15 letters P-value (vs. control)	11 (4.6%)	59 (24.8%) <0.00010	81 (33.8%) <0.00010	8 (5.6%)	50 (35.7%) <0.00010	56 (40.3%) <0.00010
Change from baseline (letters), mean (SD)	-10.5 (16.6)	6.5 (12.7)	7.2 (14.4)	-9.5 (16.4)	8.5 (14.6)	11.3 (14.6)
Approximate Snellen equivalent: 20/200 or worse	102 (42.9%)	29 (12.2%)	28 (11.7%)	86 (60.1%)	31 (22.1%)	23[a] (16.4%)
At a Starting Test Distance of 4 Meters						
n	229	229	230	141	133	139
Loss of <15 letters P-value (vs. control)	138 (60.3%)	213 (93.0%) <0.00010	209 (90.9%) <0.00010	93 (66.0%)	126 (94.7%) <0.00010	136 (97.8%) <0.00010

Continued

Visual Acuity at 12 Months	Study FVF2598g			Study FVF2587g		
	Sham (*N* = 238)	Ranibizumab		Verteporfin PDT (*N* = 143)	Ranibizumab	
		0.3 mg (*N* = 238)	0.5 mg (*N* = 240)		0.3 mg (*N* = 140)	0.5 mg (*N* = 140)
Gain of ≥15 letters	14 (6.1%)	42 (18.3%)	72 (31.3%)	15 (10.6%)	37 (27.8%)	51 (36.7%)
Change from baseline (letters), mean (SD)	-11.0 (17.9)	5.4 (13.4)	6.3 (14.1)	-8.5 (17.8)	7.2 (15.3)	11.0 (15.8)
Approximate Snellen equivalent: 20/200 or worse[b]	102 (43.0%)	29 (12.2%)	28 (11.7%)	81 (56.6%)	32 (23.0%)	23 (16.4%)

[a] *n* = 140. [b] *N* = 237, 237, 240, 143, 139 and 140 for the sham, 0.3 mg and 0.5 mg groups in Study FVF2598g and the verteporfin PDT, 0.3 mg and 0.5 mg groups in Study FVF2587g, respectively.

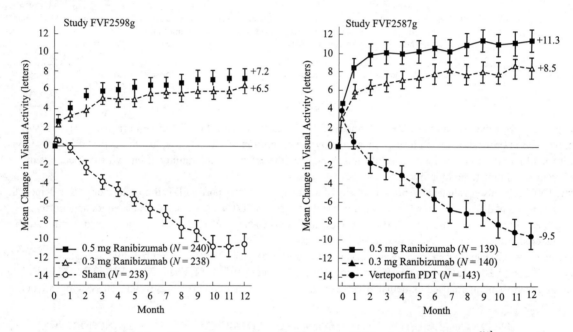

Figure 4   Mean Change from Baseline over Time up to 12 Months in Visual Acuity[21]

Table 20   Gain in VA at 12 Months in Studies FVF2598g (MARINA) and FVF2587g (ANCHOR)[21]

Gain of ≥15 Letters at 12 Months	Control	Ranibizumab	
		0.3 mg	0.5 mg
Study FVF2598g (MARINA)			
n	238	238	240
Response rate	11 (4.6%)	59 (24.8%)	81 (33.8%)
95% *CI* of the percentage	(2.0%, 7.3%)	(19.3%, 30.3%)	(27.8%, 39.7%)
P-value (vs. control)		<0.00010	<0.00010
Study FVF2587g (ANCHOR)			
N	143	140	139
Response rate	8 (5.6%)	50 (35.7%)	56 (40.3%)
95% *CI* of the percentage	(1.8%, 9.4%)	(27.8%, 43.7%)	(32.1%, 48.4%)
P-value (vs. control)		<0.00010	<0.00010

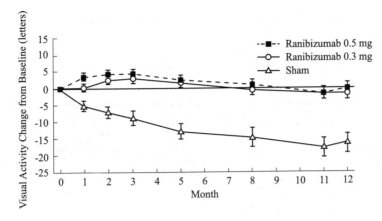

Figure 5   1-year Data from Study FVF3192 (PIER)[21]

Table 21   Visual Acuity in the Study Eye at 12 Months in Study FVF3192 (PIER) at a Starting Test Distance of 4 Meters[21]

Visual Acuity at 12 Months	Sham (N = 63)	Ranibizumab	
		0.3 mg (N = 60)	0.5 mg (N = 61)
Loss of <15 Letters from Baseline			
n (%)	31 (49.2)	50 (83.3)	55 (90.2)
95% CI for percentage[a]	(36.9%, 61.6%)	(73.9%, 92.8%)	(82.7%, 97.6%)
Difference in % (vs. sham)[b]		34.0%	37.0%
95% CI for difference[b]		(19.2%, 48.8%)	(22.5%, 51.5%)
P-value (vs. control)[c]		<0.00010	<0.00010
Gain of ≥15 Letters from Baseline			
n (%)	6 (9.5)	7 (11.7)	8 (13.1)
95% CI for percentage[a]	(2.3%, 16.8%)	(3.5%, 19.8%)	(4.6%, 21.6%)
Difference in % (vs. sham)[b]		0.90%	2.1%
95% CI for difference[b]		(-9.8%, 11.7%)	(-8.2%, 12.4%)
P-value (vs. control)[c]		0.87	0.71
Snellen Equivalent of 20/200 or Worse			
n (%)	33 (52.4)	14 (23.3)	15 (24.6)
95% CI for percentage[a]	(40.0%, 64.7%)	(12.6%, 34.0%)	(13.8%, 35.4%)
Difference in % (vs. sham)[b]		-32.5%	-26.9%
95% CI for difference[b]		(-47.5%, -17.5%)	(-41.6%, -12.3%)
P-value (vs. control)[c]		0.00020	0.0011
Distribution, n (%)			
20/200 or worse	33 (52.4)	14 (23.3)	15 (24.6)
Better than 20/200 but worse than 20/40	23 (36.5)	28 (46.7)	29 (47.5)
20/40 or better	7 (11.1)	18 (30.0)	17 (27.9)

[a] By normal approximation.   [b] Weighted estimates adjusting for the strata by using the Coohran-Mantel-Haenszel weights.   [c] From Coohran χ^2 tests adjusted for the strata.

Clinical Safety

❖ The population studied was predominantly elderly and white which is representative of the population usually affected by age-related macular degeneration.   The demographics of the patient population do not reflect problems with recruitment.

❖ Based on the population studied, there does not appear to be any difference in Lucentis's effect based on age, race, ethnicity or iris color.

❖ The most common adverse events identified are conjunctival hemorrhage, eye pain, increased intraocular pressure, retinal disorder and vitreous floaters.   These adverse events are often associated with intravitreal injections.

Table 22   Ocular Adverse Events in the Study Eye during the First Treatment Year in Studies FVF2598g and FVF2587g[21]

| Preferred Term | Study FVF2598g | | | Study FVF2587g | | |
| | Sham (N = 236) | Ranibizumab | | Verteporfin PDT (N = 143) | Ranibizumab | |
		0.3 mg (N = 238)	0.5 mg (N = 239)		0.3 mg (N = 137)	0.5 mg (N = 140)
Total cular[a]	229 (97.0%)	233 (97.9%)	233 (97.5%)	138 (96.5%)	129 (94.2%)	132 (94.3%)
Blepharitis	14 (5.9%)	16 (6.7%)	26 (10.9%)	6 (4.2%)	6 (4.4%)	7 (5.0%)
CNV	27 (11.4%)	2 (0.80%)	3 (1.3%)	14 (9.8%)	2 (1.5%)	5 (3.6%)
Conjunctival haemorrhage	139 (58.9%)	169 (71.0%)	168 (70.3%)	65 (45.5%)	92 (67.2%)	87 (62.1%)
Detachment of RPE	30 (12.7%)	24 (10.1%)	17 (7.1%)	5 (3.5%)	2 (1.5%)	5 (3.6%)
Eye irritation	43 (18. 2%)	34 (14.3%)	30 (12.7%)	30 (12.7%)	30 (12.7%)	30 (12.7%)
Eye pain	57 (24.2%)	77 (32.4%)	71 (29.7%)	24 (16.8%)	33 (24.1%)	34 (24.3%)
Eye pruritus	20 (8.5%)	18 (7.6%)	27 (11.3%)	7 (4.9%)	10 (7.3%)	12 (8.6%)
Foreign body sensation	27 (11.4%)	41 (17.2%)	39 (16.3%)	15 (10.5%)	8 (5.8%)	10 (7.1%)
IOP increased	7 (3.0%)	38 (16.0%)	39 (16.3%)	10 (7.0%)	21 (15.3%)	22 (15.7%)
Lacrimation increased	30 (12.7%)	32 (13.4%)	27 (11.3%)	6 (4.2%)	9 (6.6%)	8 (5.7%)
Macular degeneration	125 (53.0%)	88 (37.0%)	86 (36.0%)	89 (62.2%)	50 (36.5%)	50 (35.7%)
Retinal disorder	15 (6.4%)	20 (8.4%)	26 (10.9%)	2 (1.4%)	8 (5.8%)	7 (5.0%)
Retinal haemorrhage	101 (42.8%)	46 (19.3%)	40 (16.7%)	76 (53.1%)	20 (14.6%)	26 (18.6%)
Subretinal fibrosis	24 (10.2%)	18 (7.6%)	10 (4.2%)	27 (18.9%)	15 (10.9%)	18 (12.9%)
VA reduced	23 (9.7%)	15 (6.3%)	16 (6.7%)	21 (14.7%)	10 (7.3%)	5 (3.6%)
Vitreous detachment	30 (12.7%)	39 (16.4%)	40 (16.7%)	26 (18.2%)	21 (15.3%)	19 (13.6%)
Vitreous floaters	14 (5.9%)	59 (24.8%)	53 (22.2%)	6 (4.2%)	16 (11.7%)	25 (17.9%)

Multiple occurrences of the same event for a subject were counted once in the overall incidence.   IOP: Intraocular pressure.   [a] Represents the number of subjects with at least one ocular adverse event in the study eye.

Table 23   Intraocular Inflammation Adverse Events in the Study Eye during the First Treatment Year[21]

| | Study FVF2598g | | | Study FVF2587g | | |
| | Sham (N = 236) | Ranibizumab | | Verteporfin PDT (N = 143) | Ranibizumab | |
		0.3 mg (N = 238)	0.5 mg (N = 239)		0.3 mg (N = 137)	0.5 mg (N = 140)
Total[a]	23 (9.7%)	26 (10.9%)	34 (14.2%)	4 (2.8%)	14 (10.2%)	21 (15.0%)
By severity[b]						
Mild	22 (9.3%)	20 (8.4%)	30 (12.6%)	4 (2.8%)	12 (8.8%)	17 (12.1%)
By preferred term[c]						
Iridocyclitis	2 (0.80%)	1 (0.40%)	2 (0.80%)	0	0	4 (2.9%)
Iritis	16 (6.8%)	15 (6.3%)	15 (6.3%)	2 (1.4%)	7 (5.1%)	10 (7.1%)
Uveitis	2 (0.80%)	0	1 (0.40%)	0	0	1 (0.70%)
Vitritis	7 (3.0%)	13 (5.5%)	22 (9.2%)	2 (1.4%)	8 (5.8%)	12 (8.6%)

[a] Represents the number of subjects with at least one intraocular inflammation adverse event in the study eye during the first treatment year.   [b] Subjects with multiple adverse events were counted once at the maximum severity of the events experienced.   [c] Represents the number of subjects with at least one adverse event of the preferred term specified.

Table 24　Major Adverse Effects in Study FVF3192 during the First Treatment Year[21]

Category of Adverse Events	Sham (N = 62)	Ranibizumab	
		0.3 mg (N = 59)	0.5 mg (N = 61)
Ocular Events: Study Eye			
All adverse events	57 (91.9%)	51 (86.4%)	47 (77.0%)
Serious adverse events	9 (14.5%)	5 (8.5%)	3 (4.9%)
Adverse events that led to discontinuation[a]	9 (14.5%)	0	1 (1.6%)
Endophthalmitis	0	0	0
Intraocular Inflammation[b]			
Total	2 (3.2%)	3 (5.1%)	3 (4.9%)
Serious	0	0	0
Ocular Events: Fellow Eye			
All adverse events	35 (56.5%)	28 (47.5%)	36 (59.0%)
Serious adverse events	0	1 (1.7%)	2 (3.3%)
Adverse events that led to discontinuation[a]	2 (3.2%)	0	2 (3.3%)
Endophthalmitis	0	1 (1.7%)[c]	0
Intraocular Inflammation[b]			
Total	0	1 (1.7%)	0
Serious	0	0	0
Non-ocular Events			
All adverse events	40 (64.5%)	46 (78.0%)	40 (65.6%)
Serious adverse events	6 (9.7%)	8 (13.6%)	7 (11.5%)
Adverse events that led to discontinuation[a]	0	0	0

Multiple occurrences of the same event in a subject were counted once in the overall incidence.　[a] Discontinuation from either treatment or study.　[b] Intraocular inflammation reported included the preferred terms of iritis, iridocyclitis, and vitritis.　[c] Vitreous culture obtained showed growth.

Table 25　Ocular Adverse Effects in Study FVF3192 during the First Treatment Year[21]

MedDRA Preferred Terms	Sham (N = 62)	Ranibizumab	
		0.3 mg (N = 59)	0.5 mg (N = 61)
Total[a]	57 (91.9%)	51 (86.4%)	47 (77.0%)
Conjunctival hemorrhage	18 (29.0%)	27 (45.8%)	26 (42.6%)
Macular degeneration	24 (38.7%)	10 (16.9%)	14 (23.0%)
Retinal hemorrhage	23 (37.1%)	11 (18.6%)	12 (19.7%)
Visual acuity reduced	15 (24.2%)	10 (16.9%)	4 (6.6%)
Eye pain	7 (11.3%)	10 (16.9%)	11 (18.0%)
Intraocular pressure increased	3 (4.8%)	5 (8.5%)	13 (21.3%)
Vitreous detachment	11 (17.7%)	4 (6.8%)	6 (9.8%)
Subretinal fibrosis	8 (12.9%)	0	5 (8.2%)
CNV	8 (12.9%)	3 (5.1%)	0

CNV: Choroidal neovascularization.　[a] Represents the number of subjects with at least one ocular adverse event in the study eye.

Table 26　Ocular Serious Adverse Effects in Study FVF3192 during the First Treatment Year[21]

MedDRA Preferred Terms	Sham (N = 62)	Ranibizumab	
		0.3 mg (N = 59)	0.5 mg (N = 61)
Total[a]	9 (14.5%)	5 (8.5%)	3 (4.9%)
Visual acuity reduced	4 (6.5%)	1 (1.7%)	1 (1.6%)
Macular degeneration	1 (1.6%)	1 (1.7%)	1 (1.6%)
Retinal hemorrhage	2 (3.2%)	1 (1.7%)	0
Macular edema	1 (1.6%)	1 (1.7%)	0
CNV	1 (1.6%)	0	0
Eye hemorrhage	0	1 (1.7%)	0
Incorrect route of drug administration	0	0	1 (1.6%)

CNV: Choroidal neovascularization.　[a] Represents the number of subjects with at least one ocular adverse event in the study eye.

Table 27　Serious Ocular Adverse Events in the Pivotal Studies during the First Treatment Year[21]

Adverse Event Category	Study FVF2598g			Study FVF2587g		
	Sham (N = 236)	Ranibizumab		Verteporfin PDT (N = 143)	Ranibizumab	
		0.3 mg (N = 238)	0.5 mg (N = 239)		0.3 mg (N = 137)	0.5 mg (N = 140)
Ocular Events: Study Eye						
All adverse events	229 (97.0%)	233 (97.9%)	233 (97.5%)	138 (96.5%)	129 (94.2%)	132 (94.3%)
Adverse events that led to discontinuation	8 (3.4%)	3 (1.3%)	4 (1.7%)	1 (0.70%)	2 (1.5%)	4 (2.9%)
Serious adverse events	12 (5.1%)	15 (6.3%)	15 (6.3%)	6 (4.2%)	6 (4.4%)	8 (5.7%)
Key Serious Adverse Events						
Cataract traumatic	0	0	0	0	0	0
Endophthalmitis	0	1 (0.40%)	1 (0.40%)	0	0	1 (0.70%)
Intraocular inflammation	0	2 (0.80%)	2 (0.80%)	0	0	1 (0.70%)
IOP increased	0	1 (0.40%)	1 (0.40%)	0	0	0
Retinal artery occlusion	0	0	0	0	0	0
Retinal detachment[a]	0	1 (0.40%)	0	1 (0.70%)[b]	1 (0.70%)	0
Retinal tear	0	1 (0.40%)	1 (0.40%)	0	0	0
Vitreous haemorrhage	0	1 (0.40%)	1 (0.40%)	0	1 (0.70%)	0
Non-ocular Events						
All adverse events	192 (81.4%)	212 (89.1%)	200 (83.7%)	114 (79.7%)	103 (75.2%)	119 (85.0%)
Adverse events that led to discontinuation	5 (2.1%)	2 (0.80%)	5 (2.1%)	6 (4.2%)	5 (3.6%)	2 (1.4%)
Serious adverse events	39 (16.5%)	43 (18.1%)	44 (18.4%)	28 (19.6%)	20 (14.6%)	28 (20.0%)

Table entries are number (%) of subjects with at least one adverse even of the type specified.　Discontinuation refers to discontinuations from either treatment or study. Intraocular inflammation includes the preferred terms of iris, vitritis, iridocyclitis, uveitis, and anterior chamber inflammation.　IOP: Intraocular pressure.　[a] Includes one case of exudative retinal detachment in Study FVF2598g and the three cases of rhegmatogenous retinal detachments in 2 subjects in Study FVF2587g.　[b] Subject experienced two episodes.

Table 28   Non-ocular Adverse Events in the Pivotal Studies during the First Treatment Year[21]

Preferred Term	Study FVF2598g				Study FVF2587g	
	Sham (N = 236)	Ranibizumab		Verteporfin PDT (N = 143)	Ranibizumab	
		0.3 mg (N = 238)	0.5 mg (N = 239)		0.3 mg (N = 137)	0.5 mg (N = 140)
Total[a]	192 (81.4%)	212 (89.1%)	200 (83.7%)	114 (79.7%)	103 (75.2%)	119 (85.0%)
Anemia	8 (3.4%)	6 (2.5%)	10 (4.2%)	4 (2.8%)	5 (3.6%)	7 (5.0%)
Anxiety	1 (0.40%)	6 (2.5%)	8 (3.3%)	8 (5.6%)	5 (3.6%)	3 (2.1%)
Arthralgia	14 (5.9%)	15 (6.3%)	10 (4.2%)	9 (6.3%)	4 (2.9%)	8 (5.7%)
Arthritis	14 (5.9%)	7 (2.9%)	10 (4.2%)	5 (3.5%)	2 (1.5%)	2 (1.4%)
Back pain	13 (5.5%)	14 (5.9%)	13 (5.4%)	13 (9.1%)	5 (3.6%)	10 (7.1%)
Blood pressure increased	14 (5.9%)	14 (5.9%)	11 (4.6%)	3 (2.1%)	4 (2.9%)	6 (4.3%)
Bronchitis	12 (5.1%)	15 (6.3%)	13 (5.4%)	9 (6.3%)	5 (3.6%)	10 (7.1%)
Cough	10 (4.2%)	20 (8.4%)	16 (6.7%)	8 (5.6%)	12 (8.8%)	4 (2.9%)
Diarrhea	12 (5.1%)	10 (4.2%)	5 (2.1%)	6 (4.2%)	6 (4.4%)	4 (2.9%)
Dizziness	16 (6.8%)	11 (4.6%)	5 (2.1%)	4 (2.8%)	3 (2.2%)	7 (5.0%)
Gastroesophageal reflux disease	6 (2.5%)	6 (2.5%)	6 (2.5%)	8 (5.6%)	4 (2.9%)	5 (3.6%)
Headache	15 (6.4%)	24 (10.1%)	14 (5.9%)	7 (4.9%)	11 (8.0%)	11 (7.9%)
Hypertension	23 (9.7%)	20 (8.4%)	20 (8.4%)	12 (8.4%)	3 (2.2%)	9 (6.4%)
Nasopharyngitis	23 (9.7%)	21 (8.8%)	18 (7.5%)	15 (10.5%)	21 (15.3%)	14 (10.0%)
Nausea	10 (4.2%)	14 (5.9%)	13 (5.4%)	7 (4.9%)	6 (4.4%)	6 (4.3%)
Sinusitis	9 (3.8%)	13 (5.5%)	14 (5.9%)	9 (6.3%)	7 (5.1%)	7 (5.0%)
Upper respiratory tract infection	15 (6.4%)	15 (6.3%)	11 (4.6%)	6 (4.2%)	8 (5.8%)	8 (5.7%)
Urinary tract infection	12 (5.1%)	12 (5.0%)	10 (4.2%)	9 (6.3%)	9 (6.6%)	8 (5.7%)

Multiple occurrences of the same event for a subject were counted once in the overall incidence.   [a] Represents the number of subjects with at least one non-ocular adverse event.

Serious Adverse Events/Deaths/Other Significant Events

❖ Dose-dependent trend in increased arterial thromboembolic events seen in both Studies MARINA and ANCHOR, in ranibizumab-treated groups, noted during the first treatment year was reduced in the cumulative data over the 2-year treatment period (MARINA study), so the concern is no longer an issue.

Elevation in IOP

❖ Increases in IOP were reported more frequently in the active treatment arms, especially in the 0.5 mg group.   Noteworthy is the fact that this was the only AE with a notably (1.7%-6.5%) higher incidence in ranibizumab-treated patients during the last 3 months of the treatment year compared with the first 3 months of treatment, however, the incidence of elevated IOP did not increase during the 2nd year of treatment.

Anti-drug Antibody (ADA) Analysis

❖ The incidence of patients with antibodies towards ranibizumab appeared to increase during the 2nd year of treatment in the Study FVF2598g (MARINA).

❖ A relation between antibody formation to ranibizumab, and the development of intraocular inflammation can not be completely ruled out.

8   Clinical Pharmacokinetics

Summary[21, 45]

❖ A total of six clinical trials (FVF1770g, FVF2425g, FVF2128g, FVF2428g, FVF2598g, and FVF2587g) evaluated systemic ranibizumab concentrations in neovascular AMD subjects who received doses ranging from 0.05 to 2.0 mg/eye either as single-dose or in a multiple-dose regimen at a frequency ranging from every 2 weeks to every month, for up to 12 months:
  • The systemic pharmacokinetics of ranibizumab was best described in the population analysis using pooled data from five clinical trials (Studies FVF1770g, FVF2128g, FVF2425g, FVF2428g, and FVF2598g), as each study did not provide sufficient information for individual estimation of pharmacokinetic parameters.
  • The base model was a one-compartment model with a linear rate of absorption from the vitreous compartment, and a proportional error. The full covariate model included CrCL as a predictor of clearance and concomitant verteporfin PDT treatment as a predictor of the rate of absorption.

❖ Absorption
  • Following IVT administration, the time for ranibizumab to reach the maximum concentration in serum is 0.5 days, and the concentration of ranibizumab in the vitreous humor is estimated to be approximately 90,000 times of that in the systemic circulation.
  • The systemic elimination half-life was estimated to be 2 hours, whereas the vitreous elimination half-life was estimated to be approximately 9 days.
  • Because the rate of vitreous elimination is the rate-limiting step, the apparent half-life of ranibizumab in serum after IVT administration is equivalent to the vitreous elimination half-life.

❖ Distribution
  • The distribution of ranibizumab is limited to the volume of plasma (3 liters), which is expected as for drugs with high molecular weight.

❖ Elimination
  • Based on data from Study FVF1770g, ranibizumab exhibits roughly proportional kinetics in the dose range of 0.05-1 mg.

❖ Dose proportionality and time dependency
  • The predicted maximum serum concentration of ranibizumab at steadystate, 1.7 ng/mL (95th percentile), is below the ranibizumab concentration necessary to inhibit the biological activity of VEGF by 50.0%, 11-27 ng/mL, as assessed in an *in vitro* cellular proliferation assay.

❖ Special population
  • Increased exposure in patients with renal impairment and a lower systemic C_{max} in subjects receiving concomitant verteporfin PDT without any significant influence of age, gender or total body weight.

Single-Dose Pharmacokinetics

Table 29   Mean and Coefficient of Variation of Pharmacokinetic Parameters and Covariates[45]

Parameter	Study					All Studies
	FVF1770g	FVF2128g	FVF2425g	FVF2428g	FVF2598g	
No. of subjects with ≥1 measurable serum concentration	24	57	29	98	30	238
No. of subjects with ≥1 evaluable serum concentration[a]	24	54	29	97	24	228
CL/F (L/day)	23.3 (25)	23.6 (21)	25.3 (26)	25.2 (25)	23.1 (17)	24.4 (22)
V_c/F (L)	2.9 (33)	3.1 (52)	4.6 (60)	3.0 (4)	3.2 (25)	3.2 (43)
K_a (Day^{-1})	0.086 (18)	0.081 (15)	0.088 (20)	0.052 (13)	0.078 (13)	0.070 (28)
CrCL (mL/min)	67 (30)	63 (30)	57 (38)	79 (37)	65 (0)[c]	70 (35)
PDT (0/1)[b]	23/1	55/2	29/0	0/98	30/0	137/101

CL/F: Apparent systemic clearance.   CrCL: Serum creatinine clearance. K_a: Rate of systemic absorption (rate of vitreous elimination).   PDT: Photodynamic therapy. V_c/F: Apparent central compartment volume of distribution.   [a] A subject could have had all of his or her measurable serum sample(s) excluded from the analysis as outlier(s) and become unevaluable.   [b] PDT = 0: subject never received PDT during screening or treatment.   PDT = 1: subject received at least one PDT treatment during screening or the study period.   [c] CrCL for the 30 subjects with measurable serum concentration was imputed to the population median because body weight was not recorded in Study FVF2598g.

Table 30　Non-compartmental Estimates of Ranibizumab Systemic Exposure after a Single ITV Injection in Study FVF1770g[45]

Dose (mg)	n	AUC$_{0-7\,days}$ (pg·day/mL)[a]	n	AUC$_{0-14\,days}$ (pg·day/mL)[a]
0.15	2	(3,460, 4,850)[b]	0	NC[c]
0.3	4	5,770 (1,450)	3	10,200 (1,160)
0.5	7	8,260 (3,280)	5	14,500 (6,520)
1.0	2	(13,300, 14,000)[b]	2	(19,200, 20,700)[b]

NC: Not calculated.　[a] Values are mean (SD).　[b] For n = 2, the range of values is reported instead of the mean (SD).　[c] The Day 14 sample was less than reportable for these subjects.

Multiple-Dose Pharmacokinetics

Table 31　Serum Ranibizumab Concentrations (ng/mL) of Treated Subjects in Study FVF2425g[45]

Sampling Day	Time point	Group 1			Group 2			Group 3		
		n	Median	Range	n	Median	Range	n	Median	Range
Screening		9	<0.30	<0.30, <0.30	9	<0.30	<0.30, <0.30	10	<0.30	<0.30, 5.5
Day 0	Pre-dose	9	<0.30	<0.30, <0.30	10	<0.30	<0.30, 1.1	10	<0.30	<0.30, <0.30
	60 min	9	<0.30	<0.30, 0.90	10	<0.30	<0.30, 1.0	10	<0.30	<0.30, 1.2
Day 14	Pre-dose	9	0.40	<0.30, 1.1	10	<0.30	<0.30, 1.0	-	-	-
	60 min	9	0.69	<0.30, 0.90	10	<0.30	<0.30, 1.7	-	-	-
Day 28	Pre-dose	9	0.39	<0.30, 1.1	9	0.42	<0.30, 0.87	10	<0.30	<0.30, <0.30
	60 min	8	0.87	0.49, 26.5	9	1.3	0.65, 12.8	10	<0.30	<0.30, 2.3
Day 42	Pre-dose	9	0.71	<0.30, 2.1	9	0.85	<0.30, 1.3	-	-	-
	60 min	9	1.3	<0.30, 2.4	9	1.5	0.57, 5.9	-	-	-
Day 56	Pre-dose	5	1.6	1.3, 2.7	8	1.0	<0.30, 2.1	9	<0.30	<0.30, <0.30
	60 min	5	3.6	2.4, 4.8	8	1.9	0.63, 3.1	8	0.29	<0.30, 4.7
Day 70	Pre-dose	-	-	-	9	1.4	0.40, 2.0	-	-	-
	60 min	-	-	-	9	1.9	0.63, 5.4	-	-	-
Day 84	Pre-dose	9	0.74	<0.30, 4.9	8	1.7	1.4, 2.2	9	<0.30	<0.30, 0.56
	60 min	9	0.99	0.46, 3.5	8	2.5	2.0, 5.7	8	0.92	<0.30, 4.9
Day 98	Pre-dose	-	-	-	9	2.1	0.71, 6.9	-	-	-
	60 min	-	-	-	9	2.9	1.1, 10.7	-	-	-
Day 112	Pre-dose	8	0.41	<0.30, 0.69	8	2.4	1.5, 3.0	8	<0.30	<0.30, 4.6
	60 min	8	0.55	<0.30, 13.6	8	3.8	2.7, 10.9	8	1.1	<0.30, 3.6

-: No sample was collected in that group at that time point.

Table 32 Serum Ranibizumab Concentrations (ng/mL) in Part 1 of Study FVF2128g[45]

Visit	Time point	0.3 mg (N = 25)			0.5 mg (N = 28)		
		n	Median	Range	n	Median	Range
Screening		22	-	(-, 2.8)	27	-	(-, -)
Day 0	Pre-dose	22	-	(-, -)	28	-	(-, -)
	60 min	23	-	(-, 5.3)	28	-	(-, 0.77)
Day 14	2 weeks	24	-	(-, 0.40)	27	-	(-, 0.64)
Day 28	Pre-dose	25	-	(-, 0.42)	27	-	(-, 4.6)
	60 min	25	-	(-, 6.3)	27	-	(-, 2.6)
Day 42	2 weeks	25	-	(-, 4.7)	26	0.36	(-, 1.8)
Day 56	Pre-dose	24	-	(-, 1.4)	28	-	(-, 1.8)
	60 min	25	-	(-, 1.6)	26	0.33	(-, 38.2)
Day 84	Pre-dose	24	-	(-, 0.70)	24	-	(-, 0.67)
	60 min	23	-	(-, 4.4)	24	-	(-, 19.6)
Day 98[a]	2 weeks	24	-	(-, 0.64)	27	-	(-, 1.1)

-: A less than reportable value. [a] Final visit for Part 1 of study.

Table 33 Serum Ranibizumab Concentrations (ng/mL) in Part 2 by Treatment Received in Parts 1 and 2 of Study FVF2128g[45]

Visit	Time point	Usual Care/0.3 mg (N = 4)			Usual Care/0.5 mg (N = 5)			0.3 mg/0.3 mg (N = 20)			0.5 mg/0.5 mg (N = 22)		
		n	Median	Range	n	Median	Range	n	Median	Range	n	Median	Range
Day 112	Pre-dose	4	-	(-, -)	5	-	(-, -)	13	-	(-, 24.8)	18	-	(-, 2.1)
	60 min	4	-	(-, -)	4	-	(-, 1.9)	13	-	(-, 1.9)	16	-	(-, 2.8)
Day 140	Pre-dose	4	-	(-, -)	5	-	(-, -)	16	-	(-, -)	22	-	(-, 0.59)
	60 min	4	-	(-, 1.2)	4	-	(-, 2.0)	15	-	(-, 0.78)	20	-	(-, 1.6)
Day 168	Pre-dose	4	-	(-, -)	5	-	(-, -)	18	-	(-, -)	22	-	(-, 0.68)
	60 min	3	-	(-, 0.98)	5	-	(-, 0.94)	17	-	(-, 1.7)	21	-	(-, 1.9)
Day 196	Pre-dose	4	-	(-, -)	5	-	(-, -)	19	-	(-, -)	22	-	(-, 0.39)
	60 min	4	-	(-, 0.94)	5	-	(-, 0.87)	18	-	(-, 2.4)	19	-	(-, 5.3)
Final	2 weeks	4	-	(-, 0.47)	5	-	(-, 0.73)	19	-	(-, 0.82)	19	-	(-, 1.6)

-: A less than reportable value.

Table 34 Serum Ranibizumab Concentrations (ng/mL) in Study FVF2598g[45]

	Sham (N = 218)	Ranibizumab	
		0.3 mg (N = 226)	0.5 mg (N = 225)
Month 6			
No. of serum samples	132	130	139
No. of samples LTR	132 (100%)	125 (96.2%)	133 (95.7%)
Maximum concentration	LTR	2.1	2.2
Month 12			
No. of serum samples	205	221	217
No. of samples LTR	204 (99.5%)	215 (97.3%)	204 (94.0%)
Maximum concentration	1.3	2.4	2.1

LTR: Less than reportable (<0.3 ng/mL).

Table 35　Serum Ranibizumab Concentrations (ng/mL) in Study FVF2587g[45]

	Verteporfin PDT (N = 136)	Ranibizumab	
		0.3 mg (N = 135)	0.5 mg (N = 137)
Screening			
No. of serum samples	59	52	52
No. of samples LTR	59 (100%)	51 (98.1%)	52 (100%)
Maximum concentration	0	8.3[a]	0
Month 6			
No. of serum samples	115	121	116
No. of samples LTR	115 (100%)	118 (97.5%)	109 (94.0%)
Maximum concentration	LTR	16.0[b]	1.2
Month 12			
No. of serum samples	126	124	128
No. of samples LTR	126 (100%)	123 (99.2%)	123 (96.1%)
Maximum concentration	LTR	30.7[b]	0.97

LTR: Less than reportable (0.3 ng/mL).　[a] One subject (343010) had measurable ranibizumab concentration at screening.　[b] One subject (334003) received Avastin® (bevacizumab) from March 29, 2004 (treatment ongoing at the time of the Month 6 sample) to June 13, 2004 (136 days prior to the Month 12 sample).

Table 36　Vitreous Ranibizumab Concentrations (ng/mL) in Study FVF2587g[45]

Subject	Treatment Group	Timing of Sample Collection			Result (µg/mL)
		Study Day[a]	Last Prior Injection Visit[b]	Days after Last Prior Injection	
303001	0.3 mg	61	Month 1	25	0.87
339004	0.5 mg	100	Month 2	43	1.3
381008	Verteporfin PDT	149	Month 5	1	LTR
381008	Verteporfin PDT	191	Month 6	2	LTR

LTR: Less than reportable (15.6 ng/mL).　PDT: Photon dynamic treatment.　[a] Day 0 was Study Day 1.　[b] Last ranibizumab or sham injection visit prior to sample collection.

Table 37　Measurable Serum Samples of All Subjects per Study and per Sampling Time Point[45]

No. of Measurable Serum Samples/No. of All Serum Samples (%)[a, b]	Study					All Studies
	FVF1770g	FVF2425g	FVF2128g	FVF2428g	FVF2598g	
1 h (0-0.5 days)	7/24 (29.2)	142/181 (78.5)	124/371 (33.4)	2/14 (14.3)	5/21 (23.8)	280/611 (45.8)
Day 1 (0.5-4 days)	24/27 (88.9)	0/0 (NA)	0/0 (NA)	2/3 (66.7)	3/8 (37.5)	29/38 (76.3)
Day 7 (4-10 days)	15/27 (55.6)	0/1 (0.0)	5/7 (71.4)	93/101 (92.1)	1/1 (100)	114/137 (83.2)
Day 14 (11-17 days)	9/23 (39.1)	80/94 (85.1)	51/156 (32.7)	60/102 (58.8)	2/4 (50.0)	202/379 (53.3)
Day 30 (27-33 days)	0/0 (NA)	14/40 (35.0)	11/206 (5.3)	10/308 (3.2)	7/320 (2.2)	42/874 (4.8)
Day 42 (39-45 days)	0/20 (0.0)	0/1 (0.0)	0/5 (0.0)	0/15 (0.0)	1/29 (3.4)	1/70 (1.4)
Day 90 (87-93 days)	0/18 (0.0)	0/0 (NA)	0/1 (0.0)	0/0 (NA)	0/2 (0.0)	0/21 (0.0)

NA: Not applicable (no sample was collected within this time range).　[a] Includes all serum samples collected, including LTR and measurable samples from all 665 subjects in 051181_AllPatients_Final.csv.　[b] A time range was assigned to each scheduled sampling time point to account for variability in actual sampling time; not all samples were accounted for with the time range assignment.

Table 38   Median, 5th and 95th Percentiles of Model-predicted Vitreous and Serum C_{max} and C_{min} at Steady-state[45]

Steady-state Median (5th, 95th Percentiles)	C_{max} (ng/mL)	C_{min} (ng/mL)
0.3 mg/eye Monthly for 12 Doses		
Serum	0.91 (0.47; 1.7)	0.13 (0.042; 0.29)
Vitreous	87,000 (77,000; 120,000)	12,000 (2,300; 41,000)
0.5 mg/eye Monthly for 12 Doses		
Serum	1.5 (0.79; 2.9)	0.22 (0.069; 0.49)
Vitreous	140,000 (130,000; 190,000)	20,000 (3,800; 68,000)
0.3 mg/eye Monthly for 3 Doses then Quarterly for 3 Doses		
Serum	0.77 (0.34; 1.7)	0.0021 (0.000022; 0.022)
Vitreous	75,000 (75,000; 79,000)	200 (1.0; 4,000)
0.5 mg/eye Monthly for 3 Doses then Quarterly for 3 Doses		
Serum	1.3 (0.57; 2.8)	0.0035 (0.000037; 0.037)
Vitreous	120,000 (120,000; 130,000)	330 (1.7; 6,600)

Simulation values at Month 11 pre- and post-dose are summarized as steady-state C_{min} and C_{max} respectively with a vitreous elimination half-life of 9 days.   NA: Not applicable.

9   Patent

❖ Ranibizumab was approved by the U.S. Food and Drug Administration (FDA) in 2005.   It was developed and marketed as Lucentis® by Genentech (a subsidiary of Roche) and Novartis.

Summary

❖ The patent PCT applications (WO9222653A1, WO9404679A1, and WO9845331A1) related to antibodies, including ranibizumab, were filed in 1992, 1993 and 1998, separately.   The patent families of those PCT applications were granted in the United State, Europe, Japan and China, respectively.

Table 39   Originator's Key Patents of Ranibizumab in Main Countries and/or Region

Country/Region	Publication/Patent No.	Application Date	Granted Date	Estimated Expiry Date
WO	WO9222653A1	06/15/1992	/	/
US	US6407213B1	06/15/1992	06/18/2002	06/30/2020
WO	WO9404679A1	08/20/1993	/	/
US	US6054297A	05/09/1995	04/25/2000	02/26/2018
WO	WO9845331A2	04/03/1998	/	/
US	US6884879B1	08/06/1997	04/26/2005	08/06/2017
	US7365166B2	08/06/1997	04/29/2008	09/07/2017
	US7060269B1	08/06/1997	06/13/2006	07/04/2019
	US7169901B2	09/08/1997	04/25/2000	03/23/2019
	US7297334B2	08/06/1997	11/20/2007	08/06/2017
EP	EP1695985B1	04/03/1998	03/09/2001	04/03/2018
JP	JP3957765B2	04/03/1998	08/15/2007	04/03/2018
CN	CN101665536B	04/03/1998	07/03/2013	04/03/2018
	CN101210050B	04/03/1998	12/08/2010	04/03/2018

Table 40　Originator's International Patent Protection of Use and/or Method of Ranibizumab

Publication No.	Title	Publication Date
Technical Subjects	TREATMENT METHOD	
WO0037502A2	Vascular endothelial cell growth factor antagonists and uses thereof	06/29/2000
WO2010054110A2	Genetic polymorphisms in age-related macular degeneration	05/14/2010
Technical Subjects	DIAGNOSTIC METHOD	
WO2011050034A1	Genetic polymorphisms in age-related macular degeneration	04/28/2011
Technical Subjects	COMBINATION METHOD	
WO2007056470A2	Neuropilin antagonists	05/18/2007
WO2010030813A2	Methods for inhibiting ocular angiogenesis	03/18/2010
Technical Subjects	PREPARATION	
WO2004065417A2	Methods for producing humanized antibodies and improving yield of antibodies or antigen binding fragments in cell culture	08/05/2004

The data was updated until Jan 2018.

10　Reference

[1] Leung D W, Cachianes G, Kuang W J, et al. Vascular endothelial growth factor is a secreted angiogenic mitmita [J]. Science, 1989, 246(4935): 1306-1309.

[2] Keck P J, Hauser S D, Krivi G, et al. Vascular permeability factor, an endothelial cell mitogen related to PDGF [J]. Science, 1989, 246(4945): 1309-1312.

[3] Senger D R, Galli S J, Dvorak A M, et al. Tumor cells secrete a vascular permeability factor that promotes accumulation of ascites fluid [J]. Science, 1983, 219(4587): 983-985.

[4] Ferrara N, Henzel W J. Pituitary follicular cells secrete a novel heparin-binding growth factor specific for vascular endothelial cells [J]. Biochemical and Biophysical Research Communications, 1989, 161(92): 851-858.

[5] Ferrara N. VEGF and the quest for tumor angiogenesis factors [J]. Nature Reviews Cancer, 2002, 2: 795-803.

[6] Ferrara N, Gerber H P, Lecouter J. The biology of VEGF and its receptors [J]. Nature Medicine, 2003, 9(6): 669-676.

[7] Olsson A K, Dimberg A, Kreuger J, et al. VEGF receptor signaling-in control of vascular function [J]. Nature Reviews Molecular Cell Biology, 2006, 7(5): 359-371.

[8] Terman B L, Dougher-vermazen M, Carrion M, et al. Identification of the KDR tyrosine kinase as a receptor of vascular endothelial cell growth factor [J]. Biochemical and Biophysical Research Communications, 1992, 187(3): 1579-1586.

[9] http://www.ncbi.nlm.nih.gov/protein/AAK95847.1.

[10] http://www.ncbi.nlm.nih.gov/protein/XP_016811082.1.

[11] http://www.ncbi.nlm.nih.gov/protein/AFE64645.1.

[12] http://www.ncbi.nlm.nih.gov/protein/AAL07526.1.

[13] http://www.ncbi.nlm.nih.gov/protein/EDL23467.1.

[14] https://blast.ncbi.nlm.nih.gov.

[15] Herbert S P, Stainier D Y. Molecular control of endothelial cell behavior during blood vessel morphogenesis [J]. Nature Reviews Molecular Cell Biology, 2011, 12(9): 551-564.

[16] Park J E, Chen H H, Winer J, et al. Placenta growth factor. Potentiation of vascular endothelial growth factor bioactivity, in vitro and in vivo, and high affinity binding to Flt-1 but not to Flk-1/KDR [J]. Journal of Biological Chemistry, 1994, 269(41): 25646-25654.

[17] Gerber H P, Mcmurtrey A, Kowalski J, et al. VEGF regulates endothelial cell survival by the PI3K-kinase/Akt signal transduction pathway. Requirement for Flk-1/KDR activation [J]. Journal of Biological Chemistry, 1998, 273(46): 30366-30343.

[18] Broxmeyer H E, Cooper S, Li Z H, et al. Myeloid progenitor cell regulatory effects of vascular endothelial cell growth factor [J]. International Journal of Hematology, 1995, 62(4): 203-215.

[19] Dvorak H F, Brown L F, Detmar M, et al. Vascular permeability factor/vascular endothelial growth factor, microvascular hyperpermeability, and angiogenesis [J]. The American Journal of Pathology, 1995, 146(5): 1029-1039.

[20] Yang R, Thomas G R, Bunting S, et al. Effects of vascular endothelial growth factor on hemodynamics and cardiac performance [J]. Journal of Cardiovascular Pharmacology, 1996, 27(6): 838-844.

[21] European Medicines Agency (EMA) Database. http://www.ema.europa.eu/docs/en_GB/document_library/EPAR_-_Scientific_Discussion/ human/000715/WC500043550.pdf.

[22] Ellis M. Mechanism of action of bevacizumab as a component of therapy for metastatic colorectal cancer [J]. Seminars in Oncology, 2006, 33(10): S1-S7.

[23] The financial reports of Genentech; http://data.pharmacodia.com/web/homePage/index.

[24] U. S. Food and Drug Administration (FDA) Database. http://www.accessdata.fda.gov/scripts/cder/drugsatfda/index.cfm?fuseaction=Search.Label_ApprovalHistory#apphist.

[25] EMA Database. http://www.ema.europa.eu/ema/index.jsp?curl=pages/medicines/human/medicines/000715/human_med_000890.jsp&mid=WC0b01ac058001d124.

[26] FDA Database. https://www.accessdata.fda.gov/drugsatfda_docs/label/2015/125156s106lbl.pdf.

[27] EMA Database. http://www.ema.europa.eu/docs/en_GB/document_library/EPAR_-_Product_Information/human/000715/WC500043546.pdf.

[28] China Food and Drug administration (CFDA) Database. http://app1.sfda.gov.cn/datasearch/face3/base.jsp?tableId=36&tableName=TABLE36&title=进口药品&bcId=124356651564146415214424405468.

[29] Pharmaceuticals and Medical Devices (PMDA) Database. http://ss.pmda.go.jp/en_all/muv_ajax.x?u=http%3A%2F%2Fwww.pmda.go.jp%2Ffiles%2F000153061.pdf%23page%3D2&p=2&t=&q=lucentis&s=lZDVP5TqCjiWHulMrarmdVPsNIr4t4Uni4Jz95RJcR4v_-QPRzEVkRBpojf98MWRg_oBLxgDYpK-ihoSmgc7kNS71uO2_tnFId0wTwGw8s2Fik1M4WIopH3DDJyOC5xUAq7Hbq5Oq-pJTl2tb7Lu6WWWD1ZcASXuwMT0HgJXuNo.&lang=en.

[30] FDA Database. https://www.accessdata.fda.gov/scripts/cder/daf/index.cfm?event=overview.process&ApplNo=125085.

[31] FDA Database. https://www.accessdata.fda.gov/drugsatfda_docs/label/2016/125085s317lbl.pdf.

[32] FDA Database. http://www.pmda.go.jp/files/000153070.pdf.

[33] FDA Database. https://www.accessdata.fda.gov/drugsatfda_docs/nda/2012/125418_zaltrap_toc.cfm.

[34] FDA Database. https://www.accessdata.fda.gov/drugsatfda_docs/nda/2012/125418Orig1s000ChemR.pdf.

[35] FDA Database. https://www.accessdata.fda.gov/drugsatfda_docs/label/2012/125418s000lbl.pdf.

[36] FDA Database. http://www.ema.europa.eu/ema/index.jsp?curl=pages/medicines/human/medicines/002532/human_med_001617.jsp&mid=WC0b01ac058001d124.

[37] CFDA Database. http://app2.sfda.gov.cn/datasearchp/index1.do?tableId=25&tableName=TABLE25&tableView=国产药品&Id=194418.

[38] EMA Database. http://www.ema.europa.eu/ema/index.jsp?curl=pages/medicines/human/medicines/000582/human_med_000663.jsp&mid=WC0b01ac058001d124.

[39] http://www.commonchemistry.org/ChemicalDetail.aspx?ref=347396-82-1.

[40] FDA Database. https://www.accessdata.fda.gov/drugsatfda_docs/nda/2006/125156s0000_Lucentis_PharmR.pdf.

[41] Papadopoulos N, Martin J, Ruan Q, et al. Binding and neutralization of vascular endothelial growth factor (VEGF) and related ligands by VEGF trap, ranibizumab and bevacizumab [J]. Angiogenesis, 2012, 15(2): 171-185.

[42] Lowe J, Araujo J, Yang J H, et al. Ranibizumab inhibits multiple forms of biologically active vascular endothelial growth factor *in vitro* and *in vivo* [J]. Experimental Eye Research, 2007, 85(4): 425-430.

[43] https://www.drugs.com/history/ucentis.html.

[44] FDA Database. https://www.accessdata.fda.gov/drugsatfda_docs/nda/2006/125156s0000_Lucentis_MedR.pdf.

[45] FDA Database. http://101.96.10.43/www.accessdata.fda.gov/drugsatfda_docs/nda/2006/125156s0000_Lucentis_ClinPharmR.pdf.

CHAPTER

8

Rituximab

Rituximab

(Rituxan®)

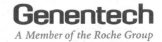

Research code: IDEC-102, IDEC-C2B8, R-105, RG-105, RO-452294

1 Target Biology

B-Cell Antigen-CD20

❖ CD20 is a B-lymphocyte surface molecule with a molecular weight of 33, 35, and 37 kDa that appears relatively late in the B-cell maturation (after the pro-B cell stage with CD45R+, CD117+) and then persists expressing before differentiating into antibody-secreting plasma cell stage.   Its molecular structure resembles to transmembrane calcium channel.[1]

❖ In humans, CD20 is encoded by the MS4A1 gene, which is located on chromosome 11 at band q12-q13.   This gene encodes a member of the membrane-spanning 4A gene family.   Members of this nascent protein family are characterized by common structural features and similar intron/exon splice boundaries and display unique expression patterns among hematopoietic cells and nonlymphoid tissues.   Alternative splicing of this gene results in two transcript variants that encode the same protein.[2]

Sequence Homology of CD20 Proteins[3-11]

Human: 297 aa.   Accession: NP_690605.1.

```
  1 MTTPRNSVNG  TFPAEPMKGP  IAMQSGPKPL  FRRMSSLVGP  TQSFFMRESK  TLGAVQIMNG
 61 LFHIALGGLL  MIPAGIYAPI  CVTVWYPLWG  GIMYIISGSL  LAATEKNSRK  CLVKGKMIMN
121 SLSLFAAISG  MILSIMDILN  IKISHFLKME  SLNFIRAHTP  YINIYNCEPA  NPSEKNSPST
181 QYCYSIQSLF  LGILSVMLIF  AFFQELVIAG  IVENEWKRTC  SRPKSNIVLL  SAEEKKEQTI
241 EIKEEVVGLT  ETSSQPKNEE  DIEIIPIQEE  EEEETETNFP  EPPQDQESSP  I E N D S S P
```

Chimpanzee: 297aa.   Accession: XP_508461.2.

❖ BLAST:
  - Max score: 504; Total score: 504; Query cover: 100%.
  - Identities: 294/297 (99.0%); Positives: 295/297 (99.0%); Gaps: 0/297 (0.0%).

```
  1 MTTPRNSVNG  TFPAEPMKGS  IAMQSGPKPL  FRRMSSLVGP  TQSFFMRESK  ALGAVQIMNG
 61 LFHIALGGLL  MIPAGIYAPI  CVTVWYPLWG  GIMYIISGSL  LAATEKNSRK  CMVKGKMIM
121 SLSLFAAISG  MILSIMDILN  IKISHFLKME  SLNFIRAHTP  YINIYNCEPA  NNPSEKNSPST
181 QYCYSIQSLF  LGILSVMLIF  AFFQELVIAG  IVENEWKRTC  SRPKSNIVLL  SAEEKKEQTI
241 EIKEEVVGLT  ETSSQPKNEE  DIEIIPIQEE  EEEETETNFP  EPPQDQESSP  I E N D S S P
```

Rhesus Monkey: 297 aa.   Accession: XP_001086364.1.

❖ BLAST:
  - Max score: 493; Total score:493; Query cover: 100%.
  - Identities: 289/297 (97.0%); Positives: 292/297 (98.0%); Gaps: 0.0% (0/297).

```
  1 MTTPRNSVNG  TFPAEPMKGP  IAMQPGPKPL  LRRMSSLVGP  TQSFFMRESK  ALGAVQIMNG
 61 LFHIALGGLL  MIPAGIYAPI  CVTVWYPLWG  GIMYIISGSL  LAATEKNSRK  CLVKGKMIMN
121 SLSLFAAISG  MILSIMDILN  IKISHFLKME  SLNFIRVHTP  YINIYNCEPA  NPSEKNSPST
181 QYCYSIQSLF  LGILSVMLIF  AFFQELVIAG  IVENEWRRTC  SRPKSSVVLL  SAEEKKEQVI
241 EIKEEVVGLT  ETSSQPKNEE  DIEIIPIQEE  EEEETETNFP  EPPQDQESSP  I E N D S S P
```

Dog: 297 aa.   Accession: NP_001041493.1.

❖ BLAST:
  - Max score: 386; Total score: 386; Query cover: 86.0%.
  - Identities: 188/258 (73.0%); Positives: 219/258 (84.0%); Gaps: 0.0% (1/258).

```
  1  MTTPRNSMSG  TLPVDPMKSP  TAMYPVQKII  PKRMPSVVGP  TQNFFMRESK  TLGAVQIMNG
 61  LFHIALGSLL  MIHTDVCAPI  CITMWYPLWG  GIMFIISGSL  LAAADKNPRK  SLVKGKMIMN
121  SLSLFAAISG  IIFLIMDIFN  ITISHFFKME  NLNLIKAPMP  YVDIHNCDPA  NPSEKNSLSI
181  QYCGSIRSVF  LGVFAVMLIF  AFFQKLVTAG  IVENEWKKLC  SKPKSDVVVL  LAAEEKKEQP
241  IETTEEMVEL  TEIASQPKKE  EDIEIIPVQE  EEGELEINFA  EPPQEQESSP  I E N D S I P
```

Cattle: 303 aa.   Accession: NP_001071322.1.

❖ BLAST:
  • Max score: 338; Total score: 338; Query cover: 100%.
  • Identities: 199/303 (66.0%); Positives: 235/303 (77.0%); Gaps: 6/303 (1.0%).

```
  1  MTTPRNSMVG  AFPAEPLKGP  IAMHAAQKVV  PRRVPVVVGP  TQSFFMREAK  ALGAVQIMNG
 61  LFHIALGSLM  LIHMDVYMPI  CVTLWYPLWG  GIMFIISGSL  LAAAEKNSTQ  SMLTGRLIMN
121  SLSLFAAISG  IIFLIMDIFN  MTISHFFKME  NLNLIKTQVP  YININNCERA  NPDENNSQSV
181  EYCARIRFVF  LSNFAVMMIF  AFLQKLVTAG  TVENEWKKLC  SRPKANVVLL  SAEEKKEQVI
241  EIKEEVVEQI  EVAEQIEISS  LPKNEEDIEI  IPVQEEEEEE  AEMNFPEPPQ  DQEDSPIEND
301  SVP
```

House Mouse: 291 aa.   Accession: NP_031667.1.

❖ BLAST:
  • Max score:387; Total score: 387; Query cover: 100%.
  • Identities: 217/291 (75.0%); Positives: 250/291 (85.0%); Gaps: 1/291 (0.0%).

```
  1  MSGPFPAEPT  KGPLAMQPAP  KVNLKRTSSL  VGPTQSFFMR  ESKALGAVQI  MNGLFHITLG
 61  GLLMIPTGVF  APICLSVWYP  LWGGIMYIIS  GSLLAAAAEK  TSRKSLVKAK  VIMSSLSLFA
121  AISGIILSIM  DILNMTLSHF  LKMRRLELIQ  TSKPYVDIYD  CEPSNSSEKN  SPSTQYCNSI
181  QSVFLGILSA  MLISAFFQKL  VTAGIVENEW  KRMCTRSKSN  VVLLSAGEKN  EQTIKMKEEI
241  IELSGVSSQP  KNEEEIEIIP  VQEEEEEEAE  INFPAPPQEQ  ESLPVENEIA  P
```

Norway Rat: 297 aa.   Accession: NP_001101048.

❖ BLAST:
  • Max score: 400; Total score: 400; Query cover: 100%.
  • Identities: 227/298 (76.0%); Positives: 258/298 (86.0%); Gaps: 2/298 (0.0%).

```
  1  MTTPRNSVSG  PFPTEPTKGP  LAMQPAQKVI  PRRPSSLVGP  TQSFFMRESK  ALGAVQIMNG
 61  LFHISLGGLL  MIPTGVFAPI  CLSVWYPLWG  GIMYIISGSL  LAAAAEKTSR  KSLATKVIMS
121  SLSLFAAISG  IILSIMDILN  ITVSHFLKME  RLELIKTPKL  YVDIYNCEPS  NSSEKNSPST
181  QYCNSVQSVF  LGILSVMLIS  AFFQKLVTAG  VVENEWKRV   SRPKSNVVLL  SAGEKKEQTI
241  KMKEEIIELS  GVSSQPKNEE  EIEIIPVQEE  CEEEEAEINFP  APPQEQESLP  V E N E I S P
```

2 General Information

Rituximab/Rituxan®

❖ Rituximab (Rituxan®; Genentech, Inc, South San Francisco, CA and IDEC Pharmaceutical Corporation, San Diego, CA) is a unique monoclonal antibody for the treatment of non-Hodgkin's lymphoma.   This chimeric mouse/human antibody was discovered in 1991 at IDEC Pharmaceuticals' laboratories, where the antibody was genetically engineered and produced utilizing high-yield expression systems.   It is a human IgG1 kappa antibody with mouse variable regions isolated from a murine anti-CD20 antibody, IDEC-2B8 that binds with high affinity to cells expressing the CD20 antigen found on the surface of malignant and normal B cells, but not on other normal tissues.   It mediates complement-dependent cell lysis in the presence of human complement, and antibody-dependent cellular cytotoxicity with human effector cells.   Also, it has been shown to induce apoptosis and to sensitize chemoresistant human lymphoma cell lines *in vitro*.   Clinical development was expedited (3 years) with the first patient entered in Phase 1 trials in March 1993 and the last patient entered in Phase 3 study in March 1996.   IDEC Pharmaceuticals began a collaboration with Genentech, Inc. in March 1995 and with F. Hoffman-LaRoche (Nutley, NJ) shortly thereafter.   Marketing approval was granted by the U.S. Food and Drug Administration on November 26, 1997 (and by the European Union on June 2, 1998) for the indication of relapsed or refractory, CD20-positive, B-cell, low-grade or follicular non-Hodgkin's lymphoma.   Rituximab is the first therapeutic monoclonal antibody approved for the treatment of cancer and the first single agent approved specifically for therapy for a lymphoma.   Substantial research has been performed over the past 8 years to further understanding this novel therapeutic.   Nevertheless, much remains to be accomplished in key areas such as mechanism of action and resistance, combinations with chemotherapy, biologics and radiotherapy/radio-immunotherapy, role within multimodality regimens, and nonmalignant applications.[12]

❖ The total sales of 7,374 million US$ for 2016; No sales data as of 2017.

World Sales[13]

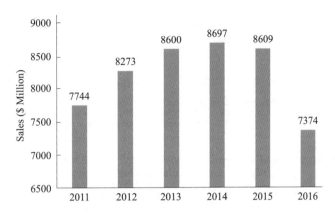

Figure 1   World Sales of Rituxan® since 2011

Approval and Indications

Table 1   Summary of the Approval of Rituximab®[13]

	US (FDA)	EU (EMA)	Japan (PMDA)	China (CFDA)
First approval date	11/26/1997	06/02/1998	06/20/2001	04/21/2008
Application or approval No.	BLA103705	EMEA/H/C/000165	21300AMY00273000	S20080044/S20080045
Brand name	Rituxan®	MabThera®	Rituxan®	MabThera®/美罗华®
Indication	NHL, CCL, RA	NHL, CCL, RA, GPA	NHL, CD20+FL, RA	NHL, CCL, RA, GPA
Authorization holder	Genentech (Roche)	Genentech (Roche)	Genentech (Roche)	Genentech (Roche)

CCL: Chronic lymphocytic leukaemia.   FL: Follicular lymphoma.   GPA: Granulomatosis with polyangiitis.   NHL: Non-Hodgkin's lymphoma.   RA: Rheumatoid arthritis.

3   CMC Profile

Product Profile[14]

Dosage route: SC injection or IV infusion.
Strength: EU: 1,400 mg, 100 mg, 500 mg.
Finished medicinal product: The complete composition of MabThera® subcutaneous formulation is 120 mg/mL rituximab in L-histidine/histidine hydrochloride, trehalose, polysorbate 80, L-methionine, and rHuPH20.   One vial of the final product contains 1,400 mg of rituximab in 11.7 mL solution (120 mg/mL).
Stability: The stability data submitted support a 24 months shelf-life when stored at -20 °C.

Amino Acid Sequence[14]

❖ Molecular formula: $C_{6426}H_{9900}N_{1700}O_{2008}S_{44}$, 144.51 kDa.

❖ Heavy chain: 1-150: Mouse derived (under line), 151-451: Human derived.

```
  1 Gln-Val-Gln-Leu-Gln-Gln-Pro-Gly-Ala-Glu-      211 Ser-Asn-Thr-Lys-Val-Asp-Lys-Lys-Ala-Glu-
 11 Leu-Val-Lys-Pro-Gly-Ala-Ser-Val-Lys-Met-      221 Pro-Lys-Ser-Cys-Asp-Lys-Thr-His-Thr-Cys-
 21 Ser-Cys-Lys-Ala-Ser-Gly-Tyr-Thr-Phe-Thr-      231 Pro-Pro-Cys-Pro-Ala-Pro-Glu-Leu-Leu-Gly-
 31 Ser-Tyr-Asn-Met-His-Trp-Val-Lys-Gln-Thr-      241 Gly-Pro-Ser-Val-Phe-Leu-Phe-Pro-Pro-Lys-
 41 Pro-Gly-Arg-Gly-Leu-Glu-Trp-Ile-Gly-Ala-      251 Pro-Lys-Asp-Thr-Leu-Met-Ile-Ser-Arg-Thr-
 51 Ile-Tyr-Pro-Gly-Asn-Gly-Asp-Thr-Ser-Tyr-      261 Pro-Glu-Val-Thr-Cys-Val-Val-Val-Asp-Val-
 61 Asn-Gln-Lys-Phe-Lys-Gly-Lys-Ala-Thr-Leu-      271 Ser-His-Glu-Asp-Pro-Glu-Val-Lys-Phe-Asn-
 71 Thr-Ala-Asp-Lys-Ser-Ser-Ser-Thr-Ala-Tyr-      281 Trp-Tyr-Val-Asp-Gly-Val-Glu-Val-His-Asn-
 81 Met-Gln-Leu-Ser-Ser-Leu-Thr-Ser-Glu-Asp-      291 Ala-Lys-Thr-Lys-Pro-Arg-Glu-Glu-Gln-Tyr-
 91 Ser-Ala-Val-Tyr-Tyr-Cys-Ala-Arg-Ser-Thr-      301 Asn*-Ser-Thr-Tyr-Arg-Val-Val-Ser-Val-Leu-
101 Tyr-Tyr-Gly-Gly-Asp-Trp-Tyr-Phe-Asn-Val-      311 Thr-Val-Leu-His-Gln-Asp-Trp-Leu-Asn-Gly-
111 Trp-Gly- Ala-Gly-Thr-Thr-Val-Thr-Val-Ser-      321 Lys-Glu-Tyr-Lys-Cys-Lys-Val-Ser-Asn-Lys-
121 Ala-Ala-Ser-Thr-Lys-Gly-Pro-Ser-Val-Phe-      331 Ala-Leu-Pro-Ala-Pro-Ile-Glu-Lys-Thr-Ile-
131 Pro-Leu-Ala-Pro-Ser-Ser-Lys-Ser-Thr-Ser-      341 Ser-Lys-Ala-Lys-Gly-Gln-Pro-Arg-Glu-Pro-
141 Gly-Gly-Thr-Ala-Ala-Leu-Gly-Gys-Leu-Val-      351 Gln-Val-Tyr-Thr-Leu -Pro-Pro-Ser-Arg-Asp-
151 Lys-Asp-Tyr-Phe-Pro-Glu-Pro-Val-Thr-Val-      361 Glu-Leu-Thr-Lys-Asn-Gln-Val-Ser-Leu-Thr-
161 Ser-Trp-Asn-Ser-Gly-Ala-Leu-Thr-Ser-Gly-      371 Cys-Leu-Val-Lys-Gly-Phe-Tyr-Pro-Ser-Asp-
171 Val-His-Thr-Phe-Pro-Ala-Val-Leu-Gln-Ser-      381 Ile-Ala-Val-Glu-Trp-Glu-Ser-Asn-Gly-Gln-
181 Ser-Gly-Leu-Tyr-Ser-Leu-Ser-Ser-Val-Val-      391 Pro-Glu-Asn-Asn-Tyr-Lys-Thr-Thr-Pro-Pro-
191 Thr-Val-Pro-Ser-Ser-Ser-Leu-Gly-Thr-Gln-      401 Val-Leu-Asp-Ser-Asp-Gly-Ser-Phe-Phe-Leu-
201 Thr-Tyr-Ile-Cys-Asn-Val-Asn-His-Lys-Pro-      411 Tyr- Ser-Lys-Leu-Thr-Val-Asp-Lys-Ser-Arg-
                                                  421 Trp-Gln-Gln-Gly-Asn-Val-Phe-Ser-Cys-Ser-
                                                  431 Val-Met-His-Glu -Ala-Leu-His-Asn-His-Tyr-
                                                  441 Thr-Gln-Lys-Ser-Leu-Ser-Leu-Ser-Pro-Gly-
                                                  451 Lys
```

❖ Glycosylation: 301*

❖ Light chain: 1-128: Mouse derived (under line); 129-213: Human derived.

```
  1 Gln-Ile-Val-Leu-Ser-Gln-Ser-Pro-Ala-Ile-      121 Asp-Glu-Gln-Leu-Lys-Ser-Gly-Thr-Ala-Ser-
 11 Leu-Ser-Ala-Ser-Pro-Gly-Glu-Lys-Val-Thr-      131 Val-Val-Cys-Leu-Leu-Asn-Asn-Phe-Tyr-Pro-
 21 Met-Thr-Cys-Arg-Ala-Ser-Ser-Ser-Val-Ser-      141 Arg-Glu-Ala-Lys-Val-Gln -Trp-Lys-Val-Asp-
 31 Tyr-Ile-His-Trp-Phe-Gln-Gln-Lys-Pro-Gly-      151 Asn-Ala-Leu-Gln-Ser-Gly-Asn-Ser-Gln-Glu-
 41 Ser-Pro-Lys-Pro-Trp-Ile-Tyr-Ala-Thr-        161 Ser-Val-Thr-Glu-Gln-Asp-Ser-Lys-Asp-Ser-
 51 Ser-Asn-Leu-Ala-Ser-Gly-Val-Pro-Val-Arg-      171 Thr-Tyr-Ser-Leu-Ser-Ser-Thr-Leu-Thr-Leu-
 61 Phe-Ser-Gly-Ser-Gly-Ser-Gly-Thr-Ser-Tyr-      181 Ser-Lys-Ala-Asp-Tyr-Glu-Lys-His-Lys-Val-
 71 Ser-Leu-Thr-Ile-Ser-Arg-Val-Glu-Ala-Glu-      191 Tyr-Ala-Cys-Glu-Val-Thr-His-Gln-Gly-Leu-
 81 Asp-Ala-Ala-Thr-Tyr-Tyr-Cys-Gln-Gln-Trp-      201 Ser-Ser-Pro-Val-Thr-Lys-Ser-Phe-Asn-Arg-
 91 Thr-Ser-Asn-Pro-Pro-Thr-Phe-Gly-Gly-Gly-      211 Gly-Glu-Cys  213
101 Thr-Lys-Leu-Glu-Ile-Lys-Arg-Thr-Val-Ala-
111 Ala-Pro-Ser-Val-Phe-Ile-Phe-Pro-Pro-Ser-
```

4 Pre-clinical Pharmacodynamics

Non-clinical Pharmacodynamics[15]

❖ Rituximab is a chimeric mouse/human monoclonal antibody, which targets an epitope CD20 on human B-lymphocytes. For primary pharmacodynamics only experiments in non-human primates are relevant. Neither rodent nor canine B cells bind rituximab. In long-term administration studies the problem of immunogenicity of rituximab in Cynomolgus monkey could make the results inconclusive. Antibodies against rituximab may appear after 2 weeks of treatment. Therefore, no xenograft experiments are feasible. No animal model is available for evaluating the antineoplastic effect. Pharmacodynamic studies consist of immunoanatomic distribution and immunopathologic analysis of rituximab. The initial *in vitro* characterisation of rituximab was performed with an early-purified antibody from first CHO-cultures. During the development, rituximab was produced at different facilities with slight modifications of the manufacturing processes. The applicant has investigated rituximab's immunoanatomic distribution with Suspension Culture Produced antibody, Hollow Fiber Produced antibody, and Stirred Tank Produced antibody at the Torreyana Facility.

❖ A number of *in vitro* studies were performed to confirm the specificity and affinity for the CD20 epitope. The apparent binding affinity constant was 5.2×10^{-9} M. The binding of human complement C1q and complement dependent cytotoxicity and antibody dependent cytotoxicity was documented by fluorescein conjugation and 51-Cr release. The tissue specificity was demonstrated in several human cross reactivity studies. Human hematopoietic progenitor cells depleted of B cells by incubation of rituximab retained their colony formation and no effect was noted on CD34+ cell population. Doses of 0.1, 0.4 or 1.6 mg/(kg·day) × 4 were equally effective for a greater than 80.0% depletion of peripheral B cells. The duration of the depletion was about 7 days after the last injection. A slow recovery of B cells was observed thereafter. Full recovery was not seen with certainty at the end of the study period (Day 90). Compared to saline treated animals a dose of 16.8 mg/kg depleted >79.0% of CD20+ bone marrow cells at the time when the animals were sacrificed and 69.0% depletion of lymph node CD20+ cells. Immuno-histochemical studies on human tissue cross-reactivity were presented. Rituximab was highly tissue restrictive.

❖ Rituximab had no effect on human haematopoietic progenitor cells. The B-cell depleting effect was demonstrated in Cynomolgus monkeys both in peripheral blood and lymphatic tissues. The major concerns were the low level of exposure in Cynomolgus monkey as compared to human level of exposure (1:1) and the lack of long-term animal studies, since B-cell recovery was not complete 90 days post dose. The only unexpected clinical sign in monkeys was nausea; otherwise rituximab appeared to be very safe. Only pharmacologic effects were observed in the laboratory parameters.

❖ No studies were performed to compare the affinity of rituximab with B cells of humans versus Cynomolgus monkeys and to determine the density of CD20 expression on monkey B cells. However, such studies are unnecessary because B cells in Cynomolgus monkeys are lysed by a single dose of rituximab, which is evidence of relevant activity even if affinity and CD20 expression may be different in humans and primates.

Overview of *in vitro* Activities[16, 17]
❖ Affinity
  • Both mouse IDEC-2B8 antibody and mouse-human chimera IDEC-C2B8 can specifically bind to human CD20 on SB cell (ATCC No. CCL120) (Figure 2A).
  • Disassociation constants of IDEC-2B8 and IDEC-C2B8 are 5.2×10^{-9} mol/L and 3.5×10^{-9} mol/L (Figure 2B).
  • IDEC-C2B8 can specifically bind to human circulating B lymphocytes (Figure 2C).
  • IDEC-C2B8 can specifically bind to human B-cell lymphoma cells (Figure 2D).
❖ CDC and ADCC activity:
  • CDC activity: Both IDEC-2B8 and IDEC-C2B8 can conjugate to CD20 on SB cells. However, only chimerical IDEC-C2B8 antibody can bind to human complement C1q (Figure 2E) and further induce CDC (Figure 2F).
  • ADCC activity: IDEC-C2B8 has the ability to induce ADCC (Figure 3A).
❖ Cell viability
  • Raji, Ramos and other leukemia cell lines (Figure 3B).

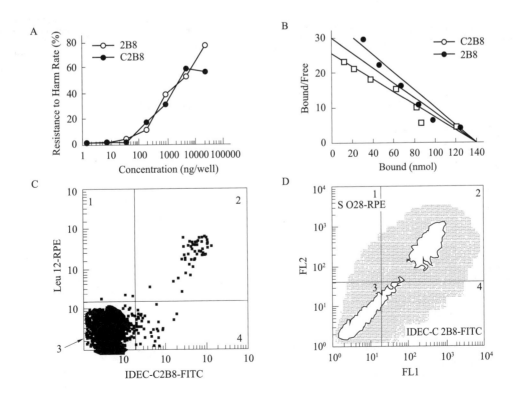

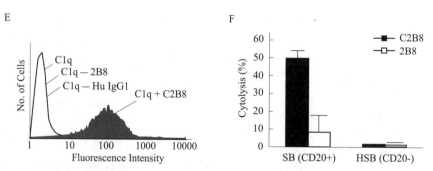

(A) Competitive inhibition assay of mouse IDEC-2B8 and mouse-human chimera IDEC-C2B8 antibodies.   (B) Scatchard analysis of the binding of CD20 and IDEC-C2B8 and IDEC-2B8.   (C) Binding specificity of IDEC-C2B8 on B lymphocytes of human peripheral blood.   (D) Specific binding of IDEC-C2B8 against tumor cells from B-cell lymphoma patients.   (E) CDC activity: Binding of the SB cells and human complement C1q via IDEC-C2B8 antibody.   (F) CDC activity: Cytolytic effect of IDEC-C2B8 and the human complement.

Figure 2   *In Vitro* Activities of Rituximab[16]

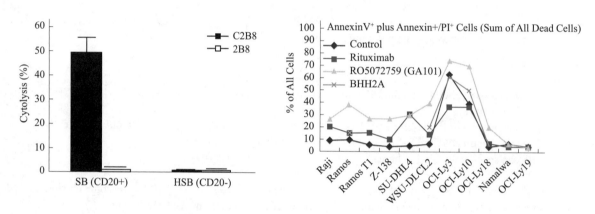

Figure 3   *In Vitro* Activities of Rituximab-ADCC and Cell Death Induction (A) (B) Cell Death Comparing GA101 and Rituximab in a Panel of Human B-cell Cancer Lines[16, 17]

Table 2   Summary of Non-clinical Primary Pharmacology Studied Findings Compared with of Ofatumumab (Anti-CD20)[18]

Biological Activity	Ofatumumab	Rituximab
Apparent affinity (ng/mL)	EC$_{50}$: 287 ± 13.0 ng/mL	ND
Epitope	Discontinuous epitope binding to small and large loop not contain A170xP172	Linear epitope binding to large loop containing A170xP172
CDC	++	+
ADCC	+	+
Translocation into Lipid Rafts	+	+
Apoptosis	-	+/-
SCID mouse tumor model	++	+

ADCC: Antibody-dependent cellular cytotoxicity.   CDC: Complement-dependent cytotoxicity.   ND: Not determined.   SCID: Severe combined immune deficiency.
+: Positive.   ++: Stronger than +.   +/-: Positive in some cell lines and negative in some cell lines.   -: Negative.

Overview of *in vivo* Activities

❖ Mouse xenograft model
- Human Z138 NHL (MCL) xenograft SCID mice model (Figure 4A).[19]
- B-cell lymphoblastic tumor (Ramos tumor cells) nude mice xenograft model (Figure 4B).[20]

❖ Cynomolgus monkey
- B lymphocyte depletion study in peripheral blood and lymph node (Figure 5 and Table 3).[16]

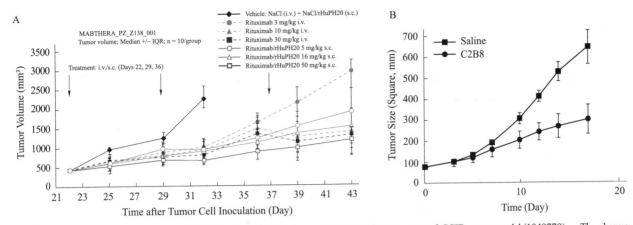

(A) Anti-tumor efficacy of i.v. and s.c. rituximab formulations in the human Z138 NHL (MCL) xenograft SCID mouse model (1049779) . The pharmacodynamic effects of the s.c. rituximab formulation (containing rHuPH20) was compared to those of rituximab administered i.v. in a xenograft model implanting Z138 mantel cell lymphoma cells into female SCID beige mice (n = 10/group). Animals were treated with s.c. and i.v. doses giving rise to similar rituximab trough levels (5, 16 and 50 mg/kg s.c. corresponding to 3, 10 and 30 mg/kg i.v., respectively) on Days 22, 29 and 36 after tumor cell inoculation. The applied s.c. rituximab formulation contained 4,600 U/mL rHuPH20 in 0.9% saline and the injection was performed s.c.. The treatment effects on tumor growth are shown in the figure above. (B) The tumoricidal impact of C2B8 in a mouse xenographic model utilizing a B-cell lymphoblastic tumor (Ramos cell line).

Figure 4 *In Vivo* Activities Studies of Rituximab in Mice Xenograft Model[19, 20]

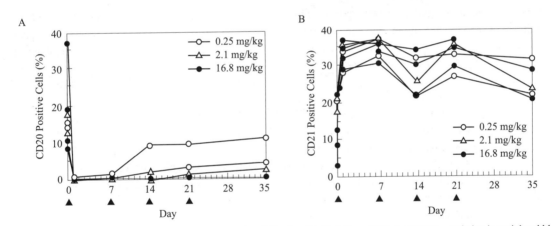

(A) Alterations in the proportion of B Cells (CD20+) in peripheral blood. (B) Variation of T Cells (CD2+) population in peripheral blood.

Figure 5 B Lymphocyte Depletion Study of Peripheral Blood and Lymph Nodes of Cynomolgus Monkeys[16]

Table 3 The Proportion of B Lymphocytes and T Lymphocytes in the Lymph Nodes and Bone Marrow[16]

	Group	Observation Date	T Lymphocytes (CD2+) %	B Lymphocytes (CD20+) %	B Lymphocytes Decrease Rate
Lymph nodes	Saline solution	Day 29	52.1	39.5	0.0
	16.8 mg/kg	Day 22, Male & female	90.0	5.3	86.6
			91.0	6.3	84.1
		Day 36, Male & female	89.9	5.0	87.4
			85.4	12.3	68.9
Bone marrow	Saline solution	Day 29	29.8	16.6	0.0
	16.8 mg/kg	Day 22, Male & female	46.7	4.3	74.1
			41.8	3.0	81.9
		Day 36, Male & Female	35.3	0.80	95.2
			25.6	4.4	73.5

5 Toxicology

Summary[15]

Toxicity

❖ Rituximab has been shown to be highly specific to the CD20 antigen on B cells. No effect other than the expected pharmacological depletion of B cells in peripheral blood as well as in lymphatic tissues was observed in toxicity studies. The B-cell population showed reconstitution after cessation of treatment. Significantly, adverse reactions unrelated to the targeted effect were seen, neither in single-nor in multiple-dose studies in the Cynomolgus monkey.

Non-clinical Single-Dose Toxicity

❖ Rituximab did not show any intrinsic toxicity when given as a single intraperitoneal injection to 5 mice (108 mg/kg) and 2 guinea pigs (66 mg/kg) as the pharmacologically non-responsive species. The results are not considered instructive for the safety characterisation of rituximab.

❖ In Cynomolgus monkeys, B-cell depletion in the peripheral blood (along with gradual depletion in peripheral lymphatic tissues) could be induced with a single i.v. injection using a dose of 0.4 and 6.5 mg/kg, with only marginal recovery by Day 35. No signs and symptoms of acute adverse reactions were observed. In a single high-dose experiment with doses of 10, 30 and 100 mg/kg (= 1,345 mg/m^2), rituximab was systemically and locally well tolerated, with only a mild transient decrease of platelets observed after dosing in the 30 and 100 mg/kg dose groups. The only adverse event involved one male monkey, which vomited one day after dosing in the 100 mg/kg dose group. Thus, serious dose limiting toxicity was not observed, even though the doses used in this study are far above a therapeutically effective dose in monkeys as well as the anticipated clinical dose.

Non-clinical Repeated-Dose Toxicity

❖ A repeated pilot pharmacology/toxicology experiment in Cynomolgus monkeys (using 16.8 mg/kg doses) demonstrated the relationship between exposure of multiple injections of rituximab to the degree of B-cell depletion in the peripheral blood and bone marrow, as well as within the lymphatic tissues. This experiment formed the basis for the initial dose escalating study in humans. Weekly dose of rituximab up to 20 mg/kg (= 276 mg/m^2) was generally well tolerated over up to 8 weeks of treatment in a further GLP toxicity study in Cynomolgus monkeys. Occasional emesis was also observed in these experiments.

❖ In addition, high plasma levels of rituximab, ranging from 137 to 438 mcg/mL were achieved in all animals 24 h after the first and second dose and persisted at significant levels (91-97 mcg/mL) during the treatment intervals.[12]

❖ An 8-week repeated-dose toxicity study was performed with the new s.c. formulation including the rHuPH20 excipient (2,000 IU/mL) to bridge to the previously performed i.v. studies with rituximab. A dose of 20 mg/(kg·week) rituximab s.c. was evaluated and the treatment period was followed by a 13-week recovery period. As in the previously submitted 8-week i.v. study, no toxicologically significant findings apart from the B-cell depletion were observed following s.c. administration of rituximab containing rHuPH20.[19]

Local Tolerance

❖ Rituximab was given in all preclinical safety studies as an i.v. injection, and the formulation was well tolerated locally. The formulation used in preclinical experiments was identical to the formulation to be marketed.

Non-clinical Immunotoxicity

❖ As described above, apart from the expected depletion of B cells, there was no other finding in clinical pathology and histopathology. Particularly, there was no evidence of toxicity to the hematopoietic system. T cells or other cells of the non-CD20+ lymphocyte lineage were not affected in any of the experiments. It does not affect the functionality of the pool of CD20 neg. antibody-producing plasma cells. However, specific experiments to demonstrate the difference between overall and B-cell specific immune-suppression have not been performed in preclinical studies. Rituximab's selectivity should result in a lower immunosuppressive potential (with lower risk and incidence of opportunistic infections). None of the rituximab-treated monkeys developed any signs of infections. No risk of neotransformation of B cells to lymphoma cells due to acute Epstein-Barr virus reactivation should be expected for rituximab. The risk for developing an immune or allergenic response under treatment of rituximab is very low. However, because rituximab does not deplete antibody-producing plasma cells, patients with an existing allergy to murine proteins should not be treated with rituximab.

Other Toxicology

❖ The monkey experiments do not provide any evidence that rituximab can fix complement and mediate ADCC *in vivo* other than a reduction in CD20 counts. Experimental proof that cell killing really occurs has not been provided. From a clinical point of view, further studies in healthy monkeys are not needed. The effects of rituximab in different B-cell populations are sufficiently documented. As pre-B cells and plasma cells do not express CD20 not all B-cell subpopulations are susceptible to the antibody.

❖ The lack of reproductive, mutagenic, genotoxic and carcinogenic studies is justified, and SPC has been amended appropriately. Findings of testicular hypospermatogenesis or aspermatogenesis and thymic lymphoid atrophy were reported in Study 204 and were analysed with respect to the negative results of the cross-reactivity studies with human tissues. Rituximab has no direct binding specificity or cytotoxicity to thymic or testicular tissue in cross-reactivity studies. The hypo- and aspermatogenesis was most likely due to sexual immaturity in the monkeys. Thymic atrophy was considered to be caused by experimental stress and is not a toxic effect of rituximab. In several studies the induction of antibodies (Monkey Anti-chimeric Antibodies) against the chimeric antibody MabThera® in Cynomolgus monkeys is reported. This is explained, as there are sequence differences between the monkey IgG and both parts of the chimeric antibody. The antigenicity of rituximab in such preclinical studies has no predictive value to humans.

Table 4   Summary Table Showing the Major Findings Made in the 8-week s.c. Repeated-Dose Toxicology Study Performed in Cynomolgus Monkeys[19]

Study ID	Species/Sex/No./Group	Dose/Route	Duration (Week)	NOAEL [mg/(kg·week)]	Major Finding
Report No. 1029890 GLP	Cynomolgus monkey 5 M/F Terminal Kill: 3 M/F Recovery Kill: 2 M/F	0, 20 mg/(kg·week), s.c.	Treatment: 8 Recovery: 13	20	20 mg/kg: B-cell depletion (Pharmacodynamic effect).

F: Female.   M: Male.   s.c.: Subcutaneous.

Table 5   Comparison of Rituximab Serum Trough Levels in the i.v. and s.c. 8-week Toxicity Studies with Rituximab in Cynomolgus Monkeys following Administration of 20 mg/(kg·week) Rituximab[19]

	Day 8 (1st Dosing Cycle)		Day 50 (7st Dosing Cycle)	
Study	Male	Female	Male	Female
i.v.	74.6-88.8 (80.9)	75.7-96.2 (87.7)	0.0-139 (84.5)	0.0-111 (64.7)
s.c.	111-120 (115)	99.0-120 (106)	<0.50-1.4 (0.28)	<0.50-274 (151)

Range and (mean) in μg/mL.   i.v.: Intravenous.   s.c.: Subcutaneous.

❖ Toxicokinetics

Table 6   Summary Table of the AUC Exposures Obtained in Cynomolgus Monkeys Negative for Anti-rituximab Antibodies Included in the 8-week s.c. Repeated-Dose Toxicity Study[19]

Study ID	Weekly Dose Rituximab (mg/kg)	Day	Animal AUC (ug·h/mL)	
			Male	Female
1029890	20	1	243,000	22,700
		43	6,590[a]	40,200[b]

[a] n = 1.   [b] n = 4.

❖ Interspecies comparison

Table 7   Summary Table Showing the Interspecies Comparison of Cynomolgus Monkey, Rabbit and Human[19]

Item	Cynomolgus Monkey	Rabbit	Patient[a]
Treatment duration	8 weeks	Single dose	Maximum of 2 years
Dosing frequency	Once weekly	Single dose	Once every 3 weeks for 8 cycles followed by a maintenance period of once every 2 months or once every 3 months
Dose	20 mg/kg corresponding to 240 mg/m²	60 mg, 20 mg/kg[b] corresponding to 240 mg/m²	1400 mg, 20 mg/kg, 736 mg/m²

Continued

Item	Cynomolgus Monkey	Rabbit	Patient[a]
Reference	Report No. 1029890	Report No. 1031874	Pivotal Study BO22334
C_{max} (µg/mL) (mean of males and females)	Day 1: 202 Day 43: 196	ND	C_{max} (geometric mean) at Cycle 7 of the induction phase with dosing every 3 weeks: 237
$AUC_{0-169\,g}$ (µg·h/mL)	Mean AUC after dosing on Day 43 calculated for a 3 weeks exposure interval: 100,500	ND	AUC (geometric mean) at Cycle 7 of the induction phase with dosing every 3 weeks: 90,694
Margin of safety for mg/m²	0.30[a]	0.30[a]	-
Margin of safety for AUC at steady-state over a 3-week interval	1.1	NA	-

NA: Not available.   ND: Not determined.   [a] Based on a maximum expected s.c. dose of 1,400 mg rituximab for 70 kg patient with a body surface area of 1.9 m². [b] Based on a 3 kg rabbit.

6   Non-clinical Pharmacokinetic

❖ The preclinical pharmacokinetics of a monoclonal antibody is of lesser relevance as the results mainly depend of the isotype of the immunoglobulin, and specific metabolic and excretory studies are not required.   Due to the binding to cellular CD20 and lysis of normal and malignant cells, plasma pharmacokinetics are influenced by the number of target cells and will depend on the size of the B lymphocyte pool at a given time point.   It may be anticipated that PK values will be different after first and subsequent doses because of the B-cell depleting effect.   In animal studies the development of antibodies to rituximab may influence the interpretation of multiple dose kinetics.   Different compartments of B lymphoid tissue may be targeted more or less easily.   Finally the kinetics of B-cell in Cynomolgus monkey and man may be different.

❖ Single-dose pharmacokinetics was performed in rats and Cynomolgus monkeys.   In both species $t_{1/2}$ was 3-7 days.   Serum concentrations increase dose-dependently in Cynomolgus monkeys.   Sex difference was also observed and could not be explained.   Multiple-dose kinetics was assessed in the Cynomolgus monkey toxicity studies.   Only C_{max} data are available suggesting that the exposure levels in the toxicity studies were similar to those attained in humans.

❖ Formal studies on absorption, metabolism and excretion are not needed.   Biodistribution was not studied, however it is clear that the antibody penetrates the lymphoid tissues.   It may also cross the placenta and deplete embryonic B cells.   It is not known whether rituximab is present in the milk.[12]

❖ Both SCID mice and Cynomolgus monkeys have been used in support of the original MAA for the i.v. formulation of rituximab via inclusion in pharmacodynamic and toxicity studies, respectively.   Rituximab shows affinity for Cynomolgus monkey CD20 and depletion of Cynomolgus monkey B cells has been demonstrated following both i.v. and s.c. administration of 10 mg/kg rituximab.

❖ An overview of the conducted studies is given in Table 8 below.

Table 8   The Pharmacokinetic Studies Performed in Support of the Current Extension Application[19]

Species and Strain	Route of Administration	Rituximab Doses (mg/kg)	rHuPH20 Doses (IU/ML)	Study No. (Report No.)
Beige SCID mouse	i.v.	30	-	1049704
	s.c.	30	6,000	
Cynomolgus monkey	s.c.	20	6,000	1036535
Gottingen minipig	i.v.	10	-	1029903
	s.c.	14, 28	2,650, 7,170	

❖ In the mouse study, 30 mg/kg rituximab with 6,000 IU/mL rHuPH20 was administered s.c..   Furthermore, a Cynomolgus monkey pharmacokinetic study applying s.c. administration of 20 mg/kg rituximab in a formulation with 6,000 IU/mL rHuPH20 was performed.   The results are summarized in Table 9 and 10 below.

Table 9   The Pharmacokinetic Parameters for Rituximab following i.v. and/or s.c. Administration to Mice and Monkeys[19]

Report No.	Species	N	Doses (mg/kg)	Route	C_{max} (μg·h/mL)	T_{max} (h)	AUC (μg·h/mL)
1049704	Beige SCID mouse	2/time/point/dose	30	i.v.	828	-	122,000
	Beige SCID mouse (female)			s.c.	300	2	76,700
1036353	Cynomolgus monkey (male)	3	20	s.c.	300	24	64,700

Table 10   The Pharmacokinetic Parameters for Rituximab following i.v. and/or s.c. Administration to Mice and Monkeys[19]

Report No.	Species	N	Doses (mg/kg)	Route	$t_{1/2}$, el (h)	V_{ss} (L/Kg)	CL^a [mL/(min·kg)]	F (%)
1049704	Beige SCID mouse	2/time point/ dose route	30	i.v.	217	0.075	0.0041	-
				s.c.	202		0.0065	62.9
1036353	Cynomolgus monkey (male)	3	20	s.c.	53.0-64.6 (329)^b	-	0.0050	-

i.v.: Intravenous.   s.c.: Subcutaneous. ^{a} CL s.c.: CL/F, tabulated in mL/min, CL i.v.: CL. ^{b} The variability of $t_{1/2}$ was large, where one animal showed $t_{1/2}$ of 329 h whereas the remaining two animals were in the range of 53.0-64.6 h.

7   Clinical Efficacy and Safety

Overview Profile[21-27]

❖ Non-Hodgkin's Lymphoma (NHL)
- In December 1997, rituximab was first approved and launched in the US and Switzerland for relapsed or refractory, low-grade or follicular B-cell NHL.
- In June 1998, EU approval as a second-line monotherapy for relapsed or refractory, low-grade or follicular B-cell NHL.
- In September 2001, rituximab was launched in Japan for the indication above.
- In August 2004, EU approval was extended to include first-line treatment of indolent NHL, in combination with conventional chemotherapy.
- In February 2006, the FDA approved rituximab in intermediate or aggressive front-line diffuse large B-cell NHL, in combination with CHOP or other anthracycline-based chemotherapy regimens.
- In September 2006, the FDA approved rituximab for first-line treatment of previously untreated follicular NHL in combination with CVP chemotherapy, and for the treatment of low-grade NHL.
- In July 2006, EU approval was granted for rituximab maintenance therapy for relapsed or refractory follicular NHL.
- In October 2010, the EMA approved the drug as a maintenance treatment in patients with advanced follicular lymphoma who responded to initial treatment with Rituxan® plus chemotherapy (induction treatment).
- In January 2011, the FDA approved the drug as a maintenance treatment in patients with advanced follicular lymphoma who responded to initial treatment with Rituxan® plus chemotherapy (induction treatment).
- In Japan, rituximab was also approved for CD20-positive B-cell lymphoma, B-cell lymphoproliferative disorder.
❖ Rheumatoid Arthritis (RA)
- In April 2006, rituximab was launched in the US for RA patients who inadequately respond to an anti-TNF therapy.
- In February 2007, launches had commenced in the EU for RA indication mentioned above.
- In December 2007, the drug had been additionally approved for RA in patients who inadequately respond to an anti-TNF therapy in the US and EU.
- In July 2010, rituximab had been approved in the US to treat patients with RA who were DMARD inadequate responders.
- In EU, rituximab had been approved for patients who have had an inadequate response to MTX, and for the prevention of joint damage across all populations according to the positive results from the IMAGE, SERENE and MIRROR trials.
❖ Chronic Lymphocytic Leukemia (CLL)
- In February 2009, EU approval was granted for rituximab in combination with chemotherapy for previously untreated CLL.
- In September 2009, EU approval was granted for rituximab in combination with chemotherapy for relapsed or refractory CLL.
- In February 2010, rituximab in combination with chemotherapy was approved in the US for treatment-experienced or

treatment-naive CLL.

❖ Granulomatosis with Ployangiitis (GPA) (Wegener's Granulomatosis) and Microscopic Polyangiitis (MPA) and other indications
   • In April 2011, the FDA approved rituximab in combination with corticosteroids for Wegener's granulomatosis and microscopic polyangiitis, two severe forms of ANCA-associated vasculitis.
   • In April 2013, rituximab was approved for ANCA-associated vasculitis in the EU.
   • In December 2014, the drug had been approved in Japan for antineutrophil cytoplasmic antibody (ANCA)-associated vasculitis.
   • In December 2014, the drug had been approved in Japan for steroid-dependent refractory nephritic syndrome.

Ongoing Development in Other Indications

❖ Ocrelizumab is a humanized monoclonal antibody from rituximab developed by Roche, and designed to selectively target CD20-positive B cells.   In 2016, US FDA grants Breakthrough Therapy Designation in primary progressive multiple sclerosis (MS).

❖ In January 2016, a Phase 3 study for thyroid eye disease was initiated.

❖ In May 2015, a Phase 3 study was initiated for pemphigus vulgaris.   At that time, the study was expected to complete in March 2019.

❖ In March 2014, Roche has also developed a subcutaneous formulation that received EU approval for DLBCL and FL.

❖ In August 2013, in Japan, Zenyaku Kogyo was investigating the drug for ITP and acquired thrombotic thrombocytopenic purpura (TTP).

❖ In July 2005, a Phase 3 SLE trial had begun, but the trial failed to meet its primary endpoint.

❖ In April 2004, a Phase 2/3 trial in ulcerative colitis began in the UK; however, no development in the indication had been reported by February 2006.

Phase 1 Trials

Table 11   The Profile of Phase 1 Clinical Trials of Rituximab[24, 25, 28]

ID	Phase	N	Population	Design	Study Posology	Endpoint
NCT00501748[a]	1	20	Neuromyelitis optica	Open, single arm	Two cycles at Month 1 and 9, Each cycle consists of two 1,000 mg infusions administered two weeks apart	Safety, efficacy
NCT00255593[a]	1	140	Renal transplantation	Randomized, double-blind, parallel assignment	ND	Safety, efficacy
NCT00930514[a]	1	281	Lymphoma, follicular	Open-label, parallel assignment	i.v. 375 mg/m^2; s.c. 1,400 mg; s.c. 375, 625, 800 mg/m^2	Pharmacokinetics
NCT0003649[a]	1/2	24	Systemic lupus erythematosus	Open, single arm	Four weekly infusions of rituximab at a dose of 375 mg/m^2	Safety, efficacy
NCT00101829[a]	1	12	Sjogren's syndrome	Open, single arm	1,000 mg intravenous infusion at study entry and at Week 2	Safety
102-01	1/2	15	B-cell lymphoma	Single dose, single agent	10-500 mg/m^2	Safety, efficacy
102-02	1/2	47	B-cell lymphoma	Multiple dose, single agent	125-375 mg/m^2	Safety, efficacy

i.v.: Intravenous.   s.c.: Subcutaneous.   [a] ClinicalTrials.gov Identifier.

Phase 2 Trials

❖ Clinical Trials for NHL

Table 12 The Profile of Phase 2 Clinical Trials of Rituximab in B-cell Lymphoma[29]

ID	Phase	N	Population	Design	Study Posology	Endpoint
102-01	1/2	15	B-cell lymphoma	Single dose Single agent	10-500 mg/m²	Safety, efficacy
102-02[a]	1/2	47	B-cell lymphoma	Multiple dose Single agent	125-375 mg/m²	Safety, efficacy
102-03	2	40	Low-grade or follicular B-cell lymphoma	Open, uncontrolled	375 mg/m² combined with CHOP 6 doses on Days 1, 6, 48, 90, 134, 141	Safety, efficacy
102-06	2	20	Relapsed low-grade or follicular B-cell lymphoma	Open, uncontrolled	Single agent, 375 mg/m² 1 dose/week for 8 doses	Safety, efficacy
102-07	2	0	Relapsed low-grade or follicular B-cell lymphoma	Open, uncontrolled	Combined with interferon α 375 mg/m² 1 dose/week for 4 doses	Safety, efficacy
102-08	2	10	Relapsed low-grade or follicular B-cell lymphoma	Open, uncontrolled	Single agent, 375 mg/m² 1 dose/week for 4 doses	Safety, efficacy

CHOP: Chemotherapy (cyclophosphamide, doxorubicin, vincristine, prednisolone). [a] Supporting study provide evidence for NHL indication.

❖ Clinical Trials for CLL

Table 13 The Profile of Phase 2 Clinical Trials of CLL[28, 30]

ID	Phase	N	Population	Design	Study Posology	Endpoint
NCT00452374[a]	2	48	PLL, or refractory/relapsed B-cell chronic lymphocytic leukemia (CLL)	Open-label, single group assignment	375 mg/m² i.v. on Day 3 of the first cycle over 4-6 h and on Day 1 on every cycle following.	Safety, efficacy
NCT00472849[a]	2	92	CLL or prolymphocytic leukemia, or Richter's transformation	Open-label, single group assignment	Rituximab 375 mg/m² i.v. on Day 3, course 1 (on Day 1, subsequent courses).	Safety, efficacy
NCT01082939[a]	2	80	CLL who have already been treated with chemotherapy	Open label, single group assignment	Cycle 1 (Week 1): 375 mg/(m²·day) i.v. on Day 2 over 4-6 h. Cycle 2-6 (Week 1): 500 mg/(m²·day) i.v. on Day 2 over 4-6 h.	Efficacy
NCT00525603[a]	2	60	High-risk previously untreated patients with CLL	Open-label, single group assignment	375 mg/(m²·day) 2 i.v. 4-6 h.	Safety, efficacy, CR, nPR, PR
NCT00074282[a]	2	110	Relapsed or refractory B-cell CLL	Open-label treatment	-	CR, nPR, PR
NCT00541034[a]	2	49	Previously untreated chronic lymphocytic leukemia	Open-label, single group assignment	Rituximab i.v. on Day 1 or on Days 1, 2.	Safety, efficacy

CLL: Chronic lymphocytic leukemia. CR: Complete remission. nPR: Nodular partial remission. PLL: Prolymphocytic leukemia. PR: Partial remission. [a] ClinicalTrials.gov Identifier.

❖ Clinical Trials for GPA and MPA

Table 14　The Profile of Phase 2 Clinical Trials of Rituximab in GPA and MPA[22]

ID	Phase	N	Population	Design	Study Posology	Endpoint
RAVE/ ITN021AI	2/3	197	WG or MPA	Randomized, double-blind, active-control, parallel group	Experimental: 375 mg/m^2 × 4 weekly doses; Control: Oral CYC 2 mg/(kg·day) for 3-6 months (+ placebo-rituximab)	BVAS/WG, ESR CRP et al.
RITUXVAS	2	44	Necrotizing glomerulonephritis	Open-label, two-group	i.v. methylprednisolone + oral glucocorticoid with or without rituximab 375 mg/m^2 weekly for 4 weeks[b]	Sustained remission[a]

BVAS/WG: Birmingham vasculitis activity score/wegener's granulomatosis.　CRP: C-reactive protein.　ESR: Erythrocyte sedimentation rate.　[a] Defined as a BVAS score of 0 that was maintained for at least 6 months.　[b] Both groups received 1 g i.v. methylprednisolone and the same oral glucocorticoid regimen (initially 1 mg/(kg·day), reduced to 5 mg/day at 6 months).　Patients were randomized 3:1 to receive rituximab 375 mg/m^2 weekly for 4 weeks, plus i.v. CYC 15 mg/kg with the first and third rituximab infusions, or i.v. CYC pulse (15 mg/kg every 2 to 3 weeks, for 3 to 6 months) followed by AZA (2 mg/(kg·day)).

Table 15　Tabular Overview of Clinical Studies of Rituximab in AAV[22]

Study	N	Patient Population	Concomitant Therapy	Study Design and Treatment Arm	Primary Endpoint
Uncontrolled Studies and Case Series					
Aries et al. 2006	8	WG with granulomatous manifestations refractory to standard therapy	CYC, MMF, MTX, GC	RTX 375 mg/m^2 every 4 weeks × 4	Remission defined as BVAS = 0. Indicating absence of signs of new/worse disease activity + persistent activity for ≤1 item.
Brihaye et al. 2007	8	Refractory WG	GC, IS	RTX 375 mg/m^2 every 4 weeks × 4	Remission defined as BVAS 2003 = 0.
Eriksson et al. 2005	9	Therapy-resistant or frequently relapsing ANCA-positive vasculitis (7 with WG and 2 with MPA)	MMF, AZA, CYC	RTX 500 mg weekly × 4 (n = 6) RTX 500 mg weekly × 2 (n = 3)	Complete remission (BVAS 1994 = 0) at 6 months after start of RTX.
Jones et al. 2009	65	Refractory AAV (46 with WG, 10 with MPA, 5 with CSS and 4 unclassified)	GC, Anti-TNF, AZA, MTX, MMF, CYC	RTX 1 g × 2, 2 weeks apart (n = 32) RTX 375 mg/m^2 weekly × 4 (n = 26)	Complete remission defined as absence of disease signs and symptoms, using the DEI, with reduction in GC.
Keogh et al. 2005	11	Severe, refractory, active AAV (10 with WG and 1 with MPA)	Plasma exchange for nephritis, GC	RTX 375 mg/m^2 weekly × 4	Complete remission defined as BVAS/WG = 0.
Keogh et al. 2006	10	Severe, active AAV refractory to CYC	GC	RTX 375 mg/m^2 weekly × 4	Complete remission defined as BVAS/WG = 0. Stable remission defined as BVAS/WG for >6 months[a].
Lovric et al. 2009	15	Refractory and relapsing AAV (13 with WG, 1 with MPA, 1 with CSS)	AZA, MMF, CYC, CsA, MTX, IFX, GC	RTX 375 mg/m^2 weekly × 4	Partial remission (reduction in BVAS 1994 >50.0%) or complete remission (BVAS 1994 = 0)[a].
Omdal et al. 2005	3	Refractory WG	GC, MTX	RTX 375 mg/m^2 weekly × 4	Remission assessed via chest radiographs, lab parameters (proteinuria, ANCA, ESR)[a].
Sanchez-Cano et al. 2008	4	Refractory WG	CYC, GC, MTX	RTX 375 mg/m^2 weekly × 4	Remission monitored using BVAS/WG[a].
Seo et al. 2008	8	Refractory, limited WG	CYC, GC	RTX 375 mg/m^2 weekly × 4	Remission monitored through sign and symptom resolution[a].
Smith et al. 2006	11	Refractory AAV (5 with WG and 5 with MPA)	MMF, GC, AZA, CYC	RTX 375 mg/m^2 weekly × 4	Complete remission defined as BVAS = 0. Partial remission defined as reduction in baseline BVAS by 50.0%[a].
Stasi et al. 2006	10	Refractory AAV (8 with WG and 2 with MPA)	GC	RTX 375 mg/m^2 weekly × 4	Complete remission defined as BVAS/WG = 0[a].

AAV: ANCA-associated vasculitis.　AZA: Azathioprine.　BVAS: Birmingham vasculitis activity score.　CsA: Cyclosporine.　CYC: Cyclophosphamide.　GC: Glucocorticosteroids.　IFX: Infliximab.　IS: Immunosuppressants.　MMF: Mycophenolate mofetil.　MPA: Microscopic polyangiitis.　MTX: Methotrexate.　RTX: Rituximab.　WG: Wegener's granulomatosis.　[a] Some of the investigator-initiated trials do not clearly define primary efficacy endpoints.

❖ Clinical Trials for RA

Table 16   The Profile of Phase 2 Clinical Trials of Rituximab in RA[28, 29]

ID	Phase	N	Population	Design	Study Posology	Endpoint
WA17043 (DANCER) NCT00074438[a]	2[b]	465	RA who had responded inadequately to DMARDs	Randomized, double-blind, double-dummy, controlled	MabThera® (2 × 1,000 mg vs. 2 × 500 mg + MTX 10-25 mg/week	ACR20 response at Week 24.
WA16291[b] NCT02693210[a]	2[a]	161	RA who had responded inadequately to DMARDs	Randomized, double-blind, parallel assignment	MabThera® (2 × 1 infusions) + CTX 2 × 750 mg i.v. or + oral MTX 10-25 mg/week	ACR50 response at Week 24, safty.

ACR: American college of rheumatology.   DMARDs: Disease-modifying anti-rheumatic drugs.   MTX: Methotrexate.   RA: Rheumatoid arthritis.   [a] ClinicalTrials.gov Identifier.   [b] Extension study protocol WA16855 for WA16291 and DANCER.

Phase 3 Trials

Table 17   The Profile of Phase 3 Clinical Trials of Rituximab[28, 31]

ID	Phase	N	Population	Design	Study Posology	Endpoint	
						Primary	Secondary
Trials for Indication: NHL							
102-05[a]	3 (pivotal)	166	Relapsed low-grade or follicular B-cell lymphoma	Open, randomized	375 mg/m², 1/week for 4 dose	ORR, TTP, PF	Safty
LNH98-5 (GELA)	3	400	Etude des lymphomes de l'Adulte (GELA)	Randomized, open-label, parallel group	1: Standard CHOP; 2: Rituximab 375 mg/m² plus standard CHOP (R-CHOP)[b]	EFS	DFS, OS, SD, PD, TTP, PF, safty
ECOG 4494	3	630	Diffuse large B-Cell lymphoma (DLBCL)	Randomized, open-label, parallel group	R-CHOP vs. CHOP with a second randomization to maintenance rituximab (MR)[c]	EFS	DFS, OS, SD, PD, TTP, PF, safty
M39021	3	318	Previously untreated patients with follicular NHL	Randomized, open-label, parallel group	8 cycles of CVP with or without rituximab 375 mg/m² on Day 1 of each 21-day cycle[d].	TTF	TTP, PF, safty, CR, Cru, PR, SD, OS
Trials for Indication: CLL							
ML17102 NCT00281918[e]	3 (pivotal)	810	Patients with previously untreated CLL	Randomized, parallel group	407 patients treated with FC; 403 patients treated with R-FC	PFS	OS, EFS, DFS, ORR, CR, PR, QoL, safty
BO17072 NCT00090051[e]	3 (pivotal)	552	Relapsed/refractory CD20-positive CLL	Open-label, comparative, parallel group, two-arm	In R-FC: Cycle 1: 375 mg/m²; Cycles 2-6: 500 mg/m² on Day 1	PFS	OS, EFS, DFS, safty
Trials for Indication: RA							
WA17042 (REFLEX)[f] NCT00468546[e]	3 (pivotal)	517	RA patients inadequate response or intolerance to one or more TNF inhibitor therapies	Randomized, double-blind, parallel group	i.v., 2 × 1,000 mg MABTHERA an interval of 15 days + i.v., 100 mg methylprednisone + oral MTX 10-25 mg/week	ACR20 response at Week 24	ACR20 response at 56 weeks, DAS28, EULAR responses, HAQ-DI, SF-36, HRQoL, FACIT-F, ESR, CRP, Safty

Continued

ID	Phase	N	Population	Design	Study Posology	Endpoint Primary	Endpoint Secondary
WA17047 (IMAGE) NCT00299104[e]	3 pivotal for indications extension	755	MTX naïve patients early in the disease course	Randomized, double-blind, parallel group	0.5 g × 2 vs. 1.0 g × 2 + MTX	Radio-graphic progression at Week 52	JSN, ACR50/70 response at Week 52, CRP, HAQ-DI et al.
WA17045 (SERENE) NCT00299130[e]	3 pivotal for indications extension	511	MTX-IR	Randomized, double-blind, parallel group placebo-controlled	Rituximab 2 × 0.5 g + MTX; Rituximab 2 × 1.0 g + MTX; placebo + MTX;	ACR20 response at 24 Weeks	ACR50/70 response at Week 24, CRP, HAQ-DI, SF-36 et al.
MIRROR (WA17044) NCT00422383[e]	3	378	MTX and anti-TNF-IR patients	Randomized, double-blind, parallel group	1: 500 mg i.v. on Days 1, 15 ,168, 182; 2: 500 mg i.v. on Days 1, 15, and 1,000 mg i.v. on Days 168, 182; 3: 1,000 mg i.v. on Days 1, 15, 168, 182	ACR20 response at 48 Weeks	ACR50/70 response at 48 weeks, DAS28-ESR, DAS28, SF-36 et al.
SUNRISE (U3384g) NCT00266227[e]	3	559	Anti-TNF-IR patients	Randomized, double-blind, placebo-controlled	Re-treatment during weeks 24-40 with or without 1,000 mg rituximab	ACR20 response at 48 weeks	ACR50/70 response at 48 weeks, DAS28-ESR, DAS28, SF-36 et al.

Trials for Indication: Vasculitis

ID	Phase	N	Population	Design	Study Posology	Endpoint Primary	Endpoint Secondary
RAVE	2/3	197	ANCA-associated vasculitis	Randomized, active-controlled, double-blind, double-dummy, parallel group	Experimental: 375 mg/m² × 4 weekly doses; Control: Oral CYC 2 mg/(kg·day) for 3-6 months (+placebo-rituximab)[g]	BVAS/WG[h]	Partial remission, ratio of patients who achieved BVAS/WG of 0 ESR, CRP et al.

Treatment failure defined as any of the following five events, 1) disease progression, 2) relapse after response, 3) institution of new lymphoma treatment during or after the randomized treatment phase, 4) stable disease after cycle 4 (SD4) or 5) death from any cause. ACR: American college of rheumatology. BVAS/WG: Birmingham vasculitis activity Score/Wegener's granulomatosis. CHOP: Chemotherapy. CR: Complete response. CRP: C-reactive protein. Cru: CR unconfirmed. CVP: Cyclophosphamide, vincristine and prednisone. DAS: Disease activity score. DFS: Disease-free survival. DLBCL: Diffuse large B-cell lymphoma. EFS: Event-free survival, defined as time from randomization date to relapse, progression, change to new therapy, or death from any cause. ESR: Erythrocyte sedimentation rate. EULAR: European league against rheumatism. FACIT-F: Functional assessment of chronic illness therapy-fatigue. FC: Fludarabine and cyclophosphamide. GELA: Groupe d'Etudes des lymphomes de l'Adulte. HAQ-DI: Health assessment questionnaire-disability index. HRQoL: Health related quality of life. MTP: Maintenance treatment program. MTX: Methotrexate. MTX-IR: Methotrexat inadequate response. NHL: Non-Hodgkin's lymphoma. ORR: Overall response rate. OS: Overall survival. PD: Progressive disease. PF: Progression free. PR: Partial response. QoL: Quality of life. REC: Response evaluation committee. RFC: Rituximab in combination with fludarabine and cyclophosphamide. SD: Stable disease. SF: Short form. TNF: Tumor necrosis factor. TNF-IR: Tumor necrosis factor-inadequate response. TTF: Time to treatment failure. TTP: Time to disease progression. [a] Pivotal Phase 3 study for first approval indication. [b] MabThera® was given together with each of the chemotherapy cycles. [c] 2 infusions of MabThera® were given before chemotherapy and then given with every other cycle of chemotherapy. [d] CVP chemotherapy: (Cyclophosphamide 750 mg/m² i.v. on Day 1; vincristine 1.4 mg/m² i.v. (max. 2 mg) on Day 1; prednisolone 40 mg/m² p.o. on Days 1 to 5. [e] ClinicalTrials.gov Identifier. [f] Extension study protocol WA17531. [g] During induction treatment phase (Month 1-6). Add on to both Experimental/Control: 1 g i.v. pulse methyl-prednisolone patients could switch to the other study arm in case of treatment failure during maintenance treatment phase (Month 7-18). Experimental: AZA-PLACEBO (from Week 4 on). Control: AZA 2 mg/(kg·day) (from Month 3-6 on). Patients were treated with rituximab in case of relapse, in each study arm. [h] Was the percentage of patients who achieved complete remission at Month 6, defined as a BVAS/WG of 0 and successful completion of the glucocorticoid taper at Month 6.

Clinical Efficacy

❖ Efficacy for NHL

Table 18 Efficacy of Phase 3 Clinical Trials for First Approval for NHL[31]

Trial ID	Study Posology	Efficacy (Median) Study Population	OR (%), [95% CI]	CR Rate	PR Rate	Median Duration of Response (Month, range)	Median Time to Progression for Responders (Month, range)
102-05 (Pivotal, Phase 3)	Weekly dosing for 4 dose 375 mg/m²	ITT (n = 166)	80/166 (48.0%) [40.0%, 56.0%]	10/166 (6.0%)	70/166 (42.0%)	9.2+ (1.9-18.8+)	11.8+ (3.6-20.5+)
		Efficacy (n = 161)	80/161 (50.0%) [40.0%, 56.0%]	10/161 (6.0%)	70/161 (43.0%)	9.2+ (1.9-18.8+)	11.8+ (3.6-20.5+)

Continued

Trial ID	Study Posology	Study Population	OR (%), [95% CI]	CR Rate	PR Rate	Median Duration of Response (Month, range)	Median Time to Progression for Responders (Month, range)
		Evaluable for efficacy (n = 151)	76/151 (50.0%) [42.0%, 59.0%]	9/151 (6.0%)	67/151 (44.0%)	9.1+ (1.9-18.8+)	11.8+ (3.6-20.5+)
102-02 (Supporting)	Weekly dosing for 4 dose 375 mg/m²	ITT (n = 37)	17 (46.0%)	3 (8.0%)	14 (38.0%)	8.6	10.2

CR: Complete response. OR: Overall response. PR: Partial response.

Table 19   Comparison of Response Rate and Duration to Most Recent Chemotherapy[24]

Population	Overall Response Rate	Complete Response Rate	Response Duration (Month)
Rituximab responders response to rituximab (n = 78)	78/161 (48.0%)	10/161 (6.0%)	9.2+
Rituximab responders response to prior chemotherapy (n = 78)	63/78 (81.0%)	41/78 (53.0%)	20.0
All patients with response to last chemotherapy (n = 117)	117/161 (73.0%)	60/161 (37.0%)	12.0

Table 20   Duration of Response, Based on the Number of Previous Chemotherapeutic Courses[31]

Prior ChemoTX Course	Overall Response Rate %, (n/N)	Complete Response Rate %, (n/N)	Median Duration of Response (Month)
0	40.0 (2/5)	0	8.6+
1	59.0 (30/51)	8.0 (4/51)	9.1+
2	31.0 (11/36)	6.0 (2/36)	9.8+
3	49.0 (24/49)	4.0 (2/49)	8.1+
≥4	52.0 (13/25)	8.0 (2/25)	9.2+
All	48.0 (80/166)	6.0 (10/166)	9.2+

❖ Efficacy for RA

Table 21   Efficacy of Phase 3 Clinical Trials for First Approval for RA[31]

Variable	MTX (N = 40)	Rit (N = 40)	Rit + CTX (N = 41)	Rit + MTX (N = 40)
Change in disease-activity score	-1.3 ± 1.2	-2.2 ± 1.4 (-1.5 to -0.31)	-2.6 ± 1.5 (-1.9 to -0.70)	-2.6 ± 1.3 (-1.9 to -0.72)[a]
Moderate or good EULAR response (%)	50.0	85.0[b]	85.0[c]	83.0[d]
Change in IgG (mg/mL)	-0.70 ± 3.1	-1.1 ± 2.6	-1.9 ± 2.2	-1.9 ± 3.1
Change in IgA (mg/mL)	-0.10 ± 0.72	-0.20 ± 0.74	-0.40 ± 0.42	-0.60 ± 0.70
Change in IgM (mg/mL)	-0.0 ± 0.37	-0.40 ± 0.37	-0.50 ± 0.30	-0.60 ± 0.72
Change in antitetanus antibody titre	-0.0 ± 0.60	-0.10 ± 0.50	-0.0 ± 0.40	-0.10 ± 0.60

Means ± SD, and values in parentheses are 95% confidence intervals for the difference in the mean change between the Rit and control group.   Changes from baseline in disease-activity score, rates of response according to EULAE criteria, and PD at Week 24.   CTX: Cyclophosphamide.   EULAR: European league against rheumatism. MTX: Methotrexate.   Rit: Rituximab.   [a] $P = 0.0020$ for the comparison with the MTX group.   [b] $P < 0.0010$ for the comparison with the MTX group   [c] $P = 0.0010$ for the comparison with the MTX group.   [d] $P = 0.0040$ for the comparison with the MTX group.

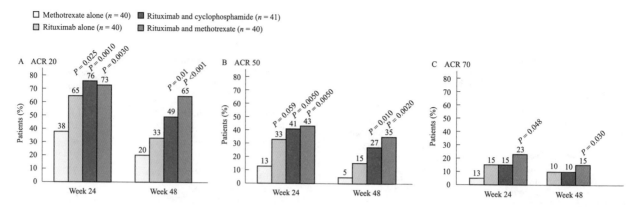

Figure 6　Median Levels of Peripheral CD19+ B cells and Median Changes in Levels of RF during the 24-Week Study Period[32]

❖ Refractory Nephrotic Syndrome

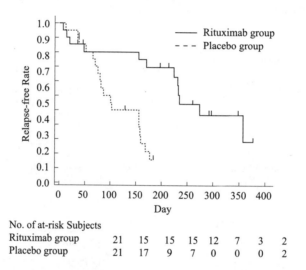

No. of at-risk Subjects

Rituximab group	21	15	15	15	12	7	3	2
Placebo group	21	17	9	7	0	0	0	2

Figure 7　Interim Analysis of Relapse-free Period[33]

Table 22　Efficacy of Phase 3 Clinical Trials for Refractory Nephrotic Syndrome[33]

	Placebo Group (*N* = 24)	Rituximab Group (*N* = 24)
No. of subjects who relapsed	23	17
Relapse-free period[a] (Day, median [95% *CI*])	101 [70.0, 155]	267 [223, 374]
Hazard ratio[b] [95% *CI*]	0.27 [0.14, 0.53]	
P-value[c]	<0.0010	

[a] Estimated by the Kaplan-Meier method.　[b] Estimated by the Cox proportional hazard model.　[c] Log-rank test, the one-sided significance level for the interim and final analyses was set to 0.25 and 2.25%, respectively, for adjustment of multiplicity.

Table 23　Efficacy of Phase 3 Clinical Trials for Refractory Nephrotic Syndrome[33]

Endpoit	Placebo Group (*N* = 24)	Rituximab Group (*N* = 24)	Hazard Ratio[a] (95% *CI*)	*P*-value
Time to treatment failure[b] (No. of cases)	163 days [70 days, 251 days] (20)	NR [287 days, NR] (10)	0.27 (0.12, 0.59)	<0.0010[c]
Incidence of relapse	4.2 times/(subject·year)	1.5 times/(subject·year)	-	<0.0010[d]

NR: Not reached.　[a] Estimated by the Cox proportional hazard model.　[b] Median (95% *CI*).　[c] Log-rank test.　[d] Sorting test.

❖ WG and MPA

Table 24 Efficacy of RAVE: Complete Remission at 6 Months after Randomization (ITT Population)[22]

	Rituximab (%)	Cyclophosphamide (%)	Difference in Rate	Two-sided 95.1% *CI* of Difference
N^a	99	98		
Complete remission (WCI)	63 (63.6)	52 (53.1)	10.6	-3.2, 24.3ᵃ *P* = 0.13 χ^2 test
95.1% *CI*	54.1, 73.2	43.1, 63.0		

The lower limit of the 95.1% *CI* for the difference, -3.2, was greater than 20 and thus met the protocol-specified non-inferiority criterion.   *CI*: Confidence interval.   ITT: Intent-to-treat.   RAVE: Rituximab in ANCA-associated vasculitis.   Source: RAVE CSR.   WCI: Worst case imputation.   ᵃ The lower limit of the 95.1% *CI* for the difference, -3.2 was greater than -20 and thus met the protocol-specified non-inferiority criterion.

Table 25 Efficacy of RAVE: Patients Who Had Complete Remission at 6 Months,
by Percentage of Protocol-defined Initial Dose Received[22]

Percentage of Protocol-defined Dose Received	*N*	No. (%) Patients Who Had Complete Remission at Month 6
≥80.0%	37	20 (54.1%)
65.0%-80.0%	31	18 (58.1%)
<65.0%	29	14 (48.3%)

The potocol-defined initial dose was adjusted for baseline weight and renal function only.   WBC count and other lab tests were not taken into account.   RAVE: Rituximab in ANCA-associated vasculitis.

Table 26 Efficacy of RAVE: Remission Rates according to Different Definitions of Prednisone Use
(Worst-case Imputation ITT Analyses)[22]

Time Point	Rituximab (*N* = 99)	Cyclophosphami (*N* = 98)	Difference (Two-sided 95.1% *CI*)
Complete Remission (%)			
6 months	63.6	53.1	10.6 (-3.2, 24.3)
12 months	47.5	38.8	8.7 (-5.1, 22.5)
18 months	39.4	32.7	6.7 (-6.6, 20.1)
BVAS of 0 on Prednisone Dose of <10 mg/(kg·day) (%)			
6 months	70.7	61.2	9.5 (-3.7, 22.7)
12 months	59.6	61.2	-1.6 (-15.3, 12.0)
18 months	54.5	53.1	1.5 (12.4, 15.4)
BVAS of 0 Irrespective of Prednisone Dose (%)			
6 months	78.8	63.3	15.5 (3.0, 28.0)
12 months	66.7	63.3	3.4 (-9.9, 16.7)
18 months	56.6	55.1	1.5 (-12.4, 15.3)

Defined as BVAS-WG = 0 and no GC use, *P <0.05.   RAVE: Rituximab in ANCA-associated vasculitis.

❖ CLL

Table 27 Efficacy of Phase 3 Clinical Trials for CLL (Trail ML17102)[30]

Endpoit		FC (*N* = 407)	R-FC (*N* = 403)
Event-free survival	Median (95% *CI*)	31.1 (25.3, 35.1)	39.8 (36.1, NR)
	P-value (long-rank)	<0.00010	
	Hazard ratio (adjusted, 95% *CI*)	0.55 (0.43, 0.70)	

Continued

Endpoit		FC (N = 407)	R-FC (N = 403)
Overall response rate	ORR	296 (72.7%)	347 (86.1%)
	P-value (Chi square)	<0.00010	
	CR	70 (17.2%)	145 (36.0%)
	PR	226 (55.5%)	202 (50.1%)
Molecular response	MRD-negative ORR	8.0% (n = 110)	18.0% (n = 74)
	MRD-negative CR	7.0% (n = 15)	25.0% (n = 24)
	MRD-negative PR[a]	8.0% (n = 95)	14.0% (n = 50)
Duration of response	DOR (n)	296	347
	Median (Month) (95% CI)	34.7 (29.5, 40.8)	40.2 (35.4, NR)
	P-value (log-Rank)	0.0040	
	Hazard ratio (adjusted, 95% CI)	0.61 (0.43, 0.85)	
Disease-free survival	DFS (n)	91	186
	Median (Month) (95% CI)	NR (NR, NR)	NR (30.9, NR)
	P-value (log-Rank)	0.79	
	Hazard ratio (adjusted, 95% CI)	0.93 (0.44, 2.0)	
Time to new treatment	Median (Month) (95% CI)	NR (NR, NR)	NR (NR, NR)
	P-value (log-Rank)	0.0052	
	Hazard ratio (adjusted, 95% CI)	0.65 (0.47, 0.90)	

CI: Confidence interval. CR: Complete response. DFS: Disease-free survival. DOR: Duration of response. EFS: Event-free survival. FC: Fludarabine and cyclophosphamide. MRD: Minimal residual disease. NR: Not reached. ORR: Overall response rate. PR: Partial response. R-FC: Rituximab in combination with fludarabine and cyclophosphamide. TTNT: Time to next treatment. [a] Includes nodular partial response (nPR).

Table 28　Efficacy of Phase 3 Clinical Trials for CLL (Trail BO17072)[34]

Efficacy		FC (N = 276)	R-FC (N = 276)
		n (%)	n (%)
Summary of composition of PFS (ITT)	Total number of events	158 (57.2)	132 (47.8)
	Death	25 (9.1)	30 (10.9)
	Progression	133 (48.2)	102 (37.0)
Summary of overall survival (ITT)	Patients with event	68 (24.6)	62 (22.5)
	Patients without event	208 (75.4)	214 (77.5)
	Time to event (Day)		
	Median[a]	1,580	
	95% CI for median	1,408	1,552
	25% and 75% ile	921	1,117
	Range	1-1,703	8-1,720
	P-value (log-Rank test)	0.29	
	Hazard ratio	0.83	
	95% CI	(0.59, 1.2)	
	P-value (Wald test)	0.29	
	2-year duration		
	No. left	141	154
	Event free rate	0.82	0.82
	95% CI for rate	(0.77, 0.87)	(0.77, 0.87)

CLL: Chronic lymphocytic leukaemia. FC: Fludarabine and cyclophosphamide. ITT: Intent-to-treat. R-FC: Rituximab in combination with fludarabine and cyclophosphamide. [a] Kaplan-Meier estimate.

Clinical Safety

Table 29　AEs Occuring in ≥10.0% of Subjects in Rit in Study 01 and All in Study 02 for Refractory Nephrotic Synbdrome[33]

	Rituximab Administration (N = 54)			Rituximab Administration (N = 54)	
	Incidence (%)	n		Incidence (%)	n
Total adverse events	100	54	Acne	16.7	9
Upper respiratory tract infection	61.1	33	Neutrophil count decreased	16.7	9
Lymphocyte count decreased	46.3	25	White blood cell count decreased	16.7	9
CRP increased	42.6	23	Influenza	14.8	8
Nasopharyngitis	31.5	17	Dyspnea	14.8	8
Gastroenteritis	25.9	14	Hordeolum	13.0	7
ALT increased	25.9	14	Arthropod sting	13.0	7
Hypertension	22.2	12	Impetigo	11.1	6
Hypoproteinemia	22.2	12	Oropharyngeal discomfort	11.1	6
Eosinophil count increased	22.2	12	Headache	11.1	6
Conjunctivitis	18.5	10	Atopic dermatitis	11.1	6
Eczema	18.5	10	Pruritus	11.1	6
Fever	16.7	9	Asteatotic eczema	11.1	6
Pharyngitis	16.7	9			

Table 30　AEs for 375mg/(m²·infusion) and 500 mg/infusion[33]

	Rituximab Administration (N = 54)		Rituximab Administration (N = 54)	
	Incidence (%)	n	Incidence (%)	n
Total AEs	100	35	100	19
Infection requiring therapy	94.3	33	84.2	16
Infusion reaction	57.1	20	73.7	14

AEs: Adverse events.

Table 31　Overview of AEs Rates for First Approval Clinical[29]

Protocol 102-05	AEs (%)	No. of Subjects Reporting Events	"Related" AEs (%)	No. Subjects Reporting "Related"AEs
Total	1,163	158	733	
During treatment	843/1,163 (72.0)	149	621/733 (85.0)	40
During follow-up	206/1,163 (18.0)	75	98/733 (13.0)	45
Pre-study/Unknown	110/1,163 (9.0)	63	14/733 (2.0)	7

AEs: Adverse events.

Table 32   All AEs W/All Grade 3/4 in Phase 3 Clinical Trail Approval for NHL (Protocol 102-05)[29]

Adverse Event by Organ System		Grade 3		Grade 4		ALL Grades	
		n	%	*n*	%	*n*	%
		36	12.8	7	2.5	263	93.3
General	Chills	6	2.1	0	0.0	98	34.8
	Headache	3	1.1	0	0.0	50	17.7
	Fever	-	-	-	-	152	53.9
Respiratory	Bronchospasm	4	1.4	0	0.0	29	10.3
	Increase in cough	1	0.40	0	0.0	24	8.5
	Dyspnea	2	0.70	0	0.0	12	4.3
Cardiovascular	Arrhythmia	1	0.40	1	0.40	5	1.8
	CPK increase (MI)	0	0.0	1	0.40	1	0.40
	Hypotension	1	0.40	1	0.40	29	10.3
	Angioedema	1	0.40	0	0.0	36	12.8
	Hypertension	1	0.40	0	0.0	13	4.6
Heme/Lymphatic system	Leukopenia	6	2.1	0	0.0	25	8.9
	Neutropenia	2	0.70	3	1.1	20	7.1
	Thrombocytopenia	3	1.1	2	0.70	26	9.2
	Anemia	4	1.4	0	0.0	13	4.6
Gastrointestinal	Nausea	2	0.70	0	0.0	66	23.4
	Pain (abdominal)	1	0.40	1	0.40	24	8.5
	Diarrhea	1	0.40	0	0.0	23	8.2
	Vomiting	1	0.40	0	0.0	31	11.0
Musculo-skeletal	Arthralgias	1	0.40	0	0.0	21	7.4
	Pain (back)	3	1.1	0	0.0	20	7.1
	Myalgia	-	-	-	-	20	7.1
Skin-appendages	Urticaria	3	1.1	0	0.0	22	7.8
	Pruritis	1	0.40	0	0.0	36	12.8
	Rash	1	0.40	0	0.0	32	11.3
Infectious disease	Infections	1	0.40	0	0.0	7	2.5
	Sinusitis	1	0.40	0	0.0	16	5.7
	Herpes simplex	1	0.40	0	0.0	12	4.3

AEs: Adverse events.   MI: Myocardial infarction.   NHL: Non-Hodgkin's lymphoma.

Table 33   Laboratory Abnormalities (Changes from Baseline) during Treatment Period in Study 102-05[29]

Laboratory Parameter	Change in Value by Toxicity Grade			
	Grade 1	Grade 2	Grade 3	Grade 4
Anemia	44/276 (31.0%)	4/276 (1.0%)	1/276 (<1.0%)	0
Leukopenia	86/276 (31.0%)	19/176 (7.0%)	0	0
Neutropenia	55/273 (20.0%)	18/273 (7.0%)	2/273 (<1.0%)	2/273 (<1.0%)
Platelet count	9/276 (3.0%)	4/276 (1.0%)	1/276 (<1.0%)	0
Lymphopenia	90/274 (33.0%)	27/274 (10.0%)	7/274 (3.0%)	2/274 (<1.0%)
Increased creatinine	8/273 (3.0%)	1/273 (<1.0%)	0	0
Increased SGOT	16/270 (6.0%)	2/270 (<1.0%)	0	0

Continued

Laboratory Parameter	Change in Value by Toxicity Grade			
	Grade 1	Grade 2	Grade 3	Grade 4
Increased SGPT	8/249 (3.0%)	0	0	0
Increased alkaline phosphatase	10/274 (4.0%)	1/274 (<1.0%)	0	0
Increased total bilirubin	1/273 (<1.0%)	7/273 (3.0%)	1/273 (<1.0%)	1/273 (<1.0%)

SGOT: Serum glutamic oxalacetic transaminase.   SGPT: Serum glutamic pyruvic transaminase.

Table 34   Laboratory Abnormalities (Changes from Baseline) during Follow-up Period in Study 102-05[29]

Laboratory Parameter	Change in Value by Toxicity Grade			
	Grade 1	Grade 2	Grade 3	Grade 4
Anemia	13/231 (6.0%)	2/231 (<1.0%)	1/231 (<1.0%)	0
Leukopenia	45/231 (19.0%)	16/231 (7.0%)	5/231 (2.0%)	0
Neutropenia	22/226 (10.0%)	15/273 (7.0%)	2/273 (<1.0%)	2/273 (<1.0%)
Platelet count	9/276 (3.0%)	4/276 (1.0%)	1/276 (<1.0%)	0
Lymphopenia	90/274 (33.0%)	27/274 (10.0%)	7/274 (3.0%)	2/274 (<1.0%)
Increased creatinine	8/273 (3.0%)	1/273 (<1.0%)	0	0
Increased SGOT	16/270 (6.0%)	2/270 (<1.0%)	0	0
Increased SGPT	8/249 (3.0%)	0	0	0
Increased alkaline phosphatase	10/274 (4.0%)	1/274 (<1.0%)	0	0
Increased total bilirubin	1/273 (<1.0%)	7/273 (3.0%)	1/273 (<1.0%)	1/273 (<1.0%)

SGOT: Serum glutamic oxalacetic transaminase.   SGPT: Serum glutamic pyruvic transaminase.

Table 35   Overview of AEs in Study ML17102 (SAP)[30]

	No. of Patients (%)	
	FC (N = 396)	R-FC (N = 397)
Grade 3 or 4 AEs	246 (62.0%)	304 (77.0%)
Serious AEs	162 (41.0%)	182 (46.0%)
AEs leading to treatment discontinuation	70 (18.0%)	71 (18.0%)
AEs leading to dose modification/interruption	80 (20.0%)	133 (34.0%)
Treatment-related death	8 (2.0%)	6 (2.0%)

AEs: Adverse events.   FC: Fludarabine and cyclophosphamide.   R-FC: Rituximab in combination with fludarabine and cyclophosphamide.

Table 36   Grade 3 or 4 AEs that Occurred with an at Least 2.0% Higher Incidence in One of the Treatment Arms[30]

	R-FC	FC
Higher Incidence in the R-FC Arm vs. the FC Arm		
Neutropenia	19.0%	30.0%
Leukopenia	12.0%	23.0%
Febrile neutrpenia	6.0%	9.0%
Pancytopenia	1.0%	3.0%
Higher Incidence in the FC Arm vs. the R-FC Arm		
Thrombocytopenia	10.0%	7.0%
Anaemia	7.0%	4.0%
Pyrexia	5.0%	3.0%

FC: Fludarabine and cyclophosphamide.   R-FC: Rituximab in combination with fludarabine and cyclophosphamide.

Table 37　Safety Summary of RAVE Study during 18 Months[21]

	Rituximab (N = 99)	CSA (N = 98)
Selected AEs		
Death (all causes)	33 (33.3%)	42 (42.9%)
Grade ≥2 leukopenia	2 (2.0%)	2 (2.0%)
Grade ≥2 thrombocytopenia	7 (7.1%)	23 (23.5%)
Grade ≥3 infections	4 (4.0%)	1 (1.0%)
Hemorrhagic cystitis	14 (14.1%)	14 (14.3%)
Malignancy	2 (2.0%)	1 (1.0%)
Venous thromboembolic event	2 (2.0%)	1 (1.0%)
Hospitalization related to disease activity or study	5 (5.1%)	8 (8.2%)
Therapy per the investigator's assessment	13 (13.1%)	5 (5.1%)
Cerebrovascular accident	0	0
Infusion reaction leading to study drug discontinuation	1 (1.0%)	0
Other AEs of special interest		
Infusion-related reaction	14 (14.1%)	12 (12.2%)
Any infection	79 (79.8%)	69 (70.4%)
Serious infection	15 (15.2%)	15 (15.3%)
Serious cardiac AEs	2 (2.0%)	2 (2.0%)

AEs: Adverse events.　CSA: Cyclophosphamide.

Table 38　Safety Summary of the Supportive Study Rituximab[22]

	Rituximab + Low-dose CSA (N = 33)	CSA (N = 11)
No. (%) of Patients Experiencing Any AE, n (%)		
Grade ≥3 AEs	25 (76.0)	7 (64.0)
SAEs	14 (42.0)	4 (36.0)
Selected Events of Special Interest, n (%)		
Death	6 (18.0)	2 (18.0)
Hospitalization	12 (36.0)	4 (36.0)
Infection	12 (36.0)	3 (27.0)
Serious infection	6 (18.0)	2 (18.0)
Malignancy	2 (6.0)[a]	0
Infusion reaction	2 (6.0)	0
Neutropenia	2 (6.0)	1 (9.0)
Anemia	2 (6.0)	2 (18.0)
Thrombocytopenia	1 (3.0)	0
Hypogammaglobulinemia	1(3.0)	0
AEs Rates/Patient-year (95% CI)		
Grade ≥3 AEs, %	1.0 (0.69-1.4)	1.1 (0.61-2.0)
Infections, %	0.66	0.60

AEs: Adverse events.　CI: Confidence interval.　CSA: Cyclophosphamide.　SAEs: Serious adverse events.　[a] One occurred after 12 months.

8   Clinical Pharmacokinetics

Summary

❖ Single-dose studies were conducted in Phase 1 and used to characterized the pharmacokinetic profile of rituximab[21, 35–37]
  • The mean half-life ($t_{1/2}$) of rituximab in the NHL patients receiving 100-500 mg/m² is 4.4 days, with a range from 1.6 to 10.5 days.
  • The mean half-life ($t_{1/2}$) of rituximab from different origin (EU or US) in the RA patients (1,000 mg doses) are 424 ± 125 h (EU) and 456 ± 145 h (US).
  • The mean V_{ss} of rituximab from EU or US in the RA patients receiving 1,000 mg doses are 5,590 ± 1,320 mL/kg and 5,810 ± 1,590 mL/kg, respectively.
  • The C_{max} of rituximab from EU or US in the RA patients receiving 1,000 mg doses are 422 ± 111 µg/mL and 430 ± 163 µg/mL, respectively.
  • The $AUC_{0-\infty}$ of rituximab from EU or US in the RA patients receiving 1,000 mg doses are 200,000 ± 74,600 µg·h/mL and 214,000 ± 95,300 µg·h/mL, respectively.

❖ The multi-dose studies were conducted in a number of clinical trials, various pharmacokinetic relationships were revealed. A fundamental conclusion of these studies is that the pharmacokinetics of rituximab are non-linear at clinically relevant doses due to: 1) saturation of elimination mechanisms; 2) interactions between rituximab with CD20-positive cells and 3) antibody degradation occurs by a non-specific catabolism of proteins which takes place in the liver and other organs and proteolytic cleavage products are eliminated by the renal route.[21, 22, 25, 38]
  • Non-Hodgkin's Lymphoma (NHL)
    ♦ The pharmacokinetic profile of NHL patients receiving 375 mg/m² q1w for 4 doses was similar to that in combination with CHOP chemotherapy for 6 doses.
    ♦ In patients receiving the 375 mg/m² dose, the mean serum half-life of rituximab was 68.1 h, the C_{max} was 238.7 µg/mL and the mean plasma clearance was 0.046 L/h after the first infusion; after the fourth infusion, the mean values for serum half-life and plasma clearance were 190 h and 0.015/h, respectively.
    ♦ The mean C_{max} following the fourth infusion was 486 µg/mL (range 77.5-997 µg/mL). C_{max} rise upon repeated dosing, about 2-3 folds accumulation on fourth-eighth infusion compared to the first infusion.
    ♦ Nonspecific clearance (CL_1), specific clearance (CL_2) and central compartment volume of distribution (V_1) were 0.14 L/day, 0.59 L/day, and 2.7 L, respectively.
    ♦ The estimated median terminal elimination half-life of rituximab was 22 days (range, 6.1-52 days).
    ♦ Patients with higher CD19-positive cell counts or tumor lesions had a higher CL_2.
    ♦ Age and gender had no effect for pre-treatment CD19 count or size of on the pharmacokinetics of rituximab.
  • Chronic Lymphocytic Leukemia (CLL)
    ♦ In CLL patients, the estimated median terminal half-life of rituximab was 32 days (range, 14-62 days).
    ♦ The mean C_{max} ($N = 15$) was 408 µg/mL (range, 97-764 µg/mL) after the fifth 500 mg/m² infusion.
  • Rheumatoid Arthritis (RA)
    ♦ Following administration of 2 doses of rituximab, concentrations after the first infusion (C_{max} first) and the second infusion (C_{max} second) were 157 µg/mL and 183 µg/mL, and 318 µg/mL and 381 µg/mL for the 2 × 500 mg and 2 × 1,000 mg doses, respectively.   Mean terminal elimination half-life ranged from 15 to 16.5 days for the 2 × 500 mg dose group and 17 to 21 days for the 2 × 1,000 mg dose group.
    ♦ The estimated clearance of rituximab was 0.34 L/day.
    ♦ The estimated volume of distribution was 3.1 L.
    ♦ Mean terminal elimination half-life was 18.0 days (range, 5.2-77.5 days).
  • Wegener's Granulomatosis (WG) and Microscopic Polyangiitis (MPA)
    ♦ 97 WG and MPA patients who received 375 mg/m² rituximab once weekly by intravenous infusion for four weeks.
    ♦ The estimated median terminal elimination half-life was 23 days (range, 9-49 days).
    ♦ Mean clearance was 0.31 L/day (range, 0.12-0.73 L/day).
    ♦ Volume of distribution was 4.5 L (range, 2.2-7.5 L).

Single-Dose Pharmacokinetics

❖ Study 102-01 was conducted in 15 NHL patients in groups of 3 with dose level 10, 50, 100, 250, 500 mg/m², following figure showed pharmacokinetic of rituximab in patients receiving 100, 250, 500 mg/m² infusions, respectively.

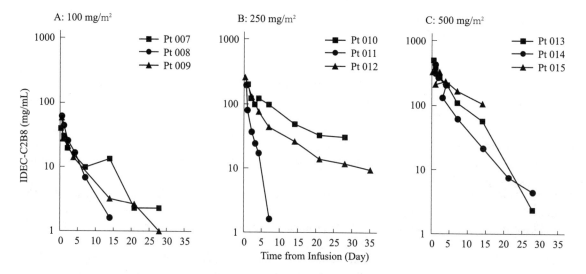

Figure 8   Single-Dose Pharmacokinetic of Rituximab in NHL Patients Receiving 100, 250, 500 mg/m² Infusions[37]

Multiple-Dose Pharmacokinetics

❖ Pharmacokinetics in Non-Hodgkin's Lymphoma (NHL) Patients

Table 39 C_{max} Values of Rituximab after Each Infusion[23]

Infusion No.	C_{max} (mean, μg/mL) ($N = 37$)	Range (μg/mL)
1	243	16.1-582
2	358	107-949
3	381	111-731
4	460	138-836
5	475	156-929
6	515	153-865
7	545	187-937
8	550	171-1,177

Non-Hodgkin's lymphoma patients treated with an intravenous infusion dose of 375mg/m², once weekly for 8 weeks.

Table 40   PK Parameters in NHL Patients Treated with 375 mg/m²[29]

	Post-1st Infusion	Post-4st Infusion
Mean $t_{1/2}$ (h)	68.1	190
Mean C_{max} (μg/mL)	239	481
Mean CL_{plasma} (L/h)	0.046	0.015

NHL: Non-Hodgkin's lymphoma.

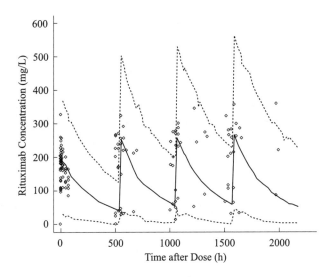

Figure 9　Mean Concentration-Time Curve of Rituximab Associated with CHOP in NHL (95% *CI*)[33]

❖ Pharmacokinetics in Refractory Nephrotic Syndrome Patients[33]

Table 41　PK Parameters in Refractory Nephrotic Syndrome Patients Treated with 375 mg/m²[33]

C_{max} (μg/mL)[a]	AUC_{all} (μg·h/mL)	$t_{1/2}$ (h)	CL (L/h)	MRT (h)	V_{ds} (L)
421 ± 84.7	366,000 ± 110,000	234 ± 86.7	0.0075 ± 0.0024	337 ± 125	2.4 ± 0.88

Mean ± SD, *n* = 22.　375 mg/(m²·infusion) (maximum of 500 mg/infusion) i.v. infusion once weekly for a total of 4 dose monitored to Day 365 after start of rituximab administration.　The highest serum concentration of the 4 values measured inmmediately after each administration.　AUC_{all}: All area under the curve.　C_{max}: Maximum concentration.　CL: Clearance.　MRT: Mean residence time.　V_{ds}: Volume at the dynamic state.

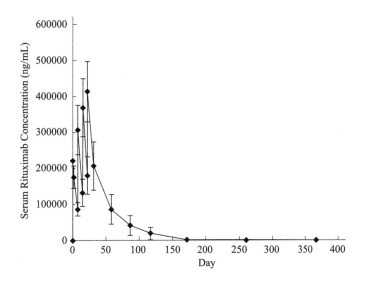

Figure 10　Changes in Serum Rituximab Concentration in Refractory Nephrotic Syndrome Patients (*N* = 22)[33]

❖ Pharmacokinetics in CLL Patients

Table 42   Exposure Parameters of Rituximab in Selected Studies Varying in Terms of Indication, Dose, Dosing Interval and Associated Drugs[39]

Type of Patients	Steady-state C_{min} Median (Range) (µg/mL)	Steady-state C_{max} Median (Range) (ng/mL)	CL Median (Range) or Mean (% CV) [mL/(h·m²) or mL/h]	V_c Median (Range) or Mean (% CV) (L/m²)	$t_{1/2}$ Median (Range) or Mean (% CV) (h)
Follicular diffuse B-cell NHL[a]	76.0 (29.0-116)	304 (176-360)	4.9 (73.9% CV)[d]	1.8 (13.0% CV)	504 (104-1,152)
Recurent low grade or follicular NHL[b]	186 (0.0-859)	460 (115-996)	9.2 ± 3.3[d]	-	206 ± 95.0
Follicular lymphoma after CHOP[b]	179 (94.0-262)	378 (266-660)	5.1 (3.8-8.1)[e]	1.8 (1.6-2.1)	513 (247-705)
Autoimmune disorders[b]	169 (43.0-499)	323 (172-559)	6.6 (3.8-11.9)[e]	2.1 (1.0-2.6)	485 (292-858)
Rheumatoid arthritis[c]	-	-	10.7 (3.4% CV)[d]	2.9 (2.1% CV)	-
Rheumatoid arthritis[c]	-	453 (261-2,400)	9.6 (3.8-27.9)[d]	-	-

CHOP: Cyclophosphamide, adriamycin, vincristine and prednisone. C_{max}: Maximum concentration. C_{min}: Minimum concentration (trough). CL: Clearance. CV: Coefficient of variation. NHL: Non-Hodgkin's lymphoma. $t_{1/2}$: Elimination half-life. V_c: Volume of the central compartment. [a] 375 mg/m² every 3 weeks. [b] 375 mg/m² weekly. [c] 750 or 1,000 mg every 2 weeks. [d] mL/h. [e] mL/(h·mp²).

Pharmacokinetics in RA patients

Table 43   The Pharmacokinetics of the Mean PK Parameters for Rituximab in RA Patients[40]

Dose	C_{first} (µg/mL)	C_{second} (µg/mL)	Ratio of C_{second}/C_{first}	C_{first} Ratio of Course 2/Course 1	C_{second} Ratio of Course 2/Course 1	$t_{1/2}$ (Day)
2 × 0.5 g in Course 1						
Image	171 ± 54.0 (32)	198 ± 58.0 (29)	1.2	NA	NA	14.8 ± 5.8 (39)
Serene	157 ± 45.9 (29)	183 ± 54.7 (30)	1.2	NA	NA	15.7 ± 5.1 (33)
Mirror	164 ± 41.0 (25)	193 ± 61.0 (32)	1.2	NA	NA	16.4 ± 6.1 (37)
2 × 0.5 g in Course 2						
Image	170 ± 38.0 (22)	ND	ND	0.99	ND	ND
Serene	ND	ND	ND	ND	ND	ND
Mirror	175 ± 41.0 (24)	207 ± 69.0 (33)	1.2	1.1	1.1	19.4 ± 6.0 (31)
2 × 1.0 g in Course 1						
Image	341 ± 84.0 (25)	404 ± 102 (25)	1.2	NA	NA	16.9 ± 5.4 (32)
Serene	318 ± 85.8 (32)	381 ± 98.3 (26)	1.2	NA	NA	18.5 ± 5.8 (31)
Mirror	312 ± 103 (33)	365 ± 126 (34)	1.1	NA	NA	18.0 ± 6.2 (32)
Sunrise	298 ± 91.2 (31)	355 ± 112 (31)	1.2	NA	NA	21.2 ± 8.2 (39)
2 × 1.0 g in Course 2						
Image	370 ± 101 (27)	ND	ND	1.1	ND	ND
Serene	ND	ND	ND	ND	ND	ND
Mirror	348 ± 89.0 (26)	386 ± 132 (34)	1.1	1.1	1.1	21.8 ± 6.4 (29)
Sunrise	317 ± 107 (34)	377 ± 120 (32)	1.2	1.1	1.1	20.9 ± 5.8 (27.6)

Mean ± SD (CV%). C_{first}: Post-infusion concentration after first infusion. C_{second}: Post-infusion concentration after second infusion. ND: Not determined. NA: Not available.

Anti-product Antibody (APA) Analysis[24-26]

❖ In 102-05 trails, one of 166 patients (0.60%) developed a human anti-chimeric antibody (HACA) response. This was detectable but below the limit of quantification on Day 50; a HACA response was not detectable on serum samples obtained on Days 43 and 99.

❖ HACA incidence in RA patients of four clinical studies at Week 24 is range 1.8%-11.9%, showed as following table.

Table 44   The HACA Incidence in RA Patients of Four Clinical Studies[22]

Study	Phase	Dosing Regimen	Patients with Positive HACA Response
Image	3	Placebo Rituximab 2 × 0.5 g Rituximab 2 × 1.0 g	1.4% (3/222) 11.9% (28/235) 7.8% (18/230)
Serene	3	Placebo 2 × 0.5 g Rituximab 2 × 0.5 g Rituximab 2 × 1.0 g	3.6% (5/137) 7.9% (12/152) 5.4% (8/149)
Sunrise	-	2 × 1.0 g, no re-treatment 2 × 1.0 g, no placebo 2 × 1.0 g, 2 × 1.0 g	6.5% (2/31) 6.7% (10/150) 5.9% (17/288)
Mirror	3	Rituximab 2 × 0.5 g Rituximab 2 × 1.0 g	6.2% (14/227) 1.8% (2/114)

A positive HACA is defined as ≥5 RU/mL and immune depletable with rituximab, a negative HACA is <5 RU/mL and not immune depletable with rituximab.   HACA: Human anti-chimeric antibody.   -: Not available.

9 Patent

❖ Rituximab was approved by the U.S. Food and Drug Administration (FDA) on Nov 26, 1997. It was developed by IDEC Pharmaceutical, and currently co-marketed by Biogen Idec and Genentech in the US, by Hoffmann-La Roche in Canada and the European Union, Chugai Pharmaceuticals, Zenyaku Kogyo in Japan, AryoGen in Iran and Roche Pharma (Schweiz) AG in China.

Summary

❖ The patent application (US5736137) related to the anti-CD20 antibody (i.e. Rituximab), nucleic acid encoding the same and therapeutic compositions thereof was filed by Biogen Idec Inc on Nov 13, 1993. Accordingly, its PCT counterpart has, among the others, been granted before USPTO (US 5736137 A), EPO (EP0669836B1), JPO (JP3095175B2) and SIPO (CN1270774C), respectively.

Table 45   Originator's Key Patent of Rituximab in Main Countries and/or Region

Country/Region	Publication/Patent No.	Application Date	Granted Date	Estimated Expiry Date
WO	WO9411026A2	11/12/1993	/	/
US	US5736137A	11/03/1993	04/07/1998	11/03/2013
	US7422739B2	25/01/2001	09/09/2008	10/10/2016
EP	EP0669836B1	11/12/1993	07/03/1996	11/12/2013
JP	JP3095175B2	11/12/1993	10/03/2000	11/12/2013
	JP4203080B2	11/12/1993	12/24/2008	11/12/2013
CN	CN1270774C	11/12/1993	08/23/2006	11/12/2013
	CN101007851B	11/12/1993	08/01/2007	11/12/2013
	CN1912111B	11/12/1993	05/26/2010	11/12/2013

Table 46   Originator's International Patent Protection of Use and/or Method of Rituximab

Publication No.	Title	Publication Date
Technical Subjects	**TREATMENT METHOD**	
WO0027433A1	Chimeric anti-CD20 antibody treatment of patients receiving BMT or PBSC transplants	05/18/2000
WO0067796A1	Treatment of autoimmune diseases with antagonists which bind to B-cell surface markers	11/16/2000
WO0103734A1	Blocking immune response to a foreign antigen using an antagonist which binds to CD20	01/18/2001
WO0110462A1	Treatment of patients having non-Hodgkin's lymphoma with bone marrow involvement with anti-CD20 antibodies	02/15/2001
WO0110460A1	Treatment of intermediate- and high-grade non-Hodgkin's lymphoma with anti-CD20 antibody	02/15/2001

Continued

Publication No.	Title	Publication Date
WO0180884A1	Intrathecal administration of rituximab for treatment of central nervous system lymphomas	11/01/2001
WO0197844A1	Bispecific fusion protein and method of use for enhancing effector cell killing of target cells	12/27/2001
WO02060485A2	Immunoregulatory antibodies and uses thereof	08/08/2002
WO03006607A2	Inhibition of apoptosis process and improvement of cell performance	01/23/2003
WO2004056312A2	Immunoglobulin variants and uses thereof	07/08/2004
WO2004091657A3	Therapy of autoimmune disease in a patient with an inadequate response to a TNF-alpha inhibitor	10/28/2004
WO2005023302A3	Anti-CD20 therapy of ocular disorders	03/17/2005
WO2005115453A3	Treatment of polychondritis and mononeuritis multiplex with anti-CD20 antibodies	12/08/2005
WO2005117972A3	Preventing autoimmune disease by using an anti-CD20 antibody	12/15/2005
WO2005117978A2	Method for treating multiple sclerosis	12/15/2005
WO2005120437A2	Method for treating lupus	12/22/2005
WO2006012508A2	Method of treating Sjögren's syndrome	02/02/2006
WO2006041680A2	Method for treating vasculitis	04/20/2006
WO2006076651A2	Treatment method	07/20/2006
WO2006093923A3	Treatment of bone disorders	09/08/2006
WO2006113308A1	Method for treating inflammatory bowel disease (IBD) by an anti-CD20 antibody	10/26/2006
WO2006116369A2	Method for treating dementia or Alzheimer's disease	11/02/2006
WO2006125140A2	Methods for treating fibrotic conditions	11/23/2006
WO2009086072A2	Therapy of rituximab-refractory rheumatoid arthritis patients	07/09/2009
WO2010033587A2	Methods for treating progressive multiple sclerosis	03/25/2010
WO2010075249A2	A method for treating rheumatoid arthritis with B-cell antagonists	07/01/2010
Technical Subjects	**DIAGNOSTIC METHOD**	
WO0110461A1	New clinical parameters for determining hematologic toxicity prior to radioimmunotherapy	02/15/2001
WO2005017529A1	Assay for human anti CD20 antibodies and uses therefor	02/24/2005
WO2005060999A3	Detection of CD20 in therapy of autoimmune diseases	07/07/2005
WO2005061542A3	Detection of CD20 in transplant rejection	07/07/2005
WO2006074076A1	Detecting human antibodies in non-human serum	07/13/2006
WO2008122007A1	Biological markers predictive of rheumatoid arthritis response to B-cell antagonists	10/09/2008
WO2008157282A1	Biological markers predictive of rheumatoid arthritis response to B-cell antagonists	12/24/2008
WO2009134738A1	Responses to immunizations in rheumatoid arthritis patients treated with a CD20 antibody	11/05/2009
Technical Subjects	**COMBINATION METHOD**	
WO0134194A1	Treatment of B-cell malignancies using anti-CD40l antibodies in combination with anti-CD20 antibodies and/or chemotherapeutics and radiotherapy	05/17/2001
WO0174388A1	Combined use of anti-cytokine antibodies or antagonists and anti-CD20 for the treatment of B-cell lymphoma	10/11/2001
WO0197858A2	Treatment of B-cell associated diseases such as malignancies and autoimmune diseases using a cold anti-CD20 antibody/radiolabeled anti-CD22 antibody combination	12/27/2001
WO0204021A1	Treatment of B-cell malignancies using combination of B-cell depleting antibody and immune modulating antibody related applications	01/17/2002
WO02078766A2	Combination therapy	10/10/2002
WO02079255A1	Recombinant antibodies coexpressed with GnT III	10/10/2002
WO2005000351A3	Combination therapy for B-cell disorders	01/06/2005
WO2006068867A1	Combination therapy for B-cell disorders	06/29/2006

Continued

Publication No.	Title	Publication Date
WO2009030368A1	Combination therapy with type I and type II anti-CD20 antibodies	03/12/2009
WO2009049841A1	Combination therapy of a type II anti-CD20 antibody with an anti-BCL-2 active agent	04/23/2009
WO2011018225A1	Combination therapy of an afucosylated CD20 antibody with fludarabine and or mitoxantrone	02/17/2011
WO2015067586A2	Combination therapy of an anti CD20 antibody with a BTK inhibitor	05/14/2015
WO2016188935A1	Combination therapy of an anti CD20 antibody with a BCL-2 inhibitor and a MDM2 inhibitor	12/01/2016
Technical Subjects	**FORMULATION**	
WO9858964A1	Methods and compositions for galactosylated glycoproteins	12/30/1998
WO9922764A1	Methods and compositions comprising glycoprotein glycoforms	05/14/1999
WO03062375A2	Stabilizing polypeptides which have been exposed to urea	07/31/2003
WO2004001007A2	Buffered formulations for concentrating antibodies and methods of use thereof	12/31/2003
WO2011029892A2	Highly concentrated pharmaceutical formulations	03/17/2011
WO2013173687A1	High-concentration monoclonal antibody formulations	11/21/2013

The data was updated until Jan 2018.

10 Reference

[1] Julius M.,Cruse M, Lewis R E. *Atlas of immunology (third edition)*, 2010.

[2] https://www.ncbi.nlm.nih.gov/gene "Entrez Gene: MS4A1 membrane-spanning 4-domains, subfamily A, member 1".

[3] http://www.ncbi.nlm.nih.gov/homologene/7259.

[4] https://blast.ncbi.nlm.nih.gov/Blast.cgi.

[5] https://www.ncbi.nlm.nih.gov/protein/118150824.

[6] https://www.ncbi.nlm.nih.gov/protein/114158610.

[7] https://www.ncbi.nlm.nih.gov/protein/109105984.

[8] https://www.ncbi.nlm.nih.gov/protein/114637776.

[9] https://www.ncbi.nlm.nih.gov/protein/23110989.

[10] https://www.ncbi.nlm.nih.gov/protein/6671710.

[11] https://www.ncbi.nlm.nih.gov/protein/157817414.

[12] Grillo-lópez A J. Rituximab: an insider's historical perspective [J]. Seminars in Oncology, 2000, 27(6 Suppl 12): 9-16.

[13] The financial reports of Genentech; http://data.pharmacodia.com/web/homePage/index.

[14] Pharmaceuticals and Medical Device Agency (PMDA) Database. http://www.pmda.go.jp/drugs/2001/P200100018/ 380101000_21300AMY00273_A100_2.pdf#page=2.

[15] European Medicines Agency (EMA) Database. http://www.ema.europa.eu/docs/en_GB/document_library/EPAR_-_ Scientific_Discussion/human/000165/WC500025817.pdf.

[16] PMDA Database. http://www.pmda.go.jp/drugs/2001/P200100018/380101000_21300AMY00273_F100_2.pdf#page=1.

[17] U.S. Food and Drug Administration (FDA) Database. http://www.accessdata.fda.gov/drugsatfda_docs/nda/2013/ 125486Orig1s000PharmR.pdf.

[18] EMA Database. http://www.ema.europa.eu/docs/en_GB/document_library/EPAR_-_Public_assessment_report/human/ 001131/WC500093094.pdf.

[19] EMA Database. http://www.ema.europa.eu/docs/en_GB/document_library/EPAR_-_Assessment_Report_-_Variation/ human/000165/WC500168097.pdf.

[20] Anderson D. Therapeutic application of chimeric and radiolabeled antibodies to human B lymphocyte restricted differentiation antigen for treatment of B cell lymphoma [P]: US6682734B1, 2004-01-27.

[21] FDA Database. http://www.accessdata.fda.gov/drugsatfda_docs/label/2011/103705s5344lbl.pdf.

[22] EMA Database. http://www.ema.europa.eu/docs/en_GB/document_library/EPAR_-_Assessment_Report_-_Variation/ human/000165/WC500150330.pdf.

[23] FDA Database. http://www.accessdata.fda.gov/drugsatfda_docs/label/2004/103737_5055lbl.pdf.

[24] FDA Database. http://www.fda.gov/Drugs/DevelopmentApprovalProcess/HowDrugsareDevelopedandApproved/ ApprovalApplications/TherapeuticBiologicApplications/ucm093352.html.

[25] Thomson-Routers Database. http://thomsonreuters.com/en/products-services/pharma-life-sciences/pharmaceutical.html.

[26] TGA Database. https://www.tga.gov.au/sites/default/files/auspar-rituximab-150827-pi.pdf.

[27] EMA Database. http://www.ema.europa.eu/docs/en_GB/document_library/EPAR_-_Assessment_Report_-_Variation/human/000165/WC500208542.pdf.

[28] https://clinicaltrials.gov.

[29] FDA Database. http://www.fda.gov/Drugs/DevelopmentApprovalProcess/HowDrugsareDevelopedandApproved/ApprovalApplications/TherapeuticBiologicApplications/ucm093345.html.

[30] EMA Database. http://www.ema.europa.eu/docs/en_GB/document_library/EPAR_-_Assessment_Report_-_Variation/human/000165/WC500025825.pdf.

[31] FDA Database. https://www.accessdata.fda.gov/scripts/cder/daf/index.cfm?event=overview.process&applno=103705.

[32] Edwards J C. Efficacy of B-cell-targeted therapy with rituximab in patients with rheumatoid arthritis [J]. The New England Journal of Medicine, 2004, 350(25): 2572-2581.

[33] PMDA Database. http://www.pmda.go.jp/files/000209810.pdf.

[34] https://www.tga.gov.au/sites/default/files/auspar-rituximab.pdf.

[35] Tobinai K, Kobayashi Y, Narabayashi M, et al. Feasibility and pharmacokinetic study of a chimeric anti-CD20 monoclonal antibody (IDEC-C2B8, rituximab) in relapsed B-cell lymphoma [J]. Annals of Oncology, 1998, 9(5): 527-534.

[36] Coben S, Emery P, Greenwald M, et al. A phase I pharmacokinetics trial comparing PF-05280586 (a potential biosimilar) and rituximab in patients with active rheumatoid arthritis [J]. British Journal of Clinical Pharmacology, 2016, 82(1): 129-138.

[37] Maloney D G; Liles T M, Czerwinski D K, et al. Phase I clinical trial using escalating single-dose infusion of chimeric anti-CD20 monoclonal antibody (IDEC-C2B8) in patients with recurrent B-cell lymphoma [J]. Blood, 1994, 84(8): 2457-2466.

[38] Cartron G, Blasco H, Paintaud G, et al. Pharmacokinetics of rituximab and its clinical use: thought for the best use? [J]. Critical Reviews in Oncology/Hematology, 2007, 62(1): 43-52.

[39] Blasco H. Pharmacokinetics of rituximab associated with CHOP chemotherapy in B-cell non-Hodgkin lymphoma [J]. Fundamental & Clinical Pharmacology 2009, 23(5): 601-608.

[40] EMA Database. http://www.ema.europa.eu/docs/en_GB/document_library/EPAR_-_Assessment_Report_-_Variation/human/000165/WC500099488.pdf.

CHAPTER

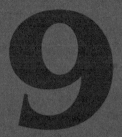

Tocilizumab

Tocilizumab

(Actemra®/RoActemra®)

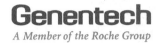

Research code: HPM-1, MRA, MRA-SC, R-1569, RG-1569, rhPM-1, RO-48775533

1 Target Biology

The IL-6 Receptor

❖ The IL-6 receptor complex mediating the biological activities of IL-6 consists of two distinct membrane-bound glycoproteins, an 80 kDa IL-6 binding type I transmembrane glycoprotein termed IL-6 receptor-α (IL-6R, CD126) and a 130 kDa type I transmembrane signal transducer protein gp130 (CD130). This ligand-receptor complex then binds to the signal-transducing protein gp130 (CD130) and activates the JAK-STAT3-signaling pathway.

❖ IL-6Rα is expressed as a membrane-bound protein in only a few cell types, whereas gp130 is expressed ubiquitously in all cell types and acts as a signaling protein for other members of the IL-6 cytokine family. In addition to the membrane-bound receptor (mIL-6R), a soluble form of the IL-6R (sIL-6R) has been purified from human serum and urine. This soluble receptor binds IL-6 with an affinity similar to that of the cognate receptor (0.5-2 nM) and prolongs its plasma half-life. More important, the (sIL-6R/IL-6) complex is capable of activating cells via interaction with membrane-bound gp130.

❖ IL-6 signaling through membrane-bound IL-6Rα is known as the classical signaling pathway or cis-signaling. In addition to the membrane-bound IL-6Rα, a soluble form of IL-6Rα (sIL-6Rα) is present in high concentration in blood and other body fluids and has an affinity for IL-6 that is similar to the membrane-bound receptor. Upon interaction with IL-6, sIL-6Rα does not act as an antagonist; instead it increases the circulating half-life of IL-6 and activates the signaling pathway in cells where the membrane-bound form of IL-6Rα is not expressed.

Sequence Homology of IL6 Receptor[1]

```
  1  MLAVGCALLA  ALLAAPGAAL  APRRCPAQEV  ARGVLTSLPG  DSVTLTCPGV  EPEDNATVHW
 61  VLRKPAAGSH  PSRWAGMGRR  LLLRSVQLHD  SGNYSCYRAG  RPAGTVHLLV  DVPPEEPQLS
121  CFRKSPLSNV  VCEWGPRSTP  SLTTKAVLLV  RKFQNSPAED  FQEPCQYSQE  SQKFSCQLAV
181  PEGDSSFYIV  SMCVASSVGS  KFSKTQTFQG  CGILQPDPPA  NITVTAVARN  PRWLSVTWQD
241  PHSWNSSFYR  LRFELRYRAE  RSKTFTTWMV  KDLQHHCVIH  DAWSGLRHVV  QLRAQEEFGQ
301  GEWSEWSPEA  MGTPWTESRS  PPAENEVSTP  MQALTTNKDD  DNILFRDSAN  ATSLPVQDSS
361  SVPLPTFLVA  GGSLAFGTLL  CIAIVLRFKK  TWKLRALKEG  KTSMHPPYSL  GQLVPERPRP
421  TPVLVPLISP  PVSPSSLGSD  NTSSHNRPDA  RDPRSPYDIS  NTDYFFPR
```

Chimpanzee: 468 aa.   Accession: XP_524889.3.

❖ BLAST:[2]
  • Max score: 862; Total score: 862; Query cover: 94.0%.
  • Identities: 99.0% (439/441); Positives: 99.0% (439/441); Gaps: 0.0% (0/441).

```
  1  MLAVGCALLA  ALLAAPGAAL  APRRCPAQEV  ARGVLTSLPG  DSVTLTCPGV  EPEDNATVHW
 61  VLRKPAAGSH  PSRWAGMGRR  LLLRSVQLHD  SGNYSCYRAG  RPAGTVHLLV  DVPPEEPQLS
121  CFRKSPLSNV  VCEWGPRSTP  S TTKAVLLV  RKFQNSPAED  FQEPCQYSQE  SQKFSCQLAV
181  PEGDSSFYIV  SMCVASSVGS  KFSKTQTFQG  CGILQPDPPA  NITVTAVARN  PRWLSVTWQD
241  PHSWNSSFYR  LRFELRYRAE  RSKTFTTWMV  KDLQHHCVIH  DAWSGLRHVV  QLRAQEEFGQ
301  GEWSEWSPEA  MGTPWTESRS  PPAENEVSTP   QALTTNKDD  DNILFRDSAN  ATSLPVQDSS
361  SVPLPTFLVA  GGSLAFGTLL  CIAIVLRFKK  TWKLRALKEG  KTSMHPPYSL  GQLVPERPRP
421  TPVLVPLISP  PVSPSSLGSD  NTSSHNRPDA  RDPRSPYDIS  NTDYFFPR
```

Rhesus monkey: 468aa.   Accession: XP_001114404.1.

❖ BLAST:
  • Max score: 844; Total score: 844; Query cover: 94.0%.
  • Identities: 98.0% (432/441); Positives: 98.0% (433/441); Gaps: 0.0% (0/441).

```
  1  MLAVGCALLA  ALLAAPGAAL  APGGCPAQEV  ARGVLTSLPG  DSVTLTCPGC  EPEDNATVHW
 61  VLRKPAMGSH  LSRWAGMGRR  LLLRSVQLHD  SGNYSCYRAG  RPAGTVHLLV  DVPPEEPQLS
121  CFRKSPLSNV  VCEWGPRSTP  SPTTKAVLLV  RKFQNSPAED  FQEPCQYSQE  SQKFSCQLAV
181  PEGDSSFYIV  SMCVASSVGS  KLSKTQTFQG  CGILQPDPPA  NITVTAVARN  PRWLSVTWQD
241  PHSWNSSFYR  LRFELRYRAE  RSKTFTTWMV  KDLQHHCVIH  DAWSGLRHVV  QLRAQEEFGQ
301  GEWSEWSPEA  MGTPWTSRSS  PPAENEVSTP  IQAPTTNKDD  DNILSRDSAN  ATSLPVQDSS
361  SVPLPTFLVA  GGSLAFGTLL  CIAIVLRFKK  TWKLRALKEG  KTSMHPPYSL  GQLVPERPRP
421  TPVLVPLISP  PVSPSSLGSD  NTSSHNRPDA  RDPRSPYDIS  N T D Y F F P R
```

Dog: 468aa.   Accession: XP_855105.1.

❖ BLAST:
  • Max score: 634; Total score: 634; Query cover: 94.0%.
  • Identities: 75.0% (329/440); Positives: 82.0% (363/440); Gaps: 0.0% (0/440).

```
  1  MLALRCALLL  ALLAAPGAAL  APWGCPAEV  MSGVMTSLPG  ASVTLTCPGC  EPEDNGTVQW
 61  LLQNLVDDSY  LGSRAAVGRL  LLLRSVQLSD  SGNYSCYQLG  RLAGTVRLLV  DAPPEEPQLA
121  CFRKSPLSMV  FCEWSPRHP  SPKTRALLV  RKFRGRPVGD  SQEPCYYAQG  LQKFSCQLAV
181  PEGDNSLYMV  SLCVTNSAGS  RSSTPQTFEG  MGILQPDPPV  NITVTAVDRN  PRWLRVTWQD
241  PLSWNSYFYR  LQFELRYRAE  RSKTFTMLMI  KEFQHHCIIH  DAWRGMRHVV  QLRAREEFGH
301  GLWSTWSQEA  MGTPWTSRSS  PAAELELPHS  IQAPTTNEDN  LNNISKDIAN  ATSLPVQDSS
361  SLPLPTFLVA  GGSLAFGTLL  CVGIVLRFKK  TWKLHALKEG  KASVHPPYSL  GQLVPERPKP
421  TPVRVPLISP  PVSPSSLGSD  NTSRHSHPDA  RGPQSPYDIS  N T D Y F F P R
```

Norway rat: 462aa.   Accession: NP_058716.2.

❖ BLAST:
  • Max score: 449; Total score: 449; Query cover: 94.0%.
  • Identities: 54.0% (241/444); Postives: 68.0% (303/444); Gaps: 3.0% (14/444).

```
  1  MLAVGCLLLM  ALLAAPAVAL  VLGSCRALEV  ANGTVTSLPG  ATVTLICPGK  EAAGNATHW
 61  VYSGSQSREW  TTTGNTLMLR  AVQVNDTGHY  LCFLDDHLVG  TVLLLVDVPP  EEPKLSCFRK
121  NPLVNAFCEW  HPSSTPSPTT  KAVMFAKKIN  ITTNGKSDFQV  PCQYSQQLKS  FSCFVEILEG
181  DKVYHIVSLC  VANSVGSRSS  HNVVFQSLKM  MQPDPPANLV  VSAIPGRPRW  LKVSWQDPES
241  WDPSYYLLQF  ELRYRPVWSK  TFTVWPLQVA  QHLCVIHDAL  RGVKHVVQMR  GKEEFDIGQW
301  SKWSPEVTGT  PWLAEPRTTP  AGIPGNPTQV  SVEDYDNHED  QYGSSTEATS  VLAPVQGSSI
361  IPLPTFLVAG  GSLAFGLLLC  VHILRLKKK  WKSQAEKESK  TLSPPPYPLG  ILKPTELLVP
421  LLTPSGSHNS  SGTDNTGSHS  CLGVRDPQCP  NDNSNRDYLF  P R
```

House mouse: 460aa.   Accession: NP_034689.2.

❖ BLAST:
  • Max score: 424; Total score: 424; Query cover: 94.0%.
  • Identities: 52.0% (233/446); Positives: 65.0% (292/446); Gaps: 4.0% (20/446).

```
  1  MLTVGCLLLM  ALLAAPAVAL  VLGSCRALEV  ANGTVTSLPG  ATVTLICPGK  EAAGNVTHW
 61  VYSGSQNREW  TTTGNTLMLR  DVQLSDTGDY  LCSLNDHLVG  TVLLLVDVPP  EEPKLSCFRK
121  NPLVNAICEW  RPSSTPSPTT  KAVLFAKKIN  ITTNGKSDFQV  PCQYSQQLKS  FSCQVEILEG
181  DKVYHIVSLC  VANSVGSKSS  HNEAFHSLKM  MQPDPPANLV  VSAIPGRPRW  LKVSWQHPET
241  WDPSYYLLQF  QLRYRPVWSK  EFTVLLLPVA  QYQCVIHDAL  RGVKHVVQMR  GKEELDLGQW
301  SEWSPEVTGT  PWLAEPRTTP  AGILWNPTQV  SVEDSANHED  QYESSTEATS  VLAPVQESSS
361  MSLPTFLVAG  GSLAFGLLLC  VHILRLKQK  WKSHALKESK  TLSPPPRYS  LGILKPTELL
421  VPLLTPHSSG  SDNTVNHSCI  GVRDAQSPYD  NSNRDYLFPR
```

Biology Activity

❖ IL-6 exerts its biological activities through two molecules: IL-6R and gp130.   IL-6R is a cognate binding receptor for IL-6, whereas gp130 is shared by cytokines of the IL-6 family including leukemia inhibitory factor, oncostatin M, ciliary neurotrophic factor, IL-11, cardiotrophin 1, cardiotrophin-like cytokine, and IL-27.

❖ IL-6 has a wide variety of functions.   IL-6 induces cell differentiation and specific gene expression.   It induces production of acute-phase proteins such as C-reactive protein, amyloid A, fibrinogen, and hepcidin, whereas it reduces synthesis of albumin and cytochrome P450 in hepatocytes.   IL-6 promotes immunoglobulin synthesis in activated B cells as well as Th17 and cytotoxic T-cell differentiation from naive T cells.   In bone marrow, IL-6 induces maturation of megakaryocytes to platelets and activation of hematopoietic stem cells.   IL-6 also acts on synovial fibroblast cells to produce RANKL (receptor activator of NF-κB ligand) and VEGF (vascular endothelial growth factor), which promote differentiation of osteoclasts and angiogenesis, respectively.   Furthermore, IL-6 stimulates dermal fibroblasts to produce collagen and the growth of cells such as myeloma/plasmacytoma cells and mesangial cells.[3]

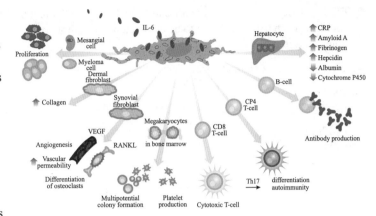

❖ After binding of IL-6 to IL-6R, the resultant IL-6/IL-6R complex associates with gp130, and the activated IL-6 receptor complex is formed as a hexameric structure that includes two molecules each of IL-6, IL-6R, and gp130.   The IL-6 signal is transduced into cells via gp130-JAK- STAT3 (signal transducer and activator of transcription 3) and gp130-JAKSHP-2 (SH2-domain containing protein tyrosine phosphatase-2) pathways.   IL-6R is a cognate binding receptor for IL-6, whereas gp130 is shared by cytokines of the IL-6 family including leukemia inhibitory factor, oncostatin M, ciliary neurotrophic factor, IL-11, cardiotrophin 1, cardiotrophin-like cytokine, and IL-27.   These cytokines often show overlapping functions with those of IL-6 via the common signal transducer gp130.

❖ IL-6 is a pleiotropic pro-inflammatory multi-functional cytokine produced by a variety of cell types including various types of lymphocyte, fibroblasts, synoviocytes, endothelial cells, neurons, adrenal glands, mast cells, keratinocytes, Langerhans cells, astrocytes, and colonic epithelial cells.   Elevated levels of IL-6 have been implicated in the disease pathology of several inflammatory and autoimmune disorders including RA.   Instrumental in RA pathophysiology, IL-6 has been shown to be involved in processes such as T-cell activation, differentiation of B cells into immunoglobulin-secreting plasma cells, maturation of megakaryocytes leading to platelet production and is now well recognized to stimulate the production of acute phase proteins by hepatocytes.   IL-6 also induces the synthesis of the iron regulatory peptide hepcidin during inflammation.[4]

2   General Information

Actemra®/RoActemra®

❖ Actemra®/RoActemra® (Tocilizumab) is a recombinant humanized monoclonal antibody of IgG1κ subclass composed of two heavy chains and two lights chains, with 12 intra-chain and 4 inter-chain disulfide bonds.   The N-linked glycol structures present in tocilizumab include complex-type oligosaccharide structures.[4]

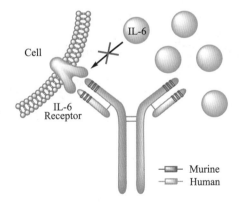

❖ Actemra®/RoActemra® is obtained by humanizing mouse antibody PM1.   CDR grafting is carried out using human NEW and REI sequences as template framework for H and L chains, respectively; however, five mouse sequence amino acids are retained in the framework as essential amino acids for maintaining the activity.[5]

❖ Actemra®/RoActemra® has been produced in a CHO cell line by recombinant DNA technology.   The fermentation process is a serum-free process.

❖ The total molecular weight of the glycoprotein is approximately 149 kDa.

❖ The total sales of 1,714 million US$ for 2016; No sales data as of 2017.

Mechanism of Action: Block Intracellular IL-6 Signal Transduction[6]
❖ Biochemical: Exerted by blocking the action of a specific protein (cytokine) called interleukin-6.

❖ Binding affinity to sIL-6R.

❖ Dissociation of IL-6 from the IL-6/sIL-6R complex: When tocilizumab was added to the complexes of recombinant human IL-6 (rhIL-6) and sIL-6R formed *in vitro*, the binding rate of rhIL-6 to sIL-6R was decreased in a MRA concentration-dependent manner and was 1 μg/mL.

❖ Effects on other cytokine signal transduction: The effects of tocilizumab on signal transduction by TNF-α, IL-1β, and IL-15, which have been shown to be involved in the pathology of RA, and IL-2, which has been shown to be involved in immune system activation.

❖ Weak/no CDC or antibody dependent cellular cytotoxicity (ADCC) effector functions (*in vitro*).

Sponsor

❖ Actemra®/RoActemra® (Tocilizumab) was developed and marketed by Genentech, Inc., a subsidiary of Roche.

World Sales[7]

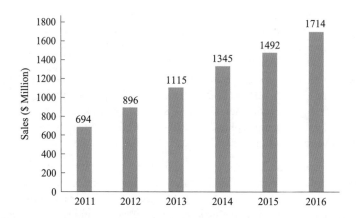

Figure 1   World Sales of Tocilizumab since 2011

Approval and Indication

Table 1   Summary of the Approved Indication[8]

Approval (Year)	Agency	Indication
2005	PMDA	Castleman's disease.
2008	PMDA	Rheumatoid arthritis, juvenile idiopathic arthritis and systemic-onset juvenile idiopathic arthritis.
2009	EMA	Rheumatoid arthritis in patients who have had an inadequate response to one or more DMARDs or TNF inhibitors.
2010	FDA	Rheumatoid arthritis in patients who have had an inadequate response to one or more DMARDs or TNF inhibitors.
	EMA	Reduction of progression of joint damage in rheumatoid arthritis.
2011	FDA	Active systemic juvenile idiopathic arthritis (sJIA); reduction or progression of joint damage in rheumatoid arthritis.
	EMA	Active sJIA to previous therapy with NSAIDs and systemic corticosteroids.
2013	PMDA	Rheumatoid arthritis in patients who have not sufficiently responded to conventional treatments.
	FDA	Polyarticular juvenile idiopathic arthritis (PJIA).
	CFDA	Severe, active and progressive rheumatoid arthritis (RA) in adults not previously treated with MTX.
	EMA	Systemic onset juvenile idiopathic arthritis and polyarticular-course juvenile idiopathic arthritis. Sc formulation for the treatment of moderate-to-severe rheumatoid arthritis.
2014	FDA	Sc formulation for the treatment of moderate-to-severe rheumatoid arthritis.

DMARDs: Disease modifying anti-rheumatic drugs.   MTX: Methotrexate.   RA: Rheumatoid arthritis.   sJIA: Systemic juvenile idiopathic arthritis.   TNF: Tumor necrosis factor.

Table 2   Summary of the Approval of Actemra®/RoActemra®[9, 10]

	Japan (PMDA)	EU (EMA)	US (FDA)	China (CFDA)
First approval date	04/11/2005	01/16/2009	01/08/2010	03/26/2013
Application or approval No.	21700AMZ00601 21900AMX01337 22000AMX00871/ 22500AMX00872	EMEA/H/C/000955	BLA125276 BLA125472	注册证号 S20130020 注册证号 S20130021 注册证号 S20130022 注册证号 S20171026 注册证号 S20171025
Brand name	Actemra®	RoActemra®	Actemra®	Actemra®/雅美罗®
Indication	Castleman's disease	Rheumatoid arthritis	Rheumatoid arthritis	Rheumatoid arthritis
Authorization holder	Chugai Pharmaceutical	Roche	Roche	Roche

Table 3   Indication and Administration[6]

No.	Administration	Indication
1	The usual dose is 8 mg/kg as an intravenous infusion every 4 weeks.	Rheumatoid arthritis (including the inhibition of progression of structural joint damage), polyarticular-course juvenile idiopathic arthritis.
2	The usual dosage is 8 mg/kg as an intravenous infusion every 2 weeks. The dosing interval may be shortened to a minimum of 1 week according to the patient's symptoms.	Systemic juvenile idiopathic arthritis, Castleman's disease.

Sourced from Japan PMDA drug label information.

Table 4   IL-6/IL-R Antagonist mAb in Development[8]

Drug	Target	Phase	Sponsor	Type	Indication
Siltuximab/Sylvant®	IL-6	Launched	Janssen Biotech	mAb	Castleman's disease.
Sarilumab	IL-6R	Pre-registered	Sanofi, Regeneron	mAb	Rheumatoid arthritis.
Sirukumab	IL-6	3	Janssen Biotech, GSK	mAb	Rheumatoid arthritis, Giant cell arteritis.
RG-6168/SA237	IL-6R	3	Roche	mAb	Neuromyelitis optica (Devic's disease).
ALX-0061	IL-6R	2	Ablynx, AbbVie	scFv, nanobody	Rheumatoid arthritis, Systemic lupus erythematosus.
Clazakizumab	IL-6	2	Alder Biopharmaceuticals	mAb	Psoriatic arthritis, Rheumatoid arthritis.
FE999301	IL-6	2	Ferring Pharmaceuticals	Peptides	Crohn's disease.
MEDI-5117	IL-6	IND Filed	AstraZeneca, WuXi MedImmune Biopharmaceutical	mAb	Rheumatoid arthritis.
EBI-031	IL-6	IND Filed	Eleven Biotherapeutics, Roche	mAb	DME and uveitis.

mAb: Monoclonal antibody.   scFv: Single chain antibody fragment.

3   CMC Profile

Product Profile

Dosage route: A sterile, preservative-free solution for IV infusion.

Strength: US, EU and JP: 80 mg/4 mL, 200 mg/10 mL, 400 mg/20 mL, and 162 mg/0.9 mL; CN: 80 mg/4 mL, 200 mg/10 mL, and 400 mg/20 mL.

Dosage form: Single-use vials of Actemra® (20 mg/mL) for intravenous administration and Prefilled Syringe (PFS) for subcutaneous administration.

Formulation: Single-use vials are available containing 80 mg/4 mL, 200 mg/10 mL, or 400 mg/20 mL of tocilizumab. Injectable solutions of tocilizumab are formulated in an aqueous solution containing disodium phosphate dodecahydrate and sodium dihydrogen phosphate dehydrate (as a 15 mmol/L phosphate buffer), polysorbate 80 (0.5 mg/L), and sucrose (50 mg/mL). A colorless to pale yellow liquid, with a pH of about 6.5.

PFS with a needle safety device is 1 mL ready-to-use, single-use. Each device delivers 0.9 mL (162 mg) of Actemra®, in a histidine buffered solution composed of Actemra® (180 mg/mL), polysorbate 80, L-histidine and L-histidine monohydrochloride, L-arginine and L-arginine hydrochloride, L-methionine, and water for injection.

Stability: In order to assess the stability of the drug product, using 3 pilot-scale lots of each fill volume of DP2, long-term testing (5 °C, inverted or upright position, 24 months), accelerated testing (25 °C, inverted or upright position, 6 months), and stress testing (temperature [40 °C, upright position, 3 months, 1 lot of each fill volume], light [upright position, 1.2 million lux·h + 200 W·h/m², 1 lot of the 200 mg preparation], vibration [upright position, 5-50 Hz, up to 60 minutes, 1 lot of the 200 mg preparation]) were conducted. In addition, using DP3 produced at commercial scale, long-term testing (5 °C, inverted position, 18 months, 3 lots of each fill volume), accelerated testing (25 °C, inverted position, 6 months, 1 lot of each fill volume), and stress testing (temperature, light, vibration, [the same number of lots as DP2]) were conducted. The test items tested in these studies are physical description, identification (SDS-PAGE [Coomassie staining and silver staining]), pH, osmotic pressure ratio, purity (GPC, IEC), foreign insoluble matter test, sterility test, bacterial endotoxins test, insoluble particulate matter test, actual volume in container, polysorbate 80 content, assay (GPC, UV, and the binding activity to IL-6 receptors), and potency (#ABC assay) (Some of the attributes were omitted in the stress testing).[6]

Real-time and accelerated stability studies were initiated in accordance with ICH guidelines and per protocol to monitor the time-temperature stability of cGMP lots of drug product. On the basis of the data provided, the approvable shelf life for the drug product is 30 months at 2-8 °C.[4]

Parenteral drug products should be inspected visually for particulate matter and discoloration prior to administration, whenever solution and container permit. If visibly opaque particles, discoloration or other foreign particles are observed, the solution should not be used.

On the basis of the stability data provided, the proposed shelf life of 24 months at ≤ -50 °C for the drug substance and 30 months at 2-8 °C for the drug product are considered acceptable.

Do not use beyond expiration date on the container. Actemra® must be refrigerated at 2-8 °C (36-46 °F). Do not freeze. Protect the vials from light by storage in the original package until time of use.

Amino Acid Sequence

❖ Tocilizumab is a recombinant humanized anti-human interleukin 6 (IL-6) receptor monoclonal antibody of the immunoglobulin IgG1κ subclass with a typical H_2L_2 polypeptide structure. Each light chain and heavy chain consists of 214 and 448 amino acids, respectively. The four polypeptide chains are linked intra- and inter-molecularly by disulfide bonds.

❖ Molecular formula:[11]
- Light chain: $C_{1033}H_{1606}N_{278}O_{337}S_6$
- Heavy chain: $C_{2181}H_{3398}N_{582}O_{672}S_{15}$

Light chain:

```
DIQMTQSPSS  LSASVGDRVT  ITCRASQDIS  SYLNWYQQKP  GKAPK
LLIYYTSRLH  SGVPSRFSGS  GSGTDFTFTI  SSLQPEDIAT  YYCQQ
GNTLPYTFGQ  GTKVEIKRTV  AAPSVFIFPP  SDEQLKSGTA  SVVCL
LNNFYPREAK  VQWKVDNALQ  SGNSQESVTE  QDSKDSTYSL  SSTLT
LSKADYEKHK  VYACEVTHQG  LSSPVTKSFN  RGEC
```

```
1                        10                        20
Asp Ile Gln Met Thr Gln Ser Pro Ser Ser Leu Ser Ala Ser Val Gly Asp Arg Val Thr
21                       30                        40
Ile Thr Cys Arg Ala Ser Gln Asp Ile Ser Ser Tyr Leu Asn Trp Tyr Gln Gln Lys Pro
41                       50                        60
Gly Lys Ala Pro Lys Leu Leu Ile Tyr Tyr Thr Ser Arg Leu His Ser Gly Val Pro Ser
61                       70                        80
Arg Phe Ser Gly Ser Gly Ser Gly Thr Asp Phe Thr Phe Thr Ile Ser Ser Leu Gln Pro
81                       90                        100
Glu Asp Ile Ala Thr Tyr Tyr Cys Gln Gln Gly Asn Thr Leu Pro Tyr Thr Phe Gly Gln
101                      110                       120
Gly Thr Lys Val Glu Ile Lys Arg Thr Val Ala Ala Pro Ser Val Phe Ile Phe Pro Pro
121                      130                       140
Ser Asp Glu Gln Leu Lys Ser Gly Thr Ala Ser Val Val Cys Leu Leu Asn Asn Phe Tyr
141                      150                       160
Pro Arg Glu Ala Lys Val Gln Trp Lys Val Asp Asn Ala Leu Gln Ser Gly Asn Ser Gln
161                      170                       180
Glu Ser Val Thr Glu Gln Asp Ser Lys Asp Ser Thr Tyr Ser Leu Ser Ser Thr Leu Thr
181                      190                       200
Leu Ser Lys Ala Asp Tyr Glu Lys His Lys Val Tyr Ala Cys Glu Val Thr His Gln Gly
201                      210
Leu Ser Ser Pro Val Thr Lys Ser Phe Asn Arg Gly Glu Cys     *1: H222-L214 disulfide bond.
```

Heavy chain:

```
VQLQESGPGL  VRPSQTLSLT  CTVSGYSITS  DHAWSWVRQP  PGRGL
EWIGYISYSG  ITTYNPSLKS  RVTMLRDTSK  NQFSLRLSSV  TAADT
AVYYCARSLA  RTTAMDYWGQ  GSLVTVSSAS  TKGPSVFPLA  PSSKS
TSGGTAALGC  LVKDYFPEPV  TVSWNSGALT  SGVHTFPAVL  QSSGL
YSLSSVVTVP  SSSLGTQTYI  CNVNHKPSNT  KVDKKVEPKS  CDKTH
TCPPCPAPEL  LGGPSVFLFP  PKPKDTLMIS  RTPEVTCVVV  DVSHE
DPEVKFNWYV  DGVEVHNAKT  KPREEQYNST  YRVVSVLTVL  HQDWL
NGKEYKCKVS  NKALPAPIEK  TISKAKGQPR  EPQVYTLPPS  RDELT
KNQVSLTCLV  KGFYPSDIAV  EWESNGQPEN  NYKTTPPVLD  SDGSF
FLYSKLTVDK  SRWQQGNVFS  CSVMHEALHN  HYTQKSLSLS  PG
```

```
1                        10                           20
pGlu Val Gln Leu Gln Glu Ser Gly Pro Gly  Leu Val Arg Pro Ser Gln Thr Leu Ser Leu
21                       30                           40
Thr Cys Thr Val Ser Gly Tyr Ser Ile Thr  Ser Asp His Ala Trp Ser Trp Val Arg Gln
41                       50                           60
Pro Pro Gly Arg Gly Leu Glu Trp Ile Gly  Tyr Ile Ser Tyr Ser Gly Ile Thr Thr Tyr
61                       70                           80
Asn Pro Ser Leu Lys Ser Arg Val Thr Met  Leu Arg Asp Thr Ser Lys Asn Gln Phe Ser
81                       90                           100
Leu Arg Leu Ser Ser Val Thr Ala Ala Asp  Thr Ala Val Tyr Tyr Cys Ala Arg Ser Leu
101                      110                          120
Ala Arg Thr Thr Ala Met Asp Tyr Trp Gly  Gln Gly Ser Leu Val Thr Val Ser Ser Ala
121                      130                          140
Ser Thr Lys Gly Pro Ser Val Phe Pro Leu  Ala Pro Ser Ser Lys Ser Thr Ser Gly Gly
141                      150                          160
Thr Ala Ala Leu Gly Cys Leu Val Lys Asp  Tyr Phe Pro Glu Pro Val Thr Val Ser Trp
161                      170                          180
Asn Ser Gly Ala Leu Thr Ser Gly Val His  Thr Phe Pro Ala Val Leu Gln Ser Ser Gly
181                      190                          200
Leu Tyr Ser Leu Ser Ser Val Val Thr Val  Pro Ser Ser Ser Leu Gly Thr Gln Thr Tyr
201                      210                          220
Ile Cys Asn Val Asn His Lys Pro Ser Asn  Thr Lys Val Asp Lys Lys Val Glu Pro Lys
221          *1           230      *3     240
Ser Cys Asp Lya Thr His Thr Cys Pro Pro  Cys Pro Ala Pro Glu Leu Leu Gly Gly Pro
             *2
241                      250                          260
Ser Val Phe Leu Phe Pro Pro Lys Pro Lys  Asp Thr Leu Met Ile Ser Arg Thr Pro Glu
261                      270                          280
Val Thr Cys Val Val Val Asp Val Ser His  Glu Asp Pro Glu Val Lys Phe Aan Trp Tyr
281                      290                  *4      300
Val Asp Gly Val Glu Val His Asn Ala Lys  Thr Lys Pro Arg Glu Glu Gln Tyr Asn Ser
301                      310                          320
Thr Tyr Arg Val Val Ser Val Leu Thr Val  Leu His Gln Asp Trp Leu Asn Gly Lys Glu
321                      330                          340
Tyr Lys Cys Lys Val Ser Asn Lys Ala Leu  Pro Ala Pro Ile Glu Lys Thr Ile Ser Lys
341                      350                          360
Ala Lys Gly Gln Pro Arg Glu Pro Gln Val  Tyr Thr Leu Pro Pro Ser Arg Asp Glu Leu
361                      370                          380
Thr Lys Asn Gln Val Ser Leu Thr Cys Leu  Val Lya Gly Phe Tyr Pro Ser Asp Ile Ala
381                      390                          400
Val Glu Trp Glu Ser Asn Gly Gln Pro Glu  Asn Asn Tyr Lys Thr Thr Pro Pro Val Leu
401                      410                          420
Asp Ser Asp Gly Ser Phe Phe Leu Tyr Ser  Lys Leu Thr Val Asp Lys Ser Arg Trp Gln
421                      430                          440
Gln Gly Asn Val Phe Ser Cys Ser Val Met  His Glu Ala Leu His Asn His Tyr Thr Gln
441                      450
Lys Ser Leu Ser Leu Ser Pro Gly
```

*1: H222-L214 disulfide bond. *2: H228-H228 disulfide bond (presumed).
*3: H231-H231 disulfide bond (presumed). *4: Glycosylation site.
pGlu: Pyroglutamic acid.

Production Process[6]

❖ Production platform
  - CHO DXB11 cells, derived from a CHO K1 strain, were transfected with an expression vector containing the genes encoding tocilizumab heavy and light chains as well as the DHFR gene.
❖ Cell bank system
  - A two-tiered cell banking system of Master Cell Bank (MCB) and Working Cell Bank (WCB) has been developed and maintained in accordance to cGMP and ICH guidelines.
  - The CHO V4 seed cells were adapted to growth in suspension culture in a serum-free medium, leading to the establishment of the original MCB (MCB-M1) and the original WCB (WCB-M1).
  - MCB-M1 was modified during development to generate a new MCB (MCB-M2971) and WCB (WCBM2971). Finally, the current WCB (WCB-M2033) was established from MCB-M2971 by replacement of animal-derived raw materials, with the exception of some bovine milk and salmon-derived additives.
  - Procedures followed for the preparation of MCB and WCB have been appropriately described. An extensive range of tests has been performed for their characterization, in accordance with ICH guidelines, including identity, viability, stability, presence of adventitious agents.
  - Transfected CHO DXB11 cells with the DHFR + phenotype were selected and then cultured in stepwise increasing concentrations of MTX. Cells were selected for resistance to MTX. By this process, an integrated copy of the DHFR sequence and the flanking regions (i.e. the tocilizumab-encoding sequence) were co-amplified. From the cells obtained, CHO V4 cells were cloned for use as seed cells for tocilizumab production.
❖ Fermentation process
  - A vial of WCB-M2033 is thawed and cells are expanded in a series of spinner flasks in a selective serum free growth medium to generate the cell inoculum. A series of bioreactors with increasing volumes is then used to expand the cell mass to generate sufficient cells for the inoculation of a production bioreactor.
  - Following the production phase, the bioreactor content is harvested using tangential flow filtration (TFF) in order to remove cells from the cell culture medium. The resulting cell culture filtrate is then further purified (see below).
  - Cell culture conditions and in-process controls (IPC) have been sufficiently described and are considered appropriate.
❖ Purification process
  - The purification process starting from the cell culture filtrate comprises the following steps, successively:
    ♦ Protein A chromatography.
    ♦ Viral inactivation step.
    ♦ Anion exchange chromatography.
    ♦ Mixed-mode ion exchange chromatography.
    ♦ Ultra-diafiltration (UF-DF).
    ♦ Nanofiltration.
    ♦ Final filling and storage.
  - Each step of the purification process has been adequately described, including description of the different buffers used, column regeneration and storage conditions of both columns and product after each step. Suitable IPC controls are in place, with acceptable limits.
❖ Manufacturing process development and process validation
  - The manufacturing process for tocilizumab drug substance has evolved over time in four main stages: "1st generation" (G1) process to "4th generation" (G4) process corresponding to the commercial process. During process development, the cell culture media used for tocilizumab fermentation process changed several times to reduce the use of components derived from animal sources.
  - The G4 process was developed to increase product yield. This included manufacturing site transfer with scale up in fermentation and purification, optimization of the cell culture media and fermentation parameters.
  - Materials obtained from the G4 process were used in Phase 3 clinical studies.
  - Manufacturing process development data were considered satisfactory. For filiation assessment, extensive structural, physicochemical and biological analyses of materials manufactured pre- and post-change were conducted prior to the implementation of each new manufacturing generation.
  - The tocilizumab manufacturing process was validated using data from commercial scale and scale-down models with respect to consistency and robustness of process performance and quality attributes, according to approved validation protocols. It was demonstrated that the G4 process consistently maintains process parameters within specified ranges and meets acceptance criteria for performance indicators. Overall, process validation was considered satisfactory.
❖ Physicochemical characterization
  - The complete amino acid sequence of tocilizumab was confirmed and the primary, secondary and tertiary structure were analyzed. It was confirmed that the disulfide linkages in tocilizumab drug substance reflect the disulfide structure known for IgG1 molecules. Monosaccharide composition was analyzed and the types and amounts of monosaccharides identified (N-acetyl glucosamine, fucose, mannose and galactose) reflect what is expected for IgG1 molecules.
  - Analysis of the oligosaccharide composition has shown that the major glycostructures are constituted by core-fucosylated biantennary complex-type oligosaccharide structures differing in the degree of terminal galactosylation, i.e. containing

two (G (2)), one (G (1)-1, G (1)-2) or no (G (0)) galactose residues. Besides the major glycostructures, afucosylated (G (0)-F, G (1)-1-F, G (1)-2-F, G (2)-F) and high mannose type oligosaccharides (M5) are present in tocilizumab. Sialylated oligosaccharides and other high mannose type structures (for example M6, M7) are present at even lower levels.

- Ion exchange chromatography (IEC) revealed the presence of several isoforms. Structural characterization of these isoforms demonstrated that differences between the isoforms are largely due to C- and N-terminal heterogeneity of the heavy chain and incomplete cleavage of the signal sequence from the N-terminus of the light chain.
- Investigation of charged-based isoforms was performed.
- The structural integrity of the tocilizumab molecule was tested.
- Size exclusion chromatography (SEC) was performed to analyze the size distribution of tocilizumab molecule. The two peaks detected in the chromatograms correspond to the monomer and dimer of tocilizumab molecule.

❖ Biological characterization
- In the cell-based bioassay, the cell growth-inhibiting activity by tocilizumab was evaluated by addition of tocilizumab and IL-6 to the cells such that they compete for the IL-6R on the cell.
- The binding activities of tocilizumab to human soluble IL-6R were also assessed.
- *In vitro* data confirmed that tocilizumab has essentially no or minimal complement dependent cytotoxicity (CDC) activity and no significant antibody-dependent cellular cytotoxicity activity.

❖ Impurities
- Product-related substances correspond to isoform peaks observed by IEC as well as the dimer and the degradation peaks observed by SEC of tocilizumab drug substance.
- Potential process-related impurities include:
  ◆ Cell substrate derived impurities: Host cell proteins (HCP) and DNA.
  ◆ Cell culture derived impurities.
  ◆ Downstream-derived impurities such as leached Protein A.
  ◆ Other impurities including endotoxin, bioburden.

❖ Pharmaceutical development
- Actemra®/RoActemra® is presented as a concentrate for solution for infusion in a single-use Type I glass vial. The concentrate is to be diluted in 0.90% sodium chloride prior to administration.
- Each vial contains 80 mg, 200 mg or 400 mg of tocilizumab formulated with sucrose, polysorbate 80, disodium phosphate dodecahydrate and sodium dihydrogen phosphate dihydrate and water for injections. These excipients are commonly used in formulating protein pharmaceuticals. Buffer, polysorbate 80 and sucrose are optimized to prevent protein aggregation that may occur in the vial on storage.
- The main changes to the formulation occurred during early clinical development and consisted of the removal of D-mannitol followed by the change of sodium chloride for sucrose.

❖ Adventitious agents
- Tocilizumab is produced in a serum-free culture medium without use of human- or animal-derived components; only fish, milk-derived and salmon-derived raw materials are added during the fermentation of tocilizumab. This minimizes a possible contamination with adventitious agents.
- Compliance with the Note for Guidance on "Minimizing the Risk of Transmitting Animal Spongiform Encephalopathy Agents via Human and Veterinary Medicinal Products" (EMEA/410/01 rev 02) has been sufficiently demonstrated.
- Extensive screening for viruses was performed. The tests did not reveal the presence of any viral contaminant in the cells used for production of tocilizumab, with the exception of intracellular A-type and C-type retroviral particles. Such particles are well known to be present in CHO cells. This is acceptable since there is sufficient capacity within the tocilizumab manufacturing process for reduction of this type of viral particles.
- The purification process of tocilizumab includes several steps for inactivation/removal of enveloped viruses. Viral safety has been sufficiently demonstrated.

❖ Protein yield: NA.
❖ Protein purity: NA.

Analytical Profile

❖ Disulfide profile

Table 5   Terminal Residue of Heavy Chain and Light Chain in Tocilizumab[11]

	N-terminal Residue	C-terminal Residue
Heavy chain	pGlul (principal component), Glnl	Gly448 (principal component), 447, Lys449
Light chain	Aspl	Cys214

Asp: Aspartic acid.   Cys: Cysteine.   Gln: Glutamine acid.   pGlu: Pyroglutamic acid.

❖ Glycosylation

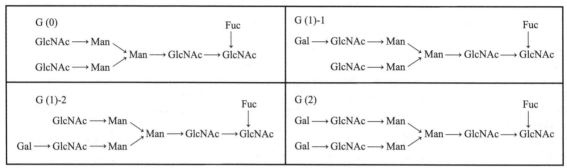

Gal: Galactosyl. GlcNAc: N-acetylglucosamine. Man: Mannose. Fuc: Fucose.

Figure 2   Glycosylation Process[11]

4   Pre-clinical Pharmacodynamics

Summary

Overview of *in vitro* Activities[6]

❖ Tocilizumab has binding affinity to membrane-bound IL-6 receptor (mIL-6R) (K_d value, about 2.5-2.8 nmol/L), the dissociation constant (K_d value) of tocilizumab to soluble form of the IL-6R (sIL-6R) was 0.71 nmol/L.

❖ When tocilizumab was added to the complexes of recombinant human IL-6 (rhIL-6) and sIL-6R formed *in vitro*, the binding rate of rhIL-6 to sIL-6R was decreased in a tocilizumab concentration-dependent manner and was <10.0% at tocilizumab concentrations >1 μg/mL.

❖ The binding rate of tocilizumab to sIL-6R was increased in a concentration-dependent manner at tocilizumab concentrations from 0.001 to 0.1 μg/mL and reached almost a plateau at >0.1 μg/mL.

❖ Tocilizumab specifically binds to the IL-6 binding site of both sIL-6R and mIL-6R with similar affinity.   Tocilizumab to the IL-6R with no direct cross-reactive inhibitory effect on TNF-α, IL-1β, IL-15 or IL-2 *in vitro*.

❖ Tocilizumab exhibits neutralizing activity against human and Cynomolgus monkey IL-6 receptors, but not against mouse or rat IL-6 receptors.

❖ The expression levels of CYP2C19 and CYP3A4 are increased following the administration of tocilizumab in RA patients, it has been inferred that the expression levels of at least CYP2C19 and CYP3A4 are lowered at the physiological concentrations of IL-6 in the intended patients for tocilizumab and the reduction of the expression levels of these enzymes is suppressed by the administration of tocilizumab.

❖ Tocilizumab undergoes the same FcRn-mediated clearance and transcytosis processes that have been described for other IgGs.   From *in vitro* binding studies at Fc-receptors on PBMC, it is assumed that binding of tocilizumab to the FcγI receptor occurs in the expected nanomolar range for an IgG.

Overview of *in vivo* Activities[6, 12]

❖ In a Cynomolgus monkey model of collagen-induced arthritis (CIA), tocilizumab was shown to prevent both the local joint and the systemic inflammatory disease manifestations.

❖ Elevations of plasma sIL-6R after the administration of tocilizumab are attributable to a slower elimination rate of the sIL-6R/tocilizumab complex compared to unbound sIL-6R.

❖ A single intraperitoneal dose of anti-mouse IL-6R antibody (MR16-1) was administered (MR16-1 was used because tocilizumab can not bind to mouse IL-6R) and then changes in the serum rhIL-6 level were examined.   As a result, the serum rhIL-6 levels were increased up to three-fold after the administration of MR16-1 (in-house data).

❖ Variations in terminal galactose content of tocilizumab do not affect its binding affinity to carbohydrate receptors and carbohydrate receptors contribute insignificantly to the elimination of tocilizumab from plasma.

❖ Tocilizumab at concentrations ranging from 1.95 to 500 μg/mL did not bind to any lectin.

❖ Tocilizumab should not affect the development of T-cell memory and T-helper cell activity.

❖ Tocilizumab was well tolerated in Cynomolgus monkeys, both as single intravenous (i.v.) doses up to 100 mg/kg and when given in multiple i.v. doses up to 50 mg/(kg·day) for 4 weeks or at i.v. doses up to 100 mg/kg/week for 6 months.

❖ Tocilizumab showed no effect on the cardiac electrophysiological performance, cardiac tissue integrity or systemic pro-thrombotic activities i.v. at doses up to 50 mg/kg.

Overview of *in vitro* Activities

Target Binding and Mechanism of Action[13]

(Japanese is presented in several tables as the first mAb was developed in Japan).

❖ The dissociation constant (K_d value) of tocilizumab to sIL-6R was 0.71 ± 0.037 nmol/L.

Table 6   List of Test Results to Support Drug Efficacy[13]

Test Item	Experiment Method/ Measurement	Concentration/Dosage/ Administration Method	Implementation Facility	Test Result
Binding to soluble IL-6 receptor	ELISA	0, 0.46-9,000 ng/mL	CSK	MRA binds to humanization request IL-6 receptor in a concentration-dependent manner.
Binding to membrane-bound IL-6 receptor	Flow cytometry analysis	10 µg/mL	CSK	MRA binds to the human membrane-bound IL-6 receptor.
	Scatchard analysis (dissociation constant)	0, 11, 33, 77, 165, 341, 11,000 nmol/L		#Y4: 2.8×10^{-9} mol/L #X7: 2.5×10^{-9} mol/L.
Neutralizing activity against various IL-6 receptors	Proliferation of PHA stimulated T lymphocytes by IL-6	Human (0, 0.02, 0.1, 0.5, 2.5 µg/mL), Cynomolgus monkey/rat/mouse (0, 0.2, 1, 5, 25 µg/mL)	CSK	It shows neutralization in humans and Cynomolgus monkeys but does not show neutralizing activity in mice and rats.
Neutralizing activity against human gp130 family cytokine receptor	Proliferation of recombinant cells proliferating depending on IL-6, IL-11, OSM, LIF, CNTF	0, 2, 10, 50, 250 µg/mL	CSK	MRA does not show neutralizing activity on human gp130 family cytokine receptor other than IL-6 receptor.

Document number at first approval.   CNTF: Ciliary neurotrophic factor.   CSK: Chugai Seiyaku Co., Ltd.   ELISA: Enzyme linked immune Sorbent Assay.   IL-6: Interleukin-6.   IL-11: Interleukin-11.   LIF: Leukemia inhibitory factor.   MRA: Tocilizumab.   OSM: Oncostatin M.   PHA: Phytohaemagglutinin.

Table 7   List of Test Results on Action Mechanism[13]

Test Item	Experiment Method/ Measurement	Concentration/Dosage/ Administration Method	Implementation Facility	Test Result
Inhibition of *in vitro* IL-6 activity	ELISA	0, 0.19 ng/mL-300 µg/mL	CSK	Inhibition of IL-6 binding to soluble IL-6 receptor.
	Proliferation of BAF-h130 cells by IL-6/soluble IL-6 receptor complex	0, 0.01, 0.1, 1, 10, 100 µg/mL	CSK	Inhibition of cellular proliferation via soluble IL-6 receptor.
	Proliferation of KPMM2 cells by IL-6	0, 0.01, 0.1, 1, 10, 100 µg/mL	CSK	Inhibition of cell proliferation mediated by membrane-bound IL-6 receptor.
Activity of MRA/soluble IL-6 receptor complex	Growth of BAF-h130 cells by MRA/soluble IL-6 receptor complex	0, 1, 10, 100 µg/mL	CSK	There is no IL-6 activity in MRA/soluble IL-6 receptor complex.
Inhibition of *in vivo* IL-6 activity	CRP and platelet count	0, 5 mg/kg single intravenous administration	CSK	Suppression of activity expression of IL-6 administered to Cynomolgus monkey.

Document number at first approval.   CRP: C-reactive protein.   CSK: Chugai Seiyaku Co., Ltd.   ELISA: Enzyme Linked Immune Sorbent Assay.   MRA: Tocilizumab (Genetical recombination).

Table 8   Pharmaceutical Efficacy Simulation Results List in Mouse Model[13]

Test Item	Experiment Method/ Measurement	Concentration/Dosage/ Administration Method	Implementation Facility	Test Result
Effect on human IL-6 transgenic mouse (reference material)	Red blood cell count IgG1 concentration, spleen weight survival rate	MR16-1 (Anti-mouse IL-6 receptor antibody): Initially, 2 mg/mouse is intravenously administered, 100 µg/mouse is administered twice a week from the following week, subcutaneously	CSK	Suppress the pathogenesis of Castleman's disease and prolong survival days.
Continuing occurrence effect in amyloidosis model (reference material)	Amyloid deposition in the spleen, liver, and kidney	Single-dose of MR 16-1 100 mg/kg intraperitoneally	CSK	Completely suppresses amyloid deposits in the spleen, liver, and kidney.

Document number at first approval.   CSK: Chugai Seiyaku Co., Ltd.

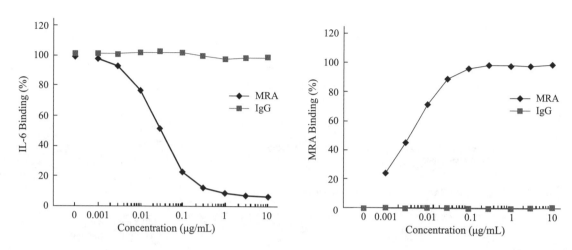

Figure 3   The Influence of IL-6/sIL-6R Complex to MRA, (mean ± SD, $n = 3$)[13]

❖ Tocilizumab binds to the IL-6R with no direct cross-reactive inhibitory effect on TNF-α, IL-1β, IL-15 or IL-2 *in vitro*.

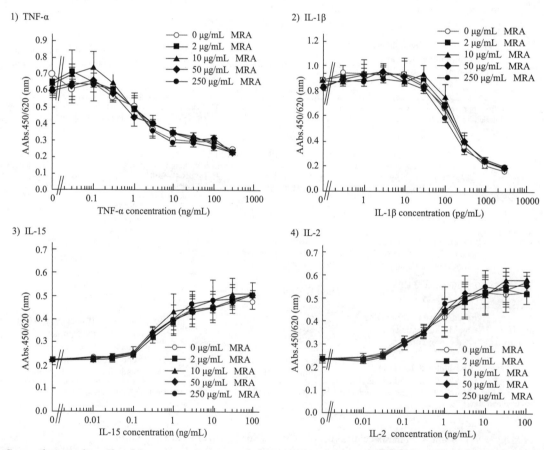

Animal: Cynomolgus monkeys (female).

Model: Arthritis was induced by immunization with bovine type II collagen twice.

Administration: The control group received PBS and the tocilizumab group received 30 mg/kg of tocilizumab intravenously once weekly for 4 weeks.

Test: Plasma MRA levels, PIP joints number, CRP and albumin.

Result: PMDA judged that the pharmacologic effects of tocilizumab against RA and similar diseases, pJIA and sJIA can be explained by the submitted data including the above study results and responses.

Figure 4   Effects of TNF-α, IL-1β, IL-15, IL-2 Biological Activity on MRA[13]

(A Cynomolgus Monkey Model of Collagen-induced Arthritis)

5 Toxicology

Summary

Non-clinical Single-Dose and Repeated-Dose Toxicology

❖ Toxicity studies have shown tocilizumab to be well tolerated in Cynomolgus monkeys, both as single intravenous (i.v.) doses up to 100 mg/kg and when given in multiple i.v. doses up to 50 mg/(kg·day) for 4 weeks or at i.v. doses up to 100 mg/(kg·week) for 6 months.

❖ Neither monkeys exposed to tocilizumab over more than 6 months, nor IL-6 k.o. mice showed morphological alterations to the primary or secondary tissues of their immune system nor in any other organ or tissues.

❖ Dose finding study for juvenile toxicity study of MR16-1 by intravenous administration in Mice.

Table 9　The 6-month Repeated-Dose Toxicology Studies of Tocilizumab in Cynomolgus Monkeys[14]

Lesion	Males (mg/kg)				Females (mg/kg)				Observation
	0	1	10	100	0	1	10	100	
Injection site, inflammation, hemorrhage	3/4 slight slight	2/4 slight slight	3/4 slight	1/5 slight	2/4 slight	1/4 slight	3/4 slight	3/5 slight	Inflammation in the injection site was noted in control and treated animals.
Recovery group	1		1	2	1	0	0	0	
Liver granuloma	0	0	0	1/4 slight	0	0	1/4 slight	0	A slight granuloma in the liver was observed and it was reversible.
Recovery group	0	0	0	0	0	0	0	0	
Skeletal muscle, femoral, degeneration of muscle fiber	0	0	1/4 slight	1/4 slight	0	0	1/4 slight	0	Degeneration of the skeletal muscle was noted and that was not completely reversible.
Recovery group	0		0	0	0	0	1/4 slight	0	

Table 10　Single-Dose and Repeated-Dose Toxicology Studies of Tocilizumab in Rats and Cynomolgus Monkeys[14]

Species	Duration (Month)	Dose [mg/(kg·day)]	Observation
Sprague Dawley rats	1	2, 10, 50 mg/kg, i.v. infusion	No treatment related mortality, injection site inflammation in placebo and drug treated animals. Antibody to MRA was noted.
Cynomolgus monkeys	Single-dose	1, 10 and 100 mg/kg	No mortality due to the treatment.
Cynomolgus monkeys	6	1, 10 and 100 mg/kg	No mortality due to the treatment. Liver granuloma and skeletal muscle degeneration at 10 and 100 mg/kg, NOEL 1 mg/kg, inflammation at injection site of placebo and drug treated animals.

Safety Pharmacology

❖ The cardiovascular safety of tocilizumab has been investigated in a series of preclinical *in vivo* studies in Cynomolgus monkeys. Tocilizumab showed no effect on the cardiac electrophysiological performance, cardiac tissue integrity or systemic pro-thrombotic activities i.v. at doses up to 50 mg/kg.

Reproductive Toxicology

❖ A reproductive teratology study was performed to address potential effects on embryo-fetal development, and supplementary data from IL-6 knock out (k.o.) and IL-6 transgenic mouse models were evaluated for functional and developmental risk assessments.

　• Pregnant Cynomolgus monkeys were treated intravenously with tocilizumab (daily doses of 2, 10, or 50 mg/kg from gestation days 20-50) during organogenesis.

　• There was no evidence for a teratogenic at any dose.

　• Tocilizumab produced an increase in the incidence of abortion/embryo-fetal death at 10 mg/kg and 50 mg/kg doses (1.25 and 6.25 times the human dose of 8 mg/kg every 2 to 4 weeks based on a mg/kg comparison).

- A higher incidence of abortion/embryo-fetal death was observed in the Cynomolgus monkeys teratology study in the 50 mg/(kg·day) high-dose group with systemic exposure of factor >100 above the human targeted efficacious plasma concentration.
- The NOAEL for this study is 10 mg/(kg·day) due to the possibly treatment-related abortion observed as statistically significant at a dose level of 50 mg/(kg·day).
- Pregnancy Category C should be designated to tocilizumab.

Table 11   Summary of Finding and Exposure in the Segment II Embryo-fetal Development Study of Tocilizumab in the Cynomolgus Monkeys[14]

	Group 1 0 mg/(kg·day)	Group 2 2 mg/(kg·day)	Group 3 10 mg(kg·day)	Group 4 50 mg/(kg·day)
Toxicokinetic data[a] Mean serum concentration	ND	320	1,646	5,814
Exposure margin based on mg/kg[b]	-	0.25	1.3	6.3
Exposure margin based on mean clinical C_{max}[c]		1.7	9.0	32.0
Fetal abortions/deaths (total)	1/10	1/10	2/10	3/10

ND: Not detected (<0.781 mcg/mL).   -: Not available.   [a] Serum measured 24 hours after final dose (GD50).   [b] Comparison made based on 8 mg/kg dose as proposed by the applicant (296 mg/m²).   [c] Clinical C trough values reported by the applicant in the proposed label are 9.7 ± 10.5 µg/mL 4-weeks after the monthly dose of 8 mg/kg. Clinical C_{max} value for the clinical study was reported as 183 ± 85.6 µg/mL.   For the table, a conservative approach comparing the clinical C_{max} to the animal concentration 24 hours post-dose was employed rather than comparison to the human C_{trough} which would produce a potentially false sense of safety.

Genotoxicity

❖ MRA was not mutagenic in either the Ames bacterial reverse mutation assay or the chromosomal aberration assay in peripheral lymphocytes from human volunteers.

Carcinogenicity

❖ The applicant did not conduct any carcinogenicity study.

Other Toxicology

❖ Tocilizumab did not affect liver enzymes in Cynomolgus monkey studies in which IL-6 was elevated due to CIA induced inflammation.   Serious hepatic events are an endpoint to be followed in pharmacovigilance and in registries.

❖ No long-term animal studies have been performed to establish the carcinogenicity potential of tocilizumab.

❖ Tocilizumab was negative for genotoxic potential in the Ames *in vitro* bacterial reverse mutation assay and the *in vitro* chromosomal aberrations assay using human peripheral blood lymphocytes.

❖ Fertility studies conducted in male and female mice using a murine analogue of tocilizumab showed no impairment of fertility.

❖ The ecotoxic potential of tocilizumab is considered to be low.

❖ The 6-month repeated-dose toxicology study for tocilizumab in Cynomolgus monkeys, liver granulomas, and skeletal muscle degeneration were noted at 10 and 100 mg/kg.

❖ Injection site inflammation was noted in control and treated animals.

Anti-product Antibody Profile

❖ Tocilizumab is immunogenic in the monkey.   The observed anti-tocilizumab response showed a clear inverse dose relationship, an effect which is frequently observed with molecules of this type.

Table 12   Immunogenicity of Tocilizumab in Cynomolgus Monkeys[14]

Special Toxicology	Species	Dose [mg/(kg·day)], Duration	Finding
Immunogenicity	Cynomolgus monkeys	0, 1, 10 and 100 mg/kg, 6-month	Anti-MRA antibody was detected at 1 and 10 mg/kg only from week 2 of the treatment up to the recovery period. No monkey at 100 mg/kg showed positive for anti-MRA antibody.
	Pregnant Cynomolgus monkeys	0, 2, 10 and 50 mg/kg between GD 20-50	Two monkeys at 2 mg/kg showed anti-MRA antibody from GD50. MRA was not neutralized during the treatment.

Table 13　Summary of Information in Cynomolgus Monkeys from Several Studies[14]

Dose (mg/kg)	Route	Frequency	$t_{1/2}$ (Day)	Conc., Week 26 though (μg/mL)	AUC (mg·h/mL)	Anti-MRA Antibody
0.5	i.v.	Single			0.39	-
1	s.c.	Single	2.8		0.73	+
5	s.c./i.v.	Single	4.6/5.6		7.8/10.4	+
5	i.v.	8 doses	9.5		9.6	+
15	s.c.	Single	9.5		55.0	-
50	i.v.	Single	8.2		256	
10	i.v.	Q weekly × 6 mo	6.8	187-244		+
100	i.v.	Q weekly × 6 mo	10.4-13.4	1,935		-

i.v.: Intravenous injection.　s.c.: Intramuscular injection.　Q weekly × 6 mo: Once weekly × 6 months.　+: Positive for anti-MRA antibody.　-: Negative for anti-MRA antibody.

6　Non-clinical Pharmacokinetic/ADME/Toxicokinetics

Summary

Non-clinical Pharmacokinetics[4, 12]

❖ Tocilizumab pharmacokinetics and metabolism are consistent with those of other IgGs, which are characterized by a slow plasma clearance and low penetration into tissues.　Both the distribution and elimination of tocilizumab was as expected for an IgG antibody.

❖ In single-dose studies in rats and Cynomolgus monkeys
  • In a single-dose intravenous study in rats values of ca. 200 h for terminal half-life, ca. 0.6 mL/(h·kg) for total CL and ca. 160 mL/kg for the distribution volume (V_{ss}) were calculated after doses of 0.5, 5 and 50 mg/kg, respectively.　Dose proportional increase in AUC was observed.
  • From single-dose intravenous studies in male Cynomolgus monkeys values of 0.5 and 0.2 mL/(h·kg) for total CL and of ca. 60 mL/kg for the distribution volume (V_{ss}) were calculated after the 5 and 50 mg/kg dose, respectively.
  • Single-dose studies in rats and monkeys show low clearance of tocilizumab with a long half-life and a low volume of distribution indicating low tissue transferability.　Non-linear pharmacokinetics were observed in Cynomolgus monkeys (as in humans), whereas linear pharmacokinetics were observed in rats.
  • A clear biphasic decline was observed.　The comparability of the results for the 5 mg/kg dose obtained in a study with female monkeys suggests that there are no pharmacokinetic differences due to gender in monkeys.　An apparent non-linear pharmacokinetic behavior in the monkeys was observed (dose dependent values for CL and over-proportional increase in AUC) which was more pronounced between the lower doses (0.5 and 5 mg/kg) than between the 5 and 50 mg/dose groups.　This resembles the findings in humans.

❖ In multiple-dose studies in Cynomolgus monkeys
  • In repeated-dose studies with weekly dosing in monkeys, steady-state was reached following the fifth or sixth administration.
  • A multiple-dose study in Cynomolgus monkeys indicated that pharmacokinetics of tocilizumab did not change upon repeated administration over 8 weeks.　Neutralizing anti-tocilizumab antibodies could be detected in plasma of Cynomolgus monkeys after single and repeated dosing which were possibly responsible for an apparently accelerated decline in plasma concentration of tocilizumab at later time points in the single-dose study.

❖ Distribution
  • Distribution studies showed no accumulation in any specific tissues, with the highest levels of radioactivity in monkeys observed in the adrenal gland, lung, kidney, liver, and the target tissues of tocilizumab, such as the synovia, membrane synovialis, bone marrow, and spleen.
  • A distribution study in Cynomolgus monkeys revealed tissue/plasma ratios of tocilizumab >1 for some tissues at Day 28 p.i..　In most cases the ratios increased from Day 7 to Day 28 suggesting slow equilibration between plasma and tissues. A 10-fold higher concentration in the synovial fluid than in plasma was observed at Day 28.　Binding to blood cells was rather low, ca. 20.0% of total tocilizumab in blood circulation seems to be bound to/in blood cells.　The extent of binding to plasma proteins, especially to the soluble receptor sIL-6R, has not been determined in animal plasma.

❖ Drug-Drug interaction

- Tocilizumab is assumed to be catabolized by endogenous proteolytic pathways and the majority of radio-labeled tocilizumab is excreted in the urine as low-molecular-weight entities.
- Pharmacodynamic drug interaction studies were not conducted with tocilizumab.

Non-clinical Pharmacokinetics

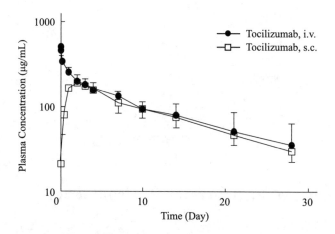

Figure 5 Time Course of Tocilizumab Plasma Concentrations in Female Göttingen Minipigs following a Single i.v. (at 20.3 mg/kg) or s.c. (at 180 mg/animal, equivalent to ca. 20.2 mg/kg) Administration of Tocilizumab (n = 3 or 5, respectively, mean ± SD)[15]

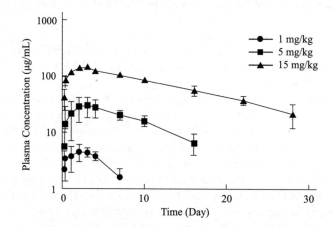

Figure 6 Time Course of Tocilizumab Plasma Concentrations in Cynomolgus Monkeys following a Single Subcutaneous Administration of Tocilizumab at Various Dose levels (n = 4/dose group, mean ± SD)[15]

Table 14 Noncompartimental Pharmacokinetic Parameters for Tocilizumab in Cynomolgus Monkeys following Single Subcutaneous Administration of Tocilizumab at Various Dose Levels[15]

Parameter	Dosing Regimen (n = 4/dose Group)		
	1 mg/kg	5 mg/kg	15 mg/kg
C_{max} (μg/mL)	4.9 ± 1.3	30.1 ± 11.8	145 ± 8.0
T_{max} (h)	50.0 ± 30.2	72.0 ± 19.8	66.0 ± 12.0
AUC_{0-inf} (μg·h/mL)	737 ± 210	7,860 ± 2,260	55,200 ± 10,200
$t_{1/2}$ (h)	68.1 ± 26.1	112 ± 9	229 ± 42.0
F (%)	NC	72.1	NC

Mean ± SD. AUC: Area under the plasma concentration-time curve. C_{max}: Maximum plasma concentration. F: Bioavailability. NC: Not calculated. T_{max}: Time to maximum plasma concentration.

Table 15 C_{min} Exposures Attained at 100 mg/kg Tocilizumab Given Intravenously or Subcutaneously in Monkey Toxicity Studies[14, 16]

Study	Time Point	Dose (mg/kg)	No. of Animals	C_{min} (µg/mL)	CV[a] or SD[b]
9-week monkey subcutaneous study (report No.1029905)	168 h after 8th weekly dose (samples taken before 9th weekly dose)	100	5 males 5 females	2,580 2,230	18.0%, 17.7%
6-month monkey intravenous study (report No. TOX02-0169)	168 h after 8th weekly dose (samples taken before 9th weekly dose)	100	5 males 5 females	1,436 1,595	135.8 87.7

[a] CV: Coefficient of variation used as the parameter in the s.c. study.   [b] SD: Standard deviation used as the parameter in the i.v. study.

PK/PD Studies

❖ The clinical pharmacology program included PK and PD data and PK-PD relationships from the following studies: Roche's pivotal study WA18221 and five supportive Chugai studies (LRO320, MRA011JP, MRA316JP, MRA317JP, and MRA324JP). In study WA18221 blood samples for PK (tocilizumab serum concentrations) and PD (IL-6, sIL-6R) were collected at pre-dose and post-dose (end of infusion) on Day 1 and at Weeks 2, 4 and 10, pre-dose at Weeks 6, 8, and 12 and at any time during the week at Weeks 1 and 11.   Anti-tocilizumab antibodies were collected at baseline (pre-dose on Day 1) and at Week 12.

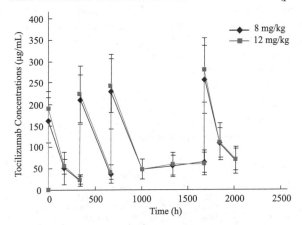

Figure 7   The Mean (± SD) Serum Tocilizumab Concentration Time Profile by Treatment Group in Study WA18221[17]

Table 16   Summary of Model-predicted Tocilizumab PK Measures at Week 12 by Dosing Groups[17]

Parameter		8 mg/kg (N = 37)	12 mg/kg (N = 38)	All patients (N = 75)
C_{max} (µg/mL)	Mean ± SD CV%	226 ± 54.5 24.1	263 ± 54.1 20.6	245 ± 57.2 23.3
C_{min} (µg/mL)	Mean ± SD CV%	54.5 ± 20.7 38.0	60.5 ± 25.5 42.1	57.5 ± 23.3 40.5
$AUC_{2\ weeks}$ (µg·day/mL)	Mean ± SD CV%	1,337 ± 409 30.5	1,346 ± 426 31.6	1,341 ± 415 30.9

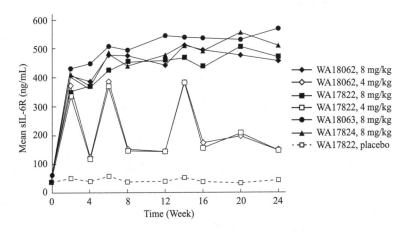

Figure 8   Mean sIL-6R Levels in Patients Treated with 4 and 8 mg/kg Tocilizumab Every 4 Weeks in Four Phase 3 Studies (WA17822, WA17824, WA18062 and WA18063)[12]

7 Clinical Efficacy and Safety

Overview Profile

❖ In January 2011, FDA approves tocilizumab for the treatment of moderately to severely active rheumatoid arthritis. In April 2011, FDA approves tocilizumab for the treatment of systemic juvenile idiopathic arthritis.

❖ In April 2013, FDA approves tocilizumab for children with polyarticular juvenile idiopathic arthritis.

❖ In October 2013, Genentech gains FDA approval for new subcutaneous formulation of tocilizumab for use in adult patients living with moderately to severely active rheumatoid arthritis.

❖ In May 2017, FDA approves tocilizumab subcutaneous injection for giant cell arteritis.

❖ In August 2017, FDA approves tocilizumab for the treatment of CAR T cell-induced cytokine release syndrome.

Rheumatoid Arthritis-Intravenous Administration[18]

❖ The efficacy and safety of intravenously administered tocilizumab was assessed in five randomized, double-blind, multi-center studies in patients greater than 18 years with active rheumatoid arthritis diagnosed according to American College of Rheumatology (ACR) criteria.

❖ Tocilizumab was given intravenously every 4 weeks as monotherapy (Study I), in combination with methotrexate (MTX) (Study II and III) or other disease-modifying anti-rheumatic drugs (DMARDs) (Study IV) in patients with an inadequate response to those drugs, or in combination with MTX in patients with an inadequate response to (Tumor Necrosis Factor) TNF antagonists (Study V).

❖ Of the 4,009 patients in this population, 3,577 received treatment for at least 6 months, 3,309 for at least one year; 2,954 received treatment for at least 2 years and 2,189 for 3 years.

❖ All patients in these studies had moderately to severely active rheumatoid arthritis with at least 8 tender and 6 swollen joints at baseline.

Clinical Efficacy

Table 17   Clinical Response at Weeks 24 and 52 in Active and Placebo Controlled Trials of Intravenous Tocilizumab in Patients with RA[18]

| | Percent of Patients | | | | | | | | | | | | |
| Response Rate | Study I | | Study II | | | Study III | | | Study IV | | Study V | | |
	MTX (N=284)	MRA[a] (N=286) (95% CI)[b]	PBO+ MTX (N=393)	MRA[c] + MTX (N=399) (95% CI)[b]	MRA[a] + MTX (N=398) (95% CI)[b]	PBO+ MTX (N=204)	MRA[c] + MTX (N=213) (95% CI)[a]	MRA[a] + MTX (N=205) (95% CI)[b]	PBO+ DMARDs (N=413)	MRA[a] (N=803) (95% CI)[b]	PBO+ MTX (N=58)	MRA[c] + MTX (N=161) (95% CI)[b]	MRA[a] + MTX (N=170) (95% CI)[b]
ACR 20													
Week 24	53.0%	70.0% (0.11, 0.27)	27.0%	51.0% (0.17, 0.29)	56.0% (0.23, 0.35)	27.0%	48.0% (0.15, 0.23)	59.0% (0.23, 0.41)	24.0%	61.0% (0.30, 0.40)	10.0%	30.0% (0.15, 0.36)	50.0% (0.36, 0.56)
Week 52	NA	NA	25.0%	47.0% (0.15, 0.28)	56.0% (0.23, 0.38)	NA	NA	NA	NA	NA	NA	NA	NA
ACR 50													
Week 24	34.0%	44.0% (0.040, 0.20)	10.0%	25.0% (0.090, 0.20)	32.0% (0.16, 0.28)	11.0%	32.0% (0.13, 0.29)	44.0% (0.25, 0.41)	9.0%	38.0% (0.23, 0.33)	4.0%	17.0% (0.050, 0.25)	29.0% (0.21, 0.41)
Week 52	NA	NA	10.0%	29.0% (0.14, 0.25)	36.0% (0.21, 0.32)	NA	NA	NA	NA	NA	NA	NA	NA
ACR 70													
Week 24	15.0%	28.0% (0.070, 0.22)	2.0%	11.0% (0.030, 0.13)	13.0% (0.050, 0.15)	2.0%	12.0% (0.040, 0.18)	22.0% (0.12, 0.27)	3.0%	21.0% (0.13, 0.21)	1.0%	5.0% (-0.060, 0.14)	12.0% (0.030, 0.22)
Week 52	NA	NA	4.0%	16.0% (0.080, 0.17)	20.0% (0.12, 0.21)	NA	NA	NA	NA	NA	NA	NA	NA
Major Clinical Responses[d]													
Week 52	NA	NA	1.0%	4.0% (0.010, 0.060)	7.0% (0.030, 0.090)	NA	NA	NA	NA	NA	NA	NA	NA

MRA: Tocilizumab.   MTX: Methotrexate.   NA: Not applicable.   PBO: Placebo.   [a] T: 8 mg/kg.   [b] CI: 95% confidence interval of the weighted difference to placebo adjusted for site (and disease duration for Study I only).   [c] T: 4 mg/kg.   [d] Major clinical response is defined as achieving an ACR 79 response for a continuous 24-week period.

Clinical Safety

Table 18   Adverse Reactions in 24-week Active or Placebo Controlled Trials of Intravenous Tocilizumab in Patients with RA[18]

	MRA[a] 8 mg/kg	MTX	MRA 4 mg/kg + DMARDs	MRA 8 mg/kg + DMARDs	PBO + DMARDs
Overall infections	119	-	133	127	112
Serious infections	3.6	1.5	4.4	5.3	3.9
Infusion reactions	-	-	8.0%	7.0%	5.0%
Neutropenia					
<1,000/mm³	-	-	1.8%	3.4%	0.10%
<500/mm³	-	-	0.40%	0.30%	0.10%
Thrombocytopenia	-	-	1.3%	1.7%	0.50%
AST (U/L)					
>ULN to 3 × ULN	22.0%	26.0%	34.0%	41.0%	17.0%
>3 × ULN to 5 × ULN	0.30%	2.0%	1.0%	2.0%	0.30%
>5 × ULN	0.70%	0.40%	0.10%	0.20%	<0.10
ALT (U/L)					
>ULN to 3 × ULN	36.0%	33.0%	45.0%	48.0%	23.0%
>3 × ULN to 5 × ULN	1.0%	4.0%	5.0%	5.0%	1.0%
>5 × ULN	0.70%	1.0%	1.3%	1.5%	0.30%
Upper respiratory tract infection	7.0%	5.0%	6.0%	8.0%	6.0%
Nasopharyngitis	7.0%	6.0%	4.0%	6.0%	4.0%
Headache	7.0%	2.0%	6.0%	5.0%	3.0%
Hypertension	6.0%	2.0%	4.0%	4.0%	3.0%
ALT increased	6.0%	4.0%	3.0%	3.0%	1.0%
Dizziness	3.0%	1.0%	2.0%	3.0%	2.0%
Bronchitis	3.0%	2.0%	4.0%	3.0%	3.0%
Rash	2.0%	1.0%	4.0%	3.0%	1.0%
Mouth ulceration	2.0%	2.0%	1.0%	2.0%	1.0%
Abdominal pain upper	2.0%	2.0%	3.0%	3.0%	2.0%
Gastritis	1.0%	2.0%	1.0%	2.0%	1.0%
Transaminase increased	1.0%	5.0%	2.0%	2.0%	1.0%

Events per 100 patient-years/%.   ALT: Alanine aminotransferase.   AST: Aspartate transaminase.   MRA: Tocilizumab.   MTX: Methotrexate.   PBO: Placebo.   RA: Rheumatoid arthritis.   ULN: Upper limit of normal.   [a] Monotherapy.

Rheumatoid Arthritis-Subcutaneous Administration[18]

❖ The efficacy and safety of subcutaneous administered tocilizumab was assessed in two double-blind, controlled, multi-center studies (Study SC-I and Study SC-II).

❖ Study SC-I was a non-inferiority study that compared the efficacy and safety of tocilizumab 162 mg administered every week subcutaneously (s.c.) and 8 mg/kg intravenously (i.v.) every 4 weeks in 1,262 adult subjects with rheumatoid arthritis.

❖ Study SC-II was a placebo controlled superiority study that evaluated the safety and efficacy of tocilizumab 162 mg administered every other week subcutaneously or placebo in 656 patients.

❖ All patients in both studies received background non-biologic DMARDs.

Clinical Efficacy

Table 19　Clinical Response at Week 24 in Trials of Subcutaneous Tocilizumab in Patients with RA[18]

	SC-I[a]		SC-II[b]	
	MRA s.c. 162 mg Every Week + DMARD (N = 558)	MRA i.v. 8 mg/kg + DMARD (N = 537)	MRA s.c. 162 mg Every Other Week + DMARD (N = 437)	PBO + DMARD (N = 219)
ACR20				
Week 24	69.0%	73.4%	61.0%	32.0%
Weighed difference (95% *CI*)	-4.0% (-9.2, 1.2)		30.0% (22.0, 37.0)	
ACR50				
Week 24	47.0%	49.0%	40.0%	12.0%
Weighted difference (95% *CI*)	-2.0% (-7.5, 4.0)		28.0% (21.5, 34.4)	
ACR70				
Week 24	24.0%	28.0%	20.0%	5.0%
Weighted difference (95% *CI*)	-4.0% (-9.0, 1.3)		15.0% (9.8, 19.9)	
Change in DAS28 (adjusted mean)				
Week 24	-3.5	-3.5	-3.1	-1.7
Adjusted mean difference (95% *CI*)	0.0 (-0.20, 0.10)		-1.4 (-1.7, -1.1)	
DAS 28 <2.6				
Week 24	38.4%	36.9%	32.0%	4.0%
Weighted difference (95% *CI*)	0.90 (-5.0, 6.8)		28.6 (22.0, 35.2)	

CI: Confidence interval.　MRA: Tocilizumab.　PBO: Placebo.　RA: Rheumatoid arthritis.　[a] Per protocol population.　[b] Intent-to-treat population.

Clinical Safety

Table 20　Summary of the Safety Data in SC-I Study[19]

	MRA s.c. 162 mg, qw (N = 631) 289.82 PY	MRA i.v. 8 mg/kg, q4w (N = 631) 288.39 PY
AE		
Total AE, *n*	1,747	1,697
Patient with ≥1 AE, *n* (%)	481 (76.2)	486 (77.0)
Discontinuation due to AE, *n* (%)	30 (4.8)	42 (6.7)
SAE		
Total SAE, *n*	34	43
Patients with ≥1 SAE, *n* (%)	29 (4.6)	33 (5.2)
SAE per 100 PY (95% *CI*)	11.7 (8.1-16.4)	14.9 (10.8-20.1)
SI		
Total SI	9	9
Patients with ≥1 SI, *n* (%)	9 (1.4)	9 (1.4)
SI per 100 PY (95% *CI*)	3.1 (1.3-5.9)	3.5 (1.7-6.4)
Serious hypersensitivity reactions[a], *n* (%)	2 (<1.0)	3[b] (<1.0)

Continued

	MRA s.c. 162 mg, qw (N = 631) 289.82 PY	MRA i.v. 8 mg/kg, q4w (N = 631) 288.39 PY
ISR		
Patients with ISR, *n* (%)	64 (10.1)	15 (2.4)
ISR, *n*	168	94
Erythema, *n* (%)	28 (4.4)	5 (0.80)
Pain, *n* (%)	12 (1.9)	5 (0.80)
Pruritus, *n* (%)	14 (2.2)	0 (0.0)
Haematoma, *n* (%)	5 (0.80)	5 (0.80)
Dose interruption or study withdrawal because of ISR, *n*	0	0
Death, *n* (%)	0 (0.0)	1 (<1.0)

AE: Adverse event.　ISR: Injection-site reaction.　i.v.: Intravenous.　MRA: Tocilizumab.　PY: Patient-years.　SAE: Serious adverse event.　SI: Serious infection.
[a] Serious hypersensitivity was defined as an SAE occurring during or within 24 h of the injection or infusion, excluding ISR, and evaluated as 'related' to study treatment by the investigator.　[b] Of the three events in the tocilizumab i.v. group, one was cellulitis and one was retinal artery occlusion; these two events were not considered consistent with a serious hypersensitivity reaction.

Table 21　Summary of the Safety Data in SC-II Study[a, 20]

	MRA s.c. 162 mg Every Other Week (N = 437)	PBO s.c. Every Other Week (N = 218)
AEs		
Total AEs, *n*	716	217
Patients with ⩾1 AEs, *n* (%)	274 (62.7)	126 (57.8)
Discontinuation due to AEs, *n* (%)	9 (2.0)	3 (1.0)
Serious AEs		
Total, *n*	25	12
Patients with ⩾1, *n* (%)	20 (4.6)	8 (3.7)
Infections		
Total, *n*	167	78
Patients with ⩾1, *n* (%)	131 (30.0)	61 (28.0)
Serious infections		
Total, *n*	12	5
Patients with ⩾1, *n* (%)	9 (2.1)	4 (1.8)
Serious hypersensitivity reactions[b], *n*	0	0
ISRs		
Total, *n*	35	9
Patients with ISRs, *n* (%)	31 (7.1)	9 (4.1)
Pain, *n* (%)	11 (2.5)	5 (2.3)
Erythema, *n* (%)	10 (2.3)	1 (0.50)
Hematoma, *n* (%)	5 (1.1)	3 (1.4)
Pruritus, *n* (%)	3 (0.70)	0 (0.0)
Dose interruption or study withdrawal because of ISRs, *n*	0	0
Death, *n* (%)	3 (<1.0)	0

AEs: Adverse events.　ISRs: Injection site-reactions.　MRA: Tocilizumab.　PBO: Placebo.　s.c.: Subcutaneous placebo.　[a] Values are the number (percentage).
[b] Serious hypersensitivity was defined as a serious AE occurring during or within 24 hours of the injection or infusion, excluding ISRs, and evaluated as related to study treatment by the investigator.

Giant Cell Arteritis-Subcutaneous Administration[18]

❖ The efficacy and safety of subcutaneously administered tocilizumab was assessed in a single, randomized, double-blind, multicenter study in patients with active GCA (Study WA28119).

❖ In Study WA28119, 251 screened patients with new-onset or relapsing GCA were randomized to one of four treatment arms: Two s.c. doses of tocilizumab (162 mg every week and 162 mg every other week) were compared to two different placebo control groups (pre-specified prednisone-taper regimen over 26 weeks and 52 weeks) randomized 2:1:1:1.

❖ All patients received background glucocorticoid (prednisone) therapy. The primary efficacy endpoint was the proportion of patients achieving sustained remission from Week 12 through Week 52.

❖ Tocilizumab 162 mg weekly and 162 mg every other week + 26 weeks prednisone taper both showed superiority in achieving sustained remission from Week 12 through Week 52 compared with placebo + 26 weeks prednisone taper.

❖ Both tocilizumab treatment arms also showed superiority compared to the placebo + 52 weeks prednisone taper.

Clinical Efficacy

Table 22   Efficacy Results from Study WA28119[18]

	PBO + 26 Weeks Prednisone Taper (N = 50)	PBO + 52 Weeks Prednisone Taper (N = 51)	MRA 162 mg s.c. qw + 26 Weeks Prednisone Taper (N = 100)	MRA 162 mg s.c. q2w + 26 Weeks Prednisone Taper (N = 49)
Sustained Remission[a]				
Responders, n (%)	7 (14.0%)	9 (17.6%)	56 (56.0%)	26 (53.1%)
Unadjusted difference in proportions vs. PBO + 26 weeks taper (99.5% CI)	NA	NA	42.0% (18.0, 66.0)	39.1% (12.5, 65.7)
Unadjusted difference in proportions vs. PBO + 52 weeks taper (99.5% CI)	NA	NA	38.4% (14.4, 62.3)	35.4% (8.6, 62.2)
Components of Sustained Remission				
Sustained absence of GCA signs and symptoms,[b] n (%)	20 (40.0%)	23 (45.1%)	69 (69.0%)	28 (57.1%)
Sustained ESR <30 mm/h,[c] n (%)	20 (40.0%)	22 (43.1%)	83 (83.0%)	37 (75.5%)
Sustained CRP normalization,[d] n (%)	17 (34.0%)	13 (25.5%)	72 (72.0%)	34 (69.4%)
Successful prednisone tapering,[e] n (%)	10 (20.0%)	20 (39.2%)	60 (60.0%)	28 (57.1%)

Patients not completing the study to Week 52 were classified as non-responders in the primary and key secondary analysis: PBO + 26: 6 (12.0%), PBO + 52: 5 (9.8%), MRA. qw: 15 (15.0%), MRA q2w: 9 (18.4%). CRP: C-reactive protein. ESR: Erythrocyte sedimentation rate. MRA: Tocilizumab. PBO: Placebo. QW: Every weekly. [a] Sustained remission was achieved by a patient meeting all of the following components: absence of GCA signs and symptoms[b], normalization of ESR[c], normalization of CRP[d] and adherence to the prednisone taper regimen[e]. [b] Patients who did not have any signs or symptoms of GCA recorded from Week 12 up to Week 52. [c] Patients who did not have an elevated ESR ≥30 mm/h which was classified as attributed to GCA from Week 12 up to Week 52. [d] Patients who did not have two or more consecutive CRP records of ≥1 mg/dL from Week 12 up to Week 52. [e] Patients who did not enter escape therapy and received ≤100 mg of additional concomitant prednisone from Week 12 up to Week 52.

Clinical Safety

Table 23   Safety Data of the Study WA28119[a, 21]

Variable	MRA Weekly (N = 100)	MRA Every Other Week (N = 49)	PBO + 26-Week Taper (N = 50)	PBO + 52-Week Taper (N = 51)
Duration in trial-patient (Year)	92.9	45.6	47.4	48.1
Patients with ≥1 adverse event, n (%)	98 (98.0)	47 (96.0)	48 (96.0)	47 (92.0)
Adverse events				
No. of events	810	432	470	486
Rate per 100 patient-year (95% CI)	872 (813-934)	948 (861-1,042)	991 (903-1,085)	1,011 (923-1,105)
Patients with ≥1 infection, n (%)				
Any	75 (75.0)	36 (73.0)	38 (76.0)	33 (65.0)
Serious	7 (7.0)	2 (4.0)	2 (4.0)	6 (12.0)
Patients withdrew from the trial because of adverse events, n (%)[b]	6 (6.0)	3 (6.0)	2 (4.0)	0

Continued

Variable	MRA Weekly (N = 100)	MRA Every Other Week (N = 49)	PBO + 26-Week Taper (N = 50)	PBO + 52-Week Taper (N = 51)
Patients with injection-site reaction, n (%)	7 (7.0)	7 (14.0)	5 (10.0)	1 (2.0)
Flare of giant-cell arteritis reported as serious adverse event, n (%)[c]	1 (1.0)	1 (2.0)[d]	1 (2.0)	1 (2.0)
Patients with ≥1 serious adverse event, n (%)				
Any	15 (15.0)	7 (14.0)	11 (22.0)	13 (25.0)
According to system organ class[e]				
Infection or infestation	7 (7.0)	2 (4.0)	2 (4.0)	6 (12.0)
Vascular disorder	4 (4.0)	2 (4.0)	2 (4.0)	1 (2.0)
Respiratory, thoracic, or mediastinal disorder	2 (2.0)	1 (2.0)	2 (4.0)	2 (4.0)
Injury, poisoning, or procedural complication	3 (3.0)	1 (2.0)	1 (2.0)	0
Nervous system disorder	1 (1.0)	1 (2.0)	2 (4.0)	1 (2.0)
Cardiac disorder	2 (2.0)	0	0	2 (4.0)
Musculoskeletal or connective-tissue disorder	1 (1.0)	0	1 (2.0)	2 (4.0)
Gastrointestinal disorder	1 (1.0)	0	2 (4.0)	0
Cancer	0	0[f]	1 (2.0)	1 (2.0)

MRA: Tocilizumab. PBO: Placebo. [a] No gastrointestinal perforations were reported, and no patients died. [b] Values are reported for the entire trial population; that is, values were included for 50 patients in the group that received tocilizumab every other week (i.e., including the patient who did not receive tocilizumab). [c] Values are for flares of giant-cell arteritis that met the protocol-defined criteria for being reported as a serious adverse event. [d] This patient had anterior ischemic optic neuropathy after randomization. [e] Values were those reported in at least 1.0% of the patients overall. Patients may have had more than one class of serious adverse event. [f] One patient in the group that received tocilizumab every other week had a benign ovarian adenoma.

Polyarticular Juvenile Idiopathic Arthritis-Intravenous Administration[18]

❖ The safety and efficacy of tocilizumab was assessed in a three-part study including an open-label extension in children 2 to 17 years of age with active polyarticular juvenile idiopathic arthritis (PJIA), who had an inadequate response to methotrexate or inability to tolerate methotrexate.

❖ Part I consisted of a 16-week active tocilizumab treatment lead-in period (N = 188) followed by Part II, a 24-week randomized double-blind placebo-controlled withdrawal period, followed by Part III, a 64-week open-label period.

❖ During part I, patients received open-label tocilizumab every 4 weeks (8 or 10 mg/kg for body weight (BW) <30 kg; 8 mg/kg for BW ≥30 kg).

❖ At Week 16, patients with ≥ JIA-American College of Rheumatology (ACR) 30 improvement entered the 24-week, double-blind part II after randomization 1:1 to placebo or tocilizumab (stratified by methotrexate and steroid background therapy) for evaluation of the primary endpoint: JIA flare, compared with Week 16.

❖ Patients flaring or completing part II received open-label tocilizumab.

Clinical Efficacy

Table 24   Improvement of All JIA-ACR Core Components at the End of Part II (Week 40) for the ITT Population Receiving Tocilizumab in Parts I and II (N = 82)[a] Compared with Baseline[22]

JIA-ACR Core Response Variables[b]	Baseline	Week 40	Week 40 (Change from Baseline)[c]
Joints with active arthritis (range, 0-71)	19.7 (14.0)	3.2 (8.1)	-14.5 (11.1)
Joints with a limitation of movement (range, 0-67)	16.5 (13.8)	3.9 (7.0)	-10.2 (9.0)
Assessment of patient overall well-being, VAS (range, 0-100)	45.5 (23.1)	8.8 (16.1)	-31.1 (28.5)
Physician global assessment of disease activity, VAS (range, 0-100)	57.8 (20.3)	6.2 (7.8)	-45.6 (21.5)
CHAQ-DI (range, 0-3)	1.2 (0.67)	0.33 (0.47)	-0.80 (0.65)
ESR (mm/h)	31.7 (22.9)	5.4 (6.1)	-25.2 (22.0)

CHAQ-DI: Childhood Health Assessment Questionnaire-disability Index.   ESR: Erythrocyte sedimentation rate.   ITT: Intent-to-treat.   JIA-ACR: Juvenile idiopathic arthritis-American College of Rheumatology.   ULN: Upper limit of normal.   VAS: Visual analogue scale (0-100 mm).   [a] Ad hoc analysis.   [b] Values are mean (SD).   [c] Change from baseline was calculated using last-observation-carried-forward imputation for missing values; in other columns, missing values were not imputed.

Clinical Safety

Table 25   Serious Adverse Events and Adverse Events Occurring in at Least 5.0% of the Patients by Treatment Group for Events[22]

Adverse Event[a]	Part I[b] Tocilizumab (N = 188)	Part II[c] All Tocilizumab (N = 82)	Part II[c] All Placebo[d] (N = 81)	All-exposure Safety Group[e] (N = 188)
Duration in study (Year)	59.9	32.3	27.4	184.4
Patients with at least one AE, n (%)	124 (66.0)	58 (70.7)	60 (74.1)	159 (84.6)
Total number of AEs[f]	365	147	141	885
Rate of AEs per 100 PY[g]	609	455	514	480
Most frequently reported (>5.0%) AEs, n (%)				
Nasopharyngitis	23 (12.2)	14 (17.1)	9 (11.1)	39 (20.7)
Headache	15 (8.0)	3 (3.7)	-	26 (13.8)
Upper respiratory infection	13 (6.9)	4 (4.9)	2 (2.5)	19 (10.1)
Cough	7 (3.7)	2 (2.4)	1 (1.2)	18 (9.6)
Pharyngitis	8 (4.3)	3 (3.7)	3 (3.7)	17 (9.0)
Nausea	12 (6.4)	2 (2.4)	2 (2.5)	16 (8.5)
Diarrhoea	7 (3.7)	2 (2.4)	3 (3.7)	14 (7.4)
Rhinitis	7 (3.7)	2 (2.4)	1 (1.2)	14 (7.4)
Vomiting	4 (2.1)	3 (3.7)	1 (1.2)	14 (7.4)
Abdominal pain	5 (2.7)	2 (2.4)	2 (2.5)	13 (6.9)
Oropharyngeal pain	8 (4.3)	1 (1.2)	5 (6.2)	13 (6.9)
Rash	3 (1.6)	4 (4.9)	1 (1.2)	10 (5.3)
SAEs, n (%)				
Patients with at least one SAE	7 (3.7)	3 (3.7)	3 (3.7)	17 (9.0)
Rate of SAEs per 100 PY	13.4	9.3	10.9	12.5
Patients with at least one infectious SAE	4 (2.1)	1 (1.2)	-	9 (4.8)
Rates of infectious SAEs per 100 PY	6.7	3.1	-	4.9

Continued

| Adverse Event[a] | Part I[b] | Part II[c] | | All-exposure Safety Group[e] |
	Tocilizumab (N = 188)	All Tocilizumab (N = 82)	All Placebo[d] (N = 81)	(N = 188)
SAEs by preferred term, *n* (%)				
Pneumonia	1 (0.50)	1 (1.2)	-	4 (2.1)
Bronchitis	2 (1.1)	-	-	2 (1.1)
Cellulitis	1 (0.50)	-	-	2 (1.1)
Varicella	-	-	-	1 (0.50)
Neck injury	-	-	-	1 (0.50)
Synovial rupture	-	-	-	1 (0.50)
Upper limb fracture	-	1 (1.2)	-	1 (0.50)
Sclerosing cholangitis	1 (0.50)	-	-	1 (0.50)
Hypertransaminasemia	1 (0.50)	-	-	1 (0.50)
Back pain	-	-	-	1 (0.50)
Osteoporosis	-	-	-	1 (0.50)
Familial mediterranean fever[h]	-	-	-	1 (0.50)
Uveitis	-	-	1 (1.2)	1 (0.50)
Constipation	1 (0.50)	-	-	1 (0.50)
Begnign intracranial hypertension	1 (0.50)	-	-	1 (0.50)
Psychosomatic disease	-	1 (1.2)	-	1 (0.50)
Urinary calculus	-	-	-	1 (0.50)
Enterocolitis	-	-	1 (1.2)	
Complicated migraine	-	-	1 (1.2)	
AEs leading to study drug discontinuation, *n* (%)				
Increased blood bilirubin level[i]	-	1 (1.2)	-	1 (0.50)
Serum sickness-like reaction	1 (0.50)	-	-	1 (0.50)
Gastroenteritis	-	-	1 (1.2)	1 (0.50)[k]
Pneumonia	1 (0.50)	-	-	1 (0.50)
Sclerosing cholangitis[j]	1 (0.50)	-	-	1 (0.50)
Benign intracranial hypertension	1 (0.50)	-	-	1 (0.50)

AE: Adverse event.   JIA: Juvenile idiopathic arthritis.   PY: Patient-years.   SAE: Serious adverse event.   [a] Values are n (%) unless stated otherwise multiple occurrences of the same AE in one individual were counted only once, except where noted.   [b] Sixteen-week, open-label, lead-in part I with all patients receiving tocilizumab. [c] Both groups received tocilizumab open-label during part I before entering part II (24-week withdrawal phase).   AE data on open-label tocilizumab escape therapy were excluded.   [d] Summarizes all AEs except those that occurred in a patient once on placebo and includes data after Week 40 because safety was based on the data cut.   [e] Multiple occurrences of the same AE in one individual were counted.   [f] Patient-year.   [g] Recurrence in patient with pcJIA, with flare of familial Mediterranean fever.   [h] Highest total bilirubin reading, 50 μmol/L (normal range, 3-24 μmol/L); two consecutive readings >51 mmol/L mandated withdrawal per protocol.   The event resolved without sequelae.   [i] Patient with serum sickness-like reaction and subcutaneous swelling on dorsum of hand, forearm and foot; the patient was discontinued from the study.   [j] The patient had transaminitis on study entry: 139 U/L aspartate aminotransferase, 147 U/L alanine aminotransferase; highest readings: 287 U/L aspartate aminotransferase, 289 U/L alanine aminotransferase.   Liver biopsy was performed on study day 134; results were compatible with sclerosing cholangitis.   The event was unresolved and considered unrelated to study medication.   [k] Occurred 46 days after the last of five doses of placebo.

Systemic Juvenile Idiopathic Arthritis-Intravenous Administration[18]

❖ The safety and efficacy of tocilizumab for the treatment of active SJIA was assessed in a 12-week randomized, double blind, placebo-controlled, parallel group, 2-arm study.

❖ Patients treated with or without MTX, were randomized (tocilizumab:placebo = 2:1) to one of two treatment groups: 75 patients received tocilizumab infusions every two weeks at either 8 mg/kg for patients at or above 30 kg or 12 mg/kg for patients less than 30 kg and 37 patients were randomized to receive placebo infusions every two weeks.

❖ After 12 weeks or at the time of escape, due to disease worsening patients were treated with tocilizumab in the open-label extension phase at weight appropriate dosing.

❖ The primary endpoint was the proportion of patients with at least 30.0% improvement in JIA ACR core set (JIA ACR 30 response) at Week 12 and absence of fever (no temperature at or above 37.5°C in the preceding 7 days).

Clinical Efficacy

Table 26   Summary of Efficacy Data for Intravenous Tocilizumab in SJIA at Week 12[18]

	Tocilizumab (*N* = 75)	Placebo (*N* = 37)
Primary Endpoint: JIA-ACR 30 Response + Absence of Fever		
Responders	85.0%	24.0%
Weighted difference (95% *CI*)	62.0 (45.0, 78.0)	-
JIA-ACR Response Rates at Week 12		
JIA-ACR 30		
Responders Weighted difference[a] (95% *CI*)[b]	91.0% 67.0 (51.0, 83.0)	24.0% -
JIA-ACR 50		
Responders Weighted difference[a] (95% *CI*)[b]	85.0% 74.0 (58.0, 90.0)	11.0% -
JIA-ACR 70		
Responders Weighted difference[a] (95% *CI*)[b]	71.0% 63.0 (46.0, 83.0)	8.0% -

JIA-ACR: Juvenile idiopathic arthritis-American College of Rheumatology.   -: Not available.   [a] The weighted difference is the difference between the tocilizumab and placebo response rates, adjusted for the stratification factors (weight, disease duration, background oral corticosteroid dose and background methotrexate use). [b] *CI*: Confidence interval of the weighted difference.

Clinical Safety

Table 27   Adverse Events of Intravenous Tocilizumab in SJIA[a, [23]]

Variable	Double-blind Phase[b]		Cumulative Data[c]
	Placebo (*N* = 37)	Tocilizumab (*N* = 75)	Tocilizumab (*N* = 112)
Exposure to Tocilizumab per Patient, (Year)	5.2	17.4	158
Adverse Events Including Fever and JIA			
No. of events	49	161	1,315
No. of events per patient-year, (Year)	9.4	9.3	8.4
Adverse Events Excluding Fever and JIA			
No. of events	38	159	1,266
No. of events per patient, (Year)	7.3	9.1	8.0
Most Frequently Reported Events, No. of Patients (%)[d]			
Upper respiratory tract infection	4 (11.0)	10 (13.0)	35 (31.0)
Pharyngitis or nasopharyngitis	3 (8.0)	10 (13.0)	35 (31.0)
Diarrhea	1 (3.0)	5 (7.0)	19 (17.0)
Headache	3 (8.0)	7 (9.0)	17 (15.0)
Serious Adverse Events			
Total, No. of events	0	4	39
Angioedema[e]	0	1	1
Urticaria	0	1	1
Varicella	0	1	4
Herpes zoster	0	0	2

Continued

| Variable | Double-blind Phase[b] | | Cumulative Data[c] |
	Placebo (N = 37)	Tocilizumab (N = 75)	Tocilizumab (N = 112)
Upper respiratory tract infection	0	0	4
Bronchopneumonia or pneumonia	0	0	4
Gastroenteritis or gastritis	0	0	5
Macrophage activation syndrome .	0	0	3
Aminotransferase increase	0	0	2
Fracture	0	0	3
Hip dislocation[f]	0	0	2
Other[g]	0	1	8
No. of events per patient, (Year)	0	0.23	0.25
Infection			
No. of events	15	60	478
No. of events per patient, (Year)	2.9	3.4	3.0
Serious Infection			
No. of events	0		18
No. of events per patient, (Year)	0		0.11
Clinical Laboratory Abnormalities, No. of Patients (%)			
Neutropenia[h]			
Grade 3	0	5 (7.0)	17 (15.0)[i]
Grade 4	0	0	2 (2.0)
Thrombocytopenia[j]			
Grade 3	0	0	1 (1.0)[i]
Grade 4	0	0	0
Increase in alanine aminotransferase[k]			
Grade 2	0	5 (7.0)	13 (12.0)
Grade 3	0	1 (1.0)	7 (6.0)
Grade 4	0	0	1 (1.0)[i]

JIA: Juvenile idiopathic arthritis. [a] Multiple occurrences of the same adverse event in one patient were counted. [b] Data on open-label tocilizumab rescue therapy were excluded. [c] Cumulative data included data for patients who received tocilizumab in the double-blind phase and subsequently received open-label tocilizumab and for patients who were assigned to placebo and made the transition to open-label tocilizumab. [d] Only adverse events that occurred in more than 5.0% of patients in either group in the double-blind phase are presented. [e] Angioedema and urticaria occurred in the same patient. [f] The two episodes of hip dislocation occurred in the same patient. [g] Eight other serious adverse events were reported: JIA, bacterial arthritis, chronic panniculitis, dehydration, pneumothorax, testicular torsion, cardiac failure, and pulmonary veno-occlusive disease. Cardiac failure related to pulmonary veno-occlusive disease was reported in the same patient, who died 13 months after withdrawing from the study. [h] Grade 3 neutropenia was defined as a neutrophil count of 0.5×10^9 to less than 1.0×10^9 per liter, and Grade 4 as a neutrophil count of less than 0.5×10^9 per liter. [i] One episode each of Grade 3 neutropenia, Grade 3 thrombocytopenia, and a Grade 4 increase in the alanine aminotransferase level occurred during the macrophage activation syndrome. [j] Grade 3 thrombocytopenia was defined as a platelet count of 25,000 to less than 50,000 per cubic millimeter, and Grade 4 as a platelet count of less than 25,000 per cubic millimeter. [k] A Grade 2 increase in the alanine aminotransferase level was defined as a level that was more than 2.5 to 5.0 times the upper limit of the normal range, Grade 3 as a level that was more than 5 to 20 times the upper limit of the normal range, and Grade 4 as a level that was more than 20 times the upper limit of the normal range.

Cytokine Release Syndrome-Intravenous Administration[18]

❖ The safety and efficacy of tocilizumab for the treatment of CRS was assessed in a retrospective analysis of pooled outcome data from clinical trials of CAR T-cell therapies for hematological malignancies.

❖ Evaluable patients had been treated with tocilizumab 8 mg/kg (12 mg/kg for patients <30 kg) with or without additional high-dose corticosteroids for severe or life-threatening CRS.

❖ The study population included 24 males and 21 females (total 45 patients) of median age 12 years (range, 3-23 years); 82.0% were Caucasian.

❖ Resolution of CRS was defined as lack of fever and off vasopressors for at least 24 hours.

❖ Patients were considered responders if CRS resolved within 14 days of the first dose of tocilizumab, no more than 2 doses of tocilizumab were needed, and no drugs other than tocilizumab and corticosteroids were used for treatment.

❖ A median of 1 dose of tocilizumab (range, 1-4 dosed) was administered.

Clinical Efficacy and Safety

❖ Thirty-one patients (69.0%; 95% *CI*: 53.0%-82.0%) achieved a response.
❖ Achievement of resolution of CRS within 14 days was confirmed in a second study using an independent cohort that included 15 patients (range: 9-75 years old) with CAR T cell-induced CRS.
❖ No adverse reactions related to tocilizumab were reported.

8 Clinical Pharmacokinetics

Summary[18]

❖ Tocilizumab's pharmacokinetic profile had been evaluated in patients with rheumatoid arthritis (RA), polyarticular juvenile idiopathic arthritis (PJIA), systemic juvenile idiopathic arthritis (SJIA), and giant cell arteritis (GCA).
❖ The dosage form of tocilizumab was an injection, used as an intravenous infusion or a subcutaneous injection.
❖ For RA patients, tocilizumab could be used as an intravenous infusion or a subcutaneous injection.
❖ For GCA patients, tocilizumab was used only as an subcutaneous injection, intravenous administration was not approved.
❖ Subcutaneous administration was not approved for PJIA and SJIA, tocilizumab was used only as the intravenous for treatment of these patients.

Rheumatoid Arthritis-Intravenous Administration[18]

❖ The total clearance of tocilizumab is concentration dependent and is the sum of the non-linear at low exposures and linear clearance (12.5 mL/h) at higher concentrations. The clearance decreased with increased doses.
❖ In RA patients the central V_d was 3.5 L, the peripheral V_d was 2.9 L, resulting in a V_{ss} of 6.4 L.
❖ The pharmacokinetic parameters (AUC, C_{max}, C_{min}) did not change with time.
❖ A more than dose proportional increase in AUC and C_{min} was observed for doses of 4 and 8 mg/kg every 4 weeks. At steady-state, predicted AUC and C_{min} were 2.7- and 6.5-fold higher at 8 mg/kg as compared to 4 mg/kg, respectively. C_{max} increased dose-proportionally.
❖ The accumulation ratio for AUC and C_{max} were small, which was higher for C_{min}.
❖ The $t_{1/2}$ is concentration-dependent. The apparent $t_{1/2}$ is up to 11 days for 4 mg/kg and up to 13 days for 8 mg/kg every 4 weeks at steady-state.
❖ Body size (body surface area, body weight, and body mass index) affected linear clearance. Tocilizumab AUC, C_{min} and C_{max} increased with increase of body weight. Tocilizumab doses exceeding 800 mg per infusion are not recommended.
❖ Tocilizumab is not metabolized via the CYP450 or the P-glycoprotein pathway. Population pharmacokinetic analysis revealed that use of concomitant medications for RA did not influence the pharmacokinetics of tocilizumab.

Table 28　Summary of Mean (SD) Predicted AUC, C_{max} and C_{min} at Steady-state following 4 and 8 mg/kg Tocilizumab i.v. q4w[18]

		AUC$_{ss}$ (µg·h/mL)	C_{max} (µg/mL)	C_{min} (µg/mL)
4 mg/kg q4wks	Mean ± SD	13,000 ± 5,800	88.3 ± 41.4	1.5 ± 2.1
	Accumulation ratios	1.1	1.0	2.0
8 mg q4wks	Mean ± SD	35,000 ± 15,500	183 ± 85.6	9.7 ± 10.5
	Accumulation ratios	1.2	2.4	1.1

SD: Standard deviation.

Rheumatoid Arthritis-Subcutaneous Administration[18]

❖ The pharmacokinetics of tocilizumab was characterized using a population pharmacokinetic analysis using a database composed of 1759 RA patients treated with 162 mg s.c. every week, 162 mg s.c. every other week, and 8 mg/kg every 4 weeks for 24 weeks.
❖ The pharmacokinetic parameters did not change with time.
❖ The absorption half-life was around 4 days.
❖ The bioavailability was 0.80.
❖ The $t_{1/2}$ is concentration-dependent. The apparent $t_{1/2}$ is up to 13 days for 162 mg every week and 5 days for 162 mg every other week at steady-state.

Table 29 Summary of Mean (SD) Predicted AUC, C_{max} and C_{min} at Steady-state following 162 mg Tocilizumab s.c. Every Week and Every Other Week[18]

		AUCₛₛ (μg·h/mL)	C_{max} (μg/mL)	C_{min} (μg/mL)
162 mg qwk	1 week	8,200 ± 3,600	50.9 ± 21.8	44.6 ± 20.6
	Accumulation ratios	6.8	5.5	6.4
	Time to steady-state (Week)	12	12	12
162 mg q2wks	1 week	3,200 ± 2,700	12.3 ± 8.7	5.6 ± 7.0
	Accumulation ratios	2.7	2.1	5.6
	Time to steady-state (Week)	12	10	12

Polyarticular Juvenile Idiopathic Arthritis-Intravenous Administration[18]

❖ The pharmacokinetics of tocilizumab was determined using a population pharmacokinetic analysis using a database composed of 188 patients with polyarticular juvenile idiopathic arthritis.
❖ The visible trend toward lower systemic exposure to tocilizumab in patients with lower body weight.
❖ The central V_d was 1.98 L, the peripheral V_d was 2.1 L, resulting in a V_{ss} of 4.1 L.
❖ The total clearance of tocilizumab is concentration dependent and is the sum of the non-linear at low exposures and linear clearance (5.8 mL/h) at higher concentrations.
❖ The $t_{1/2}$ is up to 16 days for two body weight categories during a dosing interval at steady-state.

Table 30 Summary of Mean (SD) Predicted AUC, C_{max} and C_{min} at Steady-state following Tocilizumab i.v. Every 4 Weeks[18]

		AUCₛₛ (μg·h/mL)	C_{max} (μg/mL)	C_{min} (μg/mL)
8 mg/kg q4wks	≥30 kg	29,500 ± 8,600	182 ± 37.0	7.5 ± 8.2
	Accumulation ratios	1.2	-	2.2
10 mg q4wks	<30 kg	23,200 ± 6,100	175 ± 32.0	2.4 ± 3.6
	Accumulation ratios	1.1	-	1.4

Tocilizumab: 8 mg and 10 mg.   -: No data available.

Systemic Juvenile Idiopathic Arthritis-Intravenous Administration

❖ The pharmacokinetics of tocilizumab was determined using a population pharmacokinetic analysis using a database composed of 75 patients with systemic juvenile idiopathic arthritis.
❖ The visible trend toward lower systemic exposure to tocilizumab in patients with lower body weight.
❖ Mean estimated tocilizumab exposure parameters were similar between the two dose groups defined by body weight.
❖ The central V_d was 0.94 L, the peripheral V_d was 1.6 L, resulting in a V_{ss} of 2.5 L.
❖ The total clearance of tocilizumab is concentration dependent and is the sum of the non-linear at low exposures and linear clearance (7.1 mL/h) at higher concentrations.
❖ The $t_{1/2}$ is up to 23 days for two body weight categories at Week 12.

Table 31 Summary of Mean (SD) Predicted AUC, C_{max} and C_{min} at Steady-state following Tocilizumab i.v. Every 2 Weeks[18]

		AUCₛₛ (μg·h/mL)	C_{max} (μg/mL)	C_{min} (μg/mL)
8 mg/kg q2wks (≥30 kg) or 12 mg q2wks (<30 kg)		32,200 ± 9,960	245 ± 57.2	57.5 ± 23.3
	Accumulation ratios	1.2	-	3.2 ± 1.3
	Time to stead-state (Week)	-	-	12

Tocilizumab: 8 mg and 12 mg.

Giant Cell Arteritis-Subcutaneous Administration

❖ The pharmacokinetics of tocilizumab in GCA patients was determined using a population pharmacokinetic analysis on a data set composed of 149 GCA patients treated with 162 mg every week or with 162 mg every other week.
❖ The median values of T_{max} were 3 days after the tocilizumab every week dose and 4.5 days after the tocilizumab every other week dose.

❖ The central volume of distribution was 4.1 L, the peripheral volume of distribution was 3.4 L, resulting in a volume of distribution at steady-state of 6.4 L.

❖ At steady-state, the effective $t_{1/2}$ of tocilizumab varied between 18.3 and 18.9 days for 162 mg every week dosing regimen and between 4.2 and 7.9 days for 162 mg every other week dosing regimen.

Table 32　Summary of Estimated Mean (± SD) Steady-state C_{avg}, C_{max} and C_{min} following 162 mg Tocilizumab Every Week and Every Other Week[18]

		C_{avg} (µg/mL)	C_{max} (µg/mL)	C_{min} (µg/mL)
162 mg every week	Mean ± SD	71.3 ± 30.1	73.0 ± 30.4	6,831 ± 29.5
	Accumulation ratios	10.9	8.9	9.6
162 mg every other week	Mean ± SD	16.2 ± 11.8	19.3 ± 12.8	11.1 ± 10.3
	Accumulation ratios	2.8	2.3	5.6

Summary of the Single-Dose or Multiple-Dose Pharmacokinetic Studies

Single-Dose Pharmacokinetic Studies

Table 33　Overview of Clinical Pharmacology Studies: Single-Dose Studies and Additional Studies[14]

Protocol#	Product ID /Batch	Study Objective	Study Design	Subjects No. (M/F) Type Age: Mean (Range)	Treatment (mg/kg) Infusion Duration	C_{max} (µg/mL)	AUC_{last}[a] (µg·h/mL)	CL [mL/(h·kg)]	$t_{1/2}$ (h)	V_{ss} (mL/kg)	T_{max}[b] (h)
BP19461 Part 1 only	RO4877533 /MR5C06	ST, PK ECG	DB, R, PC, two centers, SAD	36 (17/19) HV (18-61)	2 10 20 28 (1 h)	41.9 ± 3.3 242 ± 31.3 410 ± 81.3 558 ± 79.2	3,210 ± 410 37,800 ± 6,000 77,800 ± 17,100 115,000 ± 10,900	0.61 ± 0.064 0.24 ± 0.042 0.22 ± 0.052 0.19 ± 0.022	54.0 ± 10.9 201 ± 29.8 277 ± 35.5 293 ± 48.0	50.0 ± 6.5 67.5 ± 9.4 85.7 ± 20.3 81.4 ± 11.3	3.8 ± 2.7 4.1 ± 2.1 3.8 ± 2.4 3.0 ± 1.4
LRO300	RO4877533 /R7F03	ST, antigenicity PK efficacy	DB, R, PC, six centers, SAD	45 (15/30) P (35-74)	0.1 1 5 10 (1 h)	2.0 ± 1.3 17.9 ± 4.7 123 ± 21.0 273 ± 121	18.0 ± 13.0 1,180 ± 839 18,100 ± 3,530 43,600 ± 17,000	- 0.74 0.26 ± 0.039 0.26 ± 0.13	- 52.9 136 158	- 49.7 49.7 ± 7.5 58.7 ± 22.4	1.2 4.0 1.2 4.3
MRA001 JP	RO4877533 /R7F03 MRSF02	ST, PK, MTD	SB, R, PC, single center, SAD	28 (28/0) HV (20-29)	0.15 0.5 1 2 (1 h)	2.4 ± 0.61 8.5 ± 1.2 19.5 ± 2.7 37.6 ± 8.8	10.7 ± 5.7 285 ± 73.3 1,010 ± 222 2,530 ± 569	c 1.3 ± 0.21 0.83 ± 0.073 0.63 ± 0.15	17.4 ± 15.6 33.1 ± 3.7 49.4 ± 5.1 74.3 ± 9.0	c 58.4 ± 7.1 57.3 ± 10.9 65.9 ± 8.3	1.5 ± 0.60 1.6 ± 0.50 1.8 ± 1.3 2.8 ± 2.2
MRA220 JP	RO4877533 /MR4C05	ST, PK, efficacy (DDI)	OL, NR, single center	31 (6/25) P 50y (23-69)	8 (1 h)	137 ± 22.7	20,600 ± 5,750	0.40 ± 0.13	136 ± 25.7	79.9 ± 16.8	2.7 ± 1.6
MRA221 JP	RO4877533 /MR4C05	PK, ST (renal impairment)	OL, NR, multiple center	14 (3/11) P 64y (56-74)	8 Normal (2) Mild (4) Moderate (5) Severe (3) (1 h)	176 174 ± 29.1 177 ± 18.9 172 ± 35.0	23,400 20,800 ± 9,330 24,800 ± 7,710 28,700 ± 10,100	0.34 0.49 ± 0.35 0.34 ± 0.11 0.29 ± 0.10	119 101 ± 38.4 143 ± 51.5 148 ± 14.5	64.1 65.5 ± 9.6 62.5 ± 5.7 62.1 ± 16.8	NC
MRA004 JP	RO4877533 /MR9D02	ST, PK ECG	OL, NR, single center	6 (6/0) HV 22y (20-23)	2 (2 h)	26.4 ± 5.8	2,940 ± 593 (Infinity)	0.71 ± 0.17	82.1 ± 4.7	85.0 ± 19.4	6.0 ± 0.0

Mean PK parameters are rounded to 3 significant figures where appropriate, T_{max} which is rounded to 2 significant figures.　#: Parameters not reported as area extrapolated too high for all subjects (≥48.0%).　DB: Double-blind.　DDI: Drug-drug interaction.　ECG: Electrocardiogram.　HV: Healthy volunteers.　MAD: Multiple ascending doses.　M/F: Male/female.　MTD: Maximum tolerated dose.　NC: Not calculated.　NR: Non-randomized.　OL: Open label.　P: Patients.　PC: Placebo-controlled.　PD: Pharmacodynamics.　PK: Pharmacokinetics.　R: Randomized.　SAD: Single ascending dose.　SB: Single blind.　ST: Safety and tolerability.
[a] Area extrapolated very high.　[b] Time zero equal to start of 1 h infusion.　[c] Values were recalculated (i.e. normalized by body weight) for this appendix.

Chapter 9 | Tocilizumab | 261

Multiple-Dose Pharmacokinetic Studies

Table 34 Overview of Clinical Pharmacology Studies: Multiple-Dose Studies[14]

Protocol#	Study Objective	Study Design	Subjects No. (M/F) Type Age: Mean (Range)	Treatment (mg/kg) (Infusion Duration Dosing Frequency)	C_{max} (µg/mL)	AUC_{last}[a] (µg·h/mL)	CL [mL/(h·kg)]	$t_{1/2}$ (h)	V_{ss} (mL/kg)	T_{max}[b] (h)
MRA002JP[c]	Safety, PK efficacy	OL, NR, multiple center MAD	15 (4/11) P 53y (32-72)	**2**						
				1st dose	43.6 ± 10.1	3,440 ± 822	0.51 ± 0.083	74.4 ± 18.3	50.0 ± 13.0	1.9
				2nd dose	44.0 ± 9.1	3,570 ± 801		77.0 ± 13.9		2.0
				3rd dose	27.9 ± 12.3	3,010 ± 1,070		86.6 ± 18.4		3.0 ± 1.4
				4						
				1st dose	49.0 ± 12.6	4,660 ± 2,180	0.70 ± 0.53	96.9 ± 50.2	102 ± 24.0	5.7 ± 2.5
				2nd dose	55.1 ± 12.3	5,670 ± 2,750		122 ± 64.2		9.8 ± 4.3
				3rd dose	49.5 ± 10.1	6,040 ± 3,200		140 ± 71.1		15.5 ± 5.2
				8						
				1st dose	82.5 ± 32.4	10,700 ± 4,070	0.28 ± 0.095	160 ± 34.3	137 ± 31.6	14.8 ± 7.3
				2nd dose	106 ± 36.6	17,000 ± 8,230		192 ± 45.6		26.2 ± 16.3
				3rd dose	130 ± 48.1	19,900 ± 8,900		242 ± 71.4		37.1 ± 20.4
				(2 h; 2 weeks)			e		e	
MRA009JP[d]	PK, safety efficacy	DB, R, PC, PG, multiple site	162[f] (37/125) P 54y (21-74)	4	72.3 ± 16.1	9,030 ± 3,980 (Mainly 2 points only)	NC	NC	NC	NC
				8 Based on 3rd administration (1 h, 4 weeks)	160 ± 36.5	31,200 ± 10,800	0.22 ± 0.070	171 ± 41.5	52.2 ± 9.9	9.3 ± 8.7

Mean PK parameters are rounded to 3 significant figures where appropriate, except for T_{max} which is rounded to 2 significant figures.   #: Parameters not reported as area extrapolated too high for all subjects (≥48.0%).   DB: Double-blind.   HV: Healthy volunteers.   M/F: Male/female.   MAD: Multiple ascending doses.   MTD: Maximum tolerated dose.   NC: Not calculated.   NR: Non-randomized.   PC: Placebo-controlled.   PG: Parallel group.   PL: Open label.   P: Patients.   PD: Pharmacodynamics.   PK: Pharmacokinetics.   R: Randomized.   SAD: Single ascending dose.   [a] Area extrapolated very high.   [b] Time zero equal to start of 1h infusion.   [c] Product ID/Batch: RO4877533/MR9D01.   [d] Product ID/Batch: RO4877533/MR0102MR1B03MR1G02.   Values were recalculated (i.e. normalized by body weight) for this appendix.   [f] Full analysis set (FAS).

Anti-product Antibody (APA) Analysis

❖ A total of 2,876 patients with RA treated with intravenous use have been tested for anti-tocilizumab antibodies in the controlled clinical trials.   Forty-six patients (1.6%) developed positive anti-tocilizumab antibodies, of whom 5 patients had an associated medically significant hypersensitivity reaction leading to withdrawal.   In 30 patients (1.1%) who developed neutralizing antibodies, no apparent correlation to clinical response was observed.

❖ A total of 1,454 (>99.0%) patients with RA treated with subcutaneous use in the all exposure group have been tested for anti-tocilizumab antibodies.   Thirteen patients (0.90%) developed anti-tocilizumab antibodies, and, of these, 12 patients (0.80%) developed neutralizing antibodies.   The rate is consistent with intravenous experience.

❖ One patient in the 10 mg/kg less than 30 kg group in clinical studies of 188 patients with pJIA, developed positive anti-tocilizumab antibodies without developing a hypersensitivity reaction and subsequently withdrew from the study.

❖ A total of 112 patients with sJIA were tested for anti-tocilizumab at baseline.   Two patients developed positive anti-tocilizumab antibodies with one of these patients having a hypersensitivity reaction leading to withdrawal.

9 Patent

❖ Tocilizumab was approved in Japan for in Jun 2005 Castleman's disease, and for rheumatoid arthritis by European Medicines Agency (EMA) in Jan 2009 and by the U.S. Food and Drug Administration (FDA) in Jan 2010. It was developed and marketed as Actemra®/RoActemra® by Genentech Inc., a subsidiary of Roche.

Summary

❖ The patent application (WO9219759A1) related to the reconstituted human antibody against a human interleukin 6 receptors (i.e. Tocilizumab), was filed by Genentech on Apr 24, 1992. Accordingly, its PCT counterpart has, among the others, been granted before USPTO (US5795965A, US5817790A), EPO (EP0628639B1) and JPO (JP3370324B2), respectively.

Table 35 Originator's Key Patent of Tocilizumab in Main Countries and/or Region

Country/Region	Publication/Patent No.	Application Date	Granted Date	Estimated Expiry Date
WO	WO9219759A1	04/24/1992	/	/
US	US5795965A	04/24/1992	08/18/1998	08/18/2015
	US5817790A	04/24/1992	10/06/1998	10/06/2015
EP	EP0628639B1	04/24/1992	06/23/1999	04/24/2012
JP	JP3370324B2	04/24/1992	01/27/2003	04/24/2012

Table 36 Originator's International Patent Protection of Use and/or Method of Tocilizumab

Publication No.	Title	Publication Date
Technical Subjects	**TREATMENT METHOD**	
WO9611020A1	Rheumatoid arthritis remedy containing IL-6 antagonist as active ingredient	04/18/1996
WO9612503A1	Remedy for diseases caused by IL-6 production	05/02/1996
WO9842377A1	Preventives or remedies for sensitized T cell-related diseases containing IL-6 antagonists as the active ingredient	10/01/1998
WO9947170A1	Preventives or remedies for inflammatory intestinal diseases containing as the active ingredient IL-6 antagonists	09/23/1999
WO02034292A1	Preventives or remedies for psoriasis containing as the active ingredient IL-6 antagonist	05/02/2002
WO02080969A1	Remedies for infant chronic arthritis-relating diseases	10/17/2002
WO2004073741A1	Remedy for spinal injury containing interleukin-6 antagonist	09/02/2004
WO2005037315A1	Therapeutic agent for mesothelioma	04/28/2005
WO2005061000A1	Remedy for angiitis	07/07/2005
WO2007043641A1	Inhibitor of transplanted is let dysfunction in islet transplantation	04/19/2007
WO2007046489A1	Therapeutic agent for heart disease	04/26/2007
WO2007086490A1	Remedy for disease associated with choroidal angiogenesis	08/02/2007
WO2008078715A1	Therapeutic agent for inflammatory myopathy containing IL-6 antagonist as active ingredient	07/03/2008
WO2009044774A1	Remedy for graft-versus-host disease comprising interleukin-6 receptor inhibitor as the active ingredient	04/09/2009
WO2009148148A1	Neuroinvasion inhibitor	12/10/2009
Technical Subjects	**DIAGNOSTIC METHOD**	
WO2011154139A2	Gene expression markers for predicting response to interleukin-6 receptor-inhibiting monoclonal antibody drug treatment	12/15/2011
WO2012064627A2	Subcutaneously administered anti-IL-6 receptor antibody	05/18/2012
WO2015000865A1	Interference-suppressed immunoassay to detect anti-drug antibodies in serum samples	01/08/2015
WO2016068333A1	Pre-filled syringe preparation with needle, which is equipped with syringe cap	05/06/2016
WO2016136933A1	Composition for treating IL-6-related diseases	09/01/2016

Continued

Publication No.	Title	Publication Date
Technical Subjects	FORMULATION	
WO96020728A1	Antitumor agent potentiator comprising IL-6 antagonist	07/11/1996
WO03068259A1	Antibody-containing solutions pharmaceutical	08/21/2003
WO03068260A1	Antibody-containing solution pharmaceuticals	08/21/2003
WO2004096273A1	Methods for treating interleukin-6 related diseases	11/11/2004
WO2006076651A2	Treatment method	07/20/2006
WO2008135380A1	Method for stabilizing a protein	11/13/2008
WO2010106812A1	Pharmaceutical formulation containing improved antibody molecules	09/23/2010
WO2011090088A1	Solution preparation containing stabilized antibody	07/28/2011
WO2013012022A1	Stable protein-containing preparation containing argininamide or analogous compound thereof	01/24/2013
WO2016011264A1	Methods of treating cancer using TIGIT inhibitors and anti-cancer agents	01/21/2016

The date was updated until Jan 2018.

10 Reference

[1] http://www.ncbi.nlm.nih.gov/homologene/474.

[2] https://blast.ncbi.nlm.nih.gov.

[3] TANAKA T, NARAZAKI M, KISHIMOTO T. Therapeutic targeting of the interleukin-6 receptor [J]. Annual Review of Pharmacology and Toxicology, 2012, 52(1): 199-219.

[4] European Medicines Agency (EMA) Database. http://www.ema.europa.eu/docs/en_GB/document_library/EPAR_-_Public_assessment_report/human/000955/WC500054888.pdf.

[5] SATO K, TSUCHIYA M, SALDANHA J, et al. Reshaping a human antibody to inhibit the interleukin 6-dependent tumor cell growth [J]. Cancer Research, 1993, 53(4): 851-856.

[6] Pharmaceuticals and Medical Devices (PMDA) Database. http://www.pmda.go.jp/files/000153709.pdf.

[7] The financial reports of Genentech; http://data.pharmacodia.com/web/homePage/index.

[8] Thomson Integrity Database. https://integrity.thomson-pharma.com/integrity/xmlxsl/pk_prod_list.exec_form_pro_pr?p_par_pro=PRO_DRUG_NAME&p_val_pro=tocilizumab&p_origen=PROD&p_oper_pro=AND&p_par_tar=&p_val_tar=&p_oper_tar=AND&p_par_ref=&p_val_ref=&p_oper_ref=AND&p_par_pat=&p_val_pat=&p_oper_pat=AND.

[9] U. S. Food and Drug Administration (FDA) Database. http://www.accessdata.fda.gov/drugsatfda_docs/nda/2010/125276s000SumR.pdf.

[10] EMA Database. http://www.ema.europa.eu/ema/index.jsp?curl=pages/medicines/human/medicines/000955/human_med_001042.jsp&mid=WC0b01ac058001d124.

[11] PMDA Database. http://www.pmda.go.jp/drugs/2013/P201300042/index.html.

[12] FDA Database. http://www.fda.gov/ohrms/dockets/ac/08/briefing/2008-4371b1-02-roche.pdf.

[13] PMDA Database. http://www.pmda.go.jp/drugs/2008/P200800016/450045000_21900AMX01337_H100_2.pdf.

[14] FDA Database. http://www.accessdata.fda.gov/drugsatfda_docs/nda/2010/125276s000PharmR.pdf.

[15] EMA Database. http://www.ema.europa.eu/docs/en_GB/document_library/EPAR_-_Assessment_Report_-_Variation/human/000955/WC500167788.pdf.

[16] FDA Database. https://www.accessdata.fda.gov/drugsatfda_docs/nda/2013/125472orig1s000pharmr.pdf.

[17] FDA Database. http://www.fda.gov/downloads/drugs/developmentapprovalprocess/developmentresources/ucm259749.pdf.

[18] FDA Database. http://www.accessdata.fda.gov/drugsatfda_docs/nda/2010/125276s000Lable.pdf.

[19] BURMESTER G R, RUBBERT-ROTH A, CANTAGREL A, et al. A randomized, double-blind, parallel-group study of the safety and efficacy of subcutaneous tocilizumab versus intravenous tocilizumab in combination with traditional disease-modifying antirheumatic drugs in patients with moderate to severe rheumatoid arthritis (SUMMACTA study) [J]. Annals of the Rheumatic Diseases, 2014, 73(1): 69-74.

[20] KIVITZ A, OLECH E, BOROFSKY M, et al. Subcutaneous tocilizumab versus placebo in combination with disease-modifying antirheumatic drugs in patients with rheumatoid arthritis [J]. Arthritis Care & Research, 2014, 66(11): 1653-1661.

[21] STONE J H, TUCKWELL K, DIMONACO S, et al. Trial of tocilizumab in giant-cell arteritis [J]. The New England Journal of Medicine, 2017, 377(4): 317-328.

[22] Brunner HI, Ruperto N, Zuber Z, et al. Efficacy and safety of tocilizumab in patients with polyarticular-course juvenile idiopathic arthritis: results from a phase 3, randomized, double-blind withdrawal trial [J]. Annals of the Rheumatic Diseases, 2015, 74(6): 1110-1117.

[23] Ruperto N. Randomized trial of tocilizumab in systemic juvenile idiopathic arthritis [J]. The New England Journal of Medicine, 2012, 367(25): 2385-2395.

CHAPTER

10

Trastuzumab

Trastuzumab

(Herceptin®)

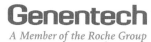

Research code: Anti-HER2/neu-Mab, huMAb4D5-8, MKC-454, R-597, RG-597, RO45-2317

1   Target Biology

The HER2 Receptor

❖ The human epidermal growth factor receptor 2 (HER2, also known as Neu, ErbB-2, CD340 or p185) is a member of the epidermal growth factor receptor (EGFR/ErbB) family encoded by the ERBB2 gene.   The family also includes the endothelial growth factor receptor (EGFR/ErbB-1), HER3, and HER4 receptors.   These receptors function by forming homo- and hetero-dimers with members of the family, with HER2 as the preferred binding partner.[1]

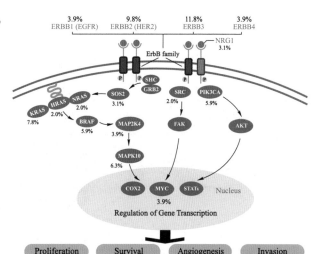

❖ HER2 binds to other members of EGF receptor family to form a heterodimer, which acts as co-receptor or a shared signaling unit, leading to stabilized ligand binding, prolonged and enhanced downstream signaling (i.e. MAPK and PI3K pathways), which regulates cell differentiation, growth and proliferation.

❖ Overexpression and amplification of HER2 is present in approximately 20.0%-25.0% of human breast cancers.[2]   Due to its kinase activity, HER2/neu overexpression results in enhanced tyrosine phosphorylation activities, and an increase in the proliferative stimuli associated with HER2, leading to increased tumor growth.

❖ Five HER2-targeting drugs have been approved and marketed (Gilotrif®, Kadcyla®, Perjeta®, Tykerb®, and Herceptin®).

Tubulin and Microtubules

❖ Tubulin is the protein that polymerizes into long chains that form microtubules, a major component of the eukaryotic cytoskeleton, found throughout the cytoplasm.[3]

❖ With the ability to shift through various formations, microtubules function in several essential cellular processes, including mitosis.   Microtubules are the major constituents of mitotic spindles and are involved in chromosome separation, facilitating cell division.[4]

❖ Tubulins are targets for anticancer drugs like Taxol®, tesetaxel and the "vinca alkaloid" drugs such as vinblastine and vincristine.   Taxol® prevents a cell from dividing by binding to tubulin and causing the proteins to lose its flexibility.[5]   In clinical, it is an effective treatment for a number of cancers including breast, lung and ovarian.

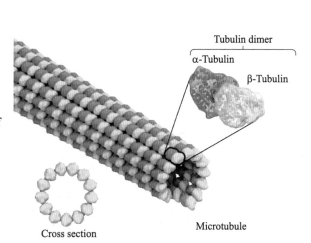

2　General Information

Herceptin®

❖ Herceptin® (Trastuzumab) is a human epidermal growth factor receptor 2 protein (HER2) antagonist, which was the first approved in Sep 1998 by US FDA.

❖ Trastuzumab is a recombinant DNA-derived humanized monoclonal antibody that targets the extracellular domain of HER2 receptor.　Herceptin® inhibits the proliferation of human tumor cells that overexpress HER2 via binding HER2 receptors and mediating antibody-dependent cell-mediated cytotoxicity (ADCC).

❖ Indicated for the treatment of HER2 overexpressing breast cancer, and HER2-overexpressing metastatic gastric or gastro-esophageal junction adenocarcinoma.

❖ The total sales of 6,851 million US$ for 2016; No sales data as of 2017.

Sponsor

❖ Herceptin® (Trastuzumab) was developed and marketed by Genentech, Inc., a subsidiary of Roche.

World Sales[6]

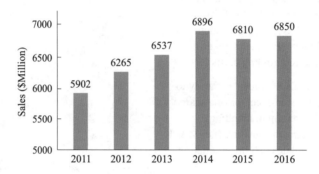

Figure 1　World Sales of Trastuzumab since 2011

Approval and Indication[6]

Table 1　Summary of the Approval of Herceptin®[6]

	US (FDA)	EU (EMA)	Japan (PMDA)	China (CFDA)
First approval date	09/25/1998	08/28/2000	04/22/2001 02/26/2004	09/05/2002
Application or approval No.	BLA103792	EMEA/H/C/000278	21600AMY00065/ 21300AMY00128	国药准字 J20110020/J20160033
Brand name	Herceptin®	Herceptin®	Herceptin®	Herceptin®/赫赛汀®
Indication	ABC, MBC, MGC	EBC, MBC, MGC	BC, MGC	ABC, MBC, MGC
Authorization holder	Roche	Roche	Roche	Roche

ABC: Adjuvant breast cancer.　BC: Breast cancer.　EBC: Early breast cancer.　MBC: Metastatic breast cancer.　MGC: Metastatic gastric cancer.

Table 2　Indication and Administration[7]

No.	Administration	Indication
1	Initial dose of 4 mg/kg over 90 min i.v. infusion, then 2 mg/kg over 30 min weekly for 52 weeks	HER2-overexpressing breast cancer, metastatic HER2-overexpressing breast cancer.
2	Initial dose of 8 mg/kg over 90 min i.v. infusion, then 6 mg/kg over 30-90 min every 3 weeks for 52 weeks	HER2-overexpressing breast cancer, metastatic HER2-overexpressing gastric cancer.

Sourced from US FDA drug label information.

3　CMC Profile

Product Profile[7]

Dosage route:　　　IV infusion.
Strength:　　　　　US: 440 mg; EU: 150 mg; JP: 60 mg, 150 mg; CN: 150 mg, 440 mg.
Dosage form:　　　Lyophilized powder for solution.
Formulation:　　　α,α-trehalose dehydrate, L-histidine hydrochloride, L-histidine, and polysorbate 20, USP.
Dissolution:　　　Reconstitution with 20 mL of the appropriate diluent
　(BWFI or SWFI) yields a solution containing 21 mg/mL trastuzumab at pH
　of approximately 6.
Stability:　　　　Stored at 2-8 °C until time of reconstitution.

Molecular Information[7]

Molecular formula:
　Light chain:　　　$C_{1032}H_{1603}N_{277}O_{335}S_6$
　Heavy chain:　　　$C_{2192}H_{3387}N_{583}O_{671}S_{16}$
　Molecular weight:　~148 kDa

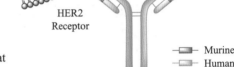

Amino Acid Sequence[8]

❖ Herceptin® is a recombinant humanized monoclonal antibody, an IgG1 that
　contains human framework regions with the CDR of a murine antibody
　that binds to HER2/neu.

```
  1  Asp-Ile-Gln-Met-Thr-Gln-Ser-Pro-Ser-Ser-Leu-Ser-Ala-Ser-Val-Gly-Asp-Arg-Val-Thr-Ile-Thr-Cys-Arg-Ala-
 26  Ser-Gln-Asp-Val-Asn-Thr-Ala-Val-Ala-Typ-Tyr-Gln-Gln-Lys-Pro-Gly-Lys-Ala-Pro-Lys-Leu-Leu-Ile-Tyr-Ser-
 51  Ala-Ser-Phe-Leu-Tyr-Ser-Gly-Val-Pro-Ser-Arg-Phe-Ser-Gly-Ser-Arg-Ser-Gly-Thr-Asp-Phe-Thr-Leu-Thr-Ile-
 76  Ser-Ser-Leu-Gln-Pro-Glu-Asp-Phe-Ala-Thr-Tyr-Tyr-Cys-Gln-Gln-His-Tyr-Thr-Thr-Pro-Pro-Thr-Phe-Gly-Gln-
101  Gly-Thr Lys-Val-Glu Ile-Lys-Arg-Thr-Val-Ala-Ala-Pro Ser-Val-Phe-Ile-Phe-Pro-Pro-Ser-Asp-Glu-Gln-Leu-
126  Lys-Ser-Gly-Thr-Ala-Ser-Val-Val-Cys-Leu-Leu-Asn-Asn-Phe-Tyr-Pro-Arg-Glu-Ala-Lys-Val-Gln-Trp-Lys-Val-
151  Asp-Asn-Ala-Leu-Gln-Ser-Gly-Asn-Ser-Gln-Glu-Ser-Val-Thr-Glu-Gln-Asp-Ser-Lys-Asp-Ser-Thr-Tyr-Ser-Leu-
176  Ser-Ser-Thr-Leu-Thr-Leu-Ser-Lys-Ala-Asp-Tyr-Glu-Lys-His-Lys-Val-Tyr-Ala-Cys-Glu-Val-Thr-His-Gln-Gly-
201  Leu-Ser-Ser-Pro-Val-Thr-Lys-Ser-Phe-Asn-Arg Gly-Glu-Cys
```

Light chain

```
  1  Glu-Val-Gln-Leu-Val-Glu-Ser-Gly-Gly-Gly-Leu-Val-Gln-Pro-Gly-Gly-Ser-Leu-Arg-Leu-Ser-Cys-Ala-Ala-Ser-
 26  Gly-Phe-Asn-Ile-Lys-Asp-Thr-Tyr-Ile-His-Trp-Val-Arg-Gln-Ala-Pro-Gly-Lys-Gly-Leu-Glu-Trp-Val-Ala-Arg-
 51  Ile-Tyr-Pro-Thr-Asn-Gly-Tyr-Thr-Arg-Tyr-Ala-Asp-Ser-Val-Lys-Gly-Arg-Phe-Thr-Ile-Ser-Ala-Asp-Thr-Ser-
 76  Lys-Asn-Thr-Ala-Tyr-Leu-Gln-Met-Asn-Ser-Leu-Arg-Ala-Glu-Asp-Thr-Ala-Val-Tyr-Tyr Cys-Ser-Arg-Trp-Gly-
101  Gly-Asp-Gly-Phe-Tyr-Ala-Met-Asp-Tyr-Trp-Gly-Gln-Gly-Thr-Leu-Val-Thr-Val-Ser-Ser-Ala-Ser-Thr-Lys-Gly-
126  Pro-Ser-Val-Phe-Pro-Leu-Ala-Pro-Ser-Ser-Lys-Ser-Thr-Ser-Gly-Gly-Thr-Ala-Ala-Leu-Gly-Cys-Leu-Val-Lys-
151  Asp-Tyr-Phe-Pro-Glu-Pro-Val-Thr-Val-Ser-Trp-Asn-Ser-Gly-Ala-Leu-Thr-Ser-Gly-Val-His-Thr-Phe-Pro-Ala-
176  Val-Lue-Gln-Ser-Ser-Gly-Leu-Tyr-Ser-Leu-Ser-Ser-Val-Val-Thr-Val-Pro-Ser-Ser-Ser-Leu-Gly-Thr-Gln-Thr-
201  Tyr-Ile-Cys-Asn-Val-Asn-His-Lys-Pro-Ser-Asn-Thr-Lys-Val-Asp-Lys-Lys-Val-Glu-Pro-Lys-Ser-Cys-Asp-Lys-
226  Thr-His-Thr-Cys*-Pro-Pro-Cys**-Pro-Ala-Pro-Glu-Leu-Leu-Gly-Gly-Pro-Ser-Val-Phe-Leu-Phe-Pro-Pro-Lys-Pro-
251  Lys-Asp-Thr-Leu-Met-Ile-Ser-Arg-Thr-Pro-Glu-Val-Thr-Cys-Val-Val-Val-Asp-Val-Ser-His-Glu-Asp-Pro-Glu-
276  Val-Lys-Phe-Asn-Trp-Tyr-Val-Asp-Gly-Val-Glu-Val-His-Asn-Aal-Lys-Thr-Lys-Pro-Arg-Glu-Glu-Gln-Tyr-Asn-
301  Ser-Thr-Tyr-Arg-Val-Val-Ser-Val-Leu-Thr-Val-Leu-His-Gln-Asp-Trp-Leu-Asn-Gly-Lys-Glu-Tyr-Lys-Cys-Lys-
326  Val-Ser-Asn-Lys-Ala-Leu-Pro-Ala-Pro-Ile-Glu-Lys-Thr-Ile-Ser-Lys-Ala-Lys-Gly-Gln-Pro-Arg-Glu-Pro-Gln-
351  Val-Tyr-Thr-Leu-Pro-Pro-Ser-Arg-Glu-Glu-Met-Thr-Lys-Asn-Gln-Val-Ser-Leu-Thr-Cys-Leu-Val-Lys-Gly-Phe-
376  Tyr-Pro-Ser-Asp-Ile-Ala-Val-Glu-Trp-Glu-Ser-Asn-Gly-Gln-Pro-Glu-Asn-Asn-Tyr-Lys-Thr-Thr-Pro-Pro-Val-
401  Leu-Asp-Ser-Asp-Gly-Ser-Phe-Phe-Leu-Tyr-Ser-Lys-Leu-Thr-Val-Asp-Lys-Ser-Arg-Typ-Gln-Gln-Gly-Asn-Val-
426  Phe-Ser-Cys-Ser-Val-Met-His-Glu-Ala-Leu-His-Asn-His-Tyr-Thr-Gln-Lys-Ser-Leu-Ser-Leu-Ser-Pro-Gly
```

Heavy chain　　　　　　　　　　Asn: Sugar chain binding site.

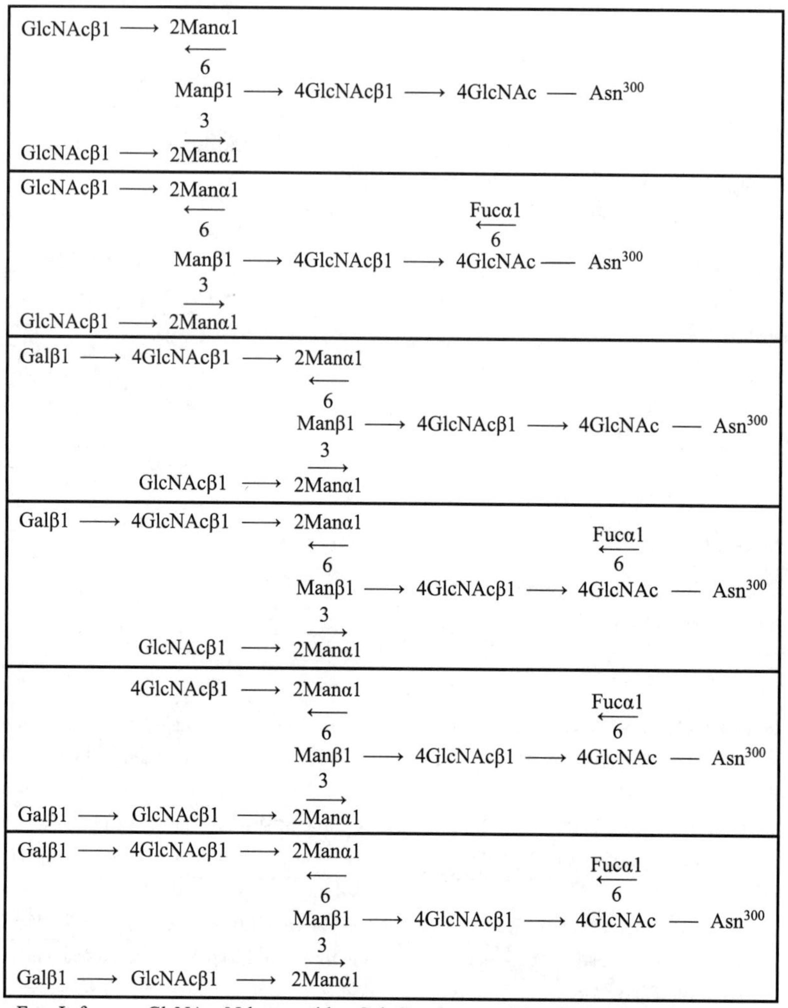

GlcNAcβ1 $\longrightarrow$ 2Manα1
$\xleftarrow{}$
6
Manβ1 $\longrightarrow$ 4GlcNAcβ1 $\longrightarrow$ 4GlcNAc $\longrightarrow$ Asn^{300}
3
$\xrightarrow{}$
GlcNAcβ1 $\longrightarrow$ 2Manα1

GlcNAcβ1 $\longrightarrow$ 2Manα1
$\xleftarrow{}$
6   Fucα1
$\xleftarrow{}$
6
Manβ1 $\longrightarrow$ 4GlcNAcβ1 $\longrightarrow$ 4GlcNAc $\longrightarrow$ Asn^{300}
3
$\xrightarrow{}$
GlcNAcβ1 $\longrightarrow$ 2Manα1

Galβ1 $\longrightarrow$ 4GlcNAcβ1 $\longrightarrow$ 2Manα1
$\xleftarrow{}$
6
Manβ1 $\longrightarrow$ 4GlcNAcβ1 $\longrightarrow$ 4GlcNAc $\longrightarrow$ Asn^{300}
3
$\xrightarrow{}$
GlcNAcβ1 $\longrightarrow$ 2Manα1

Galβ1 $\longrightarrow$ 4GlcNAcβ1 $\longrightarrow$ 2Manα1
$\xleftarrow{}$
6   Fucα1
$\xleftarrow{}$
6
Manβ1 $\longrightarrow$ 4GlcNAcβ1 $\longrightarrow$ 4GlcNAc $\longrightarrow$ Asn^{300}
3
$\xrightarrow{}$
GlcNAcβ1 $\longrightarrow$ 2Manα1

4GlcNAcβ1 $\longrightarrow$ 2Manα1
$\xleftarrow{}$
6   Fucα1
$\xleftarrow{}$
6
Manβ1 $\longrightarrow$ 4GlcNAcβ1 $\longrightarrow$ 4GlcNAc $\longrightarrow$ Asn^{300}
3
$\xrightarrow{}$
Galβ1 $\longrightarrow$ GlcNAcβ1 $\longrightarrow$ 2Manα1

Galβ1 $\longrightarrow$ 4GlcNAcβ1 $\longrightarrow$ 2Manα1
$\xleftarrow{}$
6   Fucα1
$\xleftarrow{}$
6
Manβ1 $\longrightarrow$ 4GlcNAcβ1 $\longrightarrow$ 4GlcNAc $\longrightarrow$ Asn^{300}
3
$\xrightarrow{}$
Galβ1 $\longrightarrow$ GlcNAcβ1 $\longrightarrow$ 2Manα1

Fuc: L-fucose. GlcNAc: N-hexananide. Gal: D-galactose. Man: D-mannose.

Figure 2　Heavy Chain Asn300 Site Sugar Chain Structure[8]

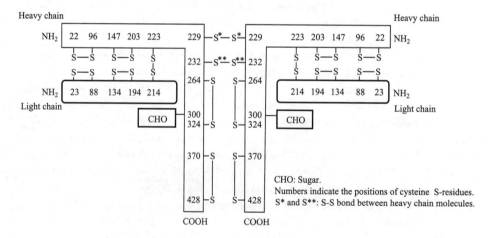

Figure 3　Trastuzumab Quadruplex Structure[9]

4 Pre-clinical Pharmacology

Summary

Mechanism of Action and *in vitro* Efficacy

❖ Herceptin® (Trastuzumab) is a recombinant DNA-derived humanized monoclonal antibody that targets the-extra cellular domain of the human epidermal growth factor receptor 2 protein (HER2) overexpressed in breast and ovarian cancer cells.

❖ Trastuzumab acts *in vitro* by a dual mechanisms of action:
  • Biochemical: Exerted by binding to the HER2p185 receptor, blocks dimer formation and induces down-regulation of the receptor, leading to the blockade of the signal transduction pathway.
  • Immunological: Exerted by Fc binding to the FcgRIII of CD16+ cells, mediating antibody-dependent cell-mediated cytotoxicity (ADCC) via recruiting immune cells to the tumor site.

❖ 4D5, the parental murine antibody of trastuzumab, downregulated the expression of HER2 receptors on cell surface.

❖ Trastuzumab induced the ADCC *in vitro* using chrome release assays.

❖ 4D5 and trastuzumab decreased the cell proliferation of HER2-overexpressing cells.

❖ Based on evidence from a variety of cell lines, antibody-coated cells are also susceptible to cytotoxic damage through binding with the FcγRIII (CD16) receptor on effector cells, NK cells and monocytes, but not neutrophils.

In vivo Efficacy

❖ Human breast cancer cell MCF7 xenograft mouse models
  • In single agent studies: Significant tumor growth inhibition at 3-30 mg/(kg·day) for 21 days.
  • In combination studies:
    ◆ Statistically superior antitumor efficacy in combination with doxorubicin, paclitaxel, cyclophosphamide, methotrexate, etoposide and vinblastine.
    ◆ Antagonistic effect of 5-fluorouracil.

❖ Human breast cancer cell BT-474 xenograft mouse models
  • In single agent studies: Significantly inhibited tumor growth and tumor regressed at ≥1 mg/(kg·day). Inhibited tumor growth in dose-dependent manner at 0.1-1 mg/(kg·day).
  • In combination studies:
    ◆ Greater inhibition of tumor growth in combination with doxorubicin or paclitaxel.
    ◆ Significantly superior complete tumor regression rate in combination with paclitaxel.

❖ Human ovary cancer cell CaOV-3-HER2 xenograft mouse models
  • Significant tumor growth inhibition at 3 mg/kg on Day 9, and at 10 mg/kg for Day 21.

❖ Human gastric cancer cell NCI-N87 xenograft mouse models
  • Trastuzumab single-dose: TGI: 62.0%.
  • Trastuzumab in combination with capecitabine, CDDP, or capecitabine/CDDP reached greater TGI: 85.0%-110%.

Mechanism of Action

Table 3 Trastuzumab-induced HER2 down Modulation on Cell Surface[8, 9]

Cell Line	Origin	HER2 Expressed on Cell Surface (Million per Cell)	Anti-HER2 Treatment (µg/mL)	HER2 Sites Decrease of Control	
				1 Day (24 h)	5 Days
SK-BR-3	Human breast cancer	1.9-2.2	muMAb 4D5ᵃ: 150	24.0%	57.0%
MCF7	Human breast cancer	~0.018	muMAb 4D5: 150	51.0%	-

ᵃ HER2-targeting antibody, the parental murine antibody of trastuzumab.

Table 4   *In vitro* ADCC Effects of Trastuzumab and IgG1 Using Chrome Release Assay[9]

Target Cell	Origin	Relative HER2 Expression[a]	Antibody	Effector Cell	Effector: Target Ratio	Finding
184A1	Human breast epithelial	0.30	TTZ[b]	PBMC	3.1-25.0	Net percent cytotoxicity: <10.0%.
MCF7	Human breast cancer	1.2	TTZ[b]	PBMC	3.1-25.0	Net percent cytotoxicity: <10.0%.
COLO201	Human colon cancer	8.3	TTZ[b]	PBMC	3.1-25.0	Net percent cytotoxicity: <20.0%.
MKN7	Human grastic cancer	16.7	TTZ[b]	PBMC	3.1-25.0	Net percent cytotoxicity: 15.0%-30.0%.
SK-BR-3	Human breast cancer	33.0	TTZ[b]	PBMC	3.1-25.0	Net percent cytotoxicity: 15.0%-50.0%.
SK-BR-3	Human breast cancer	33.0	TTZ[c]	NK	0.10-100	Cytotoxicity: >50.0% (ratio >2.0).
			TTZ[c]	Monocyte	0.10-100	Cytotoxicity: >40.0% (ratio >10.0).
			TTZ[c]	Neurophil	0.10-100	No Effect.
SK-BR-3	Human breast cancer	33.0	TTZ ± FcγR I block[d]	PBMC	NA-100	No significant change on ADCC effect.
			TTZ ± FcγR II block[e]	PBMC	NA-100	No significant change on ADCC effect.
			TTZ ± FcγR III block[f]	PBMC	NA-100	Significantly inhibited ADCC effects.
SK-BR-3	Human breast cancer	33.0	TTZ ± IgG1[g]	PBMC	0.10-100	No significant change by huIgG1.

ADCC: Antibody-dependent cell-mediated cytotoxicity.   NK: Natural killer cell.   PBMC: Peripheral blood mononuclear cell.   TTZ: Trastuzumab.   [a] HER2 expression of 184 cells as "1.0".   [b] Trastuzumab: 0.1 μg/mL.   [c] Trastuzumab: 1 μg/mL.   [d] Trastuzumab: 1 μg/mL, FcγRI block with FcγRI antibody 100 nM.   [e] Trastuzumab: 1 μg/mL, FcγRII block with FcγRI antibody 100 nM.   [f] Trastuzumab: 1 μg/mL, FcγRII block with FcγRI antibody 100 nM.   [g] Trastuzumab: 1 μg/mL, FcγRIII block with FcγRI antibody 100 nM.

Overview *in vitro* Activities

Table 5   Anti-proliferation of HER2-targeting mAb in HER2-expressing Cells[9]

Cell Line	Origin	Relative HER2 Expression[a]	Treatment	Test[b]	Relative Cell Proliferation (%)
184	Human breast epithelial	1.0	muMAb 4D5 for 5 days	Crystal violet	116
184A1	Human breast epithelial	0.30	muMAb 4D5 for 5 days	Crystal violet	100
184B5	Human breast epithelial	0.80	muMAb 4D5 for 5 days	Crystal violet	108
HBL-100	Human breast epithelial	1.0	muMAb 4D5 for 5 days	Crystal violet	104
MCF7	Human breast cancer	1.2	muMAb 4D5 for 5 days	Crystal violet	101
MDA-MB-231	Human breast cancer	1.2	muMAb 4D5 for 5 days	Crystal violet	91.0
ZR-75-1	Human breast cancer	3.3	muMAb 4D5 for 5 days	Crystal violet	102
MDA-MB-436	Human breast cancer	3.3	muMAb 4D5 for 5 days	Crystal violet	97.0
MDA-MB-175	Human breast cancer	4.5	muMAb 4D5 for 5 days	Crystal violet	62.0
MDA-MB-453	Human breast cancer	16.7	muMAb 4D5 for 5 days	Crystal violet	61.0
MDA-MB-361	Human breast cancer	16.7	muMAb 4D5 for 5 days	Crystal violet	63.0
BT474	Human breast cancer	25.0	muMAb 4D5 for 5 days	Crystal violet	27.0
SK-BR-3	Human breast cancer	33.0	muMAb 4D5 for 5 days	Crystal violet	33.0
			muMAb 4D5 for 3 days[c]	MTT	50.0-85.0
			Trastuzumab for 3 days[c]	MTT	60.0-80.0[d]
SK-OV-3	Human ovary cancer	16.7	muMAb 4D5 for 5 days	Crystal violet	77.0
MKN7	Human grastic cancer	16.7	muMAb 4D5 for 5 days	Crystal violet	99.0
KATO III	Human grastic cancer	5.0	muMAb 4D5 for 5 days	Crystal violet	91.0
COLO201	Human colon cancer	8.3	muMAb 4D5 for 5 days	Crystal violet	107
SW1417	Human colon cancer	6.7	muMAb 4D5 for 5 days	Crystal violet	98.0

MTT: 3-(4,5-dimethyl-2-thiazolyl)-2,5-diphenyl-2*H*-tetrazolium bromide.   [a] HER2 expression of human breast epithelial cell line, 184 cells as "1.0".   [b] OD was tested at 570 nm in MTT assays, or at 540 nm in crystal violet assays.   [c] 0.2-100 μg/mL.   [d] Significantly decreased in cell proliferation at 0.4-100 μg/mL (p <0.050).

Table 6　Combination of Trastuzumab with Chemotherapeutic Drugs in SK-BR-3 Cells[10]

Drug	Concentration (μM)	Trastuzumab/Drug (Molar Ratio)	Range of Trastuzumab Concentration (μM)	CI (Mean ± SEM)	P-value	Interaction
TSPA	8.3-1,260	6.4×10^{-5}	5.3×10^{-4}-6.8×10^{-2}	0.67 ± 0.12	0.00080	Synergism
CDDP	0.60-170	4.0×10^{-4}	2.6×10^{-4}-6.8×10^{-2}	0.56 ± 0.15	0.0010	Synergism
VP-16	0.26-68.0	9.9×10^{-4}	2.6×10^{-4}-6.7×10^{-2}	0.54 ± 0.15	0.00030	Synergism
DOX	0.027-6.9	9.8×10^{-3}	2.6×10^{-4}-6.8×10^{-2}	1.2 ± 0.18	0.13	Addition
TAX	0.0018-0.50	1.4×10^{-1}	2.5×10^{-4}-7.0×10^{-2}	0.91 ± 0.23	0.21	Addition
MTX	0.00080-0.20	3.3×10^{-1}	2.6×10^{-4}-6.6×10^{-2}	1.4 ± 0.17	0.21	Addition
VBL	0.00016-0.039	1.7	2.7×10^{-4}-6.6×10^{-2}	1.1 ± 0.19	0.26	Addition
5-FU	3.0-765	8.8×10^{-6}	2.6×10^{-4}-6.7×10^{-2}	2.9 ± 0.51	0.00010	Antagonize

5-FU: 5-fluorouracil, a suicide inhibitor.　CDDP: cis-Diaminedichloroplatinum.　CI: Combination index.　DOX: Doxorubicin, an anthracycline antitumor antibiotic. MTX: Methotrexate, an antimetabolite and antifolate drug.　SEM: Standard error of mean.　TAX: Paclitaxel.　TSPA: Triethylenethiophosphoramide, an alkylating agent. VBL: Vinblastine, a mitosis inhibitor.　VP-16: Etoposide, a topoisomerase II inhibitor.

Overview *in vivo* Activities

Table 7　Anti-tumor Efficacy of Trastuzumab in Xenograft Mouse Models[9]

Cell Line	Type	HER2 Status	Animal	Drug	Dose (mg/kg)	Route & Schedule	ED[a] (mg/kg)	Finding
MCF7	Human breast cancer	HER2 transfer	Swiss nude mouse (female)	Trastuzumab / Human IgG1 / muMAb 4D5	3, 10, 30, 100 / 100 / 25	i.p., Days 1, 5, 9	3	Significant tumor growth inhibition for 21 days. (Human IgG1: negative control; muMAb 4D5: positive control).
				Combined with DOX, TAX, CPA, MTX, VP-16, VBL, or 5-FU	Trastuzumab[b] 4 or 10	i.p., once or twice weekly[b]	4 or 10	Statistically superior anti-tumor efficacy in combination with DOX, TAX, CPA, MTX, VP-16, or VBL, but antagonistic for 5-FU.
BT-474	Human breast cancer	Overexpression	Nude mouse	Trastuzumab / Human IgG1	0.1-30 / 1, 30	i.p., twice a week for 4 weeks	NA	Tumor growth inhibition in a dose dependent manner for 0.1-1 mg/kg, and appeared to plateau at ≥1 mg/kg. (Human IgG1: negative control).
				Combined with DOX or/ and TAX	Trastuzumab[c]: 0.3	i.p., twice weekly for 4-5 weeks[e]	-	Greater inhibition of tumor growth in combination group. Significantly superior complete tumor regression rate compared to single agent.
CaOV3-HER2	Human ovary cancer	HER2 sensitivity	Swiss nude mouse (female)	Trastuzumab / Human IgG1 / muMAb 4D5	3, 10, 30, 100 / 100 / 25	i.p., Days 1, 5, 9	3	Significant tumor growth inhibition at 3 mg/kg on Day 9, and at 10 mg/kg for Day 21. (Human IgG1: negative control; muMAb 4D5: positive control).
NCI-N87	Human gastric cancer	HER2 overexpression	Nude mouse	Trastuzumab	20	i.p., 3 times a week	-	TGI[d] = 62.0% ($P \leqslant 0.050$)[e]
				huIgG1/ Capecitabine	359	q.d., qd × 14	-	TGI[d] = 75.0% ($P \leqslant 0.050$)[e]
				Trastuzumab/ Capecitabine	20/359[f]	Above[f]	-	TGI[d] = 110% ($P \leqslant 0.050$)[e, g]
				Trastuzumab	20	i.p., 3 times a week	-	TGI[d] = 63.0% ($P \leqslant 0.050$)[e]
				CDDP	5	i.p., 3 times a week	-	TGI[d] = 43.0% ($P \leqslant 0.050$)[e]

Continued

SC Xenograft Model				Drug	Dose (mg/kg)	Route & Schedule	Effect	
Cell Line	**Type**	**HER2 Status**	**Animal**				**ED[a] (mg/kg)**	**Finding**
NCI-N87	Human gastric cancer	HER2 overexpression	Nude mouse	Trastuzumab/ CDDP	20/5	_[h]	-	TGI[d] = 85.0% ($P \leqslant 0.050$)[e, g]
				Capecitabine/ CDDP	180/5	p.o., qd × 14[i]	-	TGI[d] = 82.0% ($P \leqslant 0.050$)[e]
				Trastuzumab/ Capecitabine/ CDDP	20/180/5	_[h]	-	TGI[d] = 106% ($P \leqslant 0.050$)[e, j]

5-FU: 5-fluorouracil, a suicide inhibitor.　CDDP: *cis*-Diaminedichloroplatinum.　CPA: Cyclophosphamide.　DOX: Doxorubicin, an anthracycline antitumor antibiotic.　HER2 : Human epidermal growth factor receptor-2.　i.p.: Intraperitoneal.　MTX: Methotrexate, an antimetabolite and antifolate drug.　p.o.: Oral.　qd: Once daily.　TAX: Paclitaxel.　TGI: Tumor growth inhibition.　VBL: Vinblastine, a mitosis inhibitor.　VP-16: Etoposide, a topoisomerase II inhibitor.　[a] The minimal effect dose of trastuzumab in those studies.　[b] Administration schedule of trastuzumab, in combination with MTX, VP-16, 5-FU, or VBL: starting dose of 8 mg/kg and then 4 mg/kg, once weekly; in combination with DOX or CPA: 10 mg/kg on Days 0, 4, 8; in combination with TAX: 10 mg/kg, i.p. twice weekly.　Administration schedule of chemotherapeutic drugs, DOX: 5 mg/(kg·day), i.p., Day 1; MTX: 2 mg/(kg·day), i.p., Days 1-5; VP-16: 20 mg/(kg·day), s.c., Days 1-3; 5-FU: 16 mg/(kg·day), i.p., Days 1-4; VBL: 0.8 mg/(kg·day), i.p., Days 1-2; CPA: 80 mg/(kg·day), i.p., Days 0, 4, and 8; TAX: 15 mg/(kg·day), i.p., Days 1-3.　[c] DOX: i.p., 10 mg/(kg·day) on Day 1 or 3.75 mg/(kg·day) on Days 1, 2, 14, 15; TAX: i.v., 5 or 10 mg/(kg·day) on Days 1, 4.　[d] TGI: Tumor growth inhibition, TGI (%) = [1 - (changes of tumor volume from Day 1 to Day 22 in treatment groups)/(changes of tumor volume from Day 1 to Day 22 in control groups).　[e] $P \leqslant 0.050$ vs. control (human IgG) group.　[f] Trastuzumab, 20 mg/kg i.p. for 3 times a week for 3 weeks.　[g] $P \leqslant 0.050$ vs. trastuzumab single.　[h] Each followed the dose schedule of single-dose.　[i] Capecitabine: 180 mg/kg, p.o., daily for 14 days.　[j] $P \leqslant 0.050$ vs. capecitabine/CDDP.　-: Not available.

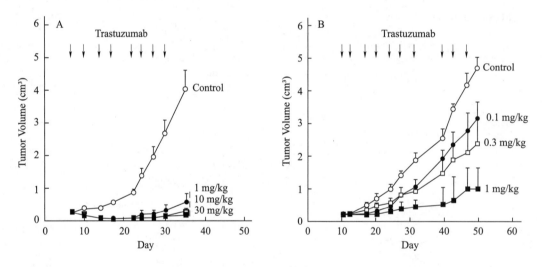

Figure 4　Effects of Trastuzumab on Human Breast Cancer BT-474 Cell Xenograft Mouse Model[9]

Study: Antitumor activities in HER2-overexpressing BT-474 human breast cancer xenograft mouse model.

Animal: Nude mouse (female).

Model: BT-474 cells were implanted into the s.c. of nude mice.

Administration: Trastuzumab: 0.1, 0.3, 1, 10, or 30 mg/(kg·day); i.p. twice a week for 4 weeks; Control: human IgG1, 1 or 30 mg/kg.

Starting: Tumors reached a size of 0.2-0.3 cm³ (Day 7 to 10 post inoculation).

Test: Measured tumor volumes.

Result: Tumor growth inhibition in a dose-dependent manner for 0.1-1 mg/kg, and appeared to plateau at ≥1 mg/kg.　Tumor regression at 1, 10, and 30 mg/kg; and 3/8, 5/10, 3/10 were complete regression.　(In 30 mg/kg group: low survival rate and significant body weight loss.)

5　Toxicology

Summary

Non-clinical Single-Dose Toxicology

❖ Acute toxicity in CD-1 mice: No lethality up to 200 mg/kg, and no APA in 2 weeks at 94 mg/kg (NOEL).

❖ Acute toxicity in monkeys: No lethality up to 200 mg/kg, and no APA in 2 weeks at 47 mg/kg (NOEL).

Non-clinical Repeated-Dose Toxicology

❖ A series of i.v. repeated-dose toxicology studies were conducted with Herceptin® in rhesus monkeys (up to 26 weeks):
  • Minimal toxic response, with the only noteworthy observations concerning injection-site trauma in the rhesus monkey.
  • Neutralising antibodies were detected from Weeks 5-26 in one low-dose female Cynomolgus monkey.

Safety Pharmacology

❖ No abnormal effect on cardiovascular, behavioral, general physiological, and respiratory function, both *in vitro* and *in vivo* safety pharmacology studies.

Genotoxicity

❖ No evidence of mutagenic activity in the standard Ames bacterial and human peripheral blood lymphocyte mutagenicity assays at concentrations of up to 5,000 µg/mL.

❖ No evidence of chromosomal damage to mouse bone marrow cells in an *in vivo* micromucleus assays following doses of up to 118 mg/kg Herceptin®.

Reproductive Toxicology

❖ No evidence of impaired or harm to the fetus in Cynomolgus monkeys at doses up to 25 times the weekly recommended human dose of 2 mg/kg.

Carcinogenicity

❖ No carcinogenicity studies were performed.

Special Toxicology

❖ No special toxicology studies were performed.

Single-Dose Toxicology

Table 8   Single-Dose Toxicology Studies of Trastuzumab[9]

Species	Dose (mg/kg)	MNLD (mg/kg)	Finding
CD-1 mouse	4.7 mg/mL: 0, 9.4, 47, 94, i.v. 20 mg/mL: 0, 200, i.v.	>200	No obvious effects. No anti-trastuzumab in 2 weeks after a dose of 94 mg/kg.
Cynomolgus monkey	4.7 mg/mL: 0, 4.7, 23.5, 47, i.v. 20 mg/mL: 0, 100, 200, i.v.	>200	No obvious effects. No anti-trastuzumab in 2 weeks after a dose of 47 mg/kg.

Formulation: 0.5% MC.   i.v.: Intravenous.   MNLD: Maximum non-lethal dose.

Repeated-Dose Toxicology

Table 9   Repeated-Dose Toxicology Studies of Trastuzumab[11]

Species	Duration (Week)	Dose [mg/(kg·day)]	Finding
IGS Wistar Hannover Rat	2	Male: 0, 10, 25, 100	25 mg/kg: ↓ BWG, ↓ reticulocyte counts, ↓ MCV and MCH, ↓ haematocrit and hemoglobin. ↓ Triglycerides, ↓ glucose and albumin, ↑ globulin. Bile duct vacuolation/hypertrophy; Adrenal gland: ↑ cortical vacuolation and/or cortical single cell necrosis; Stomach: (glandular) erosion. 100 mg/kg: Piloerection, ↓ BW, ↑ RBC# and hemoglobin, ↑ PLT#, ↑ total WBC, neutrophil and monocyte counts. ↑ AST, ↑ creatine kinase in one animal, ↓ urea, total bilirubin, and cholesterol, ↓ triglycerides, glucose, and albumin, ↑ globulin. ↓ Mean thymic and splenic weights, bile duct vacuolation/hypertrophy; focal/multifocal or single cell necrosis of hepatocytes, peri-/cholangiolitis. Hypocellularity in bone marrow (sternum), absence of haemopoiesis in spleen. Mesenteric lymph nodes: Focal/multifocal necrosis (cortex/paracortex), abscess formation (paracortex), and increase in aggregates of macrophages, subacute focal inflammation in the mesentery, reduction/absence of germinal center development. Thymus: Cortical atrophy and/or lymphocytosis; Adrenal gland: Increase in cortical vacuolation and/or cortical single cell necrosis; Small intestine: Minimal neutrophilic cell infiltration; Stomach: (glandular) erosion. NOAEL: 10 mg/kg.
	4	Male & female: 0, 7.5, 25, 75→50	≥25 mg/(kg·day): ↓ BWG, ↑ neutrophil, ↑ PLT, ↑ serum insulin concentration (male). 50 mg/(kg·day): ↓ BWG, ↓ food consumption; inflammation (↑monocyte, ↑ plasma fibrinogen), ↑ lymphocyte counts (male). ↑ Insulin (female), ↑serum liver enzyme activities (male), ↑ serum phosphorus concentration. 75 mg/(kg·day): Not tolerated and was reduced to 50 mg/kg due to adverse clinical signs. ↓ Reticulo-cyte counts, ↓ urea, ↓ phosphorus (male) and ↓ magnesium, ↑ glucose (female), ↑ calcium (male), ↑ serum AST and ALT activities (male). NOAEL: 7.5 mg/kg.

Continued

Species	Duration (Week)	Dose [mg/(kg·day)]	Finding
IGS Wistar Hannover Rat	13	Male & female: 0, 3, 10, 30	Target: Biliopancreatic duct (chronic inflammation, degeneration/necrosis, erosion, hyperplasia, dilatation, and vacuolation at all doses), the duodenum (degeneration, necrosis, hyperplasia, dilatation, inflammation, and vacuolation), liver (bile duct vacuolation), mesenteric lymph nodes (increased macrophage aggregates) and lung (macrophage aggregates). 30 mg/(kg·day): ↑ fibrinogen concentration and ↑ PLT#, ↑ total protein concentration (male), ↓ albumin concentration (female), ↑ globulin concentration and ↓ albumin-to-globulin ratio. ↑ Cholesterol concentration and ↓ triglyceride concentration. ↑ Thyroid stimulating hormone concentration. ↓ Body weight gain, ↓ food consumption and ↓ body weight. Duodenum (chronic-active inflammation, hyperplasia and luminal dilatation), mesenteric lymph node and lung (↑ number of macrophages). Exposure increased with the minor accumulation of dose following repeat dosing. NOAEL: ND.
Cynomolgus monkey	2	Male & female: 0, 10, 40, 100	≥40 mg/(kg·day): Circling, depression, cold to touch, dehydration, hunched posture, decreased locomotor activity (DLA), soft faeces/diarrhoea, emesis, thymus (lymphoid depletion), and pancreas (↓ zymogen). 100 mg/(kg·day): ↓ Neutrophils, ↓ reticulocytes, ↓ cellularity in bone marrow smears. ↑ ALT (2-3-fold), ↑ total bilirubin, ↑ urea, ↑ creatinine, bone marrow (↓ cellularity), pancreas (↓ zymogen), ↓ food consumption, ↑ neutrophils and fibrinogen, ↓ lymphocytes, and ↑ phosphorus. NOAEL: 10 mg/kg.
	4	Male & female: 0, 3, 10, 30	≥10 mg/(kg·day): ↓ Thyroid gland weights (M), small thyroid gland (M), small follicles and colloid depletion in thyroid gland (M), and sinus histiocytosis in mesenteric lymph nodes (F). 30 mg/(kg·day): ↑ Serum ALT activity, erosion and vacuolation of the lining epithelium of duodenal ampulla, associated with epithelial hyperplasia, and foamy macrophage infiltration of the submucosa. Neutrophilic inflammation in duodenal ampulla and adjacent duodenal mucosa, ↓ zymogen in the acinar pancreas. Sinus histiocytosis in mesenteric lymph nodes. Thymic lymphoid depletion. NOAEL: 10 mg/kg.
	13	Male & female: 0, 3, 10, 30	≥3 mg/(kg·day): Sporadic vomitus. 30 mg/(kg·day): Liquid faeces, ↑ ALT activity, ↑ glucose, ↑ insulin (M). Discoloured major duodenal papilla, ↑ mixed cell inflammation in the cystic bile duct (M), hepatic bile duct (M), and the common bile duct (M). Mixed cell inflammation (mononuclear cells and neutrophils) in major duodenal papilla. Fine cytoplasmic vacuoles in duct epithelium of the cystic bile duct (M), hepatic bile duct (M), common bile duct (M), and lining cells of the major duodenal papilla (M). Minimal mixed cell peribiliary inflammation in the liver. NOAEL: 10 mg/kg.

AST: Aspartate transaminase. BW: Body weight. BWG: Body weight gain. MCH: Mean cell haemoglobin. MCV: Mean cell volume. ND: No detection. NOAEL: No-observed-adverse-effect level. PLT: Platelets. RBC: Red blood cell. WBC: White blood cell.

Safety Pharmacology

Table 10   Safety Pharmacology Studies of Trastuzumab[9, 10]

Study	System	Dose (mg/kg)	Finding
Neurological effect[a]	Mouse (*n* = 10)	5.7, 17.1, 57, i.v.	No significant neurologic changes during FOB.
	Rat (*n* = 10)	5.7, 17.1, 57, i.v.	No significant neurologic changes.
Respiratory and cardiovascular effect[a]	Dog (*n* = 5)	2.28, 6.84, 22.8, i.v.	22.8 mg/kg: Significant increase on respiratory rate, and a transient decrease on heart rate.
	Monkey[b]	1, 5, 25, i.v.	No effects on respiratory rate, blood pressure, heart rate and ECG.

ECG: Electrocardiogram. FOB: Functional observation battery. [a] Vehicle: HEPES-buffered physiological saline (HB-PS) + 0.3% DMSO. [b] Positive control: Terfenadine.

Genotoxicity

Table 11　Genotoxicity Studies of Trastuzumab[11]

Assay	Species/System	Metabolism Activity	Dose	Finding
In vitro reverse mutation assay (Ames)	*S. typhimurium*: TA97, TA98, TA100, TA1535, TA102	±S9	0-1,000 µg/plate	Negative.
In vitro miniscreen Ames test	*S. typhimurium*: TA98, TA100	±S9	30-1,000 µg/well	Negative[a].
In vitro chromosome aberration assay	HPBL	3 + 17 h: ±S9 20 h: -S9	0-16 µg/mL	Negative.
			0-22 µg/mL	Incomplete[b].
In vitro micronucleus assay	HPBL	3 or 20 h: -S9 3 h: +S9	0-18.6 µg/mL	Negative.
	TK6 cell	3 or 20 h: -S9 3 h: +S9	0-125 µg/mL	Positive for 20 h treatment[c].
In vivo micronucleus assay	Rat bone marrow	-	0-2,000 mg/kg, p.o. × 2	Negative.

HPBL: Human peripheral blood lymphocytes·　[a] Positive and negative control results were not provided for comparative purposes.　[b] 2nd assay cancelled (-S9: 20 h; +S9: 3 + 17 h) by the Applicant.　[c] Increased number of cells containing micronuclei after 20 h treatment -S9, but not after 3 h treatment ± S9.

Reproductive Toxicology

Table 12　Reproductive and Developmental Toxicology Studies of Trastuzumab[12]

Study	Species	Dose [mg/(kg·day)]	Endpoint	Finding
Embryonic-fetal development	Wistar rat	0, 1, 10, 50	Maternal	Depressed gestational body weight at MD and HD.
			Fetal developmental	No embryo lethality or fetotoxicity.
	NZW rabbit	0, 2, 10, 25	Maternal	Mildly depressed gestational body weight and food consumption at HD.
			Fetal developmental	No significant embryo lethality or fetotoxicity. Significant incomplete ossification of sternebrae at all doses. Incidence of visceral anomalies in a small number of fetuses.

Vehicle: 0.5% (w/v) MC in RODI water.　HD: High Dose.　MD: Medium Dose.

6　Non-clinical Pharmacokinetic/ADME/Toxicokinetics

Summary

Non-clinical Pharmacokinetics

❖ Absorption-Bioavailability
- Exhibited non-linear pharmacokinetics in rhesus monkeys, with a pattern of supraproportional increases in AUC in the dose of 1, 10, 100 mg/kg trastuzumab.
- Was observed slowly (T_{max} = 4-15 h) in humans, mice (7 h), rats (12 h) and monkeys (13-18.3 h).
- Showed a half-life ranging between 11-39 days in mice, much longer than those in rhesus monkeys (6 days for 0.5 mg/kg dose).
- Had moderate system clearance in mice [26.6 mL/(min·kg)], rats [1.5 L/(h·kg)], but low to moderate in monkeys [0.37-0.78 L/(h·kg)], after intravenous administrations.　The CL/F in humans was 44.5-147 L/h after oral administration.
- Exhibited an extensive distribution in mice, rats and dogs, with the apparent volumes of distribution at 9.7, 19.9 and 6.5-13.5 L/kg, after intravenous administrations.　The V_z/F in humans was 1,880-6,230 L after oral administration.
- Was classified as a low passive permeability compound.
❖ Distribution
- Uptake of radioactivity was localized in tumor tissue for ^{125}I-labeled trastuzumab and not IgG1, and was shown to be saturable.　Peak tumor uptake occurred 24-48 hours after administration and ranged from 22.0%-66.0% dose/g of tissue. Extrapolation of these results to humans is compromised by the fact that the animals used do not express human p185HER2 on normal tissues.
- The corresponding tumor-to-serum radioactivity ratios ranged from 1.1 to 4.3.　Extrapolation of these results to humans

is compromised by the fact that animal used do not express human p185HER2 on normal tissues.

❖ Metabolism

- Uptake of radioactivity was localized in tumor tissue for ^{125}I-labeled trastuzumab and not IgG1, and was shown to be saturable, peak tumor uptake occurred 24-48 hours after administration and ranged from 22.0%-66.0% dose/g of tissue. Extrapolation of these results to humans is compromised by the fact that the animals used do not express human p185HER2 on normal tissues.
- The corresponding tumor-to-serum radioactivity ratios ranged from 1.1 to 4.3. Extrapolation of these results to humans is compromised by the fact that animal used do not express human p185HER2 on normal tissues.

❖ Excretion

- Was predominantly eliminated in feces in rats, monkeys and humans, with the parent drug as the significant component in rat, monkey and human feces.
- Radioactivity recovery in bile were 24.3% and 65.4% after oral and intravenous administrations.

❖ Drug-Drug interaction

- The kinetic parameters of the various chemotherapeutics were essentially unaffected by the presence of trastuzumab and vice versa, except in the case of the combination with paclitaxel where the C_{max} for trastuzumab was doubled and the clearance halved, terminal half-life being unaffected.
- Since trastuzumab is a humanized mAb, significant species differences in pharmacokinetics are to be expected: Rodent p185[neu] (corresponding receptor protein to human p185HER2) is not recognized, whereas in non-human primates trastuzumab recognizes a receptor (as yet uncharacterized) in epithelial cells. However, unlike humans these primate species do not overexpress p185HER2 or produce shed antigen.

Non-clinical Pharmacokinetics

Table 13 *In vivo* Pharmacokinetic Parameters of Trastuzumab in Mice, Minipigs and Monkeys after Single Intravenous and Oral Doses of Trastuzumab[10]

Species	Route	Dose (mg/kg)	rHuPH20 (U/mL)	T_{max} (h)	C_{max} (μg/mL)	$AUC_{0-t/inf}$ (μg·day/mL)	$t_{1/2}$ (Day)	CL or CL/F [mL/(day·kg)]	V_{ss} (mL/kg)	F (%)
Mouse (female)[a]	i.v.	1	-	NA	16.9	119	17.2	6.1	151	-
	i.v.	10	-	NA	250	1,180	39.2	3.8	215	-
	i.v.	100	-	NA	2,250	8,010	10.7	13.4	184	-
	s.c.	10	4,600	7.0	NA	NA	NA	NA	NA	83.4
Gottingen minipig (female)	i.v.	10	-	NA	NA	NA	5.7	8.9	77.6	-
	s.c.	13-14	0	67.2	101	1,529	8.6	3.4	NA	90.2
	s.c.	13-14	2,000	28.8	126	1,304	6.2	3.5	NA	81.8
	s.c.	13-14	6,000	24.0	129	1,392	6.5	3.3	NA	87.2
Rhesus monkey (female)	i.v.	2	-	NA	NA	112	2.3	18.0	56.9	-
	i.v.	10	-	NA	NA	1,312	5.6	7.7	60.2	-
Cynomolgus monkey (female)	s.c.	25	6,000	24.0	307	4,833	12.3	5.4	NA	ca. 100

CL/F (mL/h) average volume of distribution at steady-state. 108 mg per animal. i.v.: Intravenous. NA: Not available. s.c.: Subcutaneous. [a] AUC_{0-24}.

Table 14   *In vivo* Tissue Distribution of Trastuzumab and Non-specific Human IgG1
in HER2-overexpressing NIH-3T3 Xenograft Mice[9]

Tissue	^{125}I-Trastuzumab, i.v., 10 mg/kg, % of Radioactivity (% of dose/g or mL)					Tissue/ Serum Ratio	^{125}I-Non-specific IgG1, i.v., 6.4 mg/kg % of Radioactivity (% of dose/g or mL)					Tissue/ Serum Ratio
	5 min	3 h	24 h	48 h	168 h		5 min	3 h	24 h	48 h	168 h	
Serum	62.2	40.9	23.5	15.0	11.7	-	93.5	60.4	38.6	40.3	22.9	-
Blood	NS	34.8	9.4	9.3	6.8	-	41.3	26.9	24.7	23.7	14.4	-
Liver	6.3 (0.10)	4.4 (0.11)	2.6 (0.11)	1.8 (0.12)	1.3 (0.11)	<0.30	10.3 (0.11)	6.7 (0.11)	4.0 (0.10)	4.2 (0.10)	2.6 (0.11)	<0.30
Lung	10.9 (0.18)	5.6 (0.14)	4.5 (0.19)	3.3 (0.22)	2.4 (0.20)	<0.30	13.0 (0.14)	9.2 (0.15)	8.5 (0.22)	8.4 (0.21)	4.0 (0.18)	<0.30
Kidneys	8.1 (0.13)	5.9 (0.14)	3.8 (0.16)	2.5 (0.17)	1.9 (0.16)	<0.30	10.8 (0.12)	7.7 (0.13)	5.6 (0.14)	4.7 (0.12)	2.9 (0.13)	<0.30
Spleen	5.5 (0.090)	5.0 (0.12)	3.4 (0.14)	2.2 (0.14)	1.6 (0.13)	<0.30	11.2 (0.12)	7.1 (0.12)	4.5 (0.12)	5.3 (0.13)	2.7 (0.12)	<0.30
Muscle	1.0 (0.020)	1.3 (0.030)	1.6 (0.070)	1.3 (0.090)	1.1 (0.090)	<0.30	2.1 (0.020)	1.2 (0.020)	2.6 (0.070)	2.5 (0.060)	1.6 (0.070)	<0.30
Tumor	2.9 (0.050)	8.9 (0.22)	28.4 (1.2)	21.8 (1.5)	10.8 (0.92)	1.2 (24 h)	3.0 (0.030)	10.0 (0.17)	10.1 (0.060)	7.6 (0.19)	4.3 (0.19)	<0.30

i.v.: Intravenous.   NS: No sample.

Table 15   Excretion Profiles of ^{125}I-Trastuzumab in Mice after Single-Dose[10]

Gender	Dose (mg/kg)	Route	Time (Day)	Urine (% of dose)	Feces (% of dose)
Male	10	i.v.	0-7	31.0	2.0
			0-76	83.0	12.0
Female	10	i.v.	0-7	28.0	5.0
			0-76	65.0	29.0

i.v.: Intravenous.

❖ Combination with TAX significantly increased AUC of trastuzumab and decreased the CL.
❖ Trastuzumab had no significant change of the pharmacokinetic parameters of DOX, TAX, or DOX + CPA.

Table 16   *In vivo* Pharmacokinetic Parameters of Trastuzumab in Serum of Rhesus Macaque after Single or Combination Dose[10]

Administration	Trastuzumab (i.v., mg/kg)	Combination		C_{max} (μg/mL)	AUC_{0-t} (μg·day/mL)	$t_{1/2}$ (Day)	CL [mL/(day·kg)]	V_1 (mL/kg)
		Route	Dose (mg/kg)					
Trastuzumab single	1.5	-	-	39.0 ± 2.6	66.0 ± 4.4	1.7 ± 0.15	20.0 ± 1.3	50.0 ± 3.0
Trastuzumab + TAX	1.5	i.v.	4	75.0 ± 16.0	122 ± 9.8[a]	1.6 ± 0.030	12.0 ± 2.2[a]	27.0 ± 4.7
Trastuzumab + DOX	1.5	i.v.	1.5	33.0 ± 7.0	60.0 ± 1.1	1.7 ± 0.37	24.0 ± 5.0	58.0 ± 8.5
Trastuzumab + DOX + CPA	1.5	i.v.	1.5 (DOX) 15 (CPA)	46.0 ± 3.0	90.0 ± 30.0	1.9 ± 0.32	16.0 ± 4.8	43.0 ± 6.8

CPA: Cyclophosphamide.   DOX: Doxorubincin.   i.v.: Intravenous.   TAX: Paclitaxel.   [a] Significant difference compared to trastuzumab single-dose (P <0.050, ANOVA).

7   Clinical Efficacy and Safety

Overview Profile

❖ Trastuzumab is a humanized anti-HER2 monoclonal antibody that was the first launched by Genentech in 1998 as a lyophi-lized powder for intravenous administration in combination with paclitaxel in first-line treatment and as monotherapy in second- and third-line treatment of metastatic breast cancer overexpressing the HER2 protein.

❖ In 2006, the drug was approved and launched in the US and approved in the EU for adjuvant treatment of early-stage,

HER2-positive breast cancer.

❖ EU approvals have been granted for trastuzumab in combination with docetaxel (Taxotere®) and in combination with anastrozole (Arimide®) for the first-line therapy of postmenopausal women with advanced (metastatic) HER2-positive and hormone receptor-positive breast cancer.

❖ In 2010, trastuzumab in combination with chemotherapy was filed for approval in the EU and US by Roche for use in patients with HER2 positive metastatic gastric cancer.

❖ In 2011, Roche filed for the approval of trastuzumab in the EU as neoadjuvant treatment of breast cancer.

❖ In 2013, a subcutaneous injection formulated with Enhanze (TM) technology was approved in the EU for the treatment of HER2-positive early breast cancer.

❖ The clinical studies submitted to support the Biologics License Application (BLA) approval are listed as the following.

Table 17   Clinical Trials of Transtuzamab[13]

ID	Phase	N	Population	Design	Control	Treatment	Study Posology	Endpoint
Ho407g	1	16	Refractory cancer	Open	None	H	10/50/100/250/500 mg, single-dose	Safety, PK
Ho452g	1	17	Refractory cancer	Open	None	H	10/50/100/250/500 mg/w until PD	Safety, PK
Ho453g	1	15	Refractory cancer	Open	None	H + Cisplatin	10/50/100/250/500 mg/w + cisplatin until PD	Safety, PK
Ho551g	2	46	Refractory MBC	Open	None	H	250 mg LD 100 mg/w until PD	OR (REC/INV), DOR, TTP, survival
Ho552g	2	39	Refractory MBC	Open	None	H + Cisplatin	250 mg LD 100 mg/w + cisplatin until PD	OR (REC/INV), DOR, TTP
Ho648g	3 (pivotal)	469	MBC	Open, randomized, controlled	Chemo	H + Chemo	4mg/kg LD 2 mg/(kg·w) + chemo vs. chemo alone/w until PD	TTP (REC), OR, DOR, TTTF, 1-year survival, QOL
Ho649g	3	222	Refractory MBC	Open	None	H	4 mg/k LD 2 mg/(kg·w) at PD trastuzumab ± antitumor therapy	OR (REC), TTP, DOR, TTTF, survival, QOL
Ho650	NA	114	Previously untreated MBC	Open, randomized	None	H	4 mg/kg LD 2 mg/(kg·w) or 8 mg/kg LD 4 mg/(kg·w) until PD	OR (INV), DOR, TTP
M77001	2	186	Previously untreated MBC	Open-label, randomized	Docetaxel	H + Docetaxel	4 mg/k LD 2 mg/(kg·w) until PD	ORR, safety, TTP, PFS, TTF, TTR, DOR, OS
TAnDEM	3	207	Copositive MBC	Open-label randomized	Anastrozole	H + Anastrozole	4 mg/kg LD 2 mg/(kg·w) until PD	PFS, CBR, ORR, TTP, DOR, TTR, OS
BO16348	3	5,090	EBC	Open-label, randomized	None	H	6 mg/kg every 3 weeks	DFS, OS, RFS, DDFS
NSABP B-31a	3	2,130	EBC	Open-label, randomized	AC→P	AC→PH	4 mg/kg LD 2 mg/(kg·w) for 51 weeks	DFS, safety, OS
NCCTG N9831	3	3,505	EBC	Open-label, randomized	AC→P	AC→P→H AC→PH	4 mg/kg LD 2 mg/(kg·w) for 51 weeks	DFS, safety, OS
BCIRG 006	3	3,222	EBC	Open-label, randomized	AC→D	AC→DH DCarbH	4 mg/kg LD 2 mg/(kg·w), 6 mg/(kg·3w) for total 1 year.	DFS, OS, safety
MO16432	3	235	Locally advanced or inflammatory EBC	Open-label, randomized	Neoadjuvant chemo	H + Neoadjuvant chemo	8 mg/kg LD 6 mg/kg	EFS, pCR, ORR, OS, Safety
ToGA (BO18255)	3	594	Advanced gastric or gastro-oesophageal junction cancer	Open-label, randomized	Chemo	H + Chemo	8 mg/kg LD 6 mg/(kg·w) until PD	OS, PFS, TTP, ORR, DOR

AC: Anthracycline plus cyclophosphamide.   Carb: Carboplatin.   Chemo: Chemotherapy.   D: Docetaxel.   DDFS: Distant disease-free survival.   DFS: Disease-free survival.   DOR: Duration of response.   EBC: Early breast cancer.   EFS: Event-free survival.   H: Trastuzumab.   INV: Investigator response assessment.   LD: Loading dose (this is followed by a weekly maintenance dose).   MBC: Metastatic breast cancer.   NA: Not applicable/available.   OR: Overall response.   OS: Overall survival. P: Paclitaxel.   pCR: Pathological complete response.   PD: Progressive disease.   PK: Pharmacokinetics.   q1w: Weekly.   q3w: 3-weekly.   QOL: Quality of life.   REC: Response evaluation committee.   RFS: Recurrence-free survival.   TTP: Time to progression.   TTF: Time to treatment failure.

Indications 1: Metastatic Breast Cancer

Clinical Efficacy[12-14]

❖ Herceptin® is indicated for the treatment of patients with HER2 positive metastatic breast cancer.

❖ As monotherapy for the treatment of those patients who have received at least two chemotherapy regimens for their metastatic disease.   Prior chemotherapy must have included at least an anthracycline and a taxane unless patients are unsuitable for these treatments.   Hormone receptor positive patients must also have failed hormonal therapy, unless patients are unsuitable for these treatments.

❖ Study III HO649g, a non-comparative, open-label Phase 3 study, was designed to evaluate the response in patients with metastatic breast cancer overexpressing HER2, who had relapsed after one or two cytotoxic chemotherapy regimens and were then treated with Herceptin® as a single agent, in second or third line therapy.   The primary objectives of this trial were to determine the overall objective response rate to rhuMAb HER2 treatment as a single agent and to further characterize the safety profile of rhuMAb HER2.   The results of efficacy are summarized in Table 18.

❖ In combination with paclitaxel for the treatment of those patients who have not received chemotherapy for their metastatic disease and for whom an anthracycline is not suitable.

❖ The pivotal study HO648g was a phase 3 trial in which women with cancers that overexpressed HER2 who had not previously received chemotherapy for metastatic disease were randomly assigned to receive either chemotherapy alone or chemotherapy plus trastuzumab.   The chemotherapy regimen for both treatment groups was either anthracycline + cyclophosphamide (AC) or paclitaxel.   Patients who had not received anthracycline therapy in the adjuvant setting were stratified to receive AC.   Patients who had received any anthracycline therapy in the adjuvant setting were stratified to receive paclitaxel.   The primary endpoints of the study were the time to disease progression and the incidence of adverse effects.   Secondary endpoints were the rates and the duration of responses, the time to treatment failure, and overall survival.   The results of efficacy are summarized in Table 18.

❖ In combination with docetaxel for the treatment of those patients who have not received chemotherapy for their metastatic disease.

❖ M77001 is an open-label, comparative, randomized, multicenter, multinational trial comparing the efficacy and safety of first-line trastuzumab plus docetaxel with docetaxel alone in patients with HER2-positive MBC.   The results of efficacy are summarized in Table 18.

Table 18   Efficacy Results from the Monotherapy and Combination Therapy Studies[12]

Parameter	Monotherapy	Combination Therapy			
	TTZ[a] (N = 172)	TTZ + PTX[b] (N = 68)	PTX[b] (N = 77)	TTZ + DTX[c] (N = 92)	DTX[c] (N = 94)
Response rate	18.0%	49.0%	17.0%	61.0%	34.0%
95% CI	(13.0-25.0)	(36.0-61.0)	(9.0-27.0)	(50.0-71.0)	(25.0-45.0)
Median duration of response (Month, range)	9.1 (5.6-10.3)	8.3 (7.3-8.8)	4.6 (3.7-7.4)	11.7 (9.3-15.0)	5.7 (4.6-7.6)
Median TTP (Month)	3.2	7.1	3.0	11.7	6.1
95% CI	(2.6-3.5)	(6.2-12.0)	(2.0-4.4)	(9.2-13.5)	(5.4-7.2)
Median survival (Month)	16.4	24.8	17.9	31.2	22.7
95% CI	(12.3-NE)	(18.6-33.7)	(11.2-23.8)	(27.3-40.8)	(19.1-30.8)

"NE" indicates that it could not be estimated or it was not yet reached.   DTX: Docetaxel.   PTX: Paclitaxel.   TTP: Time to progression.   TTZ: Trastuzumab.
[a] Study H0649g: IHC3+ patient subset.   [b] Study H0648g: IHC3+ patient subset.   [c] Study M77001: Full analysis set (intent-to-treat), 24 months results.

❖ In combination with an aromatase inhibitor for the treatment of postmenopausal patients with hormone-receptor positive metastatic breast cancer, not previously treated with trastuzumab.

❖ TAnDEM is the first randomized Phase 3 study to combine a hormonal agent and trastuzumab without chemotherapy as treatment for human epidermal growth factor receptor 2 (HER2)/hormone receptor-copositive metastatic breast cancer (MBC).

❖ Progression-free survival was doubled in the Herceptin® plus anastrozole arm compared to anastrozole (4.8 months vs. 2.4 months).   For the other parameters the improvements seen for the combination were for overall response (16.5% vs. 6.7%); clinical benefit rate (42.7% vs. 27.9%); time to progression (4.8 months vs. 2.4 months).   For time to response and duration of response no difference could be recorded between the arms.   The median overall survival was extended by 4.6 months for patients in the combination arm.   The difference was not statistically significant, however more than half of the patients in the anastrozole alone arm crossed over to a Herceptin® containing regimen after progression of disease.

Indications 2: Early Breast Cancer

Clinical Efficacy[12, 15, 16]

❖ Herceptin® is indicated for the treatment of adult patients with HER2 positive early breast cancer (EBC).

❖ Following surgery, chemotherapy (neoadjuvant or adjuvant) and radiotherapy (if applicable):
   • Study BO16348 was an international, multicenter, randomized trial comparing one or two years of trastuzumab given every three weeks with observation in patients with HER2-positive and either node-negative or node-positive breast cancer who had completed locoregional therapy and at least four cycles of neoadjuvant or adjuvant chemotherapy. The efficacy results from the BO16348 trial following 12 months[a] and 8 years[b] median follow-up are summarized in Table 19.

Table 19   Efficacy Results from Study BO16348[12]

Parameter	Median Follow-up 12 Months[a]		Median Follow-up 8 Years[b]	
	Observation (N = 1,693)	Trastuzumab 1 Year (N = 1,693)	Observation (N = 1,697)[c]	Trastuzumab 1 Year (N = 1,702)[c]
Disease-free Survival				
No. patients with event	219 (12.9%)	127 (7.5%)	570 (33.6%)	471 (27.7%)
No. patients without event	1,474 (87.1%)	1,566 (92.5%)	1,127 (66.4%)	1,231 (72.3%)
P-value vs. observation	<0.00010		<0.00010	
Hazard ratio vs. observation	0.54		0.76	
Recurrence-free Survival				
No. patients with event	208 (12.3%)	113 (6.7%)	506 (29.8%)	399 (23.4%)
No. patients without event	1,485 (87.7%)	1,580 (93.3%)	1,191 (70.2%)	1,303 (76.6%)
P-value vs. observation	<0.00010		<0.00010	
Hazard ratio vs. observation	0.51		0.73	
Distant Disease-free Survival				
No. patients with event	184 (10.9%)	99 (5.8%)	488 (28.8%)	399 (23.4%)
No. patients without event	1,508 (89.1%)	1,594 (94.6%)	1,209 (71.2%)	1,303 (76.6%)
P-value vs. observation	<0.00010		<0.00010	
Hazard ratio vs. observation	0.50		0.76	
Overall Survival (Death)				
No. patients with event	40 (2.4%)	31 (1.8%)	350 (20.6%)	278 (16.3%)
No. patients without event	1,653 (97.6%)	1,662 (98.2%)	1,347 (79.4%)	1,424 (83.7%)
P-value vs. observation	0.24		0.00050	
Hazard ratio vs. observation	0.75		0.76	

[a] Co-primary endpoint of DFS of 1-year vs. observation met the pre-defined statistical boundary.   [b] Final analysis (including crossover of 52.0% of patients from the observation arm to Herceptin®).   [c] There is a discrepancy in the overall sample size due to a small number of patients who were randomized after the cut-off date for the 12-month median follow-up analysis.

❖ Following adjuvant chemotherapy with doxorubicin and cyclophosphamide, in combination with paclitaxel or docetaxel. NSABP B-31 was a randomized trial comparing the safety and efficacy of adriamycin and cyclophosphamide followed by Taxol® (Ac→T) to that of adriamycin and cyclophosphamide followed by Taxol® plus Herceptin® (Ac→T + H) in node-positive breast cancer patients who have tumors that overexpress HER2.[12]

❖ NCCTG N9831 was a phase 3 trial of doxorubicin and cyclophosphamide (AC) followed by weekly paclitaxel with or without trastuzumab as adjuvant treatment for women with HER2 overexpressing or amplified node positive or high-risk node negative breast cancer.[17]

❖ The efficacy results from the joint analysis of the NSABP B-31 and NCCTG 9831 trials at the time of the definitive analysis of DFS[a] are summarized in Table 20. The median duration of follow up was 1.8 years for the patients in the AC→P arm and 2.0 years for patients in the AC→PH arm. The final OS results from the joint analysis of studies NSABP B-31 and NCCTG N9831 are summarized in Table 20.[12]

Table 20   Summary of Efficacy Results from the Joint Analysis Studies NSABP B-31 and NCCTG N9831 at the Time of the Definitive DFS Analysis[a, 12]

Parameter	AC→P (N = 1,679)	AC→PH (N = 1,672)	Hazard Ratio vs. AC→P (95% CI) P-value
Disease-free Survival			
No. patients with event (%)	261 (15.5)	133 (8.0)	0.48 (0.39, 0.59) P <0.00010
Distant Recurrence			
No. patients with event	193 (11.5)	96 (5.7)	0.47 (0.37, 0.60) P <0.00010
Death (OS Event)			
No. patients with event	92 (5.5)	62 (3.7)	0.67 (0.48, 0.92) P = 0.014[b]

A: Doxorubicin.   C: Cyclophosphamide.   *CI*: Confidence interval.   H: Trastuzumab.   P: Paclitaxel.   [a] At median duration of follow up of 1.8 years for the patients in the AC→P arm and 2.0 years for patients in the AC→PH arm.   [b] P-value for OS did not cross the pre-specified statistical boundary for comparison of AC→PH vs. AC→P.

Table 21   Final Overall Survival Analysis from the Joint Analysis of Trials NSABP B-31 and NCCTG N9831[12]

Parameter	AC→P (N = 2,032)	AC→PH (N = 2,031)	P-value vs. AC→P	Hazard Ratio vs. AC→P (95% CI)
Death (OS event)	418	289		
No. patients with event (%)	20.6%	14.2%	<0.00010	0.64 (0.55, 0.74)

A: Doxorubicin.   C: Cyclophosphamide.   *CI*: Confidence interval.   H: Trastuzumab.   P: Paclitaxel.

❖ In combination with adjuvant chemotherapy consisting of docetaxel and carboplatin:
  • The BCIRG 006 was a randomized multicenter Phase 3 randomized trial conducted by the Breast Cancer International Research Group (CIRG), comparing doxorubicin and cyclophosphamide followed by docetaxel (ACide-follodoxo rubicin and cyclophosphamide and trastuzumab (Herceptin®) (ACzumab (Herceptdocetaxel, carboplatin, and trastuzumab (DCarbH) in the adjuvant treatment of node-positive and high-risk node-negative patients with operable breast cancer.[17]
  • The efficacy results from the BCIRG 006 are summarized in Tables 22 and 23.   The median duration of follow up was 2.9 years in the AC→D arm and 3.0 years in each of the AC→DH and DCarbH arms.[17]

Table 22   Overview of Efficacy Analyses BCIRG 006 AC→D versus AC→DH[12]

Parameter	AC→D (N = 1,073)	AC→DH (N = 1,074)	Hazard Ratio vs. AC→D (95% CI) P-value
Disease-free Survival			
No. patients with event	195	134	0.61 (0.49, 0.77) P <0.00010
Distant Recurrence			
No. patients with event	144	95	0.59 (0.46, 0.77) P <0.00010
Death (OS Event)			
No. patients with event	80	49	0.58 (0.40, 0.83) P = 0.0024

AC→D: Doxorubicin plus cyclophosphamide, followed by docetaxel.   AC→DH: Doxorubicin plus cyclophosphamide, followed by docetaxel plus trastuzumab.
CI: Confidence interval.

Table 23   Overview of Efficacy Analyses BCIRG 006 AC→D vs. DCarbH[12]

Parameter	AC→D (N = 1,073)	DCarbH (N = 1,074)	Hazard Ratio vs. AC→D (95% CI)
Disease-free Survival			
No. patients with event	195	145	0.67 (0.54, 0.83) P = 0.00030
Distant Recurrence			
No. patients with event	144	103	0.65 (0.50, 0.84) P = 0.00080
Death (OS Event)			
No. patients with event	80	56	0.66 (0.47, 0.93) P = 0.018

AC→D: Doxorubicin plus cyclophosphamide, followed by docetaxel.   CI: Confidence interval.   DCarbH: Docetaxel, carboplatin and trastuzumab.

❖ In combination with neoadjuvant chemotherapy followed by adjuvant Herceptin® therapy, for locally advanced (including inflammatory) disease or tumors >2 cm in diameter.[12]

❖ Clinical Study MO16432 was an international, open-label, Phase 3 trial in women with newly diagnosed locally advanced breast cancer (LABC) or inflammatory breast cancer (IBC).   Patients with HER2-positive disease (immuno histochemistry [IHC]3+ and/or HER2 amplification) were randomized to receive neoadjuvant trastuzumab plus neoadjuvant chemotherapy followed by adjuvant trastuzumab (HER2+ TC group), or neoadjuvant chemotherapy alone (HER2+ C group).   The efficacy results from Study MO16432 are summarized in Table 24.   The median duration of follow-up in the Herceptin® arm was 3.8 years.[18]

Table 24   Efficacy Results from MO16432[12]

Parameter	Chemo + Trastuzumab (N = 115)	Chemo only (N = 116)	Hazard Ratio (95% CI) P-value
Event-free Survival			
No. patients with event	46	59	0.65 (0.44, 0.96) P = 0.028
Total pathological complete response[a] (95% CI)	40.0% (31.0, 49.6)	20.7% (13.7, 29.2)	P = 0.0014
Overall Survival			
No. patients with event	22	33	0.59 (0.35, 1.0) P = 0.056

Chemo: Chemotherapy.   [a] Defined as absence of any invasive cancer both in the breast and axillary nodes.

Indications 3: Metastatic Gastric Cancer

Clinical Efficacy[10, 11]

❖ Herceptin® in combination with capecitabine or 5-fluorouracil and cisplatin is indicated for the treatment of adult patients with HER2 positive metastatic adenocarcinoma of the stomach or gastroesophageal junction who have not received prior anti-cancer treatment for their metastatic disease.[12]

❖ The ToGA trial (BO18255) is a randomized, open-label multicenter Phase 3 study of trastuzumab in combination with a fluoropyrimidine and cisplatin vs. chemotherapy alone as first-line therapy in patients with HER2 positive advanced gastric cancer.   The efficacy results from study BO18225 are summarized in Table 25.[19]

Table 25　Efficacy Results from BO18225[12]

Parameter	FP (N = 290)	FP + H (N = 294)	HR (95% CI)	P-value
Overall survival, median (Month)	11.1	13.8	0.74 (0.60-0.91)	0.0046
Progression-free survival, median (Month)	5.5	6.7	0.71 (0.59-0.85)	0.00020
Time to disease progression, median (Month)	5.6	7.1	0.70 (0.58-0.85)	0.00030
Overall response rate,%	34.5	47.3	1.7[a] (1.2, 2.4)	0.0017
Duration of response, median (Month)	4.8	6.9	0.54 (0.40-0.73)	<0.00010

FP: Fluoropyrimidine/cisplatin.　FP + H: Fluoropyrimidine/cisplatin + Herceptin®.　[a] Odds ratio.

Clinical Safety[12]

❖ The most common adverse reactions in patients receiving Herceptin® in the adjuvant and metastatic breast cancer setting are fever, nausea, vomiting, infusion reactions, diarrhea, infections, increased cough, headache, fatigue, dyspnea, rash, neutropenia, anemia, and myalgia.

❖ Adverse reactions requiring interruption or discontinuation of Herceptin® treatment include CHF, significant decline in left ventricular cardiac function, severe infusion reactions, and pulmonary toxicity.

❖ In metastatic gastric cancer setting, the most common adverse reactions (≥10.0%) that were increased (≥5.0% difference) in the Herceptin® arm as compared to the chemotherapy alone arm were neutropenia, diarrhea, fatigue, anemia, stomatitis, weight loss, upper respiratory tract infections, fever, thrombocytopenia, mucosal inflammation, nasopharyngitis, and dysgeusia.

❖ The most common adverse reactions which resulted in discontinuation of treatment on the Herceptin® containing arm in the absence of disease progression were infection, diarrhea, and febrile neutropenia.

Indications 1: Metastatic Breast Cancer

❖ The data below reflect exposure to Herceptin® in one randomized, open-label study, study Ho648g, of chemotherapy with (N = 235) or without (N = 234) trastuzumab in patients with metastatic breast cancer, and one single-arm study (Study Ho649g; N = 222) in patients with metastatic breast cancer.　Data in Table 27 are based on studies Ho648g and Ho649g.

Table 26　Per-patient Incidence of Adverse Reactions Occurring in ≥5.0% of Patients in Uncontrolled Studies or at Increased Incidence in the Trastuzumab Arm (Studies Ho648g and Ho649g)[12]

	Single Agent[a] (N = 352)	TTZ + PTX (N = 91)	PTX Alone (N = 95)	TTZ + AC[b] (N = 143)	AC[b] Alone (N = 135)
Body as a Whole					
Pain	47.0%	61.0%	62.0%	57.0%	42.0%
Asthenia	42.0%	62.0%	57.0%	54.0%	55.0%
Fever	36.0%	49.0%	23.0%	56.0%	34.0%
Chills	32.0%	41.0%	4.0%	35.0%	11.0%
Headache	26.0%	36.0%	28.0%	44.0%	31.0%
Abdominal pain	22.0%	34.0%	22.0%	23.0%	18.0%
Back pain	22.0%	34.0%	30.0%	27.0%	15.0%
Infection	20.0%	47.0%	27.0%	47.0%	31.0%
Flu syndrome	10.0%	12.0%	5.0%	12.0%	6.0%
Accidental injury	6.0%	13.0%	3.0%	9.0%	4.0%
Allergic reaction	3.0%	8.0%	2.0%	4.0%	2.0%
Cardiovascular					
Tachycardia	5.0%	12.0%	4.0%	10.0%	5.0%
Congestive heart failure	7.0%	11.0%	1.0%	28.0%	7.0%
Digestive					

Continued

	Single Agent[a] (N = 352)	TTZ + PTX (N = 91)	PTX Alone (N = 95)	TTZ + AC[b] (N = 143)	AC[b] Alone (N = 135)
Nausea	33.0%	51.0%	9.0%	76.0%	77.0%
Diarrhea	25.0%	45.0%	29.0%	45.0%	26.0%
Vomiting	23.0%	37.0%	28.0%	45.0%	26.0%
Nausea and vomiting	8.0%	14.0%	11.0%	18.0%	9.0%
Anorexia	14.0%	24.0%	16.0%	31.0%	26.0%
Heme & Lymphatic					
Anemia	4.0%	14.0%	9.0%	36.0%	26.0%
Leukopenia	3.0%	24.0%	17.0%	52.0%	34.0%
Metabolic					
Peripheral edema	10.0%	22.0%	20.0%	20.0%	17.0%
Edema	8.0%	10.0%	8.0%	11.0%	5.0%
Musculoskeletal					
Bone pain	7.0%	24.0%	18.0%	7.0%	7.0%
Arthralgia	6.0%	37.0%	21.0%	8.0%	9.0%
Nervous					
Insomnia	14.0%	25.0%	13.0%	29.0%	15.0%
Dizziness	13.0%	22.0%	24.0%	24.0%	18.0%
Paresthesia	9.0%	48.0%	39.0%	17.0%	11.0%
Depression	6.0%	12.0%	13.0%	20.0%	12.0%
Peripheral neuritis	2.0%	23.0%	16.0%	2.0%	2.0%
Neuropathy	1.0%	13.0%	5.0%	4.0%	4.0%
Respiratory					
Cough increased	26.0%	41.0%	22.0%	43.0%	29.0%
Dyspnea	22.0%	27.0%	26.0%	42.0%	25.0%
Rhinitis	14.0%	22.0%	5.0%	22.0%	16.0%
Pharyngitis	12.0%	22.0%	14.0%	30.0%	18.0%
Sinusitis	9.0%	21.0%	7.0%	13.0%	6.0%
Skin					
Rash	18.0%	38.0%	18.0%	27.0%	17.0%
Herpes simplex	2.0%	12.0%	3.0%	7.0%	9.0%
Acne	2.0%	11.0%	3.0%	3.0%	<1.0%
Urogenital					
Urinary tract infection	5.0%	18.0%	14.0%	13.0%	7.0%

AC: Anthracycline. PTX: Paclitaxel. TTZ: Trastuzumab. [a] Data for Herceptin® single agent were from 4 studies, including 213 patients from study Ho649g.
[b] Anthracycline (doxorubicin or epirubicin) and cyclophosphamide.

Indications 3: Metastatic Gastric Cancer

❖ The data below are based on the exposure of 294 patients to Herceptin® in combination with a fluoropyrimidine (capecitabine or 5-FU) and cisplatin (Study BO18255).[12]

Table 27   Study BO29 255: Per-patient Incidence of Adverse Reactions of All Grades (Incidence ≥5.0% between Arms) or Grade 3/4 (Incidence >1.0% between Arms) and Higher Incidence in Trastuzumab Arm[20]

	Trastuzumab + Chemotherapy (N = 294)		Chemotherapy Alone (N = 290)	
	All Grades	Grade 3 or 4	All Grades	Grade 3 or 4
Any Adverse Event	292 (99.0%)	201 (68.0%)	284 (98.0%)	198 (68.0%)
Gastrointestinal Disorders				
Nausea	197 (67.0%)	22 (7.0%)	184 (63.0%)	21 (7.0%)
Vomiting	147 (50.0%)	18 (6.0%)	134 (46.0%)	22 (8.0%)
Diarrhoea	109 (37.0%)	27 (9.0%)	80 (28.0%)	11 (4.0%)
Constipation	75 (26.0%)	2 (1.0%)	93 (32.0%)	5 (2.0%)
Stomatitis	72 (24.0%)	2 (1.0%)	43 (15.0%)	6 (2.0%)
Abdominal pain	66 (22.0%)	7 (2.0%)	56 (19.0%)	5 (2.0%)
Dysphagia	19 (6.0%)	7 (2.0%)	10 (3.0%)	1 (<1.0%)
Blood and Lymphatic System Disorders				
Neutropenia	157 (53.0%)	79 (27.0%)	165 (57.0%)	88 (30.0%)
Anaemia	81 (28.0%)	36 (12.0%)	61 (21.0%)	30 (10.0%)
Thrombocytopenia	47 (16.0%)	14 (5.0%)	33 (11.0%)	8 (3.0%)
Febrile neutropenia	15 (5.0%)	15 (5.0%)	8 (3.0%)	8 (3.0%)
Nausea	197 (67.0%)	22 (7.0%)	184 (63.0%)	21 (7.0%)
General, Metabolic, and Other Disorders				
Anorexia	135 (46.0%)	19 (6.0%)	133 (46.0%)	18 (6.0%)
Fatigue	102 (35.0%)	12 (4.0%)	82 (28.0%)	7 (2.0%)
Hand-foot syndrome	75 (26.0%)	4 (1.0%)	64 (22.0%)	5 (2.0%)
Weight decreased	69 (23.0%)	6 (2.0%)	40 (14.0%)	7 (2.0%)
Asthenia	55 (19.0%)	14 (5.0%)	53 (18.0%)	10 (3.0%)
Pyrexia	54 (18.0%)	3 (1.0%)	36 (12.0%)	0
Renal impairment	47 (16.0%)	2 (1.0%)	39 (13.0%)	3 (1.0%)
Mucosal inflammation	37 (13.0%)	6 (2.0%)	18 (6.0%)	2 (1.0%)
Nasopharyngitis	37 (13.0%)	0	17 (6.0%)	0
Chills	23 (8.0%)	1 (<1.0%)	0	0
Hypokalaemia	22 (7.0%)	13 (4.0%)	13 (4.0%)	7 (2.0%)
Dehydration	18 (6.0%)	7 (2.0%)	16 (6.0%)	5 (2.0%)
Dyspnoea	9 (3.0%)	1 (<1.0%)	16 (6.0%)	5 (2.0%)

Indications 4: Adjuvant Breast Cancer

❖ The data below reflect exposure to one-year Herceptin® therapy across three randomized, open-label studies, Studies NSABP B-31, NCCTG N9831, and BO16348, with (N = 3,678) or without (N = 3,363) trastuzumab in the adjuvant treatment of breast cancer.   The data summarized in Table 26 below, from Study BO16348, reflect exposure to Herceptin® in 1,678 patients; the median treatment duration was 51 weeks and median number of infusions was 18.

Table 28   Adverse Reactions for Study BO16348[a], All Grades[b, 7]

Adverse Reaction	One-year Trastuzumab (N = 1,678) n (%)	Observation (N = 1,708) n (%)
Cardiac		
Hypertension	64 (4.0)	35 (2.0)
Dizziness	60 (4.0)	29 (2.0)
Ejection fraction decreased	58 (3.5)	11 (0.60)
Palpitations	48 (3.0)	12 (0.70)
Cardiac arrhythmias[c]	40 (3.0)	17 (1.0)
Cardiac failure congestive	30 (2.0)	5 (0.30)
Cardiac failure	9 (0.50)	4 (0.20)
Cardiac disorder	5 (0.30)	0 (0.0)
Ventricular dysfunction	4 (0.20)	0 (0.0)
Respiratory Thoracic Mediastinal Disorders		
Cough	81 (5.0)	34 (2.0)
Influenza	70 (4.0)	9 (0.50)
Dyspnea	57 (3.0)	26 (2.0)
URI	46 (3.0)	20 (1.0)
Rhinitis	36 (2.0)	6 (0.40)
Pharyngolaryngeal pain	32 (2.0)	8 (0.50)
Sinusitis	26 (2.0)	5 (0.30)
Epistaxis	25 (2.0)	1 (0.060)
Pulmonary hypertension	4 (0.20)	0 (0.0)
Interstitial pneumonitis	4 (0.20)	0 (0.0)
Gastrointestinal Disorders		
Diarrhea	123 (7.0)	16 (1.0)
Nausea	108 (6.0)	19 (1.0)
Vomiting	58 (3.5)	10 (0.60)
Constipation	33 (2.0)	17 (1.0)
Dyspepsia	30 (2.0)	9 (0.50)
Upper Abdominal Pain	29 (2.0)	15 (1.0)
Musculoskeletal & Connective Tissue Disorders		
Arthralgia	137 (8.0)	98 (6.0)
Back Pain	91 (5.0)	58 (3.0)
Myalgia	63 (4.0)	17 (1.0)
Bone pain	49 (3.0)	26 (2.0)
Muscle spasm	46 (3.0)	3 (0.20)
Nervous System Disorders		
Headache	162 (10.0)	49 (3.0)
Paraesthesia	29 (2.0)	11 (0.60)
Skin & Subcutaneous Tissue Disorders		
Rash	70 (4.0)	10 (0.60)
Nail disorders	43 (2.0)	0 (0.0)
Pruritus	40 (2.0)	10 (0.60)
General Disorders		

Continued

Adverse Reaction	One-year Trastuzumab (N = 1,678) n (%)	Observation (N = 1,708) n (%)
Pyrexia	100 (6.0)	6 (0.40)
Edema peripheral	79 (5.0)	37 (2.0)
Chills	85 (5.0)	0 (0.0)
Asthenia	75 (4.5)	30 (2.0)
Influenza-like illness	40 (2.0)	3 (0.20)
Sudden death	1 (0.060)	0 (0.0)
Infections		
Nasopharyngitis	135 (8.0)	43 (3.0)
UTI	39 (3.0)	13 (0.80)
Immune System Disorders		
Hypersensitivity	10 (0.60)	1 (0.060)
Autoimmune thyroiditis	4 (0.30)	0 (0.0)

[a] Median follow-up duration of 12.6 months in the one-year Herceptin® treatment arm. [b] The incidence of Grade 3 or higher adverse reactions was <1.0% in both arms for each listed term. [c] Higher level grouping term.

8 Clinical Pharmacokinetics

Summary

Population Pharmacokinetic[7, 12]

❖ The pharmacokinetics of trastuzumab was evaluated in a pooled population pharmacokinetic (PK) model analysis of 1,582 subjects with primarily breast cancer and metastatic gastric cancer (MGC) receiving intravenous trastuzumab.

❖ Total trastuzumab clearance increases with decreasing concentrations due to parallel linear and non-linear elimination pathways.

❖ Linear clearance was 0.14 L/day for MBC, 0.11 L/day for EBC and 0.18 L/day for AGC.

❖ The non-linear elimination parameter values were 8.8 mg/day for the maximum elimination rate (V_{max}) and 8.9 µg/mL for the Michaelis-Menten constant (K_m) for the MBC, EBC, and AGC patients.

❖ The central compartment volume was 2.6 L for patients with MBC and EBC and 3.6 L for patients with AGC.

❖ In the final population PK model, in addition to primary tumor type, body-weight, serum aspartate aminotransferase and albumin were identified as a statistically significant covariates affecting the exposure of trastuzumab. However, the magnitude of effect of these covariates on trastuzumab exposure suggests that these covariates are unlikely to have a clinically meaningful effect on trastuzumab concentrations.

❖ The population predicted PK exposure values (median with 5th-95th percentiles) and PK parameter values at clinically relevant concentrations (C_{max} and C_{min}) for MBC, EBC and AGC patients treated with the approved q1w and q3w dosing regimens are shown in Table 29 (Cycle 1), Table 30 (steady-state), and Table 31 (PK parameters).

Table 29　Population Predicted Cycle 1 PK Exposure Values (Median with 5th-95th Percentiles) for Trastuzumab i.v. Dosing Regimens in MBC, EBC and AGC Patients[12]

Regimen	Primary Tumor Type	N	C_{min} (µg/mL)	C_{max} (µg/mL)	$AUC_{0-21 days}$ (µg·day/mL)
8 mg/kg + 6 mg/kg q3w	MBC	805	28.7 (2.9-46.3)	182 (134-280)	1,376 (728-1,998)
	EBC	390	30.9 (18.7-45.5)	176 (127-227)	1,390 (1,039-1,895)
	AGC	274	23.1 (6.1-50.3)	132 (84.2-225)	1,109 (588-1,938)
4 mg/kg + 2 mg/kg qw	MBC	805	37.4 (8.7-58.9)	76.5 (49.4-114)	1,073 (597-1,584)
	EBC	390	38.9 (25.3-58.8)	76.0 (54.7-104)	1,074 (783-1,502)

AGC: Advanced gastric cancer.　EBC: Early breast cancer.　MBC: Metastatic breast cancer.

Table 30   Population Predicted Steady-state PK Exposure Values (Median with 5th-95th Percentiles) for
Trastuzumab i.v. Dosing Regimens in MBC, EBC and AGC Patients[12]

Regimen	Primary Tumor Type	N	$C_{min, ss}^{a}$ (µg/mL)	$C_{max, ss}^{b}$ (µg/mL)	$AUC_{ss, 0-21 days}$ (µg·day/mL)	Time to Steady-state^{c} (Week)
8 mg/kg + 6 mg/kg q3w	MBC	805	44.2 (1.8-85.4)	179 (123-266)	1,736 (618-2,756)	12
	EBC	390	53.8 (28.7-85.8)	184 (134-247)	1,927 (1,332-2,771)	15
	AGC	274	32.9 (6.1-88.9)	131 (72.5-251)	1,338 (557-2,875)	9
4 mg/kg + 2 mg/kg qw	MBC	805	63.1 (11.7-107)	107 (54.2-164)	1,710 (581-2,715)	12
	EBC	390	72.6 (46.0-109)	115 (82.6-160)	1,893 (1,309-2,734)	14

AGC: Advanced gastric cancer.   EBC: Early breast cancer.   MBC: Metastatic breast cancer. $^{a}C_{min, ss}$: C_{min} at steady-state. $^{b}C_{max, ss}$: C_{max} at steady-state. ^{c} Time to 90.0% of steady-state.

Table 31   Population Predicted PK Parameter Values at Steady-state for Trastuzumab i.v. Dosing
Regimens in MBC, EBC and AGC Patients[12]

Regimen	Primary Tumor Type	N	Total CL Range from $C_{max, ss}$ to $C_{min, ss}$ (L/Day)	$t_{1/2}$ Range from $C_{max, ss}$ to $C_{min, ss}$ (Day)
8 mg/kg + 6 mg/kg q3w	MBC	805	0.18-0.30	15.1-23.3
	EBC	390	0.16-0.25	17.5-26.6
	AGC	274	0.19-0.34	12.6-20.6
4 mg/kg + 2 mg/kg qw	MBC	805	0.21-0.26	17.2-20.4
	EBC	390	0.18-0.22	19.7-23.2

AGC: Advanced gastric cancer.   EBC: Early breast cancer.   MBC: Metastatic breast cancer.

Immunogenicity[12]

❖ In the neoadjuvant-adjuvant EBC treatment setting, 8.1% (24/296) of patients treated with trastuzumab intravenous developed antibodies against trastuzumab (regardless of antibody presence at baseline).   Neutralizing anti-trastuzumab antibodies were detected in post-baseline samples in 2 of 24 trastuzumab intravenous patients.

❖ The clinical relevance of these antibodies is not known; nevertheless the pharmacokinetics, efficacy (determined by pathological complete response [pCR]) and safety determined by occurrence of administration related reactions (ARRs) of trastuzumab intravenous did not appear to be adversely affected by these antibodies.

❖ There are no immunogenicity data available for trastuzumab in gastric cancer.

Drug-Drug Interaction (DDI) Potential[12]

❖ No formal clinical drug-drug interaction studies have been performed.   Clinically significant interactions between Herceptin® and the concomitant medicinal products used in clinical trials have not been observed.

9   Patent

❖ Trastuzumab was approved by the U.S. Food and Drug Administration (FDA) on Sep 1998.   It was developed and marketed as Herceptin® by Genentech Inc., a subsidiary of Roche.

Summary

❖ The patent applications (WO8906692A1 and WO9222653A1) related to the monoclonal antibody specifically binding the extracellular domain of the HER2 receptor (i.e. Trastuzumab) were filed by Genentech in 1989 and 1992.   Accordingly, its PCT counterpart has, among the others, been granted by USPTO (US5821337A, US6407213B1 and US6719971B1), JPO (JP3040121B2 and JP4836147B2), respectively.

Table 32　Originator's Key Patents of Trastuzumab in Main Countries and/or Region

Country/Region	Publication/Patent No.	Application Date	Granted Date	Estimated Expiry Date
WO	WO8906692A1	01/05/1989	/	/
JP	JP3040121B2	01/05/1989	03/03/2000	01/05/2009
WO	WO9222653A1	06/15/1992	/	/
US	US5821337A	06/15/1992	10/13/1998	08/21/2012
	US6407213B1	06/15/1992	06/18/2002	06/30/2020
	US6719971B1	06/15/1992	04/13/2004	05/14/2012
JP	JP4836147B2	06/15/1992	12/14/2011	06/18/2028

Table 33　Originator's International Patent Protection of Use and/or Method of Trastuzumab

APublication No.	Title	Publication Date
Technical Subjects	TREATMENT METHOD	
WO0069460A1	Treatment with anti-ErbB2 antibodies	11/23/2000
WO0115730A1	Dosages for treatment with anti-ErbB2 antibodies	03/08/2001
WO2004048525A2	Therapy of non-malignant diseases or disorders with anti-ErbB2 antibodies	06/10/2004
Technical Subjects	DIAGNOSTIC METHOD	
WO0189566A1	Gene detection assay for improving the likelihood of an effective response to an ErbB antagonist cancer therapy	11/29/2001
WO2007019899A2	Method for predicting the response to a treatment with a HER dimerization inhibitor	02/22/2007
WO2008109440A2	Predicting response to a HER inhibitor based on low HER3 expression	09/12/2008
WO2008154249A2	Gene expression markers of tumor resistance to HER2 inhibitor treatment	12/18/2008
WO2011012280A1	A set of oligonucleotide probes as well as methods and uses related thereto	02/03/2011
WO2011146568A1	Predicting response to a HER dimerization inhibitor	11/24/2011
WO2013083810A1	Identification of non-responders to HER2 inhibitors	06/13/2013
Technical Subjects	COMBINATION METHOD	
WO9931140A1	Treatment with anti-ErbB2 antibodies	06/24/1999
WO2006063707A2	Novel pharmaceutical composition containing at least one dolastatin 10 derivative	06/22/2006
WO2006086730A2	Inhibiting HER2 shedding with matrix metalloprotease antagonists	08/17/2006
WO2007013950A2	Combination therapy of HER expressing tumors	02/01/2007
WO2007107329A1	Tumor therapy with an antibody for vascular endothelial growth factor and an antibody for human epithelial growth factor receptor type 2	09/27/2007
WO2017102789A1	Combination therapy of anti-HER3 antibodies and anti-HER2 antibodies	06/22/2017
Technical Subjects	PREPARATION	
WO2006044908A2	Reducing protein a leaching during protein an affinity chromatography	02/24/2005
Technical Subjects	FORMULATION	
WO03062375A2	Stabilizing polypeptides which have been exposed to urea	07/31/2003
WO2006044908A2	Antibody formulations	04/27/2006
WO2011012637A2	Subcutaneous anti-HER2 antibody formulation	02/03/2011

The data was updated until Jan 2018.

10 Reference

[1] Karunagaran D, Tzahar E, Beerli R R, et al. ErbB-2 is a common auxiliary subunit of NDF and EGF receptors: implications for breast cancer [J]. EMBO Journal, 1996, 15(2): 254-264.

[2] U. S. Food and Drug Administration (FDA) Database. http://www.accessdata.fda.gov/drugsatfda_docs/nda/2013/125427Orig1s000PharmR.pdf.

[3] Gunning P W, Ghoshdastider U, Whitaker S, et al. The evolution of compositionally and functionally distinct actin filaments [J]. Journal of Cell Science, 2015, 128(11): 2009-2019.

[4] Barisic M, Maiato H. The Tubulin Code: a navigation system for chromosomes during mitosis [J]. Trends in Cell Biology, 2016, 26(10): 766-775.

[5] Jordan M A, Wilson L. Microtubules as a target for anticancer drugs [J]. Nature Reviews Cancer, 2004, 4(4): 253-265.

[6] The financial reports of Genentech; http://data.pharmacodia.com/web/homePage/index.

[7] FDA Database. https://www.accessdata.fda.gov/drugsatfda_docs/label/2017/103792s5337lbl.pdf.

[8] Pharmaceuticals and Medical Device Agency (PMDA) Database. http://www.pmda.go.jp/drugs/2007/P200700066/45004500_21300AMY00128_A100_2.pdf.

[9] PMDA Database. http://www.info.pmda.go.jp/go/interview/1/450045_4291406D3021_1_020_1F.

[10] PMDA Database. http://www.pmda.go.jp/drugs/2001/P200100003/index.html.

[11] European Medicines Agency (EMA) Database. http://www.ema.europa.eu/docs/en_GB/document_library/EPAR_-_Assessment_Report_-_Uariation/human/000278/WC500153233.pdf.

[12] EMA Database. http://www.ema.europa.eu/docs/en_GB/document_library/EPAR_-_Product_Information/human/000278/WC500074922.pdf.

[13] EMA Database. http://www.ema.europa.eu/docs/en_GB/document_library/EPAR_-_Scientific_Discussion/human/000278/WC500049816.pdf.

[14] Dennis J S, Brian L-J, Steven S, et al. Use of chemotherapy plus a monoclonal antibody against HER2 for metastatic breast cancer that overexpresses HER2 [J]. The New England Journal of Medicine, 2001, 344(11): 783-792.

[15] Bellae K, John R M, Michael R C, et al. Trastuzumab plus anastrozole versus anastrozole alone for the treatment of postmenopausal women with human epidermal growth factor receptor 2-Positive, hormone receptor-positive metastatic breast cancer: results from the randomized Phase III TAnDEM study [J]. Journal of Clinical Oncology, 2009, 27(33): 5529-5537.

[16] Martine J P-G, Marion P M, Brian L-J, et al. Trastuzumab after adjuvant chemotherapy in HER2-positive breast cancer [J]. The New England Journal of Medicine, 2005, 353(16): 1659-1672.

[17] EMA Database. http://www.ema.europa.eu/docs/en_GB/document_library/EPAR_-_Assessment_Report_-_Variation/human/000278/WC500106489.pdf.

[18] EMA Database. http://www.ema.europa.eu/docs/en_GB/document_library/EPAR_-_Assessment_Report_-_Variation/human/000278/WC500126896.pdf.

[19] EMA Database. http://www.ema.europa.eu/docs/en_GB/document_library/EPAR_-_Assessment_Report_-_Variation/human/000278/WC500074921.pdf.

[20] Bang Y J, Van cutsem E, Feyereislova a, et al. Trastuzumab in combination with chemotherapy versus chemotherapy alone for treatment of HER2-positive advanced gastric or gastro-oesophageal junction cancer (ToGA): a phase 3, open-label, randomized controlled trial [J]. Lancet (London, England), 2010, 376(9742): 687-697.

Appendix

I

Abbreviation

5-FU	5-Fluorouracil
5-FU/FA	5-Fluorouracil/Folinic acid
5-FU/LV	5-Fluorouracil/Leucovorin
-	Not available

A

ABC	Adjuvant breast cancer
ACN	Acetonitrile
ACR	American College of Rheumatology
ADA	Anti-drug antibody
ADC	Antibody drug conjugates
ADCC	Antibody-dependent cell-mediated cytotoxicity
AEs	Adverse events
AGC	Advanced gastric cancer
AJCC	AmericanJoint Committee on Cancer
ALL	Acute lymphoblastic leukemia
alloHSCT	Allogeneic hematopoietic stem-cell transplantation
ALT	Alanine aminotransferase
AMD	Age-related macular degeneration
ANC	Absolute neutrophil count
APA	Aminopenicillanic acid
APCs	Antigen-presenting cells
Asp	Aspartic acid
AST	Aspartate transaminase
ATA	Anti-therapeutic antibody
AUC	Area under the plasma concentration-time curve
AUC_{all}	All area under the curve
AUC_{inf}	AUC from time zero to infinity
AVOREN	Avastin® and Roferon A® in renal cell carcinoma (BO17705)

B

BAC	Bronchoalveolar
BCR	Breakpoint cluster region
BLA	Biologics License Application
BORR	Best overall response rate
BSA	Bovine serum albumin
BSC	Best supportive care
BTD	Breakthrough Therapy Designation
BW	Body weight
BWG	Body weight gain

C

CCL	Chronic lymphocytic leukaemia
C_{max}	Maximum plasma concentration
C_{min}	Minimum concentration (trough)
CDC	Complement dependent cytotoxicity
CDDP	cis-Diaminedichloroplatinum
CDRs	Complementary-determining regions
CFDA	China Food and Drug Administration
CHAQ-DI	Childhood Health Assessment Questionnaire-Disability Index

cHL	Classical Hodgkin's lymphoma
CHO cells	Chinese hamster ovary cells
CI	Confidence interval
CIA	Collagen-induced arthritis
cIV	Continuous intravenous infusion
CL	Clearance
CL/F	Apparent systemic clearance
CLL	Chronic lymphoblastic leukaemia
CLT	Clearance rate
CML	Chronic myelogenous leukemia
CNTF	Ciliary neurotrophic factor
CNV	Choroidal neovascularization
CPA	Cyclophosphamide
CR	Complete response
CRC	Colorectal cancer
CrCL	Serum creatinine clearance
CRP	C-reactive protein
CSA	Cyclophosphamide
C_{ss}	Steady-state serum concentration
CTL	Cytotoxic T-lymphocyte
CTX	Platinum-based chemotherapy
CV	Coefficient of variation
Cys	Cysteine

D

DB	Double-blind
DCR	Disease control rate
DDFS	Distant disease-free survival
DDI	Drug-drug interaction
DFS	Disease-free survival
DLBCL	Diffuse large B-cell lymphoma
DMARDs	Disease-modifying anti-rheumatic drugs
DME	Diabetic macular edema
DOR	Duration of response
DR	Diabetic retinopathy
DTPA	Diethylene triamine pentaacetic acid

E

EBC	Early breast cancer
ECG	Electrocardiogram
ECOG	Eastern Cooperative Oncology Group
EFS	Event-free survival
EGF	Epidermal growth factor
EGFR	Epidermal growth factor receptor
ELISA	Enzyme linked immune Sorbent Assay
EMA	European Medicines Agency
ESR	Erythrocyte sedimentation rate
EU	Europe
EULAR	European league against rheumatism

F

FACIT-F	Functional assessment of chronic illness therapy-fatigue
FDA	Food and Drug Administration
FGF	Fibroblast growth factor

FL	Follicular lymphoma
FOB	Functional observation battery
FOLFIRI	Irinotecan, 5-fluorouracil, and leucovorin
FOLFOX4	Oxaliplatin plus continuous infusional 5-FU/FA
Fuc	Fucose

G

Gal	Galactose
GCA	Giant cell arteritis
GGT	Glutamyl transpeptadase
GlcNAc	N-acetylglucosamine
Gln	Glutamine acid
GPA	Granulomatosis with polyangiitis

H

HACA	Human anti-chimeric antibody
HAQ-DI	Health assessment questionnaire-disability index
HCP	Host cell proteins
HD	Hodgkin's disease
HER2	Human epidermal growth factor receptor 2
HGF	Hepatocyte growth factor
HNSCC	Head and neck squamous cell carcinoma
HPBL	Human peripheral blood lymphocytes
hPIGF 2	Human placental growth factor
HR	Hazard ratio
HRQoL	Health related quality of life
HSCT	Haempoietic stem-cell transplantation
HUVEC	Human umbilical vein endothelial cells
HV	Healthy volunteers
hVEGF	Human vascular endothelial growth factor

I

i.a.	Intra-arterial
IC	Intracameral
IC_{50}	50% inhibition concentration
IEC	Ion exchange chromatography
IFl	Irinotecan hydrochloride + 5-FU/LV
IFL	Irinotecan + 5-FU/LV
IFN	Interferon
IFP	Interstitial fluid pressure
IgG	Immunoglobulin gamma
IL-6	Interleukin-6
i.m.	Intramuscular
IN	India
INV	Investigator response assessment
IOP	Intraocular pressure
i.p.	Intraperitoneal
IPC	In-process controls
IrAE	Immune-related adverse event
IRC	Independent review committee
IRF	Independent review committee
ISR	Injection-site reaction
ITT	Intent-to-treat

ITV	Intravitreous injection
i.v.	Intravenous
IVT	Intravitral

J

JIA-ACR	Juvenile idiopathic arthritis-American College of Rheumatology

K

k.o.	Knock out
KR	Korea
KRAS	Kirsten rat sarcoma viral oncogene homolog

L

LABC	Locally advanced breast cancer
LD	Loading dose
LIF	Leukaemia inhibitory factor
LTR	Less than reportable

M

mAb	Monoclonal antibody
MAD	Multiple ascending doses
Man	Mannose
MBC	Metastatic breast cancer
MCB	Master Cell Bank
MCC	Maleimidomethyl cyclohexane-1-carboxylate linker as in T-DM1
MCH	Mean cell haemoglobin
MGC	Metastatic gastric cancer
mCRC	Metastatic colorectal cancer
MCV	Mean cell volume
MD	Medium Dose
M/F	Male/female
MI	Myocardial infarction
MMAE	Monomethyl auristatin E
MMF	Mycophenolate mofetil
MPA	Microscopic polyangiitis
mRCC	Metastatic renal cell cancer
MRD	Minimal residual disease
MRT	Mean residence time
MTC	Medullary thyroid cancer
MTD	Maximum tolerated dose
MTT	3-(4,5-dimethyl-2-thiazolyl)-2,5-diphenyl-2H-tetrazolium bromide
MTX	Methotrexate
mUC	Metastatic urothelial carcinoma

N

NA	Not applicable; Not available
NC	Not calculated
NCI-CTC	National Cancer Institute Common Terminology Criteria
ND	Not determined

NE	Not estimable		qd	Once daily
NGF	Nerve growth factor		qiw	Three times per week
NHL	Non-Hodgkin's lymphoma		QOL	Quality of life
Ni-NTA	Nickel-nitrilotriacetic acid		Qual.	Qualification
NOAEL	No-observed-adverse-effect level		QW	Every weekly
NOS	Not otherwise specified			
nPR	Nodular partial remission		**R**	
NR	Not reached			
NSCLC	Non-small cell lung cancer		RA	Rheumatoid arthritis
NSNSCLC	Non-squamous non-small cell lung cancer		RANO	Response Assessment in Neuro-oncology
NT	Not test		RBC	Red blood cell
			R/BW	Relative per body weight
O			RCC	Renal cell carcinoma
			REC	Response evaluation committee
OR	Overall response		RECIST	Response Evaluation Criteria in Solid Tumors
ORR	Objective response rate			
OS	Overall survival		RFS	Recurrence-free survival
OVCA	Ovarian carcinoma		RPLS	Reversible posterior leukoencephalopathy syndrome
P			RTK	Receptor tyrosine kinases
			RVO	Retinal vein occlusion
PBMCs	Peripheral blood mononuclear cells			
PBO	Placebo		**S**	
pCR	Pathological complete response			
PD	Pharmacodynamics		SAD	Single ascending dose
PD-1	Programmed cell death protein 1		SAE	Serious adverse event
PDGF	Platelet-derived growth factor		SALCL	Systemic anaplastic large cell lymphoma
PD-L1	Programmed death-ligand 1		s.c	Subcutaneous
PDT	Photon dynamic treatment		SCC	Squamous cell carcinoma
PE	Polyethylene		SCCHN	Squamous cell carcinoma of the head and neck
PFS	Progression-free survival			
pGlu	Pyroglutamic acid		scFv	Single chain antibody fragment
PHA	Phytohaemagglutinin		SCID	Severe combined immune deficiency
PIGF (PGF)	Placental growth factor		SCJ	Subconjunctival
PJIA	Polyarticular juvenile idiopathic arthritis		SD	Standard deviation
PK	Pharmacokinetics		SEC	Size exclusion chromatography
PLL	Prolymphocytic leukemia		SEM	Standard error of mean
PLT	Platelets		SGOT	Serum glutamic oxalacetic transaminase
PM	Pathologic myopia		SGPT	Serum glutamic pyruvic transaminase
PMDA	Pharmaceuticals and Medical Devices Agency		SI	Serious infection
			sJIA	Systemic juvenile idiopathic arthritis
p.o.	Oral		ST	Safety and tolerability
PO	Polyolefin			
PPK	Population pharmacokinetics		**T**	
PR	Partial response			
prmCC	Persistent, recurrent, or metastatic carcinoma of the cervix		$t_{1/2}$	Half-life
			TCA	Trichloracetic acid
prrEOFTPPC	Platinum-resistant recurrent epithelial ovarian, fallopian tube or primary peritoneal cancer		TCC	Transitional cell carcinoma
			TCR	T-cell receptor
			T-DM1	Trastuzumab emtansine
p.v.	Paravenous		TE	Thromboembolic event
PVC	Polyvinyl chloride		TFA	Trifluoroacetic acid
PY	Patient-years		TGD	Tumor growth delay
			TGF-α	Transforming growth factor α
Q			TGI	Tumor growth inhibition value
			TK	Toxicokinetics
q1w	Weekly		TKI	Tyrosine kinase inhibitor
q3w	Every 3 weeks		T_{max}	Time to maximum plasma concentration

TNF	Tumor necrosis factor
TSPA	Triethylenethiophosphoramide
TTF	Time to treatment failure
TTNT	Time to next treatment
TTP	Time to progression
TTR	Time to response

U

ULN	Upper limit of normal

V

VAS	Visual analogue scale
V_c	Volume of the central compartment
V_d	Apparent volume of distribution

V_{ds}	Volume at the dynamic state
VEGF	Vascular endothelial growth factor
VEGFR	Vascular endothelial growth factor receptor
VPF	Vascular permeability factor
V_{ss}	Volume of distribution at steady-state

W

wAMD	Wet age-related macular degeneration
WBC	White blood cell
WCB	Working Cell Bank
WCI	Worst case imputation
WG	Wegener's granulomatosis
WHO	World Health Organization

Appendix

II

Worldwide Approved Monoclonal Antibodies (1982-2017)

**Year
1982-1989**

Insulin human
Humulin®

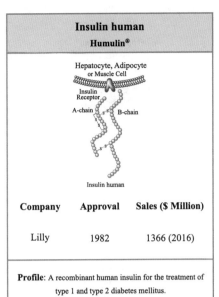

Company	Approval	Sales ($ Million)
Lilly	1982	1366 (2016)

Profile: A recombinant human insulin for the treatment of type 1 and type 2 diabetes mellitus.

Interferon alfa-2b
Intron A®

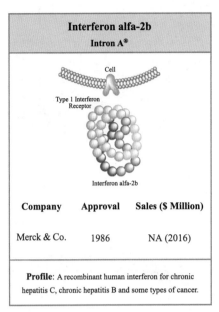

Company	Approval	Sales ($ Million)
Merck & Co.	1986	NA (2016)

Profile: A recombinant human interferon for chronic hepatitis C, chronic hepatitis B and some types of cancer.

Interferon alfa-2a
Roferon A®

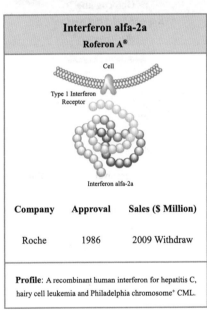

Company	Approval	Sales ($ Million)
Roche	1986	2009 Withdraw

Profile: A recombinant human interferon for hepatitis C, hairy cell leukemia and Philadelphia chromosome⁺ CML.

Muromonab-CD3
Orthoclone OKT3®

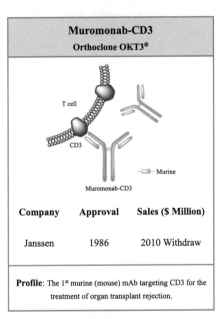

Company	Approval	Sales ($ Million)
Janssen	1986	2010 Withdraw

Profile: The 1ˢᵗ murine (mouse) mAb targeting CD3 for the treatment of organ transplant rejection.

Somatropin
Humatrope®

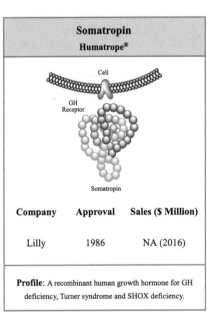

Company	Approval	Sales ($ Million)
Lilly	1986	NA (2016)

Profile: A recombinant human growth hormone for GH deficiency, Turner syndrome and SHOX deficiency.

Alteplase
Activase®/Activacin®/Grtpa®/Actilyse®

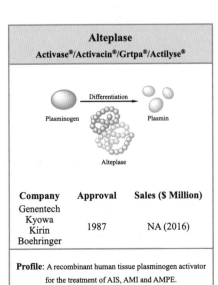

Company	Approval	Sales ($ Million)
Genentech Kyowa Kirin Boehringer	1987	NA (2016)

Profile: A recombinant human tissue plasminogen activator for the treatment of AIS, AMI and AMPE.

Epoetin alfa
Epogen®/Procrit®/Eprex®/Espo®

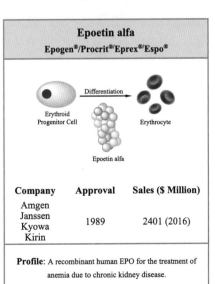

Company	Approval	Sales ($ Million)
Amgen Janssen Kyowa Kirin	1989	2401 (2016)

Profile: A recombinant human EPO for the treatment of anemia due to chronic kidney disease.

Interferon gamma-1a
Imunomax-γ®

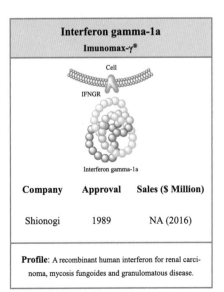

Company	Approval	Sales ($ Million)
Shionogi	1989	NA (2016)

Profile: A recombinant human interferon for renal carcinoma, mycosis fungoides and granulomatous disease.

**Year
1990-1999**

Filgrastim
Neupogen®/Gran®

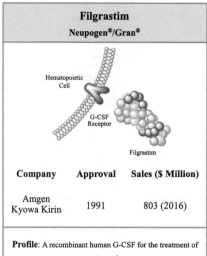

Hematopoietic Cell

G-CSF Receptor

Filgrastim

Company	Approval	Sales ($ Million)
Amgen Kyowa Kirin	1991	803 (2016)

Profile: A recombinant human G-CSF for the treatment of neutropenia.

Sargramostim
Leukine®

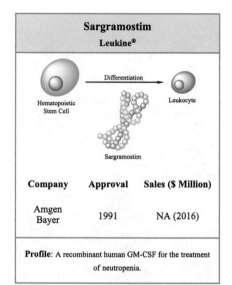

Hematopoietic Stem Cell

Differentiation

Leukocyte

Sargramostim

Company	Approval	Sales ($ Million)
Amgen Bayer	1991	NA (2016)

Profile: A recombinant human GM-CSF for the treatment of neutropenia.

Lenograstim
Neutrogin®/Granocyte®

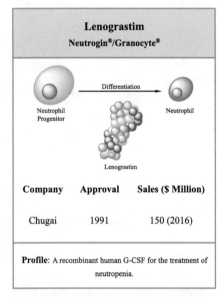

Neutrophil Progenitor

Differentiation

Neutrophil

Lenograstim

Company	Approval	Sales ($ Million)
Chugai	1991	150 (2016)

Profile: A recombinant human G-CSF for the treatment of neutropenia.

Antihemophilic factor
Recombinate®

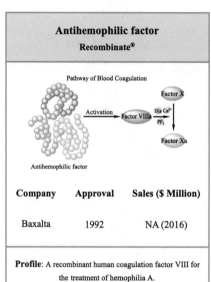

Pathway of Blood Coagulation

Activation → Factor VIIIa → IXa Ca²⁺ PF₃

Factor X

Factor Xa

Antihemophilic factor

Company	Approval	Sales ($ Million)
Baxalta	1992	NA (2016)

Profile: A recombinant human coagulation factor VIII for the treatment of hemophilia A.

Octocog alfa
Kogenate®/Helixate NexGen®/
Iblias®/Kovaltry®

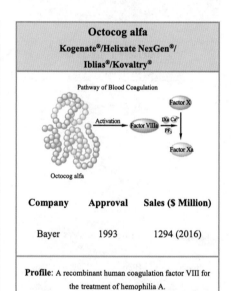

Pathway of Blood Coagulation

Activation → Factor VIIIa → IXa Ca²⁺ PF₃

Factor X

Factor Xa

Octocog alfa

Company	Approval	Sales ($ Million)
Bayer	1993	1294 (2016)

Profile: A recombinant human coagulation factor VIII for the treatment of hemophilia A.

Interferon beta-1b
Betaseron®/Betaferon®/Extavia®

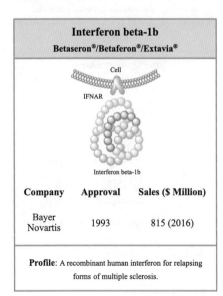

Cell

IFNAR

Interferon beta-1b

Company	Approval	Sales ($ Million)
Bayer Novartis	1993	815 (2016)

Profile: A recombinant human interferon for relapsing forms of multiple sclerosis.

Abciximab
RecoPro®

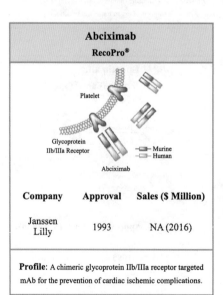

Platelet

Glycoprotein IIb/IIIa Receptor

Murine
Human

Abciximab

Company	Approval	Sales ($ Million)
Janssen Lilly	1993	NA (2016)

Profile: A chimeric glycoprotein IIb/IIIa receptor targeted mAb for the prevention of cardiac ischemic complications.

Dornase alfa
Pulmozyme®

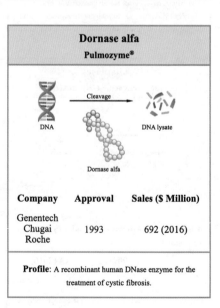

DNA

Cleavage

DNA lysate

Dornase alfa

Company	Approval	Sales ($ Million)
Genentech Chugai Roche	1993	692 (2016)

Profile: A recombinant human DNase enzyme for the treatment of cystic fibrosis.

Nartograstim
Neu-up®

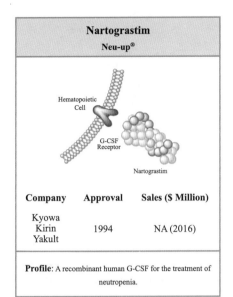

Company	Approval	Sales ($ Million)
Kyowa Kirin Yakult	1994	NA (2016)

Profile: A recombinant human G-CSF for the treatment of neutropenia.

Imiglucerase
Cerezyme®

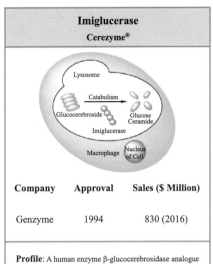

Company	Approval	Sales ($ Million)
Genzyme	1994	830 (2016)

Profile: A human enzyme β-glucocerebrosidase analogue for the treatment of Gaucher disease.

Mecasermin
Somazon®

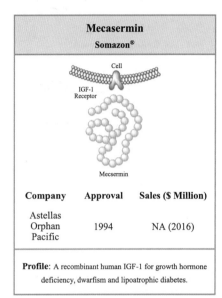

Company	Approval	Sales ($ Million)
Astellas Orphan Pacific	1994	NA (2016)

Profile: A recombinant human IGF-1 for growth hormone deficiency, dwarfism and lipoatrophic diabetes.

Follitropin alfa
Gonal-f®/Gonalef®

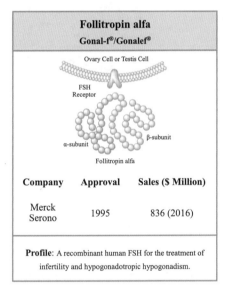

Company	Approval	Sales ($ Million)
Merck Serono	1995	836 (2016)

Profile: A recombinant human FSH for the treatment of infertility and hypogonadotropic hypogonadism.

Eptacog alfa
NovoSeven®

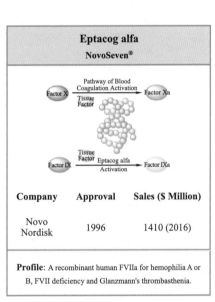

Company	Approval	Sales ($ Million)
Novo Nordisk	1996	1410 (2016)

Profile: A recombinant human FVIIa for hemophilia A or B, FVII deficiency and Glanzmann's thrombasthenia.

Insulin Lispro
Humalog®/Liprolog®

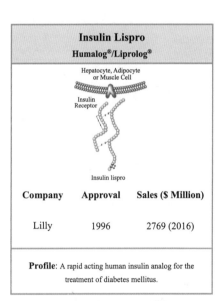

Company	Approval	Sales ($ Million)
Lilly	1996	2769 (2016)

Profile: A rapid acting human insulin analog for the treatment of diabetes mellitus.

Follitropin beta
Follistim®/Puregon®/Fertavid®

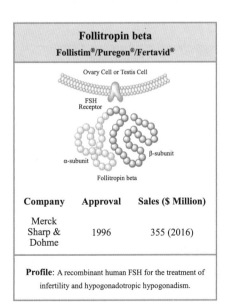

Company	Approval	Sales ($ Million)
Merck Sharp & Dohme	1996	355 (2016)

Profile: A recombinant human FSH for the treatment of infertility and hypogonadotropic hypogonadism.

Interferon beta-1a
Avonex®

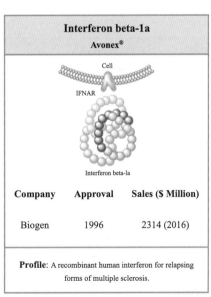

Company	Approval	Sales ($ Million)
Biogen	1996	2314 (2016)

Profile: A recombinant human interferon for relapsing forms of multiple sclerosis.

Reteplase
Retavase®/Ecokinase®/ Rapilysin®

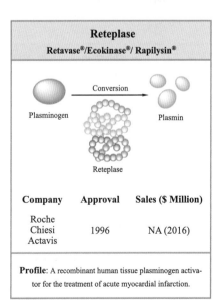

Company	Approval	Sales ($ Million)
Roche Chiesi Actavis	1996	NA (2016)

Profile: A recombinant human tissue plasminogen activator for the treatment of acute myocardial infarction.

Epoetin beta
NeoRecormon®/Epogin®

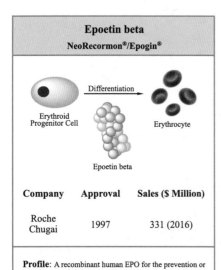

Company	Approval	Sales ($ Million)
Roche Chugai	1997	331 (2016)

Profile: A recombinant human EPO for the prevention or treatment of anemia due to kidney failure or chemotherapy.

Nonacog alfa
BeneFIX®

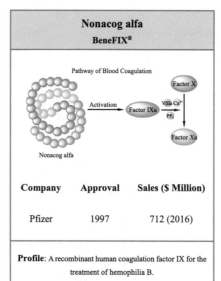

Company	Approval	Sales ($ Million)
Pfizer	1997	712 (2016)

Profile: A recombinant human coagulation factor IX for the treatment of hemophilia B.

Interferon alfacon-1
Infergen®

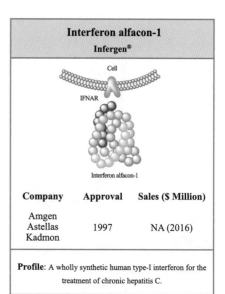

Company	Approval	Sales ($ Million)
Amgen Astellas Kadmon	1997	NA (2016)

Profile: A wholly synthetic human type-I interferon for the treatment of chronic hepatitis C.

Oprelvekin
Neumega®

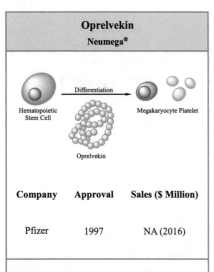

Company	Approval	Sales ($ Million)
Pfizer	1997	NA (2016)

Profile: A recombinant human IL-11 for severe thrombocytopenia in patients with nonmyeloid malignancies.

Rituximab
Rituxan®/Mab Thera®

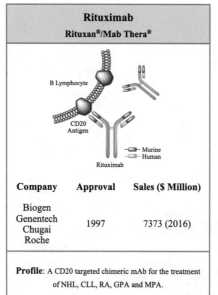

Company	Approval	Sales ($ Million)
Biogen Genentech Chugai Roche	1997	7373 (2016)

Profile: A CD20 targeted chimeric mAb for the treatment of NHL, CLL, RA, GPA and MPA.

Daclizumab
Zinbryta®/Zenapax®

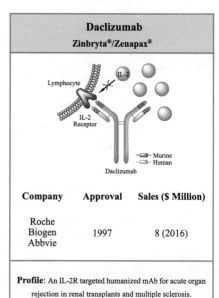

Company	Approval	Sales ($ Million)
Roche Biogen Abbvie	1997	8 (2016)

Profile: An IL-2R targeted humanized mAb for acute organ rejection in renal transplants and multiple sclerosis.

Becaplermin
Regranex®

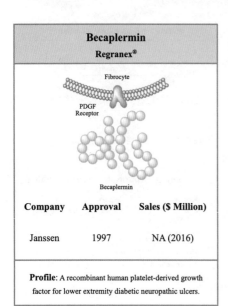

Company	Approval	Sales ($ Million)
Janssen	1997	NA (2016)

Profile: A recombinant human platelet-derived growth factor for lower extremity diabetic neuropathic ulcers.

Basiliximab
Simulect®

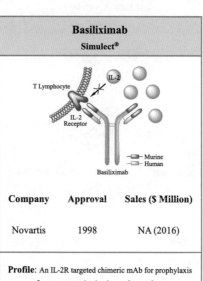

Company	Approval	Sales ($ Million)
Novartis	1998	NA (2016)

Profile: An IL-2R targeted chimeric mAb for prophylaxis of acute organ rejection in renal transplants.

Palivizumab
Synagis®

Company	Approval	Sales ($ Million)
MedImmune Abbvie	1998	1407 (2016)

Profile: A RSV protein F targeted humanized mAb for the prevention of serious RSV infection in children.

Glucagon
Glucagon G®/GlucaGen®

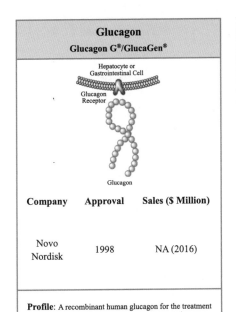

Company	Approval	Sales ($ Million)
Novo Nordisk	1998	NA (2016)

Profile: A recombinant human glucagon for the treatment of severe hypoglycemia.

Infliximab
Remicade®

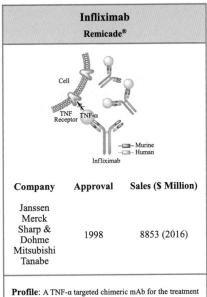

Company	Approval	Sales ($ Million)
Janssen Merck Sharp & Dohme Mitsubishi Tanabe	1998	8853 (2016)

Profile: A TNF-α targeted chimeric mAb for the treatment of Crohn's disease, RA and some other immune diseases.

Trastuzumab
Herceptin®

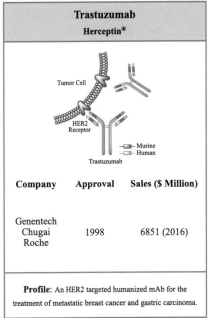

Company	Approval	Sales ($ Million)
Genentech Chugai Roche	1998	6851 (2016)

Profile: An HER2 targeted humanized mAb for the treatment of metastatic breast cancer and gastric carcinoma.

Etanercept
Enbrel®

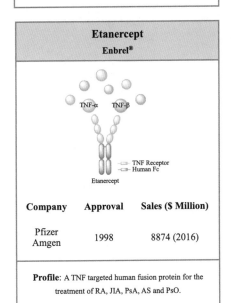

Company	Approval	Sales ($ Million)
Pfizer Amgen	1998	8874 (2016)

Profile: A TNF targeted human fusion protein for the treatment of RA, JIA, PsA, AS and PsO.

Thyrotropin alfa
Thyrogen®

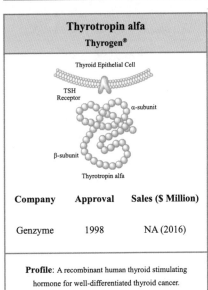

Company	Approval	Sales ($ Million)
Genzyme	1998	NA (2016)

Profile: A recombinant human thyroid stimulating hormone for well-differentiated thyroid cancer.

Monteplase
Cleactor®

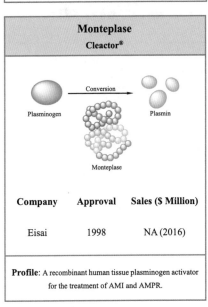

Company	Approval	Sales ($ Million)
Eisai	1998	NA (2016)

Profile: A recombinant human tissue plasminogen activator for the treatment of AMI and AMPR.

Denileukin diftitox
Ontak®

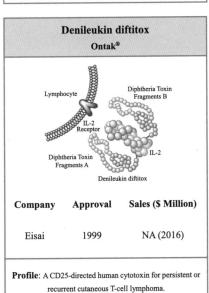

Company	Approval	Sales ($ Million)
Eisai	1999	NA (2016)

Profile: A CD25-directed human cytotoxin for persistent or recurrent cutaneous T-cell lymphoma.

Interferon gamma-1b
Actimmune®

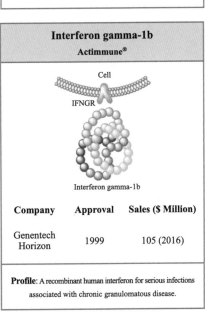

Company	Approval	Sales ($ Million)
Genentech Horizon	1999	105 (2016)

Profile: A recombinant human interferon for serious infections associated with chronic granulomatous disease.

Moroctocog alfa
ReFacto®/Xyntha®

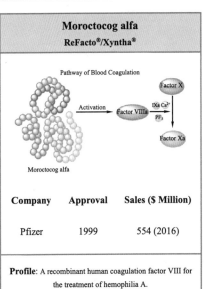

Company	Approval	Sales ($ Million)
Pfizer	1999	554 (2016)

Profile: A recombinant human coagulation factor VIII for the treatment of hemophilia A.

Insulin aspart
Novolog®/NovoRapid®/Fiasp®

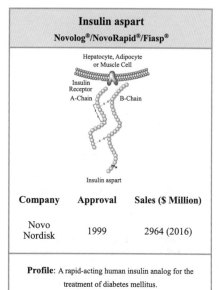

Company	Approval	Sales ($ Million)
Novo Nordisk	1999	2964 (2016)

Profile: A rapid-acting human insulin analog for the treatment of diabetes mellitus.

Year 2000-2009

Insulin glargine
Lantus®/Toujeo®

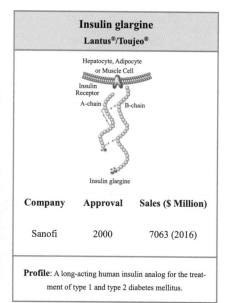

Company	Approval	Sales ($ Million)
Sanofi	2000	7063 (2016)

Profile: A long-acting human insulin analog for the treatment of type 1 and type 2 diabetes mellitus.

Gemtuzumab ozogamicin
Mylotarg®

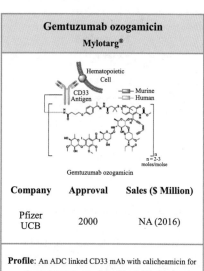

Company	Approval	Sales ($ Million)
Pfizer UCB	2000	NA (2016)

Profile: An ADC linked CD33 mAb with calicheamicin for the treatment of acute relapsed myeloid leukemia.

Peginterferon alfa-2b
PegIntron®/Sylatron®/ViraferonPeg®

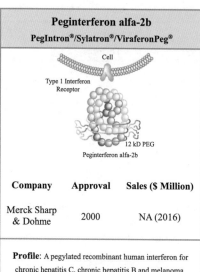

Company	Approval	Sales ($ Million)
Merck Sharp & Dohme	2000	NA (2016)

Profile: A pegylated recombinant human interferon for chronic hepatitis C, chronic hepatitis B and melanoma.

Tenecteplase
TNKase®/Metalyse®

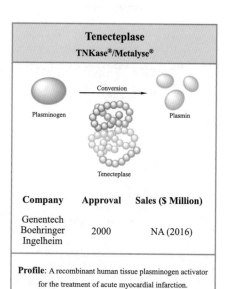

Company	Approval	Sales ($ Million)
Genentech Boehringer Ingelheim	2000	NA (2016)

Profile: A recombinant human tissue plasminogen activator for the treatment of acute myocardial infarction.

Choriogonadotropin alfa
Ovidrel®/Ovitrelle®

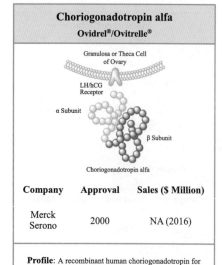

Company	Approval	Sales ($ Million)
Merck Serono	2000	NA (2016)

Profile: A recombinant human choriogonadotropin for ovulation induction and infertility treatment.

Lutropin alfa
Luveris®

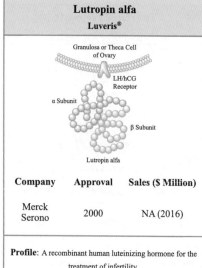

Company	Approval	Sales ($ Million)
Merck Serono	2000	NA (2016)

Profile: A recombinant human luteinizing hormone for the treatment of infertility.

Rasburicase
Elitek®/Fasturtec®/Rasuritek®

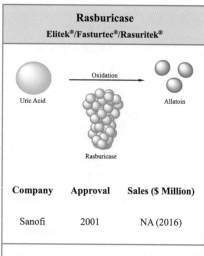

Company	Approval	Sales ($ Million)
Sanofi	2001	NA (2016)

Profile: A recombinant Aspergillus flavus urate-oxidase for initial management of plasma uric acid levels.

Trafermin
Fiblast®/Regroth®

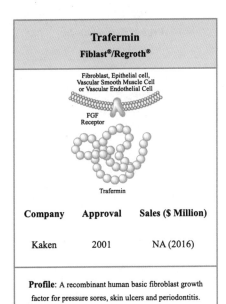

Company	Approval	Sales ($ Million)
Kaken	2001	NA (2016)

Profile: A recombinant human basic fibroblast growth factor for pressure sores, skin ulcers and periodontitis.

Alemtuzumab
Campath®/MabCampath®/Lemtrada®

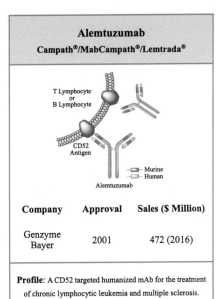

Company	Approval	Sales ($ Million)
Genzyme Bayer	2001	472 (2016)

Profile: A CD52 targeted humanized mAb for the treatment of chronic lymphocytic leukemia and multiple sclerosis.

Eptotermin alfa
Osigraft®/OP-1 Implant®/Opgenra®/OP-1 Putty®

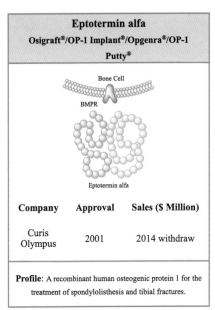

Company	Approval	Sales ($ Million)
Curis Olympus	2001	2014 withdraw

Profile: A recombinant human osteogenic protein 1 for the treatment of spondylolisthesis and tibial fractures.

Darbepoetin alfa
Aranesp®/Nesp®/Nespo®

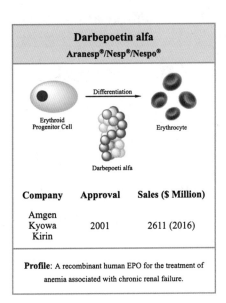

Company	Approval	Sales ($ Million)
Amgen Kyowa Kirin	2001	2611 (2016)

Profile: A recombinant human EPO for the treatment of anemia associated with chronic renal failure.

Agalsidase beta
Fabrazyme®

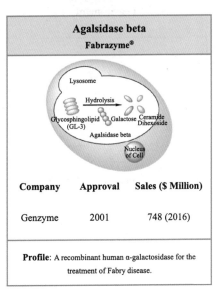

Company	Approval	Sales ($ Million)
Genzyme	2001	748 (2016)

Profile: A recombinant human α-galactosidase for the treatment of Fabry disease.

Agalsidase alfa
Replagal®

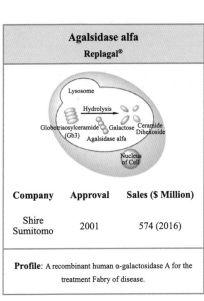

Company	Approval	Sales ($ Million)
Shire Sumitomo	2001	574 (2016)

Profile: A recombinant human α-galactosidase A for the treatment Fabry of disease.

Nesiritide
Natrecor®

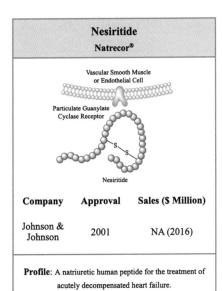

Company	Approval	Sales ($ Million)
Johnson & Johnson	2001	NA (2016)

Profile: A natriuretic human peptide for the treatment of acutely decompensated heart failure.

Anakinra
Kineret®

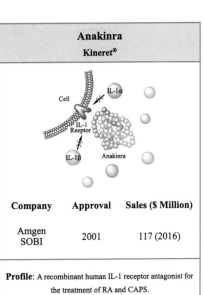

Company	Approval	Sales ($ Million)
Amgen SOBI	2001	117 (2016)

Profile: A recombinant human IL-1 receptor antagonist for the treatment of RA and CAPS.

Drotrecogin alfa
Xigris®

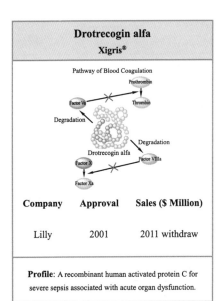

Company	Approval	Sales ($ Million)
Lilly	2001	2011 withdraw

Profile: A recombinant human activated protein C for severe sepsis associated with acute organ dysfunction.

Pegfilgrastim
Neulasta®/Ristempa®/G-Lasta®

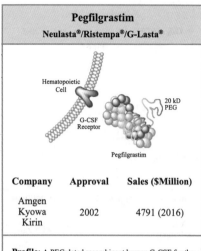

Company	Approval	Sales ($Million)
Amgen Kyowa Kirin	2002	4791 (2016)

Profile: A PEGylated recombinant human G-CSF for the treatment of neutropenia.

Ibritumomab tiuxetan
Zevalin®

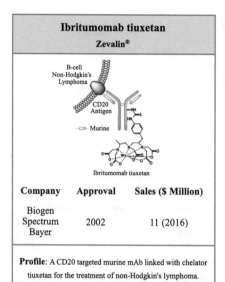

Company	Approval	Sales ($ Million)
Biogen Spectrum Bayer	2002	11 (2016)

Profile: A CD20 targeted murine mAb linked with chelator tiuxetan for the treatment of non-Hodgkin's lymphoma.

Peginterferon alfa-2a
Pegasys®

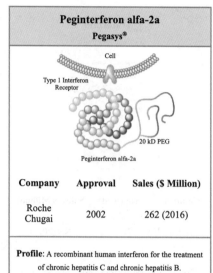

Company	Approval	Sales ($ Million)
Roche Chugai	2002	262 (2016)

Profile: A recombinant human interferon for the treatment of chronic hepatitis C and chronic hepatitis B.

Dibotermin alfa
Inductos®

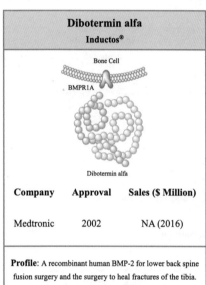
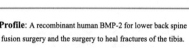

Company	Approval	Sales ($ Million)
Medtronic	2002	NA (2016)

Profile: A recombinant human BMP-2 for lower back spine fusion surgery and the surgery to heal fractures of the tibia.

Pegvisomant
Somavert®

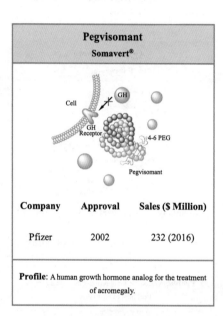

Company	Approval	Sales ($ Million)
Pfizer	2002	232 (2016)

Profile: A human growth hormone analog for the treatment of acromegaly.

Teriparatide
Forteo®/Forsteo®

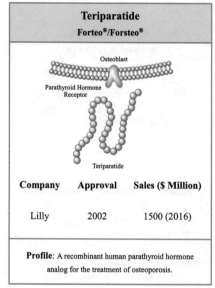

Company	Approval	Sales ($ Million)
Lilly	2002	1500 (2016)

Profile: A recombinant human parathyroid hormone analog for the treatment of osteoporosis.

Adalimumab
Humira®

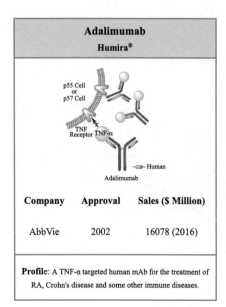

Company	Approval	Sales ($ Million)
AbbVie	2002	16078 (2016)

Profile: A TNF-α targeted human mAb for the treatment of RA, Crohn's disease and some other immune diseases.

Alefacept
Amevive®

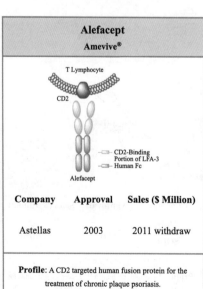

Company	Approval	Sales ($ Million)
Astellas	2003	2011 withdraw

Profile: A CD2 targeted human fusion protein for the treatment of chronic plaque psoriasis.

Laronidase
Aldurazyme®

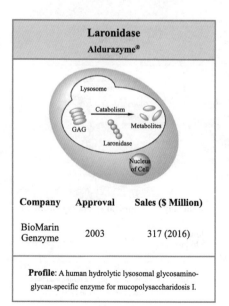

Company	Approval	Sales ($ Million)
BioMarin Genzyme	2003	317 (2016)

Profile: A human hydrolytic lysosomal glycosamino-glycan-specific enzyme for mucopolysaccharidosis I.

Omalizumab
Xolair®

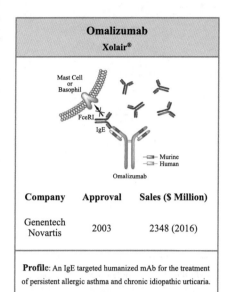

Company	Approval	Sales ($ Million)
Genentech Novartis	2003	2348 (2016)

Profile: An IgE targeted humanized mAb for the treatment of persistent allergic asthma and chronic idiopathic urticaria.

Iodine 131 tositumomab
Bexxar®

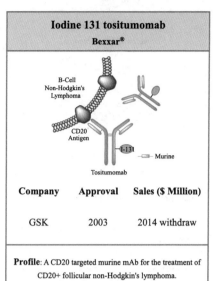

Company	Approval	Sales ($ Million)
GSK	2003	2014 withdraw

Profile: A CD20 targeted murine mAb for the treatment of CD20+ follicular non-Hodgkin's lymphoma.

Rurioctocog alfa
Advate®

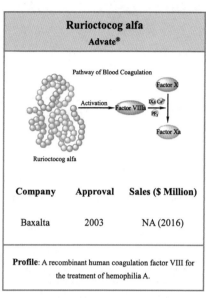

Company	Approval	Sales ($ Million)
Baxalta	2003	NA (2016)

Profile: A recombinant human coagulation factor VIII for the treatment of hemophilia A.

Efalizumab
Raptiva®

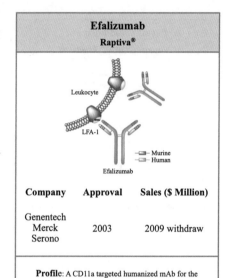

Company	Approval	Sales ($ Million)
Genentech Merck Serono	2003	2009 withdraw

Profile: A CD11a targeted humanized mAb for the treatment of plaque psoriasis.

Cetuximab
Erbitux®

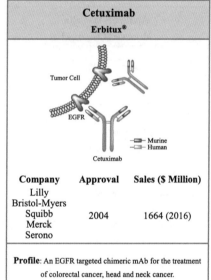

Company	Approval	Sales ($ Million)
Lilly Bristol-Myers Squibb Merck Serono	2004	1664 (2016)

Profile: An EGFR targeted chimeric mAb for the treatment of colorectal cancer, head and neck cancer.

Bevacizumab
Avastin®

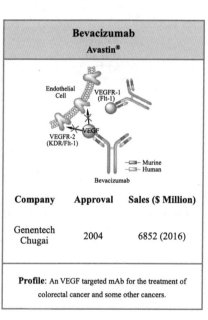

Company	Approval	Sales ($ Million)
Genentech Chugai	2004	6852 (2016)

Profile: An VEGF targeted mAb for the treatment of colorectal cancer and some other cancers.

Insulin glulisine
Apidra®

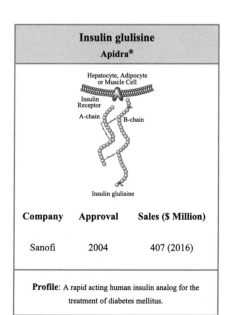

Company	Approval	Sales ($ Million)
Sanofi	2004	407 (2016)

Profile: A rapid acting human insulin analog for the treatment of diabetes mellitus.

Insulin detemir
Levemir®

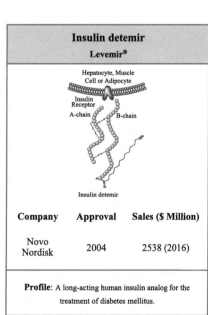

Company	Approval	Sales ($ Million)
Novo Nordisk	2004	2538 (2016)

Profile: A long-acting human insulin analog for the treatment of diabetes mellitus.

Natalizumab
Tysabri®

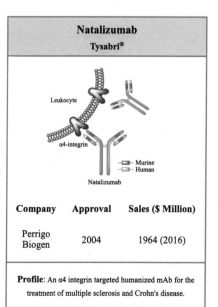

Company	Approval	Sales ($ Million)
Perrigo Biogen	2004	1964 (2016)

Profile: An α4 integrin targeted humanized mAb for the treatment of multiple sclerosis and Crohn's disease.

Palifermin
Kepivance®

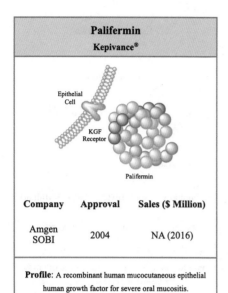

Company	Approval	Sales ($ Million)
Amgen SOBI	2004	NA (2016)

Profile: A recombinant human mucocutaneous epithelial human growth factor for severe oral mucositis.

Tocilizumab
Actemra®/RoActemra®

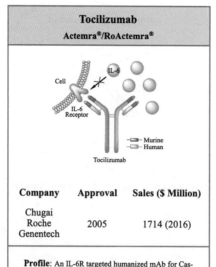

Company	Approval	Sales ($ Million)
Chugai Roche Genentech	2005	1714 (2016)

Profile: An IL-6R targeted humanized mAb for Castleman's disease, RA and some other autoimmune disease.

Galsulfase
Naglazyme®

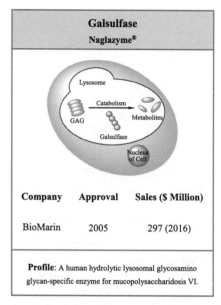

Company	Approval	Sales ($ Million)
BioMarin	2005	297 (2016)

Profile: A human hydrolytic lysosomal glycosamino glycan-specific enzyme for mucopolysaccharidosis VI.

Abatacept
Orencia®

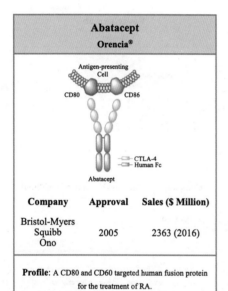

Company	Approval	Sales ($ Million)
Bristol-Myers Squibb Ono	2005	2363 (2016)

Profile: A CD80 and CD60 targeted human fusion protein for the treatment of RA.

Alglucosidase alfa
Myozyme®/Lumizyme®

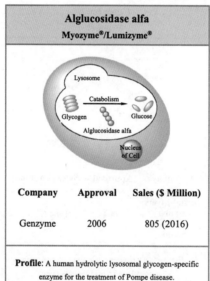

Company	Approval	Sales ($ Million)
Genzyme	2006	805 (2016)

Profile: A human hydrolytic lysosomal glycogen-specific enzyme for the treatment of Pompe disease.

Parathyroid hormone
Natpara®/Natpar®/Preotact®

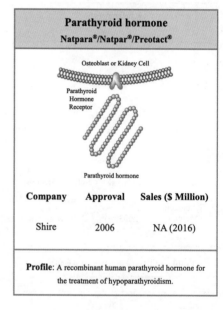

Company	Approval	Sales ($ Million)
Shire	2006	NA (2016)

Profile: A recombinant human parathyroid hormone for the treatment of hypoparathyroidism.

Ranibizumab
Lucentis®

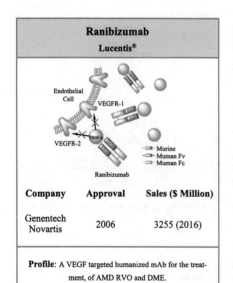

Company	Approval	Sales ($ Million)
Genentech Novartis	2006	3255 (2016)

Profile: A VEGF targeted humanized mAb for the treatment, of AMD RVO and DME.

Nimotuzumab
BioMAb-EGFR®

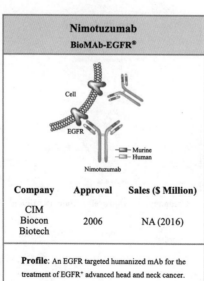

Company	Approval	Sales ($ Million)
CIM Biocon Biotech	2006	NA (2016)

Profile: An EGFR targeted humanized mAb for the treatment of EGFR+ advanced head and neck cancer.

Idursulfase
Elaprase®

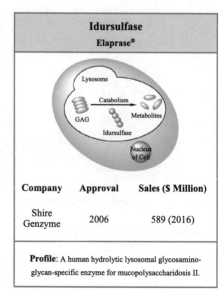

Company	Approval	Sales ($ Million)
Shire Genzyme	2006	589 (2016)

Profile: A human hydrolytic lysosomal glycosamino-glycan-specific enzyme for mucopolysaccharidosis II.

Antithrombin alfa
ATryn®

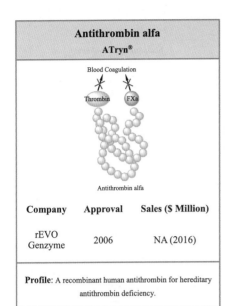

Company	Approval	Sales ($ Million)
rEVO Genzyme	2006	NA (2016)

Profile: A recombinant human antithrombin for hereditary antithrombin deficiency.

Panitumumab
Vectibix®

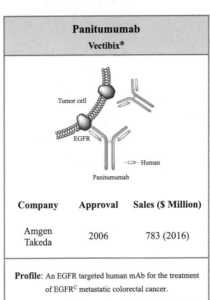

Company	Approval	Sales ($ Million)
Amgen Takeda	2006	783 (2016)

Profile: An EGFR targeted human mAb for the treatment of EGFR[C] metastatic colorectal cancer.

Eculizumab
Soliris®

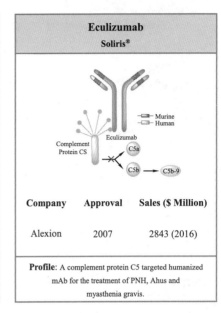

Company	Approval	Sales ($ Million)
Alexion	2007	2843 (2016)

Profile: A complement protein C5 targeted humanized mAb for the treatment of PNH, Ahus and myasthenia gravis.

Methoxy polyethylene glycol-epoetin beta
Mircera®

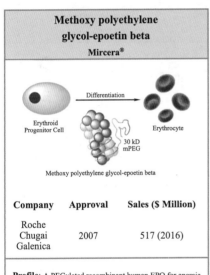
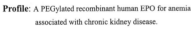

Company	Approval	Sales ($ Million)
Roche Chugai Galenica	2007	517 (2016)

Profile: A PEGylated recombinant human EPO for anemia associated with chronic kidney disease.

Thrombin topical
Recothrom®

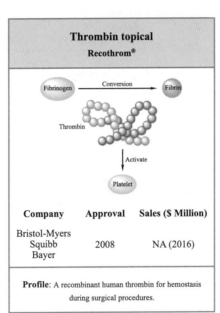

Company	Approval	Sales ($ Million)
Bristol-Myers Squibb Bayer	2008	NA (2016)

Profile: A recombinant human thrombin for hemostasis during surgical procedures.

Thrombomodulin alfa
Recomodulin®

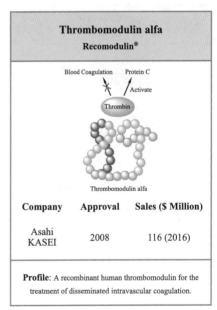

Company	Approval	Sales ($ Million)
Asahi KASEI	2008	116 (2016)

Profile: A recombinant human thrombomodulin for the treatment of disseminated intravascular coagulation.

Rilonacept
Arcalyst®

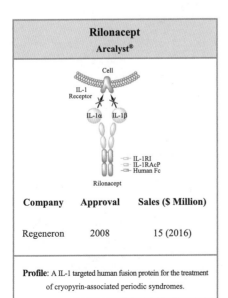

Company	Approval	Sales ($ Million)
Regeneron	2008	15 (2016)

Profile: A IL-1 targeted human fusion protein for the treatment of cryopyrin-associated periodic syndromes.

Certolizumab Pegol
Cimzia®

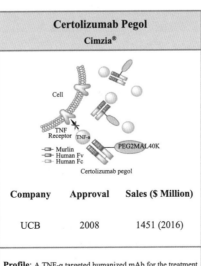

Company	Approval	Sales ($ Million)
UCB	2008	1451 (2016)

Profile: A TNF-α targeted humanized mAb for the treatment of Crohn's disease, RA and some other immune diseases.

Romiplostim
Nplate®/Romiplate®

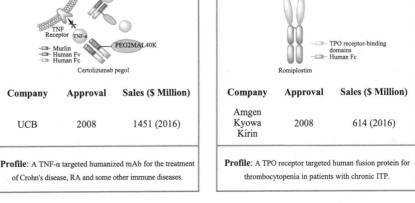

Company	Approval	Sales ($ Million)
Amgen Kyowa Kirin	2008	614 (2016)

Profile: A TPO receptor targeted human fusion protein for thrombocytopenia in patients with chronic ITP.

Ustekinumab
Stelara®

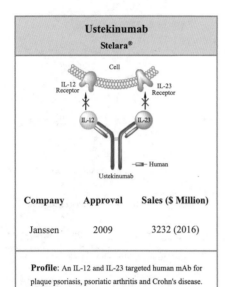

Company	Approval	Sales ($ Million)
Janssen	2009	3232 (2016)

Profile: An IL-12 and IL-23 targeted human mAb for plaque psoriasis, psoriatic arthritis and Crohn's disease.

Catumaxomab
Removab®

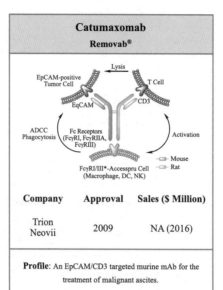

Company	Approval	Sales ($ Million)
Trion Neovii	2009	NA (2016)

Profile: An EpCAM/CD3 targeted murine mAb for the treatment of malignant ascites.

Golimumab
Simponi®/Simponi aria®

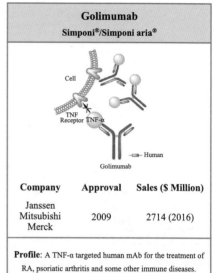

Company	Approval	Sales ($ Million)
Janssen Mitsubishi Merck	2009	2714 (2016)

Profile: A TNF-α targeted human mAb for the treatment of RA, psoriatic arthritis and some other immune diseases.

Canakinumab
Ilaris®

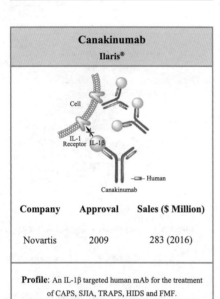

Company	Approval	Sales ($ Million)
Novartis	2009	283 (2016)

Profile: An IL-1β targeted human mAb for the treatment of CAPS, SJIA, TRAPS, HIDS and FMF.

Liraglutide
Victoza®/Saxenda®

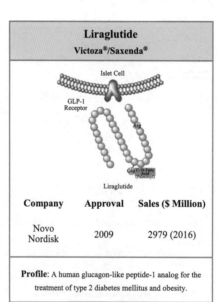

Company	Approval	Sales ($ Million)
Novo Nordisk	2009	2979 (2016)

Profile: A human glucagon-like peptide-1 analog for the treatment of type 2 diabetes mellitus and obesity.

Epoetin theta
Biopoin®/Eporatio®

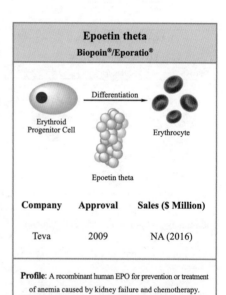

Company	Approval	Sales ($ Million)
Teva	2009	NA (2016)

Profile: A recombinant human EPO for prevention or treatment of anemia caused by kidney failure and chemotherapy.

Ofatumumab
Arzerra®

Company	Approval	Sales ($ Million)
Genmab GSK Novartis	2009	NA (2016)

Profile: A CD20 targeted human mAb for the treatment of chronic lymphocytic leukemia.

Ecallantide
Kalbitor®

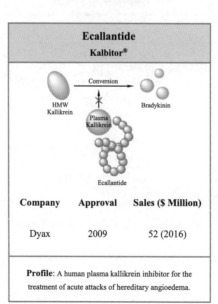

Company	Approval	Sales ($ Million)
Dyax	2009	52 (2016)

Profile: A human plasma kallikrein inhibitor for the treatment of acute attacks of hereditary angioedema.

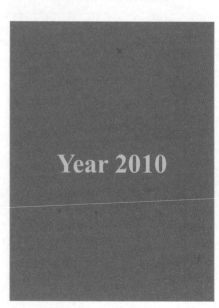

Year 2010

Corifollitropin alfa
Elonva®

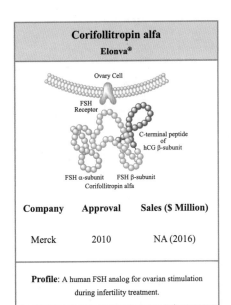

Company	Approval	Sales ($ Million)
Merck	2010	NA (2016)

Profile: A human FSH analog for ovarian stimulation during infertility treatment.

Velaglucerase alfa
Vpriv®

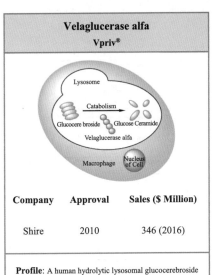

Company	Approval	Sales ($ Million)
Shire	2010	346 (2016)

Profile: A human hydrolytic lysosomal glucocerebroside specific enzyme for the treatment of type 1 Gaucher disease.

Denosumab
Prolia®/Xgeva®/Ranmark®/Pralia®

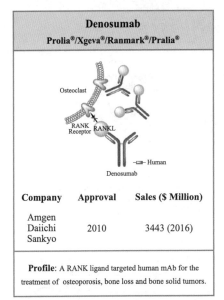

Company	Approval	Sales ($ Million)
Amgen Daiichi Sankyo	2010	3443 (2016)

Profile: A RANK ligand targeted human mAb for the treatment of osteoporosis, bone loss and bone solid tumors.

Pegloticase
Krystexxa®

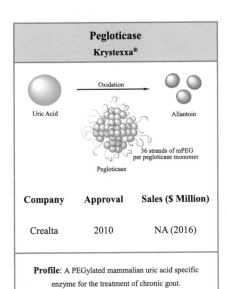

Company	Approval	Sales ($ Million)
Crealta	2010	NA (2016)

Profile: A PEGylated mammalian uric acid specific enzyme for the treatment of chronic gout.

Conestat alfa
Ruconest®

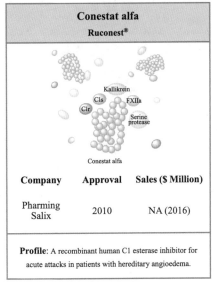

Company	Approval	Sales ($ Million)
Pharming Salix	2010	NA (2016)

Profile: A recombinant human C1 esterase inhibitor for acute attacks in patients with hereditary angioedema.

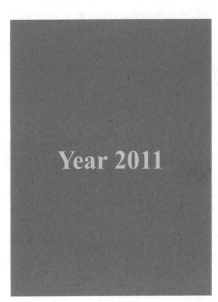

Year 2011

Belimumab
Benlysta®

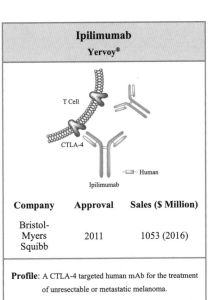

Company	Approval	Sales ($ Million)
GSK	2011	416 (2016)

Profile: A BLyS targeted human mAb for the treatment of systemic lupus erythematosus.

Ipilimumab
Yervoy®

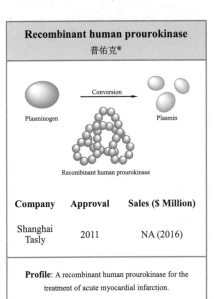

Company	Approval	Sales ($ Million)
Bristol-Myers Squibb	2011	1053 (2016)

Profile: A CTLA-4 targeted human mAb for the treatment of unresectable or metastatic melanoma.

Recombinant human prourokinase
普佑克®

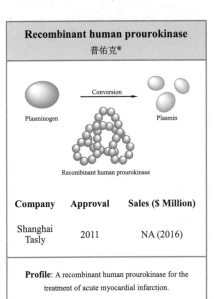

Company	Approval	Sales ($ Million)
Shanghai Tasly	2011	NA (2016)

Profile: A recombinant human prourokinase for the treatment of acute myocardial infarction.

Belatacept
Nulojix®

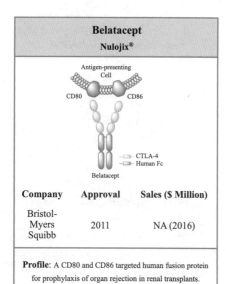

Company	Approval	Sales ($ Million)
Bristol-Myers Squibb	2011	NA (2016)

Profile: A CD80 and CD86 targeted human fusion protein for prophylaxis of organ rejection in renal transplants.

Brentuximab Vedotin
Adcetris®

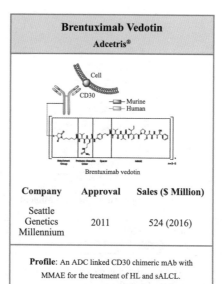

Company	Approval	Sales ($ Million)
Seattle Genetics Millennium	2011	524 (2016)

Profile: An ADC linked CD30 chimeric mAb with MMAE for the treatment of HL and sALCL.

Aflibercept
Eylea®

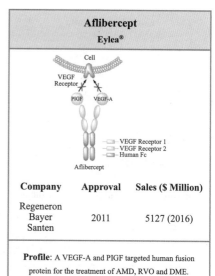

Company	Approval	Sales ($ Million)
Regeneron Bayer Santen	2011	5127 (2016)

Profile: A VEGF-A and PIGF targeted human fusion protein for the treatment of AMD, RVO and DME.

Year 2012

Glucarpidase
Voraxaze®

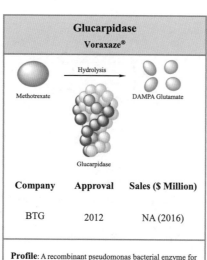

Company	Approval	Sales ($ Million)
BTG	2012	NA (2016)

Profile: A recombinant pseudomonas bacterial enzyme for toxic plasma methotrexate concentrations (>1 μmol/L).

Mogamulizumab
Poteligeo®

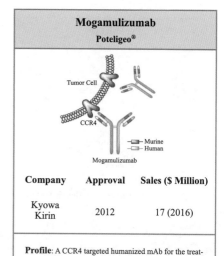

Company	Approval	Sales ($ Million)
Kyowa Kirin	2012	17 (2016)

Profile: A CCR4 targeted humanized mAb for the treatment of relapsed or refractory T-cell leukemia/lymphoma.

Taliglucerase alfa
Elelyso®

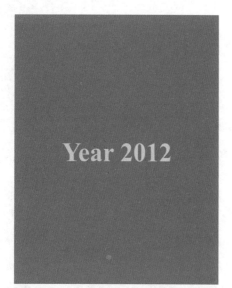

Company	Approval	Sales ($ Million)
Protalix Pfizer	2012	NA (2016)

Profile: A human hydrolytic lysosomal glucocerebroside-specific enzyme for type 1 Gaucher disease.

Pertuzumab
Perjeta®

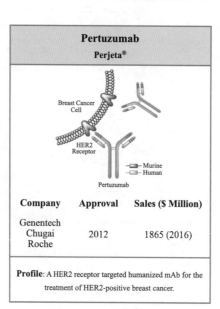

Company	Approval	Sales ($ Million)
Genentech Chugai Roche	2012	1865 (2016)

Profile: A HER2 receptor targeted humanized mAb for the treatment of HER2-positive breast cancer.

Ziv-aflibercept
Zaltrap®

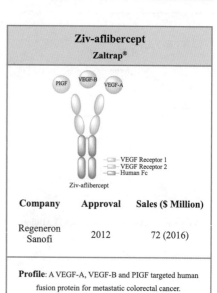

Company	Approval	Sales ($ Million)
Regeneron Sanofi	2012	72 (2016)

Profile: A VEGF-A, VEGF-B and PIGF targeted human fusion protein for metastatic colorectal cancer.

Teduglutide
Gattex®/Revestive®

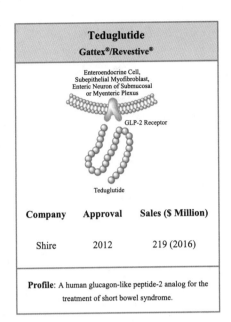

Company	Approval	Sales ($ Million)
Shire	2012	219 (2016)

Profile: A human glucagon-like peptide-2 analog for the treatment of short bowel syndrome.

Catridecacog
NovoThirteen®/Tretten®

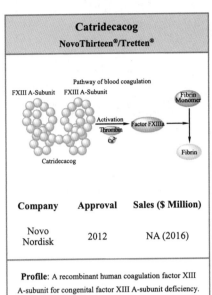

Company	Approval	Sales ($ Million)
Novo Nordisk	2012	NA (2016)

Profile: A recombinant human coagulation factor XIII A-subunit for congenital factor XIII A-subunit deficiency.

Insulin degludec
Tresiba®

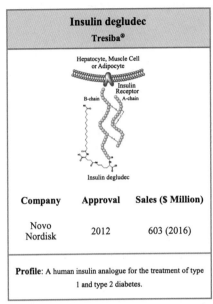

Company	Approval	Sales ($ Million)
Novo Nordisk	2012	603 (2016)

Profile: A human insulin analogue for the treatment of type 1 and type 2 diabetes.

Ocriplasmin
Jetrea®

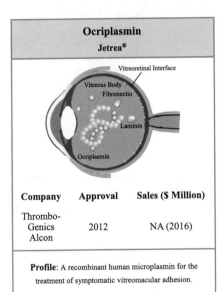

Company	Approval	Sales ($ Million)
Thrombo-Genics Alcon	2012	NA (2016)

Profile: A recombinant human microplasmin for the treatment of symptomatic vitreomacular adhesion.

Raxibacumab
Abthrax®

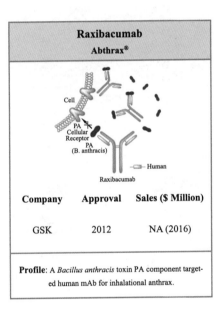

Company	Approval	Sales ($ Million)
GSK	2012	NA (2016)

Profile: A *Bacillus anthracis* toxin PA component targeted human mAb for inhalational anthrax.

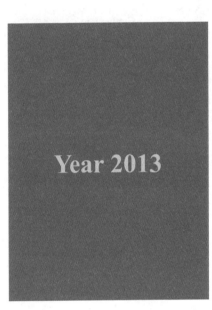

Year 2013

Ado-trastuzumab emtansine
Kadcyla®

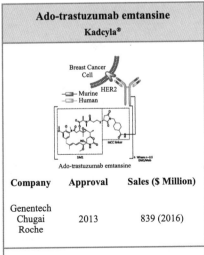

Company	Approval	Sales ($ Million)
Genentech Chugai Roche	2013	839 (2016)

Profile: An ADC linked HER2 humanized mAb with DM1 for the treatment of HER2+ metastatic breast cancer.

Metreleptin
Myalept®/Metreleptin [SHIONOGI]®

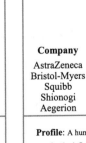
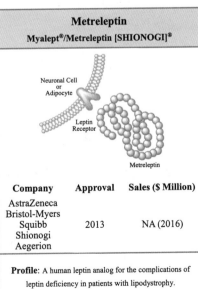

Company	Approval	Sales ($ Million)
AstraZeneca Bristol-Myers Squibb Shionogi Aegerion	2013	NA (2016)

Profile: A human leptin analog for the complications of leptin deficiency in patients with lipodystrophy.

Nonacog gamma
Rixubis®

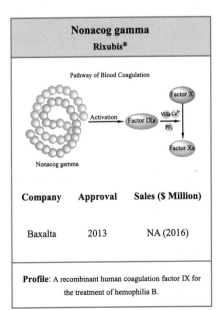

Company	Approval	Sales ($ Million)
Baxalta	2013	NA (2016)

Profile: A recombinant human coagulation factor IX for the treatment of hemophilia B.

Lipegfilgrastim
Lonquex®

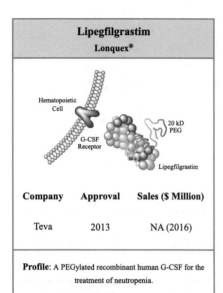

Company	Approval	Sales ($ Million)
Teva	2013	NA (2016)

Profile: A PEGylated recombinant human G-CSF for the treatment of neutropenia.

Turoctocog alfa
Novoeight®

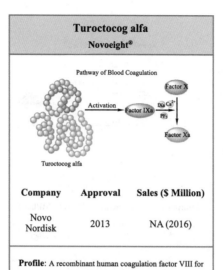

Company	Approval	Sales ($ Million)
Novo Nordisk	2013	NA (2016)

Profile: A recombinant human coagulation factor VIII for the treatment of hemophilia A.

Obinutuzumab
Gazyva®/Gazyvaro®

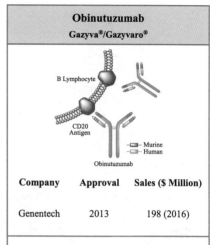

Company	Approval	Sales ($ Million)
Genentech	2013	198 (2016)

Profile: A CD20 targeted human mAb for the treatment of chronic lymphocytic leukemia and follicular lymphoma.

Conbercept
朗沐®

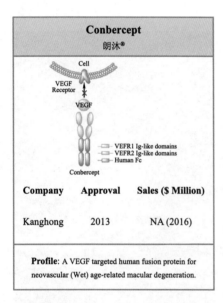

Company	Approval	Sales ($ Million)
Kanghong	2013	NA (2016)

Profile: A VEGF targeted human fusion protein for neovascular (Wet) age-related macular degeneration.

Year 2014

Elosulfase alfa
Vimizim®

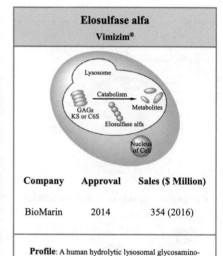

Company	Approval	Sales ($ Million)
BioMarin	2014	354 (2016)

Profile: A human hydrolytic lysosomal glycosamino-glycan-specific enzyme for mucopolysaccharidosis IVA.

Albiglutide
Tanzeum®/Eperzan®

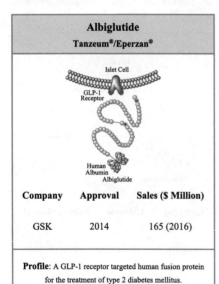

Company	Approval	Sales ($ Million)
GSK	2014	165 (2016)

Profile: A GLP-1 receptor targeted human fusion protein for the treatment of type 2 diabetes mellitus.

Eftrenonacog alfa
Alprolix®

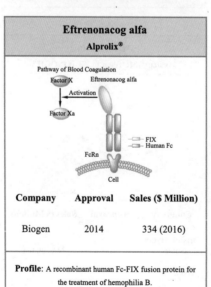

Company	Approval	Sales ($ Million)
Biogen	2014	334 (2016)

Profile: A recombinant human Fc-FIX fusion protein for the treatment of hemophilia B.

Ramucirumab
Cyramza®

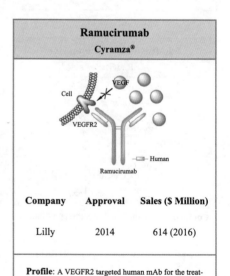

Company	Approval	Sales ($ Million)
Lilly	2014	614 (2016)

Profile: A VEGFR2 targeted human mAb for the treatment of gastric cancer and non-small cell lung cancer.

Siltuximab
Sylvant®

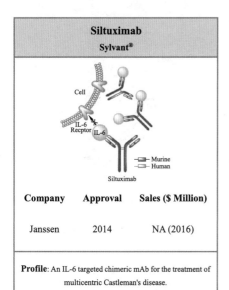

Company	Approval	Sales ($ Million)
Janssen	2014	NA (2016)

Profile: An IL-6 targeted chimeric mAb for the treatment of multicentric Castleman's disease.

Vedolizumab
Entyvio®

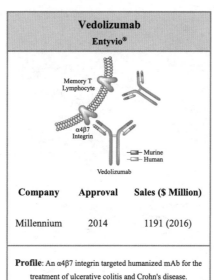

Company	Approval	Sales ($ Million)
Millennium	2014	1191 (2016)

Profile: An α4β7 integrin targeted humanized mAb for the treatment of ulcerative colitis and Crohn's disease.

Efmoroctocog alfa
Elocta®/Eloctate®

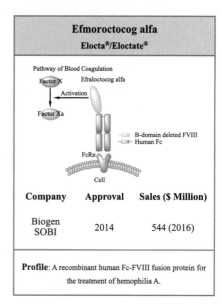

Company	Approval	Sales ($ Million)
Biogen SOBI	2014	544 (2016)

Profile: A recombinant human Fc-FVIII fusion protein for the treatment of hemophilia A.

Nivolumab
Opdivo®

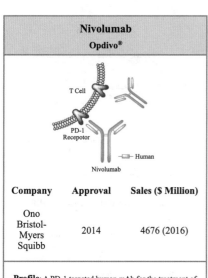
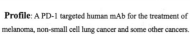

Company	Approval	Sales ($ Million)
Ono Bristol-Myers Squibb	2014	4676 (2016)

Profile: A PD-1 targeted human mAb for the treatment of melanoma, non-small cell lung cancer and some other cancers.

Peginterferon beta-1a
Plegridy®

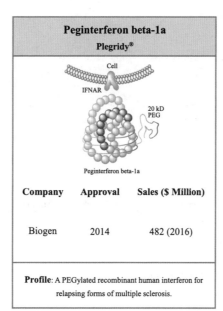

Company	Approval	Sales ($ Million)
Biogen	2014	482 (2016)

Profile: A PEGylated recombinant human interferon for relapsing forms of multiple sclerosis.

Simoctocog alfa
Nuwiq®/Vihuma®

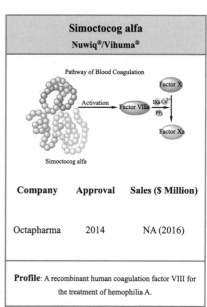

Company	Approval	Sales ($ Million)
Octapharma	2014	NA (2016)

Profile: A recombinant human coagulation factor VIII for the treatment of hemophilia A.

Pembrolizumab
Keytruda®

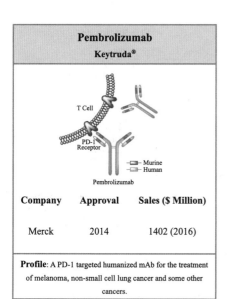

Company	Approval	Sales ($ Million)
Merck	2014	1402 (2016)

Profile: A PD-1 targeted humanized mAb for the treatment of melanoma, non-small cell lung cancer and some other cancers.

Dulaglutide
Trulicity®

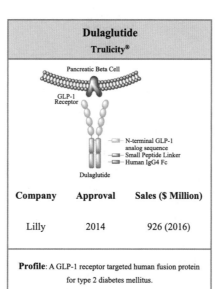

Company	Approval	Sales ($ Million)
Lilly	2014	926 (2016)

Profile: A GLP-1 receptor targeted human fusion protein for type 2 diabetes mellitus.

Blinatumomab
Blincyto®

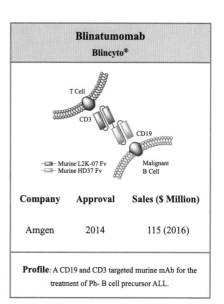

Company	Approval	Sales ($ Million)
Amgen	2014	115 (2016)

Profile: A CD19 and CD3 targeted murine mAb for the treatment of Ph- B cell precursor ALL.

Secukinumab
Cosentyx®

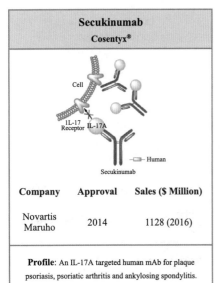

Company	Approval	Sales ($ Million)
Novartis Maruho	2014	1128 (2016)

Profile: An IL-17A targeted human mAb for plaque psoriasis, psoriatic arthritis and ankylosing spondylitis.

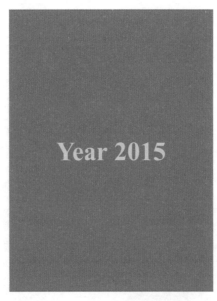

Year 2015

Dinutuximab
Unituxin®

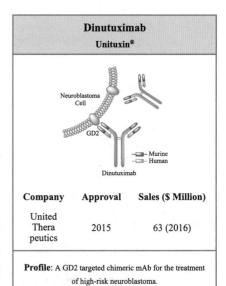

Company	Approval	Sales ($ Million)
United Therapeutics	2015	63 (2016)

Profile: A GD2 targeted chimeric mAb for the treatment of high-risk neuroblastoma.

Trenonacog alfa
Ixinity®

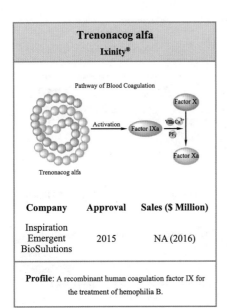

Company	Approval	Sales ($ Million)
Inspiration Emergent BioSulutions	2015	NA (2016)

Profile: A recombinant human coagulation factor IX for the treatment of hemophilia B.

Antithrombin gamma
Acoalan®

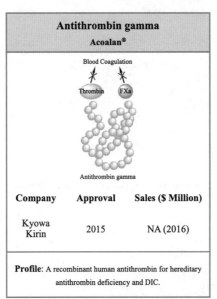

Company	Approval	Sales ($ Million)
Kyowa Kirin	2015	NA (2016)

Profile: A recombinant human antithrombin for hereditary antithrombin deficiency and DIC.

Asfotase alfa
Strensiq®

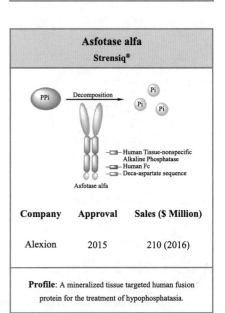

Company	Approval	Sales ($ Million)
Alexion	2015	210 (2016)

Profile: A mineralized tissue targeted human fusion protein for the treatment of hypophosphatasia.

Evolocumab
Repatha®

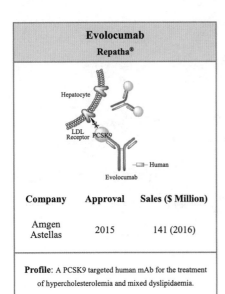

Company	Approval	Sales ($ Million)
Amgen Astellas	2015	141 (2016)

Profile: A PCSK9 targeted human mAb for the treatment of hypercholesterolemia and mixed dyslipidaemia.

Alirocumab
Praluent®

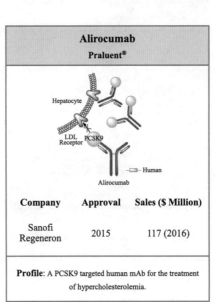

Company	Approval	Sales ($ Million)
Sanofi Regeneron	2015	117 (2016)

Profile: A PCSK9 targeted human mAb for the treatment of hypercholesterolemia.

Sebelipase alfa
Kanuma®

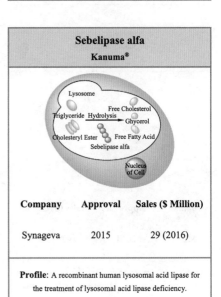

Company	Approval	Sales ($ Million)
Synageva	2015	29 (2016)

Profile: A recombinant human lysosomal acid lipase for the treatment of lysosomal acid lipase deficiency.

Idarucizumab
Praxbind®/Prizbind®

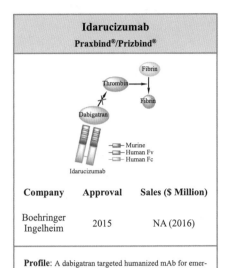

Company	Approval	Sales ($ Million)
Boehringer Ingelheim	2015	NA (2016)

Profile: A dabigatran targeted humanized mAb for emergency surgery and bleeding in patients treated with dabigatran.

Mepolizumab
Nucala®

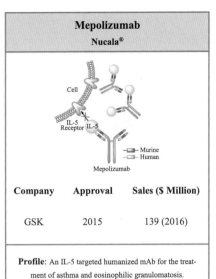

Company	Approval	Sales ($ Million)
GSK	2015	139 (2016)

Profile: An IL-5 targeted humanized mAb for the treatment of asthma and eosinophilic granulomatosis.

Daratumumab
Darzalex®

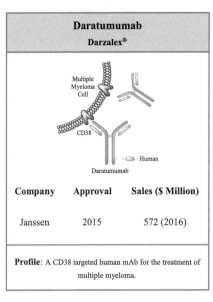

Company	Approval	Sales ($ Million)
Janssen	2015	572 (2016)

Profile: A CD38 targeted human mAb for the treatment of multiple myeloma.

Necitumumab
Portrazza®

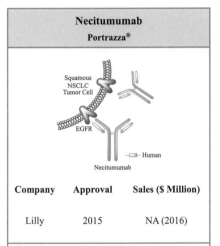

Company	Approval	Sales ($ Million)
Lilly	2015	NA (2016)

Profile: An EGFR targeted human mAb for the treatment of metastatic squamous non-small cell lung cancer.

Elotuzumab
Empliciti®

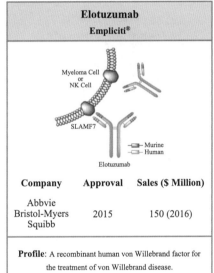

Company	Approval	Sales ($ Million)
Abbvie Bristol-Myers Squibb	2015	150 (2016)

Profile: A recombinant human von Willebrand factor for the treatment of von Willebrand disease.

Von Willebrand factor (Recombinant)
Vonvendi®

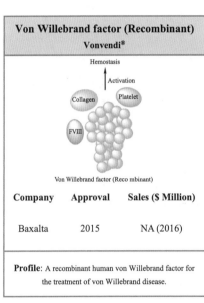

Company	Approval	Sales ($ Million)
Baxalta	2015	NA (2016)

Profile: A recombinant human von Willebrand factor for the treatment of von Willebrand disease.

Year 2016

Asparaginase (Recombinant)
Spectrila®

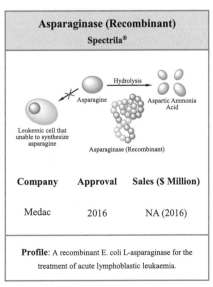

Company	Approval	Sales ($ Million)
Medac	2016	NA (2016)

Profile: A recombinant E. coli L-asparaginase for the treatment of acute lymphoblastic leukaemia.

Albutrepenonacog alfa
Idelvion®

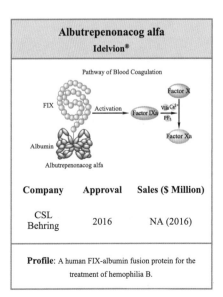

Company	Approval	Sales ($ Million)
CSL Behring	2016	NA (2016)

Profile: A human FIX-albumin fusion protein for the treatment of hemophilia B.

Obiltoxaximab
Anthim®

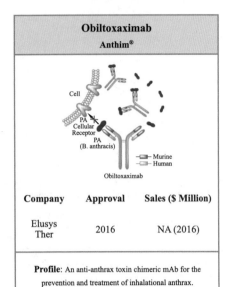

Company	Approval	Sales ($ Million)
Elusys Ther	2016	NA (2016)

Profile: An anti-anthrax toxin chimeric mAb for the prevention and treatment of inhalational anthrax.

Ixekizumab
Taltz®

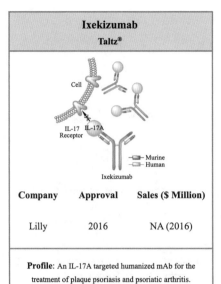

Company	Approval	Sales ($ Million)
Lilly	2016	NA (2016)

Profile: An IL-17A targeted humanized mAb for the treatment of plaque psoriasis and psoriatic arthritis.

Reslizumab
Cinqair®/Cinqaero®

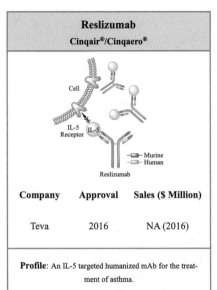

Company	Approval	Sales ($ Million)
Teva	2016	NA (2016)

Profile: An IL-5 targeted humanized mAb for the treatment of asthma.

Atezolizumab
Tecentriq®

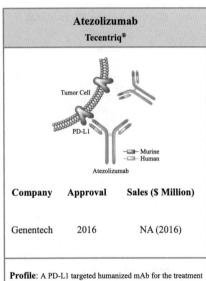

Company	Approval	Sales ($ Million)
Genentech	2016	NA (2016)

Profile: A PD-L1 targeted humanized mAb for the treatment of urothelial carcinoma and non-small cell lung cancer.

Brodalumab
Lumicer®/Siliq®/Kyntheum®

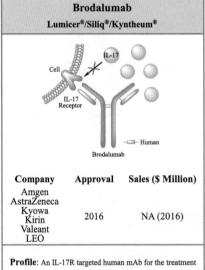

Company	Approval	Sales ($ Million)
Amgen AstraZeneca Kyowa Kirin Valeant LEO	2016	NA (2016)

Profile: An IL-17R targeted human mAb for the treatment of psoriasis and psoriatic arthritis.

Olaratumab
Lartruvo®

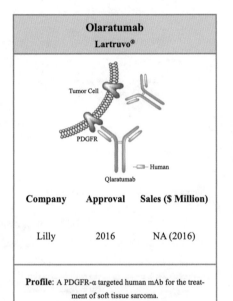

Company	Approval	Sales ($ Million)
Lilly	2016	NA (2016)

Profile: A PDGFR-α targeted human mAb for the treatment of soft tissue sarcoma.

Bezlotoxumab
Zinplava®

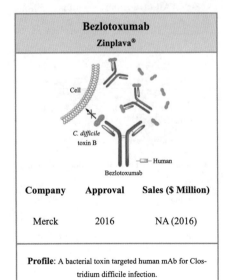

Company	Approval	Sales ($ Million)
Merck	2016	NA (2016)

Profile: A bacterial toxin targeted human mAb for Clostridium difficile infection.

Lonoctocog alfa
Afstyla®

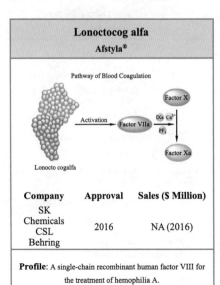

Company	Approval	Sales ($ Million)
SK Chemicals CSL Behring	2016	NA (2016)

Profile: A single-chain recombinant human factor VIII for the treatment of hemophilia A.

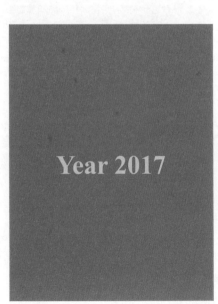

Year 2017

Guselkumab
Tremfya®

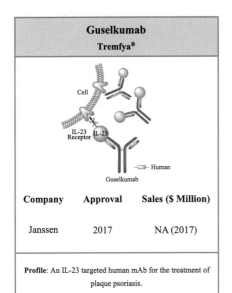

Company	Approval	Sales ($ Million)
Janssen	2017	NA (2017)

Profile: An IL-23 targeted human mAb for the treatment of plaque psoriasis.

Durvalumab
Imfinzi®

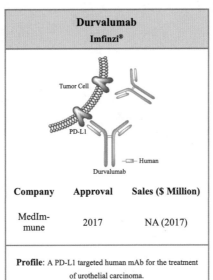

Company	Approval	Sales ($ Million)
MedIm-mune	2017	NA (2017)

Profile: A PD-L1 targeted human mAb for the treatment of urothelial carcinoma.

Benralizumab
Fasenra®

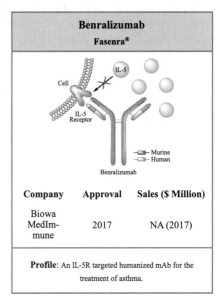

Company	Approval	Sales ($ Million)
Biowa MedIm-mune	2017	NA (2017)

Profile: An IL-5R targeted humanized mAb for the treatment of asthma.

Avelumab
Bavencio®

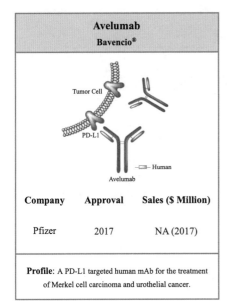

Company	Approval	Sales ($ Million)
Pfizer	2017	NA (2017)

Profile: A PD-L1 targeted human mAb for the treatment of Merkel cell carcinoma and urothelial cancer.

Emicizumab
Hemlibra®

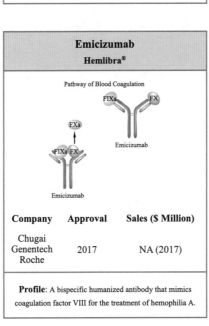

Company	Approval	Sales ($ Million)
Chugai Genentech Roche	2017	NA (2017)

Profile: A bispecific humanized antibody that mimics coagulation factor VIII for the treatment of hemophilia A.

Nonacog beta pegol
Refixia®/Rebinyn®

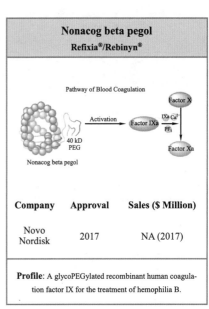

Company	Approval	Sales ($ Million)
Novo Nordisk	2017	NA (2017)

Profile: A glycoPEGylated recombinant human coagulation factor IX for the treatment of hemophilia B.

Dupilumab
Dupixent®

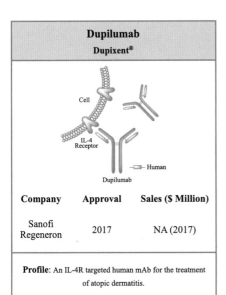

Company	Approval	Sales ($ Million)
Sanofi Regeneron	2017	NA (2017)

Profile: An IL-4R targeted human mAb for the treatment of atopic dermatitis.

Inotuzumab ozogamicin
Besponsa®

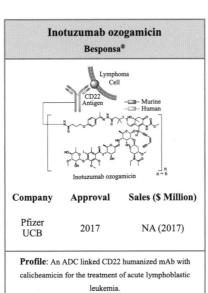

Company	Approval	Sales ($ Million)
Pfizer UCB	2017	NA (2017)

Profile: An ADC linked CD22 humanized mAb with calicheamicin for the treatment of acute lymphoblastic leukemia.

Vestronidase alfa-vjbk
Mepsevii®

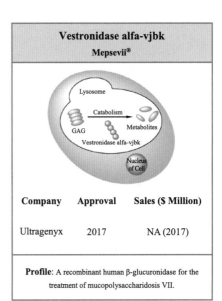

Company	Approval	Sales ($ Million)
Ultragenyx	2017	NA (2017)

Profile: A recombinant human β-glucuronidase for the treatment of mucopolysaccharidosis VII.

Dinutuximab beta
Dinutuximab beta EUSA®

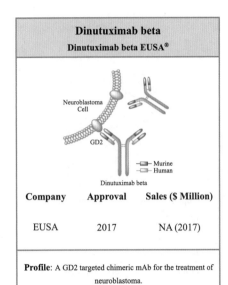

Company	Approval	Sales ($ Million)
EUSA	2017	NA (2017)

Profile: A GD2 targeted chimeric mAb for the treatment of neuroblastoma.

Ocrelizumab
Ocrevus®

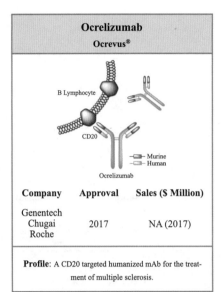

Company	Approval	Sales ($ Million)
Genentech Chugai Roche	2017	NA (2017)

Profile: A CD20 targeted humanized mAb for the treatment of multiple sclerosis.

Cenegermin
Oxervate®

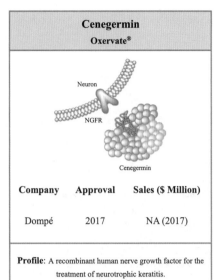

Company	Approval	Sales ($ Million)
Dompé	2017	NA (2017)

Profile: A recombinant human nerve growth factor for the treatment of neurotrophic keratitis.

Sarilumab
Kevzara®

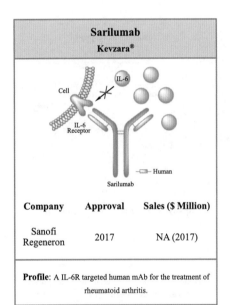

Company	Approval	Sales ($ Million)
Sanofi Regeneron	2017	NA (2017)

Profile: A IL-6R targeted human mAb for the treatment of rheumatoid arthritis.

Cerliponase alfa
Brineura®

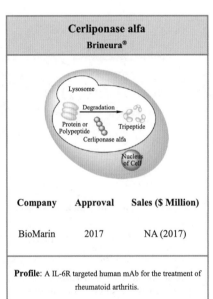

Company	Approval	Sales ($ Million)
BioMarin	2017	NA (2017)

Profile: A IL-6R targeted human mAb for the treatment of rheumatoid arthritis.

Semaglutide
Ozempic®

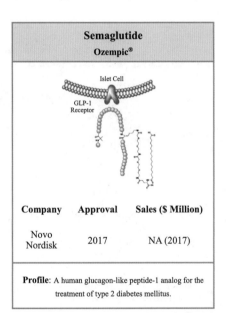

Company	Approval	Sales ($ Million)
Novo Nordisk	2017	NA (2017)

Profile: A human glucagon-like peptide-1 analog for the treatment of type 2 diabetes mellitus.